PLASTIC RECONSTRUCTIVE AND AESTHETIC SURGERY
The Essentials

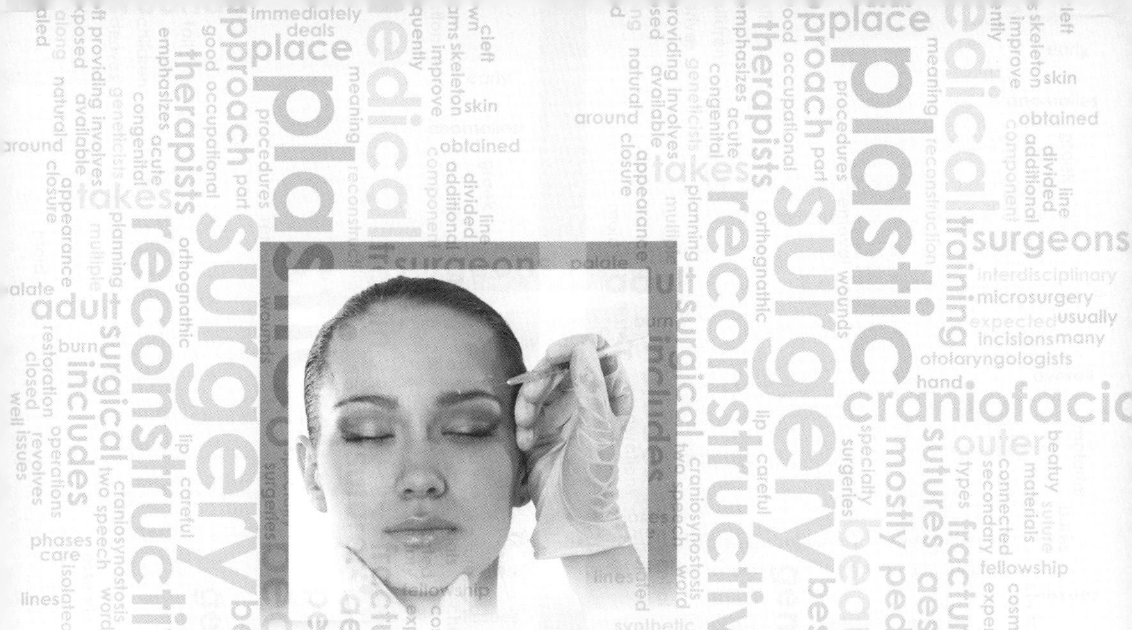

PLASTIC RECONSTRUCTIVE AND AESTHETIC SURGERY

The Essentials

Edited by

Deniz Dayicioglu

University of South Florida, USA

John C Oeltjen

Kenneth L Fan

Seth R Thaller

University of Miami, USA

World Scientific

NEW JERSEY • LONDON • SINGAPORE • BEIJING • SHANGHAI • HONG KONG • TAIPEI • CHENNAI

Published by

World Scientific Publishing Co. Pte. Ltd.
5 Toh Tuck Link, Singapore 596224
USA office: 27 Warren Street, Suite 401-402, Hackensack, NJ 07601
UK office: 57 Shelton Street, Covent Garden, London WC2H 9HE

British Library Cataloguing-in-Publication Data
A catalogue record for this book is available from the British Library.

PLASTIC RECONSTRUCTIVE AND AESTHETIC SURGERY
The Essentials

ISBN 978-981-4307-10-9

Typeset by Stallion Press
Email: enquiries@stallionpress.com

Printed in Singapore by Mainland Press Pte Ltd.

"I would like to dedicate this book to my father Vedat,
my mother Nilgun and my sister Ceren Dayicioglu
for bringing me to this day."

~~ Deniz Dayicioglu

"I would like to dedicate the following to my wife, Stacey,
and children, Christopher and Nicole,
whose love and support inspire only the best in me."

~~ John C. Oeltjen

"To Mom and Dad, for being the single and greatest constants."

~~ Kenneth Fan

"I would like to dedicate this book to my wife and children
who allow me the opportunity to practice this
exceptional field of plastic surgery.
To my parents who gave me the opportunity to become a physician.
To my mentors who help make a plastic surgeon and
to the many residents and medical students
with whom I have had the pleasure of
expanding my knowledge of plastic surgery."

~~ Seth R. Thaller

CONTENTS

EDITORS

Deniz Dayicioglu, MD
Assistant Professor
Department of Surgery
Division of Plastic Surgery
University of South Florida
12902 USF Magnolia Drive
Tampa, FL 33612, USA

John C. Oeltjen MD, PhD, FACS
Assistant Professor
The DeWitt Daughtry Family Department of Surgery
Division of Plastic Surgery
University of Miami/Miller School of Medicine
Clinical Research Building
1120 NW 14th ST., 4th Floor
Miami, FL 33136, USA

Kenneth L. Fan MS
Division of Plastic Surgery
University of Miami/Miller School of Medicine
Clinical Research Building
1120 NW 14th ST., 4th Floor
Miami, FL 33136, USA

Seth R. Thaller, MD, DMD, FACS
Chief and Professor
The Dewitt Daughtry Family Department of Surgery
Division of Plastic Surgery
University of Miami/Miller School of Medicine
Clinical Research Building
1120 NW 14th ST., 4th Floor
Miami, FL 33136, USA

CONTRIBUTORS

Joshua M. Adkinson
Division of Plastic Surgery
Lehigh Valley Health Network
Cedar Crest and I-78, P.O Box 689
Allentown, PA 18105-1556, USA

Anuja K. Antony
Department of Surgery
Division of Plastic Surgery
University of Illinois at Chicago (UIC)
m/c 958, 820 W. Wood, 515 CSN
Chicago, IL 60612, USA

Milton B. Armstrong
Professor of Surgery
Department of Surgery
Division of Plastic Surgery
Medical University of South Carolina
96 Jonathan Lucas Street
MSC 613/CSB 404
Charleston, SC 29425, USA

Yash Avasha
Department of Surgery
Division of Plastic Surgery
University of Miami/Miller School of Medicine
Clinical Research Building
1120 NW 14th ST., 4th Floor
Miami, FL 33136, USA

John R. Barbour
Division of Plastic and Reconstructive Surgery
Washington University School of Medicine
660 South Euclid Avenue, NWT 1150
Saint Louis, MO 63110, USA

Harvey W.-M. Chim
Department of Plastic Surgery
Case Western Reserve University
11100 Euclid Avenue
Cleveland, OH 44106, USA

Jessica A. Ching
Department of Surgery
Division of Plastic Surgery
University of South Florida
2 Tampa General Circle
7th floor
Tampa, FL 33606, USA

Miguel Cobas
Department of Anesthesiology
University of Miami Hospital
Miller School of Medicine
P.O. Box 016370
Miami, Fl 33136, USA

Paul G. Cofnas
Department of Surgery
Division of Plastic, Aesthetic, and Reconstructive Surgery
University of Miami/Miller School of Medicine
Clinical Research Building
1120 NW 14th ST., 4th Floor
Miami, FL 33136, USA

Mimis N. Cohen
Department of Surgery
Division of Plastic Surgery
University of Illinois at Chicago (UIC)
m/c 958, 820 W. Wood, 515 CSN
Chicago, IL 60612, USA

Patrick Cole
Division of Plastic Surgery
Michael E. DeBakey Department of Surgery
Baylor College of Medicine
Texas Children's Hospital
Clinical Care Center
6701 Fannin, Suite 610
Houston, TX 77030, USA

C. Wayne Cruse
Professor
Department of Surgery
Division of Plastic Surgery
University of South Florida
2 Tampa General Circle
7th floor
Tampa, FL 33606, USA

Deniz Dayicioglu
Assistant Professor
Department of Surgery
Division of Plastic Surgery
University of South Florida
12902 USF Magnolia Drive
Tampa, FL 33612, USA

Kevin O. Delaney
Assistant Professor of Surgery
Department of Surgery
Division of Plastic Surgery
Medical University of South Carolina
96 Jonathan Lucas Street
MSC 613/CSB 404
Charleston, SC 29425, USA

Ulvila Derek
Department of Surgery
Division of Plastic Surgery
University of Miami/Miller School of Medicine
Clinical Research Building
1120 NW 14th ST., 4th Floor
Miami, FL 33136, USA

Michelle De Souza
Assistant Professor
Department of Plastic and Reconstructive Surgery
University of Kansas Medical Center
3901 Rainbow Boulevard
Mail Stop 3015
Kansas City, KS 66160, USA

Kenneth L. Fan
Division of Plastic Surgery
University of Miami/Miller School of Medicine
Clinical Research Building
1120 NW 14th ST., 4th Floor
Miami, FL 33136, USA

Victor J. Hassid
Department of Surgery
Division of Plastic Surgery
University of Illinois at Chicago (UIC)
m/c 958, 820 W. Wood, 515 CSN
Chicago, IL 60612, USA

Stacy R. Henderson
Department of Surgery
Division of Plastic Surgery
Indiana University School of Medicine
340 West 10th Street
Indianapolis, IN 46202, USA

Larry Hollier, Jr.
Professor and Residency Program Director
Division of Plastic Surgery
Michael E. DeBakey Department of Surgery
Baylor College of Medicine
Texas Children's Hospital
Clinical Care Center
6701 Fannin, Suite 610
Houston, TX 77030, USA

Wrood Kassira
Assistant Professor of Clinical Surgery
Dewitt Daughtry Department of Surgery
Division of Plastic, Aesthetic, and Reconstructive Surgery
University of Miami/Miller School of Medicine
Clinical Research Building
1120 NW 14th ST., 4th Floor
Miami, FL 33136, USA

Benjamin Lemelman
Department of Surgery
Division of Plastic, Aesthetic, and Reconstructive Surgery
University of Miami/Miller School of Medicine
Clinical Research Building
1120 NW 14th ST., 4th Floor
Miami, FL 33136, USA

Umbareen Mahmood
Department of Surgery
Division of Plastic Surgery

University of South Florida
1 Tampa General Circle
Tampa, FL 33606, USA

Erick Martell
Department of Surgery
Division of Plastic Surgery
University of Miami/Miller School of Medicine
Clinical Research Building
1120 NW 14th ST., 4th Floor
Miami, FL 33136, USA

Garry Martin II
Department of Plastic and Reconstructive Surgery
University of Kansas Medical Center
3901 Rainbow Boulevard
Mail Stop 3015
Kansas City, KS 66160, USA

Alan Matarasso
Department of Plastic Surgery
Manhattan Eye, Ear & Throat Hospital
Lenox Hill Hospital/North Shore — Long Island
Jewish Health System
1009 Park Avenue
New York, NY 10028, USA

Haaris S. Mir
Assistant Professor
Department of Surgery
Division of Plastic Surgery
University of Miami/Miller School of Medicine
Clinical Research Building
1120 NW 14th ST., 4th Floor
Miami, FL 33136, USA

Raja Mohan
Division of Plastic Surgery
University of Miami/Miller School of Medicine
Clinical Research Building
1120 NW 14th ST., 4th Floor
Miami, FL 33136, USA

Askari Morad
Assistant Profesor
Department of Surgery
Division of Plastic Surgery
University of Miami/Miller School of Medicine
Clinical Research Building
1120 NW 14th ST., 4th Floor
Miami, FL 33136, USA

Robert X. Murphy Jr.
Assistant Chief Medical Officer
Division of Plastic Surgery
Lehigh Valley Health Network — Muhlenberg
2597 Schoenersville Road
Administrative Suite, 4th Floor
Bethlehem, PA 18017, USA

David Nesky
Division of Otolaryngology, Head and Neck Surgery
University of Miami/Miller School of Medicine
Clinical Research Building
1120 NW 14th ST., 4th Floor
Miami, FL 33136, USA

Mark S. Nestor
Director, Center for Cosmetic Enhancement
Director, Center for Clinical and Cosmetic Research
2925 Aventura Blvd, Suite 205
Aventura, FL 33180, USA

Voluntary Associate Professor
Department of Dermatology and Cutaneous Surgery
University of Miami/Miller School of Medicine
1295 N.W. 14th Street, Suite K-M
Miami, FL 33136, USA

John C. Oeltjen
Assistant Professor
The DeWitt Daughtry Family Department of Surgery
Division of Plastic Surgery
University of Miami/Miller School of Medicine
Clinical Research Building
1120 NW 14th ST., 4th Floor
Miami, FL 33136, USA

Zubin J. Panthaki
Associate Professor
The DeWitt Daughtry Family Department of Surgery
Department of Surgery
Division of Plastic Surgery
University of Miami/Miller School of Medicine
Clinical Research Building
1120 NW 14th ST., 4th Floor
Miami, FL 33136, USA

Gian Paparcuri
Department of Anesthesiology
University of Miami Hospital
Miller School of Medicine
P.O. Box 016370
Miami, Fl 33136, USA

Rajiv P. Parikh
Department of Surgery
Division of Plastic Surgery
University of South Florida
2 Tampa General Circle
7th floor
Tampa, FL 33606, USA

Steven Rueda
University of Miami/Miller School of Medicine
31 SE 5th ST., Apt 2502
Miami, FL 33131, USA

Karim W. Sadik
Department of General Surgery
Division of Plastic Surgery
Indiana University School of Medicine
545 Barn Hill Drive
Emerson Hall 232
Indianapolis, IN 46202, USA

Christopher J. Salgado
Associate Professor of Surgery
Division of Plastic Surgery
University of Miami/Miller School of Medicine
Clinical Research Building
1120 NW 14th ST., 4th Floor
Miami, FL 33136, USA

Dennis K. Schimpf
Assistant Professor of Surgery
Director of MUSC Advanced Breast Reconstructive Program
Associate Program Director Plastic and
Reconstructive Surgery Residency
Department of Surgery

Division of Plastic Surgery
Medical University of South Carolina
96 Jonathan Lucas Street
MSC 613/CSB 404
Charleston, SC 29425, USA

Jessica S. Suber
Department of Surgery
Division of Plastic Surgery
University of South Florida
2 Tampa General Circle
7th floor
Tampa, FL 33606, USA

Seth R. Thaller
Chief and Professor
The Dewitt Daughtry Family Department of Surgery
Division of Plastic Surgery
University of Miami/Miller School of Medicine
Clinical Research Building
1120 NW 14th ST., 4th Floor
Miami, FL 33136, USA

Jason P. Ulm
Department of Surgery
Division of Plastic Surgery
Medical University of South Carolina
96 Jonathan Lucas Street
MSC 613/CSB 404
Charleston, SC 29425, USA

Donald Weed
Division of Otolaryngology, Head and Neck Surgery
University of Miami/Miller School of Medicine
Clinical Research Building
1120 NW 14th ST., 4th Floor
Miami, FL 33136, USA

Sara Yegiyants
Department of Surgery
Division of Plastic Surgery
University of Illinois, Chicago
820 South Wood Street, 515 CSN
Chicago, IL 60612, USA

Matthew B. Zarraga
Dermatology Fellow
Center for Clinical and Cosmetic Research
2925 Aventura Blvd, Suite 205
Aventura, FL 33180, USA

FOREWORD

The practice of Plastic Surgery is a joyous endeavor. The breadth of the specialty provides an opportunity to work with patients of all ages with a wide range of congenital and acquired deformities. No two patients are identical; no two reconstructive challenges are ever the same. Each new case requires the surgeon to use his imagination and skill in developing the best options to solve clinical problems. From this flows innovation and adaptation of techniques to obtain the best result. It also is the opportunity for interaction with a patient over the course of surgical planning and treatment in a mutually valued relationship.

The same features that make Plastic Surgery a fulfilling career also make it a challenging field for a learner of the specialty. The challenge is not only the acquisition of a large body of knowledge, but also the personal processing and integration of this mass of data so that it is accessible for optimal use in the clinical setting.

Essentials of Plastic Surgery takes on the challenges facing the student of Plastic Surgery and is organized to link basic concepts with surgical management. Chapters are organized to cover the breadth of the specialty. Each chapter opens with a clinical case, provides information about anatomy, physiology and pathology, and concisely reviews associated mechanisms of treatment. Technical methods are discussed, psychological considerations are raised, and selected experts keep the focus on what is important to know.

Different from electronic search results, *Essentials of Plastic Surgery* is not merely a storage repository for bits of information. It does more than make knowledge available. The text provides structure, which could be called a curriculum, to inform the reader's thinking and aid with integration, retention, and utility of what is learned.

This book meets the need for a comprehensive yet concise source of information for Plastic Surgery practice. For study, or as a tool when preparing for surgery, *Essentials of Plastic Surgery* reflects current knowledge in a relatively compact volume that is still a comprehensive textbook of plastic surgery. It emphasizes the important conditions faced by contemporary plastic surgeons, and describes what all plastic surgeons need to know, including preoperative care, operative technique and postoperative care.

For the resident or medical student, *Essentials of Plastic Surgery* is a key text for identifying core matters of surgical principles and patient care, both operative and nonoperative. For the practicing surgeon dedicated to continuing education, it is a trove of usefully organized information in a single source.

Mary H. McGrath, MD MPH
Professor of Surgery, Division of Plastic Surgery
University of California San Francisco

PREFACE

This handbook was initiated primarily for plastic surgery residents in their training and other house officers who will be rotating on a plastic surgery service. In addition, this textbook will serve as a readily accessible resource for practicing plastic surgeons that will be facing their daily clinical challenges.

The overall goal of this manuscript is to present the extensive field of plastic surgery in a concise, practical, and comprehensive, practicable arrangement emphasizing the basic essential principles of our specialty incorporating significant plastic, reconstructive and aesthetic surgery components.

Contributors were selected for their expertise and clinical experience in their specific assigned topic. Each chapter will be uniquely organized by a seasoned clinician to provide the reader with a contemporary and balanced approach to the clinical practice of plastic surgery. This unique approach should provide the reader with a novel assessment of topics within our specialty and allow a broader appreciation of how a specific procedure should be approached.

Our book will be specifically directed towards procedural topics focusing on both preparation and execution of the procedure in the operating room. This will therefore serve as a portable handbook that can be employed throughout the perioperative period in preparation for actual cases particularly the most commonly encountered cases. There will be a distinct emphasis on patient safety.

Seth R. Thaller
University of Miami/Miller School of Medicine, USA

CORE KNOWLEDGE AND GENERAL PRINCIPLES

CHAPTER 1

WOUND REPAIR

Jason P. Ulm and Kevin O. Delaney

Illustrative Case

67 yo male suffered large facial laceration while playing tennis 45 minutes ago (Fig. 1)
Denies LOC
ALL-NKDA
Meds-Lipitor
PMH-HTN, Hypercholesterolemia
PE:GCS 15
Large frontoparietal laceration extending to dorsum of nose, exposed calvarium
Copiously irrigated and closed in layers using principles below

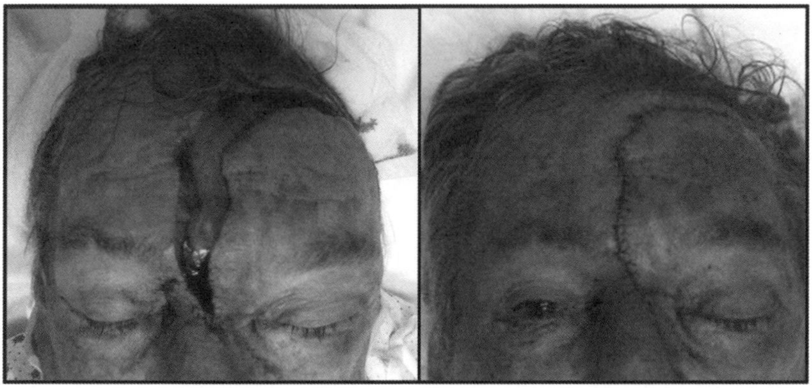

Fig. 1. Sixty-seven year old male with large facial laceration.

"I dress the wound, God heals it."
Ambroise Paré, Surgeon
16th century

I. Basic Principles of Wound Repair

- Adequate debridement and irrigation of the wound prior to closure is critically important and unfortunately often overlooked
- Take all steps necessary to eliminate or minimize tension at the closure site
  - Repair wound in layers to minimize tension at the epidermal layer
  - In full thickness wounds, place deep dermal sutures in order to absorb any tension which may exist thereby minimizing tension more superficially
- Attempt to eliminate any significant wound dead space by performing a layered closure or placing a temporary drain
- Evert the wound edges during approximation in order to minimize a depressed scar with contour abnormalities
- Gently approximate the wound edges during closure……DO NOT STRANGULATE
  - The wound will likely develop inflammatory edema and tight sutures will become ligatures at the wound edge thereby causing ischemia and poor perfusion
  - The goal should be gentle apposition of the wound edges
- Adhere to the principles of atraumatic tissue technique throughout the entire wound repair

II. Preparation of the Patient

- Always begin with a focused history and physical examination; remember that you are treating the patient and not just the wound
- Identify any acute or chronic medical conditions that may prevent or alter surgical intervention
- Determine the medical stability of the patient and whether or not their condition is amenable to treatment at this point in time

- Decide upon a treatment plan for wound repair which includes but is not limited to:
    - Type of repair (primary closure, delayed primary closure, closure by second intention)
    - Timing of repair (acute vs. delayed)
        - Setting (office, emergency room, operating room)
        - Type of anesthesia (Local, Regional, MAC, Concious Sedation, General)
- Always obtain surgical consent
- Consider taking photos of the wound with necessary measurements prior to intervention
- Obtain all necessary supplies, instruments, and assistants prior to beginning repair
- Properly position the patient to optimize surgical repair and minimize surgeon fatigue

III. Wound Preparation

- Preparation of the wound prior to treatment is critical
- Sterile preparation and draping of the wound in the standard fashion while providing adequate exposure is of paramount importance
- Provide excellent anesthesia before beginning debridement because insufficient anesthesia will likely prevent an optimal outcome
- One must perform appropriate and adequate debridement of any necrotic tissue
- Evaluation for associated foreign bodies in the wound must be completed
- If foreign bodies are identified in the wound, they must be removed
- Copious irrigation with sterile saline must follow debridement and foreign body removal in order to eliminate any residual debris in the wound
- The presence of infection must be identified and adequately treated prior to any consideration of primary closure
- Don't forget to take cultures of infected wounds and treat with appropriate empiric antibiotics followed by culture-specific antibiotics

- If infection or contamination are present, then consider alternative wound closure techniques including delayed primary closure or closure by second intention
- Obtain meticulous hemostasis following irrigation and debridement in order to minimize hematoma formation, wound infection, and inflammation

IV. Suturing Techniques

- Simple Interrupted Suture (Fig. 2)
  - The most commonly used suture technique
  - Easy technique to learn and apply
  - Good for optimal alignment of the wound edge
  - The needle should enter the skin at an angle which allows it enter the deeper tissue at a point farther from the wound edge than the entry site of the needle at the skin level
  - The path of the suture resembles a trapezoid or triangle after exiting the skin on the opposite side of the wound

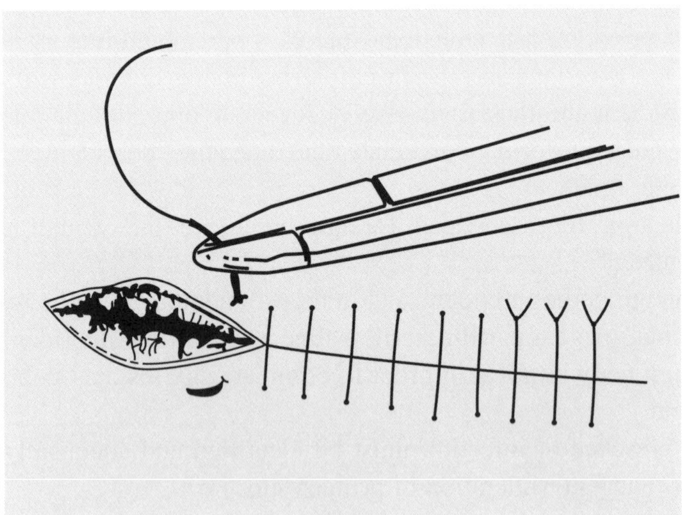

Fig. 2. Simple interrupted suture.

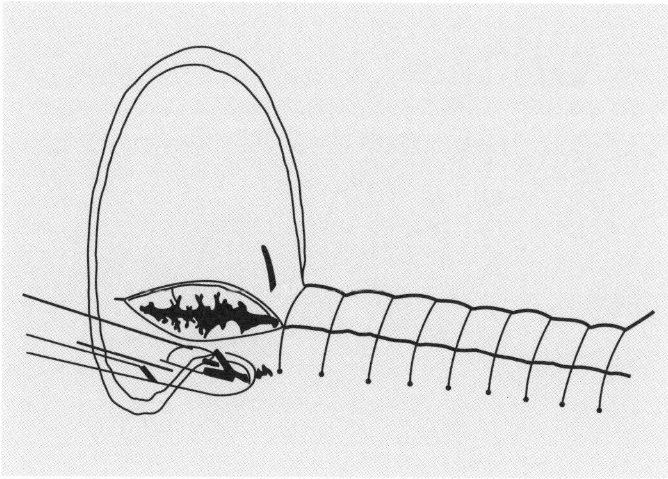

Fig. 3. Continuous running simple suture.

- Continuous Running Simple Suture (Fig. 3)
  - Fast technique which is easy to learn, similar to the simple interrupted suture
  - Often employed in wound closures without any tension
  - Can also be used for obtaining hemostasis at the wound edges by locking it along its route
- Horizontal Mattress Suture (Fig. 4)
  - Very effective for optimal wound edge eversion
  - Frequently used for wound closure in areas of the body with thick skin (glaborous skin of the hands and feet)
  - Some consider them to be potentially ischemic sutures especially if tied too tightly
- Vertical Mattress Suture (Fig. 5)
  - Very effective for optimal wound edge eversion
  - Frequently used for wound closure in areas of the body with thick skin (glaborous skin of the hands and feet)
  - Considered less likely to cause wound edge ischemia than horizontal mattress sutures

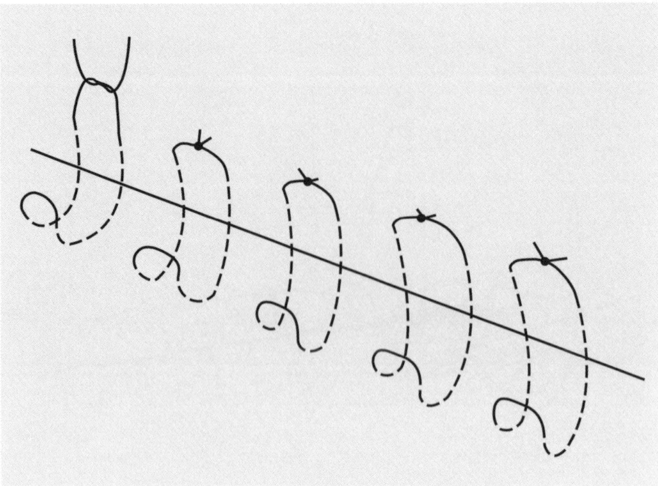

Fig. 4. Horizontal mattress suture.

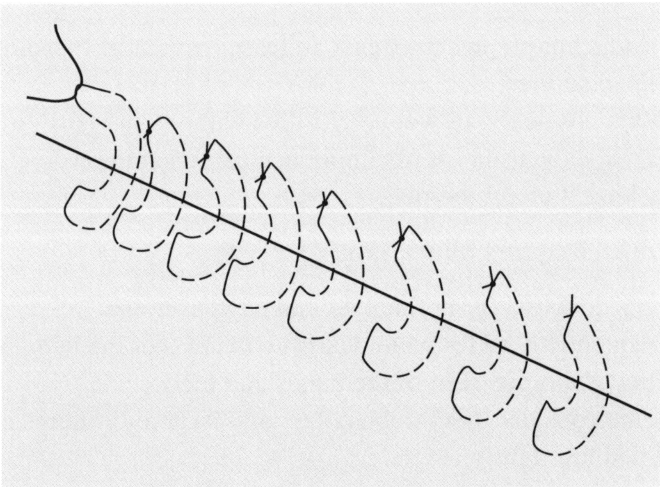

Fig. 5. Vertical mattress suture.

- Subcuticular Suture (Intradermal Suture) (Fig. 6)
  - Commonly used for skin edge approximation in conjunction with buried deep dermal sutures

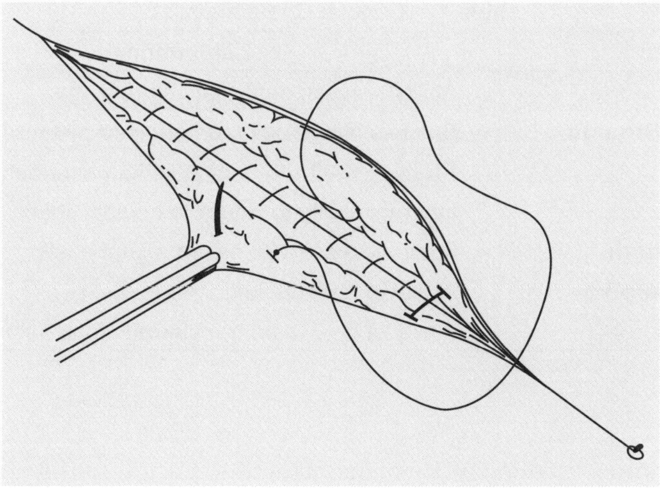

Fig. 6. Subcuticular suture (intradermal suture).

- ○ The suture is a running, intradermal suture at the level of the superficial dermis immediately deep to the epidermal-dermal junction
- ○ Every attempt to maintain placement of the suture at the same depth on each side of the wound is made
- ○ Provides excellent cosmesis by eliminating the need for external sutures and the possibility of permanent suture marks in the skin ("railroad tracks")

V. Suturing Materials

History

- Earliest reports of surgical suturing from ancient Egypt 3000 BC
- Oldest known suture harvested from Mummy's abdomen from 1100 BC
- Sushruta (500 BC) — first detailed description of wound suture and materials
- Joseph Lister first endorsed sterilizing suture materials in 1860s
- First synthetic suture manufactured in early 1930s

Table 1. General Characteristics.

	Definitions
Tensile Strength	Ability to resist deformation/breakage
Breaking Strength	Suture's failure point, determined by tensile strength
Elasticity	Ability to return to original length after deformation
Memory	Inherent ability to return to original shape
Knot Strength	Force necessary to cause a knot to slip
Fluid Absorption	Ability to take up fluid
Capillarity	Ability of fluid to be transferred along suture

- All sutures used today are manufactured to ensure sterility, pliability, and uniform size and tensile strength
- United States Pharmacopeia (USP) rating system is used:
  - Given in **#–0** intervals, where higher number denotes smaller diameter
  - Based on diameter of given material that equates with ***breaking strength***
    - Ex. 3-0 polypropylene and 3-0 silk will have same breaking strength, but not same diameter
- **The quality of a given suture is dependent on its permanence, origin, structure, size, and tensile strength (Table 1)**
- Permanence:
  - **Absorbable (Table 2)**
    - Hydrolytic degredation — synthetic sutures
    - Proleolytic degredation — natural sutures
      - — Cell mediated
      - — More inflammation/scarring (reactivity)
    - At 4 weeks ~50% strength
    - Wound infection accelerates absorption

- **Non-absorbable (Table 3)**
  - Will become encapsulated by fibroblasts

- Origin:
  - **Natural** (gut, cotton, silk, steel)
  - **Synthetic** (everything else)

- Structure:
  - **Monofilament** — generally have more memory, less friction and capillarity
  - **Multifilament** (braided or twisted) — generally have more knot strength/security (less throws needed)

Needles

- General Characteristics (Table 4)
  - Most are made from stainless steel alloys which decrease corrosion
  - Should be smallest diameter possible, but stable enough to carry suture material through tissue
  - Appropriate sharpness for desired tissue dissection

Table 2. Absorbable Sutures.

Material	Trade Name	Structure	50% Strength	Memory	Reactivity
Plain gut		Natural	~7 days	Low	High
Chromic gut		Natural	~14 days	Low	High
Poliglecaprone 25	Monocryl	Monofilament	7 days	Medium	Low
Polyglytone	Caprosyn	Monofilament	5–7 days	Medium	Low
Glycolide	Biosyn	Monofilament	2–3 wks	Medium	Low
Polyglycolic acid	Dexon	Braided	2–3 wks	Low	Low
Glycolide/lactide polymer	Vicryl, Polysorb	Braided	2–3 wks	Low	Moderate
Polyglyconate	Maxon	Monofilament	4 wks	High	Moderate
Polydioxanone	PDS	Monofilament	4 wks	High	Low

Table 3. Non-Absorbable Sutures.

Material	Trade Name	Structure	Memory	Reactivity
Cotton		Twisted	Low	High
Silk	Sofsilk (coated)	Braided	Low	High
Polypropylene	Prolene, Surgipro	Monofilament	High	Low
Polybutester (coated)	Novafil (Vascufil)	Monofilament	High	Low
Nylon	Ethilon, Dermalon, Monosoft	Monofilament	High	Low
Nylon	Nurolon, Surgilon	Braided	Low	Moderate
Polyester	Mersilene, Surgidac	Braided	Low	Moderate
Polyester coated	Ethibond, Ti-Cron	Braided	Low	Moderate
Steel		Monofilament	High	Low

Source: Modified from Refs. 1 and 2.

    - Ductility — resistance of a needle to deform under tensile stress
    - Clamping moment — stability of needle while grasped by needle holder

- Anatomy
    - Point-tip of needle, may be blunt or sharp
    - Body — majority of needle, ideal needle holder grasp is $\frac{1}{2}$ to $\frac{2}{3}$ from point
    - Swage — end of needle connected to suture-secure or pop-off
- Size
    - Chord length — straight line distance from point to swage (bite width)
    - Needle length — distance along needle from point to swage-on suture package
    - Diameter — thickness or gauge, typically smallest possible allowed by suture material
    - Radius — distance from center of curvature to body (bite depth)
- Shape
    - Straight (Keith, Brunnel) — typically hand

- Half-curved (Ski) — difficult to handle, rarely used
- Curved
  - 1/4 circle
  - 3/8 circle
  - 1/2 circle
  - 5/8 circle
- Compound curved

Table 4. Needle characteristics.

Type	Description	Benefit	Applications	Examples
Cutting	Triangular, third sharp edge on interior arc of needle	For tough tissue, but may cause weak point in suture tract	Skin	PC
Reverse Cutting	Triangular, third sharp edge on exterior arc of needle	Stronger, suture tract NOT weakened by cutting surface	Skin Fascia Tendon/ ligament Oropharynx	P PS PC FS C
Side Cutting	Flat on top and bottom, sharp edge on sides of needle	Reduced tissue injury, maximum ease of penetration	Eye Micro	S SS
Tapercutting	Sharp cutting point, blunt body		Oropharynx Trachea/ bronchus Periosteum/ sternum	CC V MVK
Taper Point	Sharp point, blunt body	Does not cut tissue Good for soft tissues, less bleeding	Abdominal viscera Dura/nerve muscle Fascia Micro	SH UR CT BV CV MV
Blunt	Blunt point and body	Good for soft parenchymal tissues	Liver/kidney OB/GYN Micro	CTX BP BTX

- Points:
    - Cutting
    - Reverse cutting
    - X-cutting — 4-sided, for subcuticular approximation
    - Side cutting (spatula)
    - Tapercutting
    - Taper
    - Blunt

Suture Choice

- Dictated by wound and patient factors
    - Infected or contaminated wounds should be closed with monofilament sutures
    - Pt wound healing ability (nutritional status, systemic co-morbidities), reliability, and age
    - Wound location
        - Joints, glaborous skin, or high tension will require heavier suture
        - Face — smaller suture
- Avoid "Railroad track" scar — skin layer closure must NOT be under tension

Suture Removal

- Eyelid — 3–5 days
- Face — 5–7 days
- Trunk — 7–10 days
- Extremity — 10–14 days

Microsutures and Needles

- Monofilament polypropylene or nylon
- 8–0 to 11–0 caliber, dictated by size of vessels

- Needles BV-3 (3 mm chord length) to BV-5
    - Use 8–0 on a BV-5 for 4 mm vessels (Radial artery)
    - Use 11–0 on a BV-3 for <1 mm vessels (Child)

Acknowledgments

Illustrations in this chapter are by Robert L. Smith (robertlawrencesmith@gmail.com).

References

1. Kryger Z, Howard M. (2007) Basic concepts in wound repair. In: Kryger Z, Sisco M (eds.), *Practical Plastic Surgery*. Landes Bioscience, Austin, Texas, pp. 4–11.
2. Mosser S. (2006) Suture and needles. In: Janis J (ed.), *Essentials of Plastic Surgery*. Quality Medical Publishing, St. Louis, pp. 13–19.

CHAPTER 2

GRAFTS AND FLAPS

Jason P. Ulm and Dennis K. Schimpf

Illustrative Case

68 year old male referred by neurosurgeon for evaluation of scalp wound with underlying osteomyelitis. Pt is 10 yrs post craniotomy for brain tumor resection and subsequent XRT. He recently suffered minor blunt trauma to the top of his head and developed a non-healing wound.

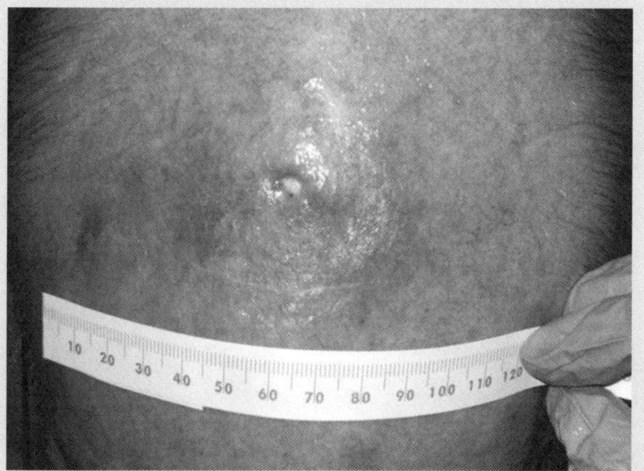

First procedure — Pt refused free flap reconstruction. The outer table of calvarium was burred down and a wound vac was placed with subsequent Integra placement in preparation for skin graft.

(Continued)

(*Continued*)

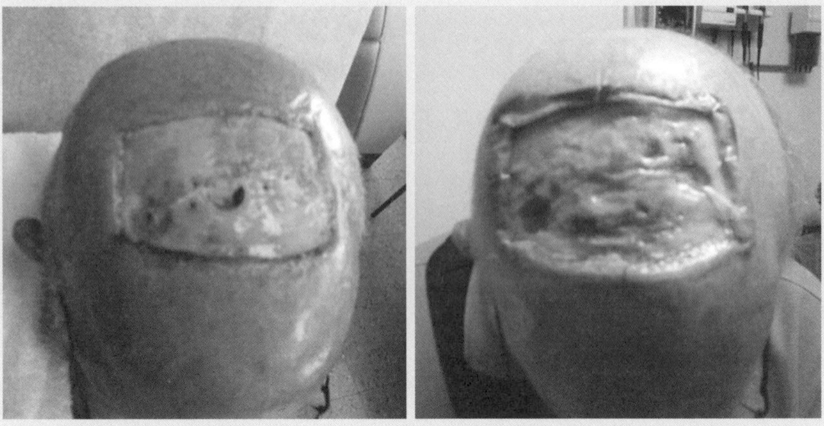

There was poor granulation and wound bed preparation, with persistent osteomyelitis and areas of radiation necrosis. Pt now agreed to free flap reconstruction. Debridement with craniectomy was done with a free rectus abdominis and STSG reconstruction.

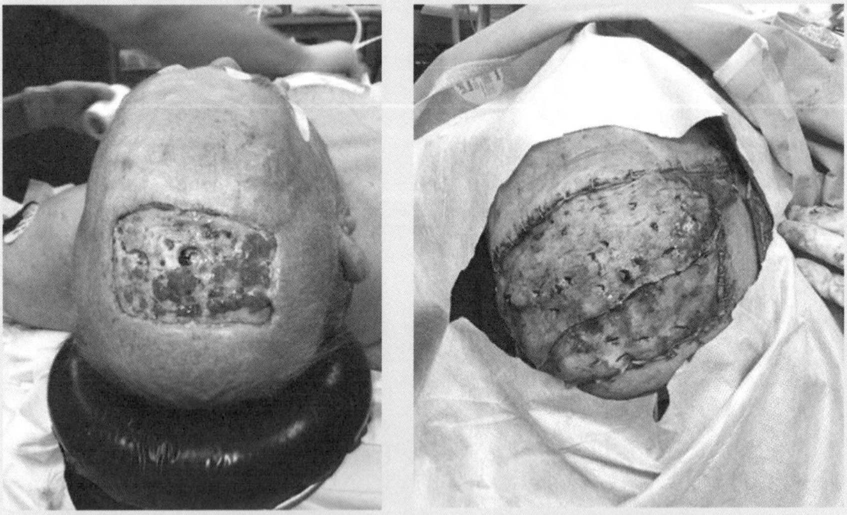

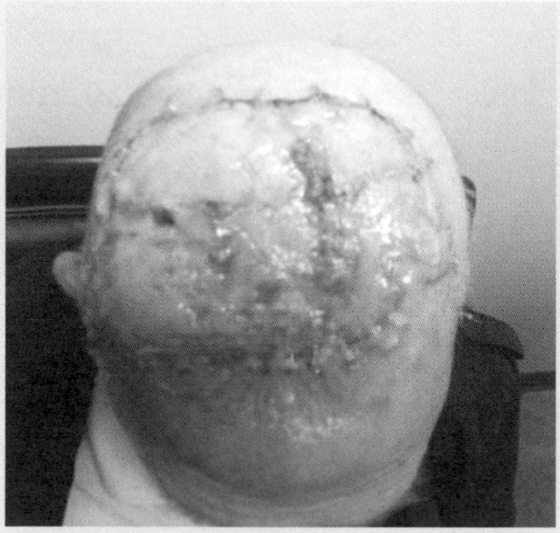

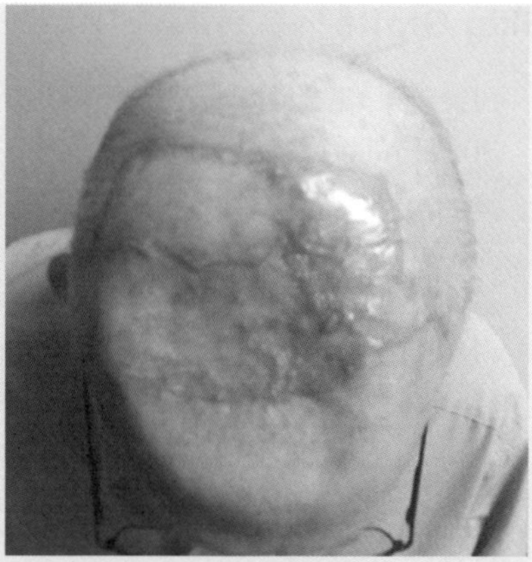

Pt healed well and was pleased with the results. A contour deformity remained, however he declined subsequent calvarium reconstruction.

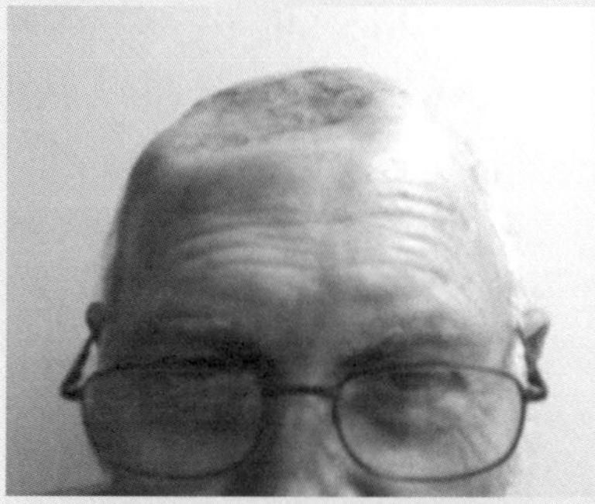

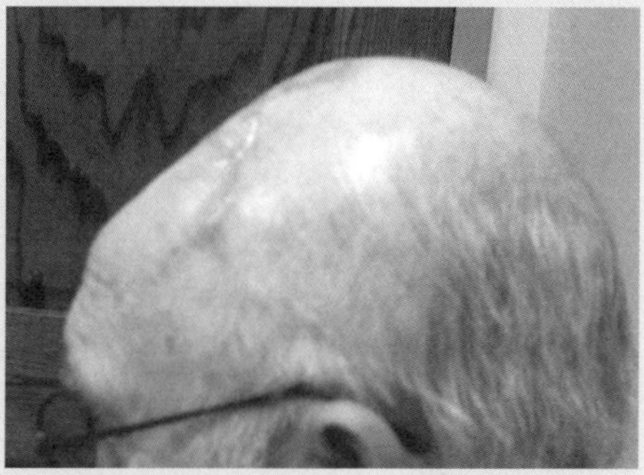

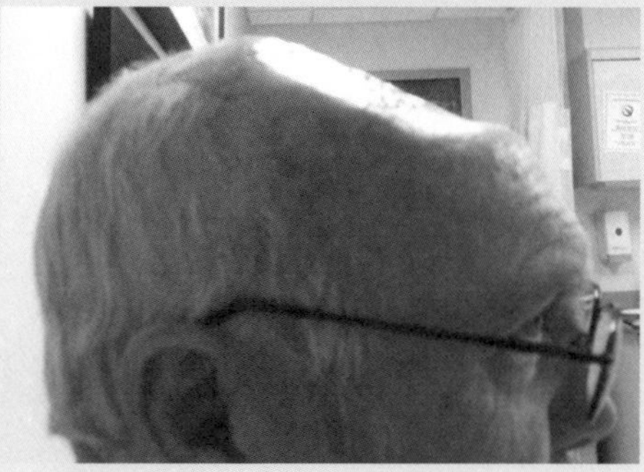

Skin Grafts

- Devascularized epidermis and some (split-thickness) or all (full-thickness) of dermis, detached and transferred from one body part to another
- Low on the reconstruction ladder, often next option if primary closure not possible
- Rely on a vascularized wound bed for ingrowth and graft survival
    - Will generally **NOT** take on exposed **bone/tendon/cartilage**
    - **Will** take on periosteum, peritenon, perichondrium, granulation tissue, fascia
- Three Phases
    - **Imbibition** (24–48 hrs) — diffusion of nutrients by capillary action
    - **Inosculation** — graft and recipient capillaries align
    - **Neo- or Revascularization** — vascular ingrowth of graft from recipient site
- Successful "Take"
    - **Graft adherence** — initially from fibrin deposition (<72 hrs), then ingrowth of fibrous tissue
    - Failure
        - **Hematomas, seromas**, shearing, and infection are the common causes of failure
- Contracture
    - Primary
        - Initial recoil seen when harvested
        - Secondary to **elastin in dermis**
        - **↑graft thickness** = **↑primary contracture**
    - Secondary — **WORSE**
        - Occurs later in healing (6–18 months)
        - Likely from **myofibroblast** activity

    - **↓ graft thickness = ↑ secondary contracture**
    - Splinting/compression dressings may help

- Unmeshed (more cosmetic) or Meshed (1:1.5 increases surface area by 50%; 1:3 — 200%)
- STSG typically 0.012–0.018 inch (range 0.005–0.28), check dermatome with #15 blade (0.015)
- Apply saline with epinephrine soaked lap pad to donor site immediately after harvest, then use semi occlusive dressing (i.e. tegaderm/opsite) for ↓ pain and faster healing
- Use bolster dressing or VAC to adhere graft to recipient site

Bone Grafts

- **Cancellous** — porous, trabeculae; osteoblasts stimulates healing, for smaller defects with minimal structural support
- **Cortical** — non-porous, lamellar bone; for larger defects requiring structural support
- **Corticocancellous** — provides elements of both
- Can be vascularized or nonvascularized
- **Osteoconduction** — graft acts as scaffold for new ingrowth from native bone
- **Osteoinduction** — graft stimulates host osteoprogenitor cells to differentiate and make new bone
- Donor sites: Fibula, Ilium, Radius, Ribs, Cranium

Tissue Expansion

I. Tissue expansion physiology

- Increased surface area achieved by growth of new tissue, not stretching
- **Creep**
    - Mechanical — morphologic changes to cell
    - Biological — processes involved in cellular proliferation

  - **Stretch-induced signal transduction pathway** — "stretching" of tissue initiates a complex biomechanical process in which cellular proliferation and ECM restructuring occurs
    - Growth Factors (EGF, TGF, PDGF, bFGF), ion channels, membrane proteins/adhesion complexes (Integrins), actin, protein kinases, and second messenger systems (cAMP) have all been shown to play active roles

- **Increased vascularity**

II. Uses

- Scalp
- Face/neck
- Breast
- Trunk
- Extremities

III. Methods

- Can be standard or custom made
  - Usually round, rectangle, or crescent in shape
  - Size — 100–2,000 cm^3
  - Port-integrated or remote
- Try to place via incision that will eventually be excised
- Avoid placing in infected/contaminated field, or area with recent trauma or scarring

IV. Complications — ~10% rate

- Infection
- Implant exposure/extrusion/deflation
- Flap ischemia
- Seroma
- Poor scarring/dog ears

Implants

- Ideally should be biologically inert, sterile, resistant to microbes, non-allergenic, noncarcinogenic, and illicits no foreign-body response from recipient
- Traditionally four categories: **Metals, Polymers, Calcium ceramics**, and **Biologics**

I. Metals

- Titanium
- Vitallium
- Stainless steel
- Gold

II. Polymers

- Polymethylmethacrylate
- Polypropylene (prolene, marlex)
- Polyesters (Dacron, Mersilene)
- Polytetrafluoroethylene (Teflon, Gore-tex)
- Polyethylene (Medpor)
- Biodegradable polyesters (polyglycolic acid, poly-L-lactic acid)

III. Calcium ceramics

- Hydroxyapatite
- Tricalcium phosphate
- Bioactive glass

IV. Biologic materials

- Acellular Dermal Matrix
- Collagen

Flaps

I. Definition

- Transplanted tissue that maintains its own blood supply

II. Classification

***May be categorized by vascular supply, composition, relation to defect, or method of movement**

- Vascularity
  - Random Pattern
  - Axial
- Composition
  - Cutaneous
  - Fasciocutaneous
  - Musculocutaneous
  - Osteocutaneous/Osteomusculocutaneous
  - Visceral
  - Innervated (Functional)
- Relation/Proximity to defect
  - Local
  - Regional
  - Distant
  - Free
- "Method of Movement"
  - Rotation
  - Advancement
  - Transposition
    - Z-plasty
    - Limberg (Rhomboid) flap
    - Dufourmental flap
  - Island/Interpolation
  - Distant
    - Groin, Cross-leg, Thenar
    - Tubed
    - Free

Table 1. Common Muscle/Musculocutaneous Flaps.

Flap	Blood Supply Type Vessel	Reliability	Donor Site Morbidity	Dissection (Easy, Mod, Hard)	Pedicle Caliber	Pedicle Length
Pectoralis Major	V Thoracoacromial	Very good	Some	Easy	Moderate	Short
Latissimus Dorsi	V Thoracodorsal	Excellent	Minimal	Easy	Large	Long
Serratus	III Thoracodorsal	Good	Minimal	Easy	Large	Long
Rectus Abdominus	III Superior and Deep Inferior Epigastric	Good	Some	Easy	Large	Long
Gluteus Maximus	V Sup/Inf Gluteal	Good	Significant	Moderate	Large	Long
Gracilis	II Medial Fem Cir	Very good	None	Easy	Moderate	Medium
Sartorius	IV SFA	Poor	None	Easy	Moderate	Short
Tensor Fascia Lata	I Lateral Fem Cir	Very good	Some	Difficult	Moderate	Medium
Vastus Lateralis	II Lateral Fem Cir	Very good	Some	Moderate	Moderate	Medium
Rectus Femoris	II Lateral Fem Cir	Very good	Some	Easy	Moderate	Medium
Gastrocnemius	I Sural	Excellent	Some	Moderate	Moderate	Short
Soleus	II Popliteal, PT, Peroneal	Good	Some	Moderate	Moderate	Short

III. Muscle/musculocutaneous (Table 1)

- *Mathes and Nahai classification*
  Type I: Single vascular pedicle
  Type II: Dominant vascular pedicle(s) and minor vascular pedicle(s)
  Type III: Two dominant pedicles
  Type IV: Segmental vascular pedicles
  Type V: Dominant vascular pedicle and secondary vascular pedicles
  Mnemonic: **Ten Graceful Glutes Sat on Latrines** (TFL, gracilis, gluteus maximus, sartorius, latissmus dorsi)

IV. Fasciocutaneous flaps (Tables 2 and 3)

Classifications:

- *Mathes and Nahai*
  - Type A: Direct cutaneous perforator
  - Type B: Septocutaneous
  - Type C: Musculocutaneous
- *Cormack and Lamberty*
  - Type A: Multiple perforators
  - Type B: Solitary perforators
  - Type C: Segmental perforators

Table 2. Common Fasciocutaneous Flaps.

Flap	Dissection	Donor Site Morbidity	Pedicle Caliber	Pedicle Length
Radial forearm	Easy	Significant	Large	Long
Lateral arm	Moderate	Minimal	Small	Short
Scapular	Easy	Minimal	Large	Medium
Parascapular	Easy	Minimal	Large	Medium
Temporoparietal	Moderate	Moderate	Small	Short
Deltopectoral	Moderate	Significant	Large	Variable

Table 3. Common Perforator Flaps.

Flap	Source Artery	Dissection	Donor Site Morbidity	Pedicle Caliber	Pedicle Length
Anterolateral thigh (ALT)	Lateral Circ Fem	Moderate	Moderate	Large	Long
DIEP	Deep Inf Epigastric	Easy	Minimal	Large	Long
GAP	Sup/Inf Gluteal	Mod/Difficult	Moderate	Large	Short
TUG/TMG	Med Fem Cir	Easy	Moderate	Small	Short
TAP	Thoracodorsal	Easy	Minimal	Large	Long
PAP	Profunda Femoris	Moderate	Minimal	Large	Long

- *Nakajima*
- *Taylor* — "angiosome" concept- distinct area of tissue supplied by same source artery

Further Reading

1. De Filippo RE, Atala A. (2002) Stretch and growth: the molecular and physiologic influences of tissue expansion. *Plast Reconstr Surg* **109**(7): 2450–2460.
2. Takei T, *et al.* (1998) Molecular basis for tissue expansion: clinical implications for the surgeon. *Plast Reconstr Surg* **102**(1): 247–258.
3. Bauer B. (2007) Tissue expansion. In: Thorne CH, *et al.* (eds.), *Grabb and Smith's Plastic Surgery*, 6th Edn. Lippincott Williams & Wilkins, Philadelphia, PA, pp. 84–90.
4. Hallock G. (2009) Classification of flaps. In: Wei F, Mardini S (eds.), *Flaps and Reconstructive Surgery*. Saunders, Elsevier, New York, pp. 7–15.
5. Hallock G. (2009) Flap selection. In: Wei F, Mardini S (eds.), *Flaps and Reconstructive Surgery*. Saunders Elsevier, New York, pp. 17–27.
6. Allen RJ, *et al.* (2012) Breast reconstruction with the profunda artery perforator flap. *Plast Reconstr Surg* **129**(1): 16e–23e.

CHAPTER 3

ANESTHETIC IMPLICATIONS IN COSMETIC SURGERY

Gian Paparcuri and Miguel Cobas

Introduction

Anesthesiologists providing care for plastic surgery face several challenges. In this consumer driven medical care business of cosmetic surgery, elective procedures are performed for the convenience and wishes of the buyer patient. These unique patients have extremely high standards and expectations as the procedure itself is expected to be a life changing experience.

Cosmetic surgery is mainly an elective procedure with no clear medical indication. Most of the times performed in otherwise healthy ASA 1 or 2 patients who are willing to undergo the stress associated with anesthesia and surgery in order to experience improvement in their physical appearance.

Although efforts should be made to maximize service, anesthesiologists should never compromise the prevailing anesthetic standards of care. Meeting the standard of care is the minimum requirement of our practice.

The American Society of Anesthesiologists (ASA) has issued practice guidelines, standards of care, positions, and statements regarding the safe practice of anesthesia. Providers are encouraged and invited to review and practice "safe anesthesia" under these parameters.

Preoperative Evaluation

> Patients coming for elective plastic surgery are usually healthy
>
> Most cosmetic procedures constitute elective surgeries and mandates appropriate patient optimization
>
> Preoperative patient evaluation includes a thorough history and physical examination
>
> Diligent perioperative care avoids postoperative complications

ASA basic standards for preanesthesia care and goals[1]

- Reduce patient's psychological and physiological anxiety
- Review available medical records
- Assess health status and physical readiness for scheduled surgery
- Order and review pertinent available tests and consultations
- Define therapeutic and monitoring strategies for the proposed anesthesia and surgery
- Plan postoperative care and pain therapy
- Order appropriate preoperative medications
- Obtain informed consent for anesthesia (include type of anesthesia and the most common and severe possible complications)
- Document in the chart that the above has been performed
- Coordinate patient care in a way that decreases total cost and improves outcomes

Although most of these patients have been cleared by their primary care physicians, regardless of what the surgeon has planned or what the specialists have cleared the patient for, the ultimate decision of whether or not to proceed with the case is always in the hands of the person in charge of the anesthetic care. The anesthesiologist is ultimately responsible for the pre and postoperative management of the patient. From the medico-legal perspective, the anesthesiologist is the final gatekeeper.

Pertinent preoperative patient information

1. Age and weight
2. Allergies to medication and the specific reaction (i.e., urticaria, rash, and anaphylaxis)
3. Current medications, including herbal supplements like Ginko Biloba, Garlic, Ginseng, Echinacea, Ephedra, or St John's Wort (coagulopathy, interference with anesthesia, and cardiovascular disturbances). Inquire about estrogen therapy, like oral contraceptive pills (OCP) and hormonal replacement therapy (HRT) which increases thromboembolism perioperative risk
4. Pregnancy
5. Tobacco exposure, pack per year history, time from last cigarette
6. History of asthma. Assess most recent attack, current medication, and consider preinduction inhalers
7. Coagulation abnormalities
8. History of motion sickness
9. Previous anesthetic experiences (i.e., prolonged emergence or PONV)
10. Personal or familiar history of malignant hyperthermia (use non trigger anesthetics)
11. History of recent weight changes that suggest anorexia and electrolyte imbalance
12. Any other pertinent medical information (i.e., obstructive sleep apnea with compromised cardiopulmonary reserve, hepatitis, HIV/AIDS)

Smokers and those exposed to second hand smoke are subject to the perioperative implications of tobacco exposure[2]:

- Increases wound infections
- Decreases macrophage function
- Negatively affects coronary flow reserve
- Causes vascular endothelial dysfunction, hypertension, and ischemia
- Increases respiratory or airway complications (including oxygen desaturation), and severe coughing
- Smokers require longer hospital stay than nonsmokers do and often need postoperative intensive care admission
- Females smokers receiving estrogen therapy have an increased risk for thromboembolism
- Additionally, smoking increases plastic surgery complications, including flap survival/viability[3]

The most common and widespread classification of preoperative physical status is the ASA classification:

	ASA Physical Status Classification	Example
I	Normal healthy patient; no systemic disease; not at extremes of age	Healthy 21 year old patient
II	Controlled medical conditions with mild systemic effects. No functional limitation	Controlled DM, controlled HTN, smoker, obesity
III	Disease with severe functional limitation or systemic effects	Stable angina, controlled CHF, morbid obesity, COPD, CRF
IV	Poorly controlled severe medical condition associated with significant impairment in functional ability and constant threat to life	Unstable angina, symptomatic COPD, symptomatic CHF
V	Moribund patient, critical condition, not expected to survive without operation	Ruptured aortic aneurysm
VI	Organ donor	Declared brain death
E	Emergency surgery for any class, trauma	GSW, GI perforation

One of the most deciding factors in determining whether patients can undergo surgery safely is their functional capacity estimated in metabolic equivalent of task (MET). As a general rule patients able to generate equal or more than 4 MET can undergo most procedures without further testing given the fact that most, if not all, cosmetic surgeries are considered low or intermediate risk.

ACC/AHA 2007 Guidelines on Perioperative Cardiovascular Evaluation and Care for Noncardiac Surgery.[4]

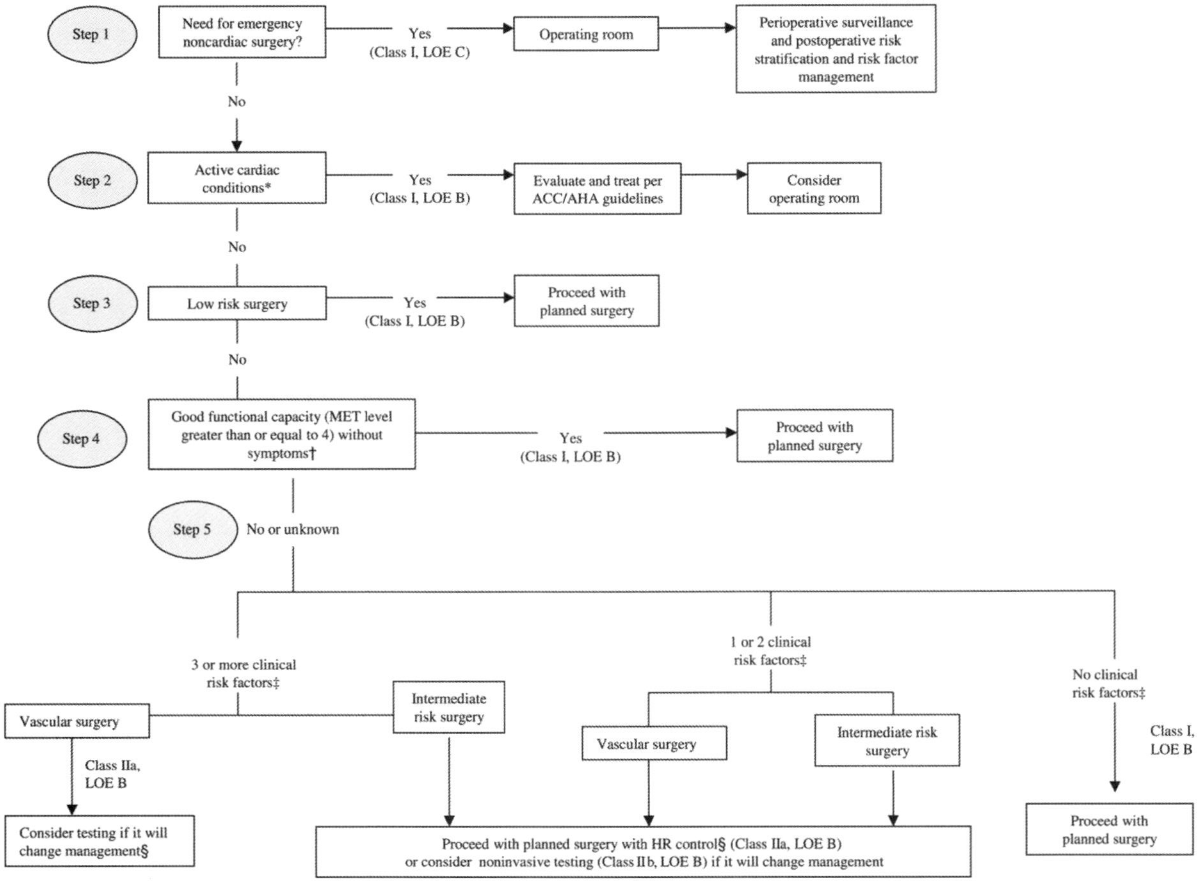

Estimated energy requirements for various activities

	Can you...
1 MET	Take care of yourself?
	Eat, dress, or use the toilet?
	Walk indoors around the house?
	Walk a block or 2 on level ground at 2 to 3 mph (3.2 to 4.8 kph)?
4 MET	Do light work around the house like dusting or washing dishes?
	Climb a flight of stairs or walk up a hill?
	Walk on level ground at 4 mph (6.4 kph)?
	Run a short distance?
	Do heavy work around the house like scrubbing floors or lifting or moving heavy furniture?
	Participate in moderate recreational activities like golf, bowling, dancing, doubles tennis, or throwing a baseball or football?
Greater than 10 MET	Participate in strenuous sports like swimming, single tennis, football, basketball, or skiing?

Fasting recommendations

Summary of ASA Fasting Recommendations to Reduce the Risk of Pulmonary Aspiration:*[5]

Ingested material	Minimum fasting period (h)
Clear liquids‡	2
Breast milk	4
Infant formula	6
Non human milk	6
Light meal¶	6

*These recommendations apply for healthy patients who are undergoing elective procedures. Following the Guidelines does not guarantee complete gastric emptying.
‡Examples of clear liquids include water, fruit juices without pulp, carbonated beverages, clear tea, and black coffee.
¶A light meal typically consists of toast and clear liquids. Meals that include fried or fatty foods or meat may prolong gastric emptying time. Both the amount and type of foods ingested must be considered when determining an appropriate fasting period.

Patients who regularly consume caffeinated beverages who experience caffeine withdrawal headache without their morning coffee are encouraged to drink their cup of black coffee WITHOUT any dairy product. Non dairy creamers are acceptable, if needed. An alternative is OTC caffeine table

Patients who are scheduled for afternoon surgery may have a light breakfast not closer than 6 hours prior to their surgery. Again, "light" means NO DAIRY PRODUCTS (i.e., milk, cream, butter, yogurt, or cheese)

Following this rules the patient the stomach will be empty without having the risk of hypoglycemia before surgery

Patients are encourage to void before getting on the OR table

Airway

Failure of the anesthesiologist to monitor and maintain patent airway of patient undergoing cosmetic surgery, is one of the most common causes of anesthesia related morbidity and mortality

Signs of potentially difficult airway ("LEMON")

- Look externally for: abnormal face shape, facial trauma, sunken cheeks, narrow mouth, edentulous, "buck teeth" (large incisors), large tongue, receding mandible, beard or moustache, facial/neck pathology, obesity, upper lip bite test
- Evaluate the 3–3-2 rule:
  - Mouth opening (incisors distance) less than 3 fingerbreadths
  - Hyoid/chin (mental) distance less than 3 fingerbreadths
  - Thyroid cartilage to mouth floor (thyromental) distance less than 2 fingerbreadths

- **M**allampati score (see below): classes III and IV
- **O**bstruction: presence of any condition that could cause an obstructed airway. Pathology around upper airway (peritonsillar abscess)
- **N**eck mobility: limited range of motion (cervical spine flexion/ extension). Examine pt for decreased range of motion that might limit head movement into sniffing position during intubation

Mallampati Scoring System

Pt in an upright position, mouth open as wide as possible, not sticking tongue out

Grade view	Visible structures	Intubation
1	Tonsillar pillars, soft palate, entire uvula	Unlikely difficult
2	Pillars and soft palate, only part of uvula	Unlikely difficult
3	Soft palate and base of uvula	Possible difficult
4	Hard palate only	Difficult/impossible

Perioperative instructions

Patients stable on their preoperative regimen of medications should continue taking those medications with the following possible exceptions:

- Instruct patients taking diuretics not to take their a.m. dose as this will tend to cause their bladder to become full under anesthesia. A full bladder can cause enuresis (spontaneous voiding) and high blood pressure. A short (less than 4 hours) elective cosmetic surgery does not routinely require bladder catheterization. Not requiring catheterization eliminates the risk of iatrogenic bladder infection
- Schedule insulin dependent diabetics as first case in the morning. Avoid their full a.m. dose of insulin; instead one half to one third of their usual morning insulin dose should be enough for short morning case. Hourly check of their blood sugars during anesthesia is strongly recommended
- Avoid herbal remedies for at least two weeks prior to surgery and one week after surgery

Instruct asthmatic patients to bring their inhalers to surgery
Patients with obstructive sleep apnea (OSA) on non-invasive positive pressure ventilation should bring their CPAP machine with them the day of surgery
Follow ASA fasting guidelines to reduce the risk of pulmonary aspiration
Outpatients should be notified that they require a responsible caregiver to accompany them to and from surgery and to stay with them the night of surgery

Preoperative testing

Preoperative tests, as component of the preanesthesia evaluation, are indicated to diagnose or assess an already known disorder which may affect perioperative anesthetic care. They also help to formulate specific plans and alternatives for perioperative care. No routine laboratory is necessary. Appropriate indications for ordering test include the identification during preoperative evaluation of specific risk factors, like age, preexisting medical conditions, and magnitude of the surgical procedure (i.e., ECG in patients with a known cardiac disease and chest radiographs for those with acute pulmonary symptoms).

Complications During Elective Outpatient Cosmetic Surgery

Providing anesthesia in the office based setting deserves special consideration since this practice often has little or no regulation compared with hospitals and licensed ambulatory surgical facilities.

The ASA, recognizing the unique needs of this growing practice, and has issued guidelines for the practice of anesthesia in the office setting.

These are minimal guidelines intended to assist anesthesia providers considering OBA and may be exceeded at any time based on the judgment of the involved anesthesia personnel. Compromising safety for improved results can lead to devastating problems:

- PONV
- Postoperative pain
- Hemorrhage
- Fluid overload
- Local anesthetic toxicity
- Intraoperative fire
- Thromboembolism (i.e., pulmonary embolism and deep venous thrombosis)
- Malignant hyperthermia

ASA guidelines for office based anesthesia (OBA)[6]

The anesthesiologist should be satisfied that the procedure is within the scope of practice of the health care practitioners and the capabilities of the facility
The procedure should be of a duration and degree of complexity that will permit the patient to recover and be discharged from the facility
Patients who by reason of preexisting medical or other conditions may be at undue risk for complications should be referred to an appropriate facility for performance of the procedure and the administration of anesthesia
The anesthesiologist should be physically present during the intraoperative period and immediately available until the patient has been discharged from anesthesia care
Discharge of the patient is the physician's responsibility and should be documented in the medical record
Personnel with training in advance resuscitation techniques should be immediately available until all patients are discharged home
Facilities should have a reliable source of oxygen, suction, resuscitation equipment and emergency drugs
Back up power to ensure patient protection in the event of an emergency should be available
In any location in which anesthesia is administered, there should be appropriate anesthesia apparatus and equipment which allow monitoring consistent with ASA standards
Facility personnel should be appropriately trained in the facility's written emergency protocols
The facility should have medications, equipment and written protocols to treat emergencies disasters such as cardiopulmonary arrest, fire, malignant hyperthermia (specially when triggering agents are used)
The facility should have written protocols for the safe and timely transfer of patients to a prespecified alternate care facility when extended or emergency services are needed
Policies and procedures. Including fire, safety, drugs, emergencies, staffing, training, and unanticipated patient transfers. These policies and procedures should be written and reviewed on an annual basis
All health care providers should be qualified and hold a valid license to perform their assigned duties
Maintain continuous communication with the surgeon. Never disable alarms. Never let your guard down
Hope for the best, prepare for the worst

In this section, major complications like intraoperative fires, malignant hyperthermia, and thromboembolism will be discussed. Anesthetic implications of postoperative nausea and vomiting and pain management will be reviewed in detail in following sections.

Intraoperative fire

To start a fire it is necessary to have three components:

1. Increased oxidative environment (i.e., oxygen pool around the face)
2. Flammable substance (i.e., paper drape)
3. Heat source (i.e., surgical cautery device)

Described preventing measures include:

- Discontinuing the oxygen supply or switching to compressed air, while a cautery or laser device is in use (decrease oxidative environment)
- If patient requires uninterrupted supplemental oxygen because of partial obstruction or desaturation, consider using supraglottic airway device (i.e., LMA) or endotracheal intubation
- Avoid using drapes as a tent, enriching the entire area with oxygen
- Flammable agents such as alcohol or tinctured based products should be avoided as skin preparation
- Keeping electrocautery device in a holster when not in use
- Avoiding foot pedal controls that might accidentally be deployed by stepping on them
- Use moist sponges and towels to drape off the surgical field

Thromboembolism

The American Society of Plastic Surgery has formulated a task force on Deep Venous Thrombosis Prophylaxis and has established some guidelines.

It is recommended that patients be stratified according to their risk of deep venous thrombosis and pulmonary embolus[7]:

Low risk Patients under the age of forty without known risk factors Surgical procedures of thirty minutes or less	Comfortable positioning on the OR table, with slight knee flexion provided with a pillow under the knees, to enhance popliteal venous return External pressure on the legs or constricting garments should be avoided
Moderate risk Patients aged forty or older, taking OCP or HRT Procedures longer than thirty minutes GA greater than one hour	Same measures, plus intermittent pneumatic compression garments worn before, during, and after general anesthesia until fully awake These patients are asked if possible to stop taking risky medications at least 1 week before surgery
High risk Patients falling into the moderate risk category but have additional risk factors such as malignancy, immobilization, obesity, and hypercoagulable states	Same measures as the other two previous categories, plus a preoperative hematology consultation Consider LMWH 2 hours before surgery and daily until the patient is ambulating

Risk factors for deep venous thrombosis and pulmonary embolism	
Virchow's triad: hypercoagulability, vascular injury, and stasis	Obesity (BMI greater than 30) Recent MI or CVA
Immobilization (i.e., surgery or fracture)	Previous history of deep vein thrombosis
Malignancy	History of radiation therapy (especially pelvic)
Thrombophlebitis	Antiphospholipid antibody syndrome
Pregnancy and for six to twelve weeks postpartum	Homocystinemia
Extremity trauma	Polycythemia
Estrogen therapy (i.e., HRT or OCP) Smoking	Other hypercoagulable states: abnormal protein C or S, factor V Leiden

Malignant hyperthermia

Malignant hyperthermia (MH) is a life threatening, inherited, pharmacogenetic disorder of the skeletal muscle, triggered by halogenated volatile anesthetics and depolarizing muscle relaxants in susceptible individuals.

Emergency therapy for malignant hyperthermia (adapted from MHAUS)

DIAGNOSIS vs. ASSOCIATED PROBLEMS		
Signs of MH: ·Increasing $EtCO_2$ ·Trunk or total body rigidity ·Masseter spasm or trismus ·Tachycardia/tachypnea ·Mixed respiratory and metabolic acidosis ·Increased temperature (may be late sign) ·Myoglobinuria	**Sudden/unexpected cardiac arrest in young patients:** ·Presume Hyperkalemia and initiate treatment (see #6) ·Measure CK, myoglobin, ABGs, until normalized ·Consider Dantrolene ·Usually secondary to occult myopathy (e.g., muscular dystrophy) ·Resuscitation may be difficult and prolonged	**Trismus or masseter spasm with succinylcholine:** ·Early sign of MH in many patients ·If limb muscle rigidity, begin treatment with Dantrolene ·For emergent procedures, continue with non triggering agents, evaluate and monitor the patient, and consider dantrolene treatment ·Follow CK and urine myoglobin for 36 hours ·Check CK immediately and at 6 hours intervals until returning to normal. Observe for dark or cola colored urine. If present, liberalize fluid intake and test for myoglobin ·Observe in PACU or ICU for at least 12 hours
ACUTE PHASE TREATMENT		
1. GET HELP. GET DANTROLENE – Notify Surgeon ·Discontinue volatile agents and succinylcholine ·Hyperventilate with 100% oxygen at flows of 10 L/min or more ·Halt the procedure as soon as possible; if emergent, continue with non-triggering anesthetic technique ·Don't waste time changing the circle system and CO_2 absorbant **2. Dantrolene 2.5 mg/kg rapidly IV through large bore IV, if possible** *To convert kg to lbs for amount of dantrolene, give patient 1 mg/lb (2.5 mg/kg approximates 1 mg/lb)* ·Dissolve the 20 mg in each vial with 60 ml sterile, preservative free water for injection. Prewarming (not to exceed 39°C) the sterile water may expedite solublization of dantrolene. However to date, there is no evidence that such warming improves clinical outcome	·Repeat until signs of MH are reversed Sometimes more than 10 mg/kg (up to 30 mg/kg) is necessary ·Each 20 mg bottle has 3 gm mannitol for isotonicity. The pH of solution is 9 **3. Bicarbonate for metabolic acidosis** ·1 – 2 mEl/kg if blood gas values are not yet available **4. Cool** the patient with core temperature >39 °C. Lavage open body cavities, stomach, bladder, or rectum. Apply ice to surface. Infuse cold saline IV. Stop cooling if temp. <38 °C and falling to prevent drift <36°C **5. Dysrhythmias** usually respond to treatment of acidosis and Hyperkalemia ·Use standard drug therapy **except calcium channel blockers, which may cause Hyperkalemia or cardiac arrest in the presence of dantrolene**	**6. Hyperkalemia** – Treat with hyperventilation, bicarbonate, glucose/insulin, calcium ·Bicarbonate 1 – 2 mEq/kg IV ·For **pediatric**, 0.1 U/kg and 1 ml/kg 50% glucose or for **adult**, 10 U regular insulin IV and 50 ml 50% glucose ·Calcium chloride 10 mg/kg or calcium gluconate 10 – 50 mg/kg for life threatening Hyperkalemia ·Check glucose levels hourly **7. Follow** ETCO2, electrolytes, blood gases, CK, core temperature, urine output and color, coagulation studies. If CK an/or K+ rise more than transiently or urine falls to less than 0.5 ml/kg/hr, induce diuresis to > 1 ml/kg/hr and give bicarbonate to alkalinize urine to prevent Myoglobinuria induced renal failure (see D below) ·Venous blood gas (e.g., femoral vein) values may document hypermetabolism better than arterial values ·Central venous or PA monitoring as needed and recorded minute ventilation ·Place Foley catheter and monitor urine output
POST ACUTE PHASE		
A Observe the patient in an ICU for at least 24 hours, due to the risk of recrudescence **B** Dantrolene 1 mg/kg q4-6 hours or 0.25 mg/kg/hr by infusion for at least 24 hours. Further doses may be indicated **C** Follow vitals and labs as above (see #7) ·Frequent ABG as per clinical signs ·CK every 8 – 12 hours; less often as the values trend downward	**D** Follow urine myoglobin and institute therapy to prevent myoglobin precipitation in renal tubules and the subsequent development of Ac Renal Failure. CK levels above 10.000 IU/L is a presumptive sign of rhabdomyolysis and Myoglobinuria. Follow standard intensive care therapy for acute rhabdomyolysis and Myoglobinuria (urine output >2 ml/kg/hr by hydration and diuretics along with alkalinization of urine with Na – bicarbonate infusion with careful attention to both urine and serum pH values) **E** Counsel the patient and family regarding MH and further precautions; refer them to MHAUS. Fill out and send in the Adverse Metabolic Reaction to Anesthesia (AMRA) from (www.mhreg.org) and send a letter to the patient and her/his physician. Refer patient to the nearest Biopsy Center for follow up	

http://www.mhaus.org/

MH Hotline 1-800-644-9737

Outside the US: 1-315-464-7079

The incidence of MH has been calculated to be between 1:5.000 and 1:100.000; however, the frequency has increased in recent years.[8]

The Malignant Hyperthermia Association of the United States (MHAUS) has recently established diagnostic criteria and management protocols (see below) to prevent perioperative deaths.

Intraoperative Monitoring

A vigilant anesthesiologist constitutes the most important intraoperative monitor.

ASA standard monitors

Oxygenation	Circulation
Inspired oxygen concentration	ECG: leads II and V5
Pulse oximetry (SpO_2)	Noninvasive blood pressure monitoring (NIABP)
Ventilation	HR
Exhaled or end tidal carbon dioxide ($EtCO_2$): especially when opioids have been given or patient is draped	Temperature especially when MH triggering agents are in use

Intraoperative awareness

Incidence of awareness under general anesthesia is a very significant concern for many patients, with a reported incidence of 0.2 to 1.5%.[9] In 2003 a study published by Tong *et al.* patients were willing to pay out of their pockets US$34 for a monitor that would assist an anesthesia care provider assess the depth of anesthesia in an effort to avoid awareness. This increased to US$43, if the insurance company was making the payment.[10]

The bispectral index (BIS) is a variable derived from the EEG that represents a measure of the hypnotic effect of anesthetic agents, predicting depth of consciousness. Calculation of the BIS integrates several complex signals from EEG into a single variable. These signals or parameters were selected from EEG data collected from thousands of anesthetics and then correlated with patient's level of consciousness and response to surgical stimuli. Finally, these parameters are ranked from 0 to 100. BIS values of less than 60 appear to predict absence of consciousness.

Several studies have shown good correlation between the BIS and the level of sedation, loss of consciousness, and the probability of recall. During surgical procedures performed under monitored anesthesia care (MAC), it is imperative to understand that the BIS will not be able to predict movement in response to pain. Motor response to incision may be mediated by subcortical structures, which are not measured by the BIS.[11]

BIS monitor...

Constitutes a processed EEG. BIS algorithm processing lacks behind real time (delay of 15–30 seconds)

Uses: monitor anesthesia depth in order to prevent intraoperative awareness

Does not predict patient movement

Not yet an ASA standard monitor

Under MAC anesthesia, by being able to demonstrate adequate sedation levels (BIS 60–75) during patient movement, the surgeon can be educated to inject more analgesia (more local) instead of deepening the anesthetic plane

Intraoperative Management

Premedication

Patients having lower anxiety levels preoperatively, tend to have less pain postoperatively.

Midazolam: 2 mg IV. Anxiolysis and sedation

Clonidine (α2 agonist): 0.1–0.3 mg PO (30–60 min preoperatively). Anxiolysis, sedation, propofol/opioid sparring effect, and antiadrenergic effects

Glycopyrrolate: 0.2 mg IV. May be used to minimize secretions (relevant when using ketamine)

Commonly used intravenous sedatives and anesthetics

Drug	Induction (mg/kg)	Maintenance (mcg/kg/min)	Sedation (mcg/kg/min)	Pharmacodynamic effects
Propofol	2–2.5	100–200	25–75	Sedation, amnesia, ↓ pruritus, ↓ PONV, anticonvulsant Pain on injection, respiratory depression, hypotension
Ketamine	1–2	10–100	5–20	Dissociative state, amnesia, sedation, analgesia, maintains pharyngeal and laryngeal reflexes, bronchodilation Laryngospasm‡, tachycardia¶, HTN, colorful dreams, emergence delirium, ↑ salivary secretions, psychosis, hallucinations¶, horizontal nystagmus
Midazolam	0.15–0.35	0.25–1.5	0.25–1	Sedation, anxiolysis, anterograde amnesia, anticonvulsant, skeletal muscle relaxation Respiratory depression, prolonged sedation, paradoxical excitement
Dexmedetomidine (Precedex)	n/a	0.2–1 mcg/kg/h		Sedation, analgesia, anxiolysis, minimal respiratory depression Hypotension, bradycardia
Thiopental	3–5	200–300 (1st 20 min) 30–70 (thereafter)	30–80	Anticonvulsant Hypoventilation
Etomidate	0.2–0.6	10	2.5–7.5	Nausea, vomiting, adrenocortical suppression
Fentanyl	5–40 mcg/kg	0.03–1	0.01–0.04	Sedation, analgesia PONV, pruritus, respiratory depression, requires supplemental oxygen (fire hazard), urinary retention, constipation, muscle rigidity, depression of laryngeal reflexes with increased risk of aspiration
Remifentanil (Ultiva)	0.5–3 mcg/kg/min	0.05–2	0.025–0.2	
Sufentanil	2–10 mcg/kg	0.01–0.1	0.005–0.01	

‡Management of ketamine induced laryngospasm includes early diagnosis and prompt therapy: positive pressure, jaw thrust, lidocaine 2 mg/kg IVB or propofol 50 mg IVB; administering succinylcholine (SCH) adds unnecessary risks as an MH triggering agent and further myalgias associated with SCH.

¶Hypnotic doses of propofol or midazolam block ketamine induced hallucinations as well as hemodynamic sequellae ± judicious use of beta blockers (labetalol, esmolol, propanolol). Beta blockers might be contraindicated in asthmatic patients.

Sedation continuum

Minimal sedation (anxiolysis)

- Drug induced cognitive function and coordination impairment
- Patients respond normally to verbal commands
- Ventilatory and cardiovascular functions are unaffected

Moderate sedation/analgesia (conscious sedation)

- Drug induced depression of consciousness
- Patients respond purposefully to verbal commands, either alone or accompanied by light tactile stimulation
- No *interventions*† are required to maintain a patent airway, and spontaneous ventilation is adequate
- Cardiovascular functions is usually maintained
- A second physician is involved in: deep sedation analgesia

Deep sedation/analgesia

- Drug induced depression of consciousness
- Patients cannot be easily aroused but respond purposefully to following repeated or painful stimulation
- The ability to independently maintain ventilatory function may be impaired
- Patient may require *assistance*‡ in maintaining a patent airway, and spontaneous ventilation may be inadequate
- Cardiovascular functions is usually maintained
- Reflex withdrawal from painful stimulus is NOT considered a purposeful response

GA

- Drug induced loss of consciousness
- Patients are not arousable, even by painful stimulation
- The ability to independently maintain ventilatory function is often impaired
- Patients often require assistance in maintaining a patent airway, and positive pressure ventilation may be required because of depressed spontaneous ventilation or drug induced depression of neuromuscular function
- Cardiovascular functions may be impaired
- Reflex withdrawal from painful stimulus is NOT considered a purposeful response

†Neck extension with or without lateral rotation, placement of a shoulder roll, chin lift.
‡Supraglottic mechanical device (nasal airway, oral airway, LMA, combitube).

Most OBA procedures are performed under sedation (MAC) and not under GA. It is crucial to differentiate among these 2 techniques, as many drugs in the anesthesia armament are useful for both. Regardless of the initial intention, if the patient loses consciousness and the ability to respond purposefully, the anesthesia care is a general anesthetic, irrespective of whatever airway instrumentation is required. Anesthesia providers have to be ready to support vital functions and to convert to general or regional when necessary.[12]

Minimally invasive anesthesia

If patient and surgeon are willing, elective cosmetic procedures could be performed under just local anesthesia with some form of sedation. This technique known as monitored anesthesia care or MAC offers several advantages over general anesthesia (GA) in today's cosmetic surgery practice, like

Clinical pathway for MIA technique[13]

1. Clonidine 0.2 mg PO 30–60 min preop (systolic >100, body weight >100 pounds)
2. Glycopyrrolate 0.2 mg IV with 2 mL 1% lidocaine plain
3. Incrementally titrate propofol to BIS <75 with multiple, sequential 150 mcg/kg every 20 sec mini boluses or set initial rate to 450 mcg/kg/min and reduce rate toward 50 as soon as the EMG begins to decrease
4. Basal propofol infusion rate 50 mcg/kg/min (BEFORE ketamine to prevent hallucinations)
5. Ketamine 50 m IVP at BIS <75 2–3 min prior to injection of local anesthesia (AFTER propofol)†
6. Adjust basal propofol rate upward to maintain BIS 60–75 if Ketamine causes an increase
7. Inject adequate local analgesia
8. Administer more ketamine (25–50 mg) only after two reinjections (total of three) of the field fail to eliminate patient movement
9. Maintain propofol at BIS 60–75, EMG 0 on BIS scale, 30 on EMG scale
10. Bupivacaine in field before closure, especially for browlift, subpectoralis augmentation, and abdominoplasty

†Do not administer ketamine until the BIS is less than 75 in the context of a gradual propofol induction (not propofol bolus).

short recovery, better postoperative analgesia, and minimization of postoperative complications (i.e., postoperative nausea and vomiting or PONV), timely postoperative discharge, and patient satisfaction.

Furthermore, some authors have modified and adapted MAC techniques to the strong exigencies of the office based anesthesia (OBA) practice. Entire texts of anesthesia for cosmetic surgery are based on what is known today as minimally invasive anesthesia (MIA), providing safe, gratifying, expedite, and sustainable care for cosmetic surgery patients.[13]

Basically MIA consist in providing conscious sedation with short acting intravenous anesthetics and the concomitant administration of local analgesics (LA) to prevent patient movement by the surgeon.

Neuromuscular blockers

- Indicated only for specific procedures (i.e., breast surgery and abdominoplasty)
- Can be avoided in most cases of cosmetic surgery
- If they ever need it carefully titrate to avoid residual paralysis, delayed awakening, or postoperative airway complications
- Neostigmine used as reversal agent is associated with PONV

Intravenous anesthetics antagonists

- Specific antagonist must be available whenever benzodiazepines and opioids are administered but should not be used routinely. When given to antagonize respiratory depression and sedation, patients should be observed long enough to ensure that cardiorespiratory depression does not recur.

Agent	Indications	Dosage
Flumazenil (romazicon)	Benzodiazepine overdose	0.2 mg IVP up to 5 mg†
Naloxone (narcan)	Opioid overdose (short acting)¶	0.4–2 mg IV

†Black box warning: seizure risk when benzodiazepine use for long term sedation. Prepare for seizure management.

¶Following reversal, consider continuous infusion at 2.5 mcg/kg/h IV.

Fluid management

- Healthy patients scheduled for elective cosmetic surgery are not significantly "dry" or "behind" on fluid volume despite been "nothing per oral" (NPO) after midnight
- In most cosmetic procedures vasodilating inhaled anesthetic are no longer being used
- Large fluids shifts and blood loss are not expected or contemplated
- Lastly "third space" created by the aspiration of fat is functionally obliterated by the use of compression garments
- Restrict IVF to avoid fluid overload:
  - Edema (i.e., tissue and pulmonary)
  - Bleeding disorder (i.e., platelet dilution, coagulopathy)
  - Bladder distention, enuresis on OR table, patient embarrassment
  - Bladder catheterization, exposure to urinary tract infection

Post Anesthesia Care Unit (PACU)

Postanesthetic care is defined as those activities undertaken to manage the patient following completion of a surgical procedure.[14] Any time an anesthetic is administered, proper PACU care must be established.

Perioperative management allows routinely and periodic assessment and monitoring of:

- Respiratory function: respiratory rate, airway patency, and oxygen saturation. Perioperative use of pulse oximetry is associated with early detection of hypoxemia. Evidence supports the use of supplemental oxygen during patient transportation or in the recovery room to reduce the incidence of hypoxemia
- Cardiovascular function: pulse rate, blood pressure and in selected patients electrocardiographic monitoring should be immediately available
- Neuromuscular function: should be performed for patients who have received nondepolarizing neuromuscular clocking agents or who have medical conditions associated with neuromuscular dysfunction.

Includes physical examination and in selected patients nerve stimulator

- Mental status
- Temperature. Options to prevent and treat hypothermia and shivering are forced air warming devices and meperidine
- Pain
- Nausea and vomiting. Antiemetic agents should be used for the prevention and treatment of PONV when indicated
- Fluids: certain procedures involving significant loss of blood or fluids may require additional fluid management
- Urine output, drainage and bleeding

In the PACU, surgical patients must remain under continuous, close observation until they are no longer at increased risk for cardiorespiratory depression, meeting discharge criteria. The patient should also have a responsible individual accompany them home.

Patient discharge constitutes a medical act and should be performed only by a physician followed by proper documentation on the record.

Postoperative pain management

- Postoperative pain management starts intraoperatively
- Dissociative effect of ketamine constitutes the base for preemptive analgesia: preventing noxious signals from reaching the cortex by affecting midbrain thalamoneocortical projection system. Remember, ketamine should be given before any noxious stimulus, including field infiltration
- Assuring adequate local analgesia during the case minimizes most postoperative pain issues
- Use long acting local anesthetic, such as bupivacaine, before closing
- Concerns about increase risk of bleeding has limited the use of NSAIDs (ketorolac toradol)
- Nubain (nalbuphine) 5–10 mg IV. Is a mixed agonist/antagonist opioid with good analgesic profile and a respiratory ceiling
- Pain management solutions may include continuous infusion pumps and intercostal and incisional blocks

- By treating postoperative pain with generous local anesthetics infiltration, instead of more IV opioids, pain relief is more efficient, patient ambulates sooner, minimizing the risks of thromboembolic phenomena, and lastly is less prone to PONV

Safe Administration of Local Anesthesia

- Local anesthetics (LA) are weak bases, hydrophilic, tertiary amines
- Exert their action by binding to Na channel, thereby blocking depolarization induced influx of Na and blocking propagation of nerve impulses

Classification

Local anesthetics have a lipophilic benzene ring linked to an amine group by a hydrocarbon chain or amide or ester linkage. This linkage separates local analgesics into two groups:

Esters	Amides
Undergo hydrolysis by plasma cholinesterases	Undergo hepatic microsomal metabolism
Their pKa is usually higher than 8	Their pKa is usually lower than 8
Allergic reaction are caused by PABA (metabolite)	Contain antibacterial preservative (methylparaben) Allergic reactions are less common

Pharmacodynamic properties

- Onset of action (ionization). Local anesthetics exist in both charged or ionized and neutral or unionized forms
    - Uncharged (lipid soluble) form penetrates nerve membrane

- Charged (water soluble) form binds to Na receptor and exerts blockade
- Since local anesthetics are weak bases, the lower their pKa, the greater the fraction of uncharged (permeable) form at a given pH
- To expedite onset of action, bicarbonate is added to local anesthetic solutions. Alkalinization increases the uncharged form resulting in a quicker onset time
- Acidosis (i.e., infection) increases charged forms, delaying onset of action
- Increasing concentration and total dose of local also speeds up onset of action
- Potency (lipid solubility): the higher the solubility, the greater the potency
- Duration of action (protein binding): only the unbound form is active and susceptible to degradation (liver metabolism or plasma pseudocholinesterase)
- Sites with more vascular supply tend to have shorter duration (more systemic absorption)
- By adding epinephrine (or any other vasoconstrictor) systemic absorption is limited, duration of action is prolonged and risk of systemic toxicity decreases

Epinephrine 1:1000 contains 1 mg of epinephrine per mL
1:10.000 solution = 0.1 mg/mL (or 100 mcg/mL)
1:100.000 solution = 10 mcg/mL
1:200.000 solution = 5 mcg/mL
1:400.000 solution = 2.5 mcg/mL

Commonly used local anesthetics

	pKa	Relative potency	Onset (min)	Duration (hr)	Max dose (mg/kg)	Concentrations with clinical uses
Esters						
Chloroprocaine	8.7	2	5–10	0.5–1	9, 15 (with epi)	Epidural 2–3% Infiltration 1% Peripheral nerve block 2%
Tetracaine	8.5	8	5–10	3	1.5, 2.5 (with epi)	Spinal 0.5% Topical 2%
Amides						
Bupivacaine†	8.1	8	5–10	4–8 (long acting)†	2.5, 3 (with epi)	Epidural/Spinal 0.5–0.75% Infiltration 0.25% Peripheral nerve block 0.25–0.5%
Lidocaine	7.9	2	<2	1–2 (short acting)‡	4.5, 7 (with epi)	Epidural/Spinal 1.5–2% Infiltration 0.5–1 % IV regional 0.25–0.5% Peripheral nerve block 1–1.5% Topical 4%
Mepivacaine	7.6	2	3–5	1.5–3	5, 7 (with epi)	Epidural/Spinal 1.5–2% Infiltration 0.5–1 % IV regional 0.25–0.5% Peripheral nerve block 1–2%
Ropivacaine	8.1	6	10–15	4–8	2.5, 3 (with epi)	Epidural 0.5–1% Infiltration 0.2–0.5% Peripheral nerve block 0.5–1%

† Bupivacaine is more cardiotoxic than ropivacaine.

‡ Lidocaine provides intraoperative analgesia with bupivacaine providing postoperative analgesia.

Tumescent technique for liposuction involves infiltration of large volumes of diluted lidocaine and epinephrine

Frequently, injectate volumes equal the volume of fat aspirated with a maximum of 4–5 liters

During tumescent liposuction doses of lidocaine in the range of 35–55 mg/kg and epinephrine of 0.055 mg/kg are used

These doses are substantially greater than the recommended maximum for other routes of administration

It is believed that these larger doses are well tolerated with this technique because of decreased lidocaine uptake due to:

- Drug sequestration in adipose tissue
- Vasoconstriction associated with epinephrine
- Reduced vascularity of adipose tissue

Systemic absorption and toxicity

Toxicity results from excessive plasma concentrations secondary to absorption from tissue or accidental intravascular injection.

Variables related to local anesthetic absorption include:

1. Dose
2. Addition of vasoconstrictors
3. Degree of vasodilation
4. Local anesthetic lipid solubility
5. Presence of concomitant renal, hepatic, or cardiac disease
6. Site of injection

Intravascular > intercostal > caudal > epidural > brachial plexus > subcutaneous

- Toxicity mainly affects CV system and CNS
- CNS is more sensitive and usually affected first

- Signs of local anesthetic toxicity with increasing plasma concentrations include:

Light headedness → circumoral numbness → facial tingling → tinnitus → metallic taste on the tongue → slurred speech → delirium → disorientation → seizures → unconsciousness → respiratory arrest → cardiovascular depression → circulatory arrest

Blood lidocaine levels and manifestations of toxicity

mcg/ml	Clinical state in the awake patient
1.5–5.0	Therapeutic
5–10	Dizziness, tinnitus, patient complaint of metallic taste on the tongue, lethargy
10–20	Delirium, disorientation, eventually seizures and coma
>20	Probable cardiac arrest

Local anesthetic toxicity treatment

1. Stop local anesthetic administration
2. Get help
3. Maintain airway. Intubate if necessary
4. Provide 100% oxygen
5. Consider hyperventilation in presence of metabolic acidosis
6. Treat seizures. Options include: benzodiazepines, propofol, or thiopental
7. For cardiac arrest:
   a. Start CPR and follow ACLS protocols
   b. Consider cardiopulmonary bypass and lipid emulsion (intralipid 20%):

Loading dose: 1.5 ml/kg over 1 min (≈ 100 ml in 70 kg pt)
Infusion rate: 0.25 ml/kg/min (17.5 ml/min for 70 kg pt)
May repeat bolus (1.5 ml/kg) x2 at 5 min intervals
After 15 min, increase infusion to 0.5 ml/kg/min (35 ml/min for 70 kg pt) if circulation not restored
Continue CPR throughout intralipid infusion
Recovery from local anesthetic induced cardiac arrest may take as long as 1 hr

LA tips

- A blanched surgical field from epinephrine does not guarantee adequate surgical anesthesia
- Patient movement in the presence of adequate sedation (BIS 60–75) usually constitutes an indication for more local analgesia injection
- More local analgesia resolves patient movement 99% of the time

Antiemetic Therapy

Postoperative nausea and vomiting (PONV) are very unpleasant experiences for most patients undergoing elective procedures. In a published study from 2001, patients were willing to pay US$56 out of their pockets for a hypothetical new drug that would eliminate PONV.[15]

PONV risk factors[16]

- Patient factors: female, nonsmoker, history of PONV or motion sickness
- Anesthetic factors: volatile anesthetics (including nitrous oxide), opioids
- Surgical factors: emetogenic procedures (i.e., ophthalmic, gynecologic, laparoscopic, breast), surgical duration (each additional 30 min raises PONV risk by 60%)

Simplified risk score for PONV

Risk Factors	Points
Female	1
History of PONV/motion sickness	1
Nonsmoker	1
Perioperative opioids	1

Prediction and prophylaxis of PONV[17]

No. of points	% Risk of PONV	Prophylaxis
0	10% (low risk)	No prophylaxis
1	21% (low risk)	
2	39% (mod risk)	Monotherapy
3	61% (high risk)	Multimodal therapy/consider TIVA
4	79% (high risk)	

High risk patient has been defined as nonsmoking, female with a previous PONV/motion sickness history having elective cosmetic surgery greater than two hours in duration

- Prophylaxis is better than treatment. It is far more desirable to prevent the problem altogether than to have to deal with the consequences
- Avoidance of opioids is the single largest factor in preventing PONV
- Make certain patients are well hydrated. Encourage clear liquids up to three hours before surgery
- If a cosmetic surgery patient who is considered high risk for PONV must receive opioids, he or she should have multimodal therapy
- All of the anesthesiologist's efforts to prevent PONV and effect adequate pain management may be for naught if the surgeon discharges the patient home with an opioids containing analgesic

Antiemetic drugs classes

5HT3 (to be given at the end of surgery)
Ondansetron (Zofram): 4 mg IV
Granisetron (Kytril): 1 mg IV
Dolasetron (Anzemet): 12.5 mg IV

- Mechanism of action (5HT3 receptor antagonists): centrally (chemoreceptor trigger zone) and peripherally (abdominal vagal nerve terminals)
- Comments: side effects include headaches

Steroids

Dexametasone (Decadron): 4–8 mg IV (prior to induction)

- Mechanism of action (corticosteroids): unknown, likely centrally mediated

Butyrophenones (to be given at the end of surgery)
Droperidol (Inapsine): 0.625–1.25 mg IV

- Mechanism of action (butyrophenones/antipsychotic): dopamine antagonist in chemoreceptor trigger zone. Centrally, also interferes with transmission of NE, 5HT, GABA. Peripherally exerts some $\alpha 1$ blockade
- Comments: QT prolongation (black box warning), hypotension, drowsiness, rare extrapiramidal side effects (can be treated with diphenhydramine 25–50 mg IV)

Phenothiazines

Promethazine (Phenergan): 12.5–25 mg IV
Prochlorperazine (Compazine): 2.5–10 mg IV

- Mechanism of action (phenothiazines/antipsychotic): H1 receptor antagonist, antidopaminergic and α adrenergic blocking properties
- Comments: respiratory depression (avoid in patients with COPD, OSA), CNS depression, drowsiness, agitation, rare neuroleptic malignant syndrome, severe tissue damage with venous extravasation, contraindicated in children less than 2 years old owing to risk of fatal respiratory depression

Antihistamine

Dimenhydrinate: 1 mg/kg

Anticholinergics

Scopolamine patch: 4 hours before end of surgery

Prokinetics

Metoclopramide (Reglam): 10–20 mg IV (1 hour before end of surgery)

- Mechanism of action (prokinetics): central dopaminergic antagonist, peripheral cholinomimetic (increases LES tone, enhances peristalsis, decreases pyloric sphincter tone)
- Comments: rare extrapiramidal side effects, neuroleptic malignant syndrome, contraindicated in patients with intestinal obstruction

Others

Propofol: 20 mg IV (to be given in PACU). Monitor for respiratory depression
Ephedrine: 0.5 mg/kg IM (to be given at the end of surgery)

Nonpharmacologic therapy

P6 accupoint stimulation

Anesthesia for Specific Plastic Surgery Procedures

Liposuction

- Invented in Rome, Italy by two Italo-American surgeons in 1974. Constitutes the most commonly performed plastic surgery procedure
- Also known as lipoplasty (fat modeling), liposculture, suction lipectomy or simply lipo
- Constitutes a contouring procedure (not indicated for weight loss) performed by inserting hollow rods into the skin in order to suction subcutaneous fat (up to 5.000 mL per operative visit)
- The procedure may be performed under general or local ("tumescent") analgesia, allowing the procedure to be done safely in the office based setting, under IV sedation
- Removal of very large volumes of fat is complex and increases surgical risk
- Most plastic surgery literature defines "large" volume as being either total fat removed during the procedure of more than 4 liters or total

volume removed during the procedure (fat plus wetting solution) of 5 liters[18]

- Large volume liposuction may require admission for overnight stay in order to optimize pain management and for appropriate fluid balance and blood loss monitoring
- Removing too much fat can also cause unusual contour irregularities, "lumpiness" or "dents" in the skin of "over suctioned" patients

Tumescent liposuction

Described in 1985, constitutes the most common form of liposuction

Implies injecting large volume of fluid containing local anesthetic into the subcutaneous fat. This "wetting solution" contains up to 500 mg of lidocaine, 1 mg of epinephrine, and 12.5 meq of NaHCO3 in 1.000 mL of NSS (local analgesic "megadose")

Safe tumescent liposuction with lidocaine megadoses (as high as 35–55 mg/kg) relies on:

1. Administration of diluted local analgesic (500–1000 mg of lidocaine in 1.000 mL of crystalloid)
2. Use of epinephrine to delay absorption
3. Concomitant use of propofol which increases the seizure threshold
4. Removing some of the injectate with the aspirate solution

Blood loss reduction constitutes an additional benefit of epinephrine use

Offers sustained postoperative analgesia

Concerns over the high volume of fluid and potential local analgesic toxicity with tumescent technique led to the concept of lower volume (dry, wet, super wet) techniques.

Described recommendations to avoid complications after liposuction

- ASA III and IV patients with uncontrolled medical problems should not be candidates for large volume liposuction
- Candidates for large volume liposuction should have their weight stable or decreasing with diet and exercise. Over the counter and prescription diet medications should be discontinued at least 2–3 weeks prior to surgery

- Restrict IVF and consider urine output monitoring with Foley catheter in case of large volume liposuction
- Keep tract of wetting solution infused, fat and saline aspirated, blood loss, and urine output
- Do not hesitate to discuss with surgeon whether the case should be staged if it has exceeded the time and blood losses anticipated
- Limit lidocaine dose to 35–55 mg/kg for tumescent liposuction, it might be lower in patients with low protein and other medical conditions
- Limit epinephrine dose to 0.05 mg/kg
- Avoid combined procedures (i.e., large volume liposuction and abdominoplasty)
- Not to exceed a volume liposuction greater than 5.000 mL, especially in outpatient facilities
- By performing large volume liposuctions under GA concerns about lidocaine toxicity are minimized

Fluid balance is calculated using the residual volume theory. The residual volume is the difference between all fluids received by the patient (IVFs, wetting solution, and any post treatment bupivacaine solution) and the total saline portion of the aspirate (do not include fat) and urine output of the patient. The difference is the residual crystalloid volume that remains in the patient, which acts as the fluid resuscitation source for the postoperative period. Divide this number by the patient's preoperative weight (in kg to obtain a value in ml/kg. This number is usually in the range of 90–120 ml/kg. Healthy patients within this range do not exhibit signs of intravascular volume depletion or overload.[19]

Animal studies have shown that hemodynamic parameters return to baseline 20 hours following tumescent fluid infiltration.[20]

Complications associated with liposuction

- Following a census survey among cosmetic surgeons, Grazer *et al.* reported in 2000 a mortality of 19 per 100.000 liposuctions[21]
- Thromboembolism constitutes the most common cause of death. High risk patients for deep venous thrombosis and pulmonary embolism are females smokers on OCP

- Fat embolism
- Major infection
- Skin or soft tissue necrosis
- Fluid overload
- Hemorrhage
- Vascular or organ perforation (penetration injuries)
- Drug toxicity (i.e., lidocaine or epinephrine)
- Unplanned blood transfusion
- Hypothermia. Large areas of tissue exposed to convective loss

Practice advisory on anesthetic infiltration solutions[22]

Wetting solutions with local anesthetics may provide sufficient pain relief without additional anesthesia for small volume liposuction

Avoid bupivacaine (marcaine) as additive to infiltration solution

Lidocaine given in large volumes may cause systemic toxicity. Preventive measures include:

- Limit lidocaine dose to 35–55 mg/kg, although this dose may not be safe in patients with hypoalbuminemia
- Utilize lower volume
- Reduce lidocaine dose if procedure is done under GA or regional anesthesia

Avoid epinephrine in patients with pheochromocytoma, hyperthyroidism, severe hypertension, cardiac disease, or peripheral vascular disease

Consider staged infiltration of various sites to decrease effects of excessive epinephrine

Breast augmentation

- Extremely popular procedure
- Implants have been used since at least 1895 to augment the size or shape of women's breast
- Patients seeking breast augmentation have been reported as being usually younger and less educated than those who seek other plastic surgeries. These women are more likely to have undergone psychotherapy, have low levels of self esteem, and have higher prevalence of depression, suicide attempts, and mental illness as compared to the general population

- During preoperative interview address postprocedure pain management strategy:
  - As weight is added to the chest and many will have a firm circumferential pressure dressing, pain is expected
  - The quality of the pain is that of acute pressure and heaviness
  - Stretching of skin is often felt as a deep ache in the shoulders and back
  - Submuscular dissection and implant placement will also involve postprocedure deep muscular pain
  - Postoperative oral diazepam can be very helpful in relieving pain secondary to muscle spasm
- Anesthesia technique is usually GA (separation of pectoralis muscle may require paralysis) but MAC with local anesthesia could also be used
- Implant placement requires position changes intraprocedurally from supine to sitting. Airway circuits and IV lines of sufficient length should enable a smooth and timely transition
- Check pressure points and abduction angles. Ensure safely transition from supine to sitting as placement of the implants is confirmed
- Consider the effects of position as pertains to vascular tone and blood pressure. Be prepared to treat
- Awareness of serious surgical complications would encompass pneumothorax and uncontrolled bleeding from the thoracic vessels
- One of the key factors for a good surgical result is to have control of the bleeding and oozing in the breast pocket
- A plan for transfer and admission to an acute care facility should be in place in the event that complications cannot be definitively addressed in the office surgical suite setting
- Dressing will involve wound covering as well as bras and elastic bands or bandages
- The ideal awakening would involve extubation without coughing as increases in venous pressure may increase the chance of bleeding and oozing in the pocket
- Consider antiemetic prophylaxis

Blepharoplasty (surgical modification of the eyelid)

- Excess tissue such as skin and fat are removed or repositioned, and surrounding muscles and tendons may be reinforced
- Anesthesia technique is usually local anesthesia with MAC. In case of general anesthesia, less cough or buck is obtained with a LMA compared to an endotracheal tube
- Avoid bucking and coughing during emergence (may increase risk of bleeding)
- Keeping the head elevated 30° will aid in reducing the venous pressure impacting on the surgical field

Abdominoplasty ("tummy tuck")

- Cosmetic surgery procedure used to make the abdomen firmer by removing excess skin and fat. Usually sought by patients with loose tissues after pregnancy or individuals with sagging skin after major weight loss
- Anesthesia technique is GA with muscle paralysis for imbrication of the rectus muscle sheath
- Because sutures are closed under tension, efforts should be made during extubation to avoid coughing or bucking
- Abdominoplasty has one of the highest rates of deep venous thrombosis and pulmonary embolus in plastic surgery

Rhinoplasty

- Surgical procedure usually performed in order to improve the function or the appearance of a human nose
- Airway is secured with an oral Ring Adair Elwin endotracheal tube (RAE) or an armored flexible style LMA taped to the patient's chin
- Blood in the stomach is a well recognize cause of PONV following rhinoplasty
- LMA offers the advantage of reducing the amount of blood that drips down of the esophagus

- To minimize the amount of blood going down the esophagus surgeons can throat packing. Attention must be paid to see that the throat packs are removed
- Awakening is challenging because the patient should not cough, and yet must be awake to guard against aspiration
- In addition, since anesthesia providers should not exert proper mask pressure with a "new nose" to avoid injuring the repair, the patient has to be awake at extubation to minimize the laryngospasm risk

Rhytidectomy (surgical removal of wrinkles or facelift)

- Cosmetic surgery procedure used to give a more youthful appearance. Usually involves the removal of excess facial skin, with or without the tightening of underlying tissues, and the redraping of the skin on the patient's face and neck
- The first facelift was performed in Berlin in 1901. Currently is one of the most popular aesthetic surgeries performed in the United States
- Patients coming for facelifts are usually over the age of 45, requiring evaluation and proper optimization of existing comorbid conditions
- The most common complication can be bleeding which usually requires a return to the operating room. Less common, but potentially serious, complications may include damage to the facial nerves and necrosis of the skin flaps, or infection
- The risk of postoperative complications is increased in cigarette smokers and patients with hypertension and diabetes
- Anesthesia technique is usually GA with ETT, RAE, or LMA. Securing the airway to the chin or to the teeth avoids distortion of the face
- Beware of airway fire when performing the procedure under MAC with supplemental oxygen
- Protect the eyes with gel or eye shields during the entire case
- In order to minimize blood losses maintain the blood pressure within the lower 20–30% range of baseline during resection and bring it back up close to baseline prior to closing to assess hemostasis
- Keep fluid load to a minimum as excess can contribute significantly to facial edema

- Anticipate surgeon request for dexamethasone
- During emergence avoid bucking and coughing as this may increase the risk of bleeding
- The head dressing will be circumferential to the face and neck. Make sure is not too constricting around the neck
- Elevate the head as soon as it is feasible as it helps with postprocedure swelling

Conclusions

Anesthesia for cosmetic surgery is a challenging and rewarding area of the anesthetic practice: the patients are healthy and the procedures are designed to embellish people's bodies and minds. Perhaps in no other area of our specialty the need for close collaboration between surgeon and anesthesiologist is as important, as most of these procedures are done outside the hospital settings, only counting on the expertise of a single person for an integral perioperative care. This may be minor surgery, but there's never minor anesthesia and it is very true that in these cases an ounce of prevention is worth a pound of cure.

At the end of the day the patient expects (and needs to have) an adequate perioperative evaluation, a concierge level of care, a safe anesthesia, a painless and smooth wake up, and uneventful (and specially nausea free) postoperative period.

References

1. American Society of Anesthesiologists. Basic standards for preanesthesia care (October 2005).
2. Miller RD. (2010) *Miller's Anesthesia*, 7th Edn. Churchill Livingstone Elsevier, Philadelphia, PA.
3. Manchio JV, Litchfield CR, Sati S, Bryan DJ, Weinzweig J, Vernadakis AJ. (2009) Duration of smoking cessation and its impact on skin flap survival. *Plast Reconstr Surg* **124**(4): 1105–1117.
4. Fleisher LA, *et al.* (2007) ACC/AHA 2007 Guidelines on perioperative cardiovascular evaluation and care for noncardiac surgery: executive summary. *J Am Coll Cardiol* **50**(17): 1707–1732.

5. Practice guidelines for preoperative fasting and the use of pharmacologic agents to reduce the risk of pulmonary aspiration: a report by the American Society of Anesthesiologists Task Force on Preoperative Fasting. *Anesthesiology* **90**(3): 896–905 (March 1999).
6. American Society of Anesthesiologists. Standards for basic anesthesia monitoring (October 2005).
7. Most D, Koslow J, Heller J, Shermak MA. (2005) Thromboembolism in plastic surgery. *Plast Reconst Surg* **115**(2): 20e–30e.
8. Wappler F. (2010) Anesthesia for a patient with a history of malignant hyperthermia. *Curr Opin Anesthesiol* **23**(3): 417–422.
9. Ranta SO, Laurilla R, Saario J, Ali-Melkkila T, Hynynen M. (1998) Awareness with recall during general anesthesia: incidence and risk factors. *Anesth Analg* **86**: 1084–1089.
10. Tong TJ, Ing RJ, Dear G, Wright D, El-Moalem HE, Lubarsky DA. (2003) How much are patients willing to pay to avoid intraoperative awareness? *J Clin Anesth* **15**(2): 108–112.
11. Barash P. (2001) *Clinical Anesthesia*, 5th Edn. Lippincott Williams & Wilkins, Philadelphia, PA.
12. American Society of Anesthesiologists. Position on monitored anesthesia care (September 2008).
13. Friedberg BL. (2007) *Anesthesia in Cosmetic Surgery*. Cambridge University Press, New York, NY.
14. American Society of Anesthesiologists. (2002) Practice guidelines for postanesthetic care. *Anesthesiology* **96**: 742–752.
15. Gan T, Sloan F, Dear Gde L, El-Moalem HE, Lubarsky DA. (2001) How much are patient willing to pay to avoid postoperative nausea and vomiting? *Anesth Analg* **92**(2): 393–400.
16. Gan T, *et al.* (2007) Society for Ambulatory anesthesia guidelines for the management of postoperative nausea and vomiting. *Anesth Analg* **105**(6): 1615–1628.
17. Apfel CC, Laara R, Koivuranta M, Greim CA, Roewer N. (1999) A simplified risk score for predicting PONV: conclusions from cross validations between two centers. *Anesthesiology* **91**(3): 693–700.
18. Saleh Y, El-Oteify M, Abd El-Salam AE, Tohamy A, Abd-Elsayed AA. (2009) Safety and benefits of large volume liposuction: a single center experience. *Int Arch Med* **2**(1): 4.
19. Gabriel A, Gingrass MK. (2010) Large volume liposuction, safety and indications. Emedicine.medscape.com.

20. Ozmen S, Kusza K, Ulusal BG, Pryor L, Siemionow M, Zins JE. (2009) Hemodynamic changes and fluid shifts after large volume fluid infiltration: results from a porcine model. *Ann Plast Surg* **64**(1): 83–88.
21. Grazer FM, de Jong RH. (2000) Fatal outcomes from liposuction: census survey of cosmetic surgeons. *Plast Reconstr Surg* **105**(1): 436–446; discussion 447–448.
22. Iverson R, Lynch D. (2004) the ASPS Committee on Patient Safety. Practice Advisory on liposuction. *Plast Reconstr Surg* **113**(5): 1478–1490; discussion 1491–1495.

CHAPTER 4

LASERS AND AESTHETIC DEVICES

Mark S. Nestor and Matthew B. Zarraga

Illustrative Case

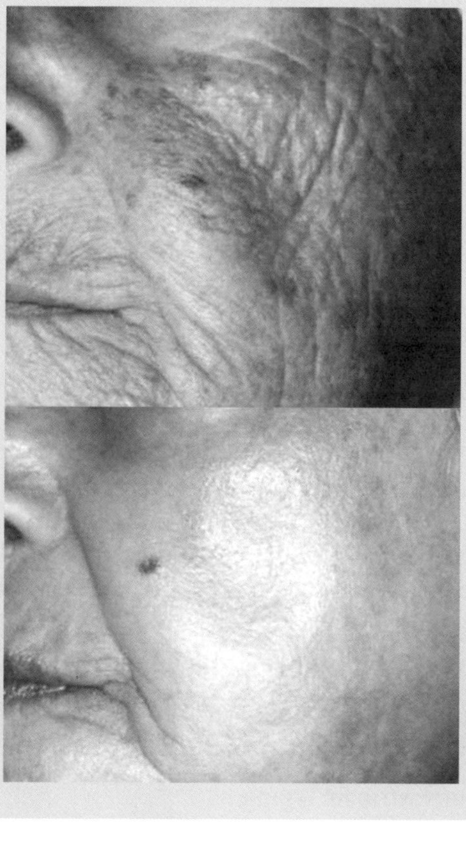

A 78 year old female patient came in for an initial consultation regarding extensive and deep rhytids. The patient was given an overall outline of the procedure and what to expect in terms of the process itself. Risks of the procedure were also outlined including pain, infection, scarring, hyper- and hypopigmentation, and delayed healing.

The patient was placed on preoperative antibiotics including cefdinir 300 mg BID and famciclovir 250 mg BID one day and two days prior to the procedure respectively.

The procedure was performed as follows: topical anesthesia was used as well as necessary blocks of intralesional anesthesia. We used the Sciton erbium laser set at an energy of 150 microns for ablation and 50 microns for coagulation; two passes were conducted. Post-operatively, the patient was dressed with Aquaphor and was given full post-operative instructions; these included returning to the office three times over the course of 10 days for application of saline-soaked sterile gauze to remove any crusting. Above are the before and 3-month post-procedure pictures.

I. Introduction

A. Aging

  i. A complex and multifactorial process that causes many "undesirable" changes
  ii. Body composition changes with a redistribution of fat
  iii. Clinically-aged skin is characterized by laxness, wrinkling, dryness, roughness, atrophy and changes in pigmentation[1]

B. Intrinsic versus Extrinsic Aging

  i. Both intrinsic and extrinsic aging cause the clinical signs of aging[2–4]

ii. Intrinsic aging: time and genetics
iii. Extrinsic aging: overexposure to the sun
iv. Extrinsic aging can become superimposed on intrinsic aging resulting in more rapid alterations of the skin

C. Histological appearance of aged skin[1,5]:

i. Thinning of the epidermis with dermal atrophy
ii. Loss of the elastic tissue in the dermis
iii. Dermal elastosis
iv. Actinic changes with fragmentation of the dermal collagen matrix composed primarily of proteins, fibroblasts, proteoglycans and glycosaminoglycans with loss of structural integrity[6]

D. Minimally-invasive procedures

i. Designed to reverse the signs of aging
ii. Have increased exponentially in popularity over the past decade[7]
iii. Treatment modalities include:

1. Botulinum toxin
2. Fillers
3. Laser devices
4. Light devices
5. Radiofrequency devices
6. Ultrasound devices
7. Cryolipolysis systems
8. Chemical peels
9. Cosmeceuticals
10. Prescription medications

E. Benefits of minimally-invasive procedures:

i. Minimal recovery
ii. Fewer risks
iii. Decreased cost
iv. Less time-consuming — can be completed in less time than the typical lunch hour

v. May also benefit medical conditions such as rosacea, acne, melasma, psoriasis, warts and actinic damage

F. Ensuring patient satisfaction

i. Must evaluate the needs, desires and expectations
ii. Goals must be realistic
iii. Limitations of the treatment(s) must be thoroughly explained
iv. Drastic improvement may only be accomplished by surgical or other invasive procedures
v. Significant adverse reactions are rare but patients must fully understand both the risks involved and the recovery time associated with the procedure(s)

II. Lasers

A. Laser: an acronym for Light Amplification by Stimulated Emission of Radiation
B. Lasers have become an effective treatment modality for a variety of dermatologic conditions

a. New lasers are constantly being developed while existing technology continues to be refined

C. History of lasers

a. 1959: Theodore Maiman invented the laser[8]
b. 1960s: Leon Goldman first pioneered its use for dermatologic applications[8]
c. 1980s: Anderson and Parrish revolutionized laser surgery with the concept of "selective photothermolysis", which states that destruction of a specific target in the skin can be accomplished without significant thermal damage to surrounding normal tissue[9]

D. All laser systems are comprised of four essential components[10]:

a. Delivery system
b. Medium (gas, liquid or solid)
c. Energy source
d. Mirrors to reflect photons of light

E. All laser systems share three distinct characteristics[10]:

a. Monochromaticity — the emitted light is of a single, discrete wavelength determined by the lasing medium which can be solid (ruby crystal), liquid (dye) or gas (CO_2 or argon)
b. Collimation — there is an emission of a narrow, intense beam of light that travels in a parallel fashion over long distances without light divergence
c. Coherence — laser light is considered in phase with its peaks and troughs aligned with respect to both space and time

 i. Allows lasers to be focused to extremely small spot sizes

F. Cutaneous applications of lasers

a. Laser light can be absorbed, transmitted or reflected by the target.
b. For a clinical effect to take place, the first law of photobiology (the Grotthus-Draper law) states that light must be absorbed

 i. Light has no effect when it is transmitted or reflected[11]

c. Lasers are chosen by matching their particular wavelength with the absorption spectrum of the particular target or chromophore

 i. The first pulse dye laser (PDL) emitted a wavelength of 577 nm, coinciding with the last absorption peak of oxyhemoglobin[9]
 ii. This was later increased to 585 nm in order to penetrate more deeply while maintaining vascular specificity[12]

d. Ideal laser-tissue interaction would include:

 i. Delivery of a wavelength specifically absorbed by the chromophore
 ii. Induction of heat buildup
 iii. Destruction of the target with minimal unwanted thermal injury to the surrounding normal tissue[11]

G. Laser terminology[11,13,14]

a. Energy — fundamental unit of work

 i. Spread of thermal energy to adjacent tissue is proportional to the time it is exposed to laser energy

b. Fluence — the energy absorbed by the chromophore is measured in joules per square centimeter
c. Chromophore — medium that exhibits characteristic bands of absorption at certain wavelengths

    i. Three primary chromophores in the skin: water, hemoglobin and melanin

d. Thermal relaxation time (TRT) — the time required for the heated tissue to lose half of its heat
e. Pulse duration (pulse width) — laser exposure duration time

    i. A pulse duration shorter than or approximately equal to the TRT of the target allows the amount of heat buildup to be confined to the desired target
    ii. An example of when pulse duration is particularly important occurs when PDL is used for vascular lesions

        1. By increasing the pulse duration, there is a slower, more uniform heating of the targeted vessels, resulting in reduced or absent post-treatment purpura

f. Laser power — the rate at which energy is delivered may be increased to limit exposure time for a given fluence
g. Spot size — diameter of the laser beam on the skin surface
h. Depth of penetration — because the depths of targets vary, the depth of penetration is important

    i. In practical terms, the longer the wavelength and the larger the spot size, the deeper the laser energy penetrates
    ii. To achieve the greatest effective penetration depth, a combination of the appropriate wavelength and spot size is necessary

H. Types of lasers[10,14]

a. Lasers used for dermatologic applications can be divided into continuous wave (CW) and pulsed devices
b. CW lasers (argon and CO_2)

    i. Emit a constant beam of light

ii. Usually have a limited peak power
iii. With long exposure durations, nonselective tissue injury may occur

c. Quasi-CW lasers (copper vapor and KTP)

i. Produce interrupted emissions of constant laser energy usually with low energy pulses

d. Pulsed lasers (ruby, alexandrite, Nd:YAG, diode, etc.)

i. Can achieve very high peak power in ultrashort pulse durations
ii. Q-switched ruby laser has an electro-optical shutter that permits release of stored energy within the laser cavity in short high-energy bursts

1. Q refers to a quality factor of energy storage in the lasing medium, which is changed suddenly to produce a short, intense burst of light

e. Lasers should be selected based on the individual absorption characteristics of the target chromophore

III. Ablative Lasers

A. Ablative lasers create confluent, uniform patches of epidermal or dermal injury
B. CO_2 lasers[10]

a. First developed in 1964, and used primarily as a surgical cutting tool
b. The CW CO_2 laser has a wavelength of 10,600 nm

i. All water in tissue absorbs this wavelength
ii. Absorption is not dependent on selective absorption by any biologic tissue
iii. As the water absorbs energy, the temperature rises quickly, resulting in vaporization of tissue.

c. Its use in the aesthetic patient was limited by the undesired damage it caused to surrounding tissue

    i. Due to uncontrollable delivery and absorption of energy, it caused excessive heat deposition and subsequent char formation

d. High-energy, short-pulsed and focused, scanned CO_2 lasers were developed in the early 1990s

    i. Considered the gold standard for facial rejuvenation
    ii. Ablates the epidermis and papillary dermis before a significant amount of heat spreads to the adjacent tissue

        1. Results in collagen shrinkage and remodeling

    iii. Produces the most dramatic improvements in the clinical and histologic appearance of photodamaged facial skin and superficial rhytides
    iv. Can effectively and dramatically improve fine and deep lines, wrinkles and acne scars

e. Disadvantages of CO_2 lasers[15–17]:

    i. Significant amount of downtime
    ii. Risks including scarring, post-operative viral and bacterial infections and/or hyper-/hypopigmentation

C. Erbium:YAG laser[18]

a. The erbium:YAG laser has a wavelength of 2,940 nm

    i. The target chromophore is water
    ii. Erbium energy is 12–18x more efficiently absorbed by water-containing tissues than CO_2 energy

b. Benefits of Erbium: YAG laser over CO_2 lasers

    i. Decrease the associated downtime and risk due to its more shallow depth of penetration.
    ii. Causes less erythema and less residual thermal injury

c. Hemostasis with the erbium:YAG laser

i. The short pulsed Er:YAG has the disadvantage of not allowing for hemostasis because collateral thermal damage is reduced
ii. The long pulsed Er:YAG laser allows for hemostasis and improved outcomes but is associated with greater downtime and risk

d. A series of superficial erbium laser treatments (microlaserpeels) can improve outcome with minimal recovery for each treatment although the patient had to undergo a series of "weekends with a red peeling face"[19]

D. Recently, CO_2 and erbium lasers have made a resurgence, both being used as mediums for fractionated laser treatments, with the hope of being more effective with minimal downtime and fewer risks[20]

IV. Fractionated Lasers

A. Ablative and non-ablative fractionated lasers have been developed and found in effective in treating acne scarring,[21] wrinkle reduction and skin resurfacing[17,22]

B. Ablative fractionated lasers[20,23]

i. Create a confluent column of ablation and thermal injury that extends from the dermis and epidermis through the stratum corneum

1. Induce the body's wound healing responses
2. Stimulate fibroblasts to produce new collagen and elastin
3. The unaffected surrounding tissue serves as a reservoir of cells that promote safe and speedy re-epithelialization and long-term collagen remodeling

ii. Cause tissue vaporization resulting in a greater degree of heating, leading to thermal molecular changes and subsequent tissue tightening
iii. Produce more dramatic results than non-ablative fractionated lasers but also require more downtime
iv. Examples: ProFractional (Sciton), Pixel CO_2 (Alma), and Matrix Fractional CO_2 (SandStone)

C. Non-ablative fractionated lasers
    i. Have inherent advantages of minimal downtime and fewer complications[24]
    ii. Have been proven effective for photodamage, mild to moderate periorbital wrinkles, acne scars,[25–27] surgical scars, melisma,[28–30] and actinic damage[22,25,31]
    iii. Induce collagen remodeling by producing an array of microthermal zones and creating small columns of thermal injury to the dermis without epidermal disruption[32]
        1. Dermal heating results in contraction and remodeling of the dermis with synthesis of new collagen[33]
    iv. Examples: Fraxel Restore (Solta) and Artisan 1540 (Palomar)
    v. Advantages: faster recovery, fewer side effects, and less need for physician oversight
    vi. Disadvantages and side effects[34]:
        1. Require a series of treatments to obtain the desired clinical effect
        2. The most common SEs include mild edema and erythema with resolution occurring within a few days in most patients

V. Vascular Lasers

A. Non-ablative vascular lasers have revolutionized the treatment of congenital and acquired vascular lesions
B. Target intravascular oxyhemoglobin
    i. Three primary absorption peaks for oxyhemoglobin: 418, 542 and 577 nm
C. In general, very superficial vessels respond to potassium titanyl phosphate (KTP), intense pulsed light (IPL) or pulse dye lasers (PDL) while larger leg veins may respond to long-pulsed neodymium-doped yttrium aluminium garnet (Nd:YAG) 1064 nm lasers[10]
D. Large caliber leg veins
    i. Sclerotherapy is the treatment of choice for large caliber leg veins

1. Side effects include scarring, ulceration, allergic reactions to the injected sclerosant and telangiectatic matting[35,36]

ii. Many different laser systems[35–41] have been evaluated for the treatment of leg veins

E. PDL[11]

i. First laser developed specifically for the treatment of vascular lesions
ii. Commonly use rhodamine dye as the active medium and a flash-lamp to energize the laser
iii. Produces wavelengths that range from 585 to 600 nm
iv. Currently the standard of treatment for port-wine stains, facial telangiectasias, cherry angiomas, poikiloderma of Civatte, warts, and scars
v. Main side effect: purpura

1. Dependent on fluence and spot size
2. Results from immediate microvascular hemorrhage, subsequent thrombosis and delayed appearance of vasculitis (inflammation of the blood vessels)
3. To prevent formation, pulse duration can be increased to heat the vessel more gently

a. The vessels instead collapse and tend to disappear immediately after treatment

4. Delayed purpura can still occur due to a phase of vasculitis that may occur several days after treatment

vi. Other complications include vesiculation, crusting, pigmentary changes and scarring
vii. Associated with use of excessive fluences and overlapping laser spots[42,43]

F. KTP[10]

i. Produces a 532 nm wavelength by using a Nd:YAG crystal (1064 nm) to produce light that is passed through a KTP crystal that doubles the frequency

ii. Frequently used to treat facial telangiectasias
iii. Because of its inherent shorter wavelength, penetration is more superficial
iv. Main advantages:
    1. High efficacy
    2. Rapid healing time
    3. Resolution of mild to moderate erythema within 1–2 weeks
v. Main disadvantages:
    1. Time- and labor-intensiveness (each vessel must be individually traced)
    2. Cannot be used in darker skin types since the 532 nm wavelength is more readily absorbed by melanin
vi. Most common side effects: mild erythema, edema and transient crusting
    1. Purpura is avoided due to the slow heating of blood vessels at longer pulse durations, allowing for cooling of the vessels without microvascular hemorrhage.

G. Long-pulsed Nd:YAG[38]
    i. The most commonly used laser for larger-caliber leg veins and port-wine stains with a deeper component
    ii. Emits a standard wavelength of 1064 nm
    iii. Main advantage: can be used in both fair and more darkly pigmented skin
    iv. Main disadvantage: the energy it produces is absorbed much less by hemoglobin than other vascular specific lasers
        1. Treatment requires multiple sessions to obtain the desired result

VI. Intense Pulsed Light

A. Developed in the mid 1990s[44]

B. Improves vascular and pigmented conditions such as lentigines,[45,46] acne,[47] diffuse telangiectasias,[48] and hair removal[44]
C. Has some effect on fine lines, wrinkles and tightening
D. Uses a flashlamp to produce polychromatic, incoherent, high-intensity pulsed light with an emission spectrum from 500 to 1300 nm

   i. Because IPLs are polychromatic, convertible cut-off filters can be used to obtain the desired wavelength by preventing the emission of the lower wavelengths

E. Mechanism of action: delivers a wavelength, which is absorbed by the target chromophore causing heat to build up resulting in the destruction of the target
F. A cooling gel is applied on the skin prior to exposure to the IPL

   i. Decreases epidermal damage and increases efficiency of light energy to deeper vessels

G. Advantages over lasers:

   i. Larger spot size
   ii. High skin coverage rate
   iii. High versatility

H. Disadvantages of IPL:

   i. Inconsistence of emitted spectrum and fluence
   ii. Necessary application of gel to the skin and direct contact of the handpiece to the skin both hamper the ability to observe an immediate local response

I. Side effects: blistering, purpura, crusting, erythema, hypo-/hyperpigmentation, atrophy, scarring, and risk of infection

   i. Most can be prevented by adjusting wavelengths, pulse durations and fluences customized to each patient's needs

J. Photorejuvenation with IPL[45,49]

   i. Has become a very popular option for aesthetic enhancement

ii. IPL produces a range of wavelengths of light in one pulse

1. Allows for treatment of pigmented and vascular lesions, and collagen stimulation concurrently

iii. Usually done in a series allowing for maximal improvement with minimal downtime

iv. Dozens of IPL systems are currently available

1. There is a broad range of clinical effectiveness seen with varied consistencies in results

VII. Pigment Specific Lasers

A. Multiple types of lasers have been employed to specifically treat pigmented lesions[50–52]

i. Such lasers include Q-switched ruby, Q-switched YAG, and Q-switched alexandrite

B. Absorb in the superficial pigment spectrum from UV to near-IR

i. The targeted chromophore in endogenous pigmented lesions is melanin

C. Effective in treating epidermal lesions (solar lentigines, ephelides, café-au-lait macules), dermal and mixed epidermal/dermal lesions (melanocytic nevi, blue nevi, nevi of Ota/Ita, drug-induced hyperpigmentation, Becker's nevi, and nevus spilus) and exogenous tattoo pigment

D. Q-switched ruby lasers

i. Have a wavelength of 694 nm that is well absorbed by melanin

ii. Useful in treatment of tattoo pigment except for bright shades of red and yellow

E. Q-switched alexandrite lasers

i. Emit a light with a wavelength of 755 nm

ii. Similar in function and effectiveness as the Q-switched ruby lasers

F. Q-switched KTP Nd:YAG lasers

  i. Produce a wavelength of 532 nm
  ii. Effective against melanin
  iii. Unlike the other Q-switched lasers, also can remove red and yellow tattoo ink
  iv. Not effective on green ink

G. Most common side effects of all of the Q-switched lasers are transient pigmentary alterations and textural changes at higher fluences
H. Other rare complications include:

  i. Scarring
  ii. Darkening of cosmetic tattoos
  iii. Allergic reactions to the liberated pigments

VIII. Laser Hair Removal

A. Laser hair removal has become one of the most popular procedures in aesthetic medicine
B. It is necessary to choose a laser specifically based on each individual patient's skin type to enhance clinical benefit and minimize risk
C. The target chromophore in laser hair removal is the pigment present within the hair shaft
D. High-energy lasers with wavelengths in the red to near-IR region of the spectrum must be used

  i. Long-pulsed ruby,[53] long-pulsed alexandrite,[54] long-pulsed diode[55] and long-pulsed Nd:YAG lasers[34]

E. Mechanism of action:

  i. Permanent hair removal requires damage to follicular stem cells and/or dermal papilla at the base of the hair follicle, both of which are non-pigmented targets
  ii. Heat must diffuse from the primary target, the pigmented follicular melanin, to the amelanotic stem cells
  iii. Pulse durations longer than the TRT must be employed[8,56]

F. Laser hair removal in darker skin types can now be done safely

   i. The alexandrite (755 nm), diode (810 nm) and Nd:YAG (1064 nm) lasers work well on darker skin types due to their longer wavelengths[57]

G. Most common adverse reactions of laser hair removal systems include pain during treatment, erythema, and perifollicular edema

   i. Blistering, crusting scarring and dyspigmentation have also been observed
   ii. Risk can be reduced with effective cooling by using gels, cryogenic sprays or contact cooling devices

IX. Radiofrequency

A. Radiofrequency (RF) devices have been FDA-approved within the last decade for facial skin tightening[58]
B. Compared to laser-based systems, radiofrequency (RF)-based technologies produce higher volumetric heating via tissue impedance with resultant heat diffusion to deeper tissues[59]
C. The first nonsurgical technique developed for facial skin tightening employed the use of monopolar RF
D. Mechanism of action of RF systems:

   i. Unlike lasers, non-ablative RF systems use electric current to selectively heat zones of the dermis and deeper tissues[60]
   ii. The energy produced causes direct collagen contraction and immediate skin tightening[61]
   iii. Long-term effects include remodeling and reorientation of collagen bundles and the formation of new collagen[62]

E. Main advantage of RF systems: safe to use in patients with all skin types[60]

   i. The energy produced is not absorbed by epidermal melanin

F. Monopolar and bipolar RF systems

i. Monopolar systems — current is delivered through a single contact point with an accompanying grounding pad that completes the electrical circuit by serving as a low resistance path for current flow[63]

1. Example device: Thermage (Solta)[64,65]

ii. Bipolar devices — electrical current passes between two positioned electrodes that are directly applied to the skin

1. No current flows through the rest of the body
2. A grounding pad is not necessary with these systems[66]
3. Example device: eMatrix (Syneron)

G. Fractionated bipolar RF[59,67]

i. The newest RF technology, eMatrix (Syneron), utilizes fractionated bipolar RF energy to induce sublative facial rejuvenation
ii. Can cause skin ablation/coagulation/necrosis and resurfacing impacts[67]
iii. Difference as compared to other RF systems:

1. Energy produced creates a cone-shaped thermal injury zone, with the tip of the cone at the surface of the epidermis then expanding out to a wider area deep within the dermis

iv. Benefits of the sublative rejuvenation technique:

1. Traditional fractional ablative laser treatments typically disrupt up to 70% of the epidermis while having little effect on the dermis
2. The sublative rejuvenation technique minimally affects the epidermis (up to 5%) with majority of its impact contained within the dermis

a. Results in faster healing times and minimized downtimes

H. Most common side effects of all RF systems are[67]:

i. Swelling
ii. Erythema

iii. Transient crusting
iv. Heat sensation and discomfort during the procedure

X. Light-Emitting Diodes (LED)

A. Nonablative, non-thermal device that utilizes light at a variety of wavelengths
B. LED systems include:

i. Omnilux (Phototherapeutics)
ii. Gentlewaves (Light BioScience)

C. Used for the treatment of photodamaged skin[68]
D. Studies have demonstrated moderate but significant improvement in peri-ocular wrinkles, reduction in Fitzpatrick photoaging classification, global skin texture and background erythema, and pigmentation
E. Exact mechanism of action has yet to be defined

i. Hypothesized that the skin absorbs specific LED light wavelengths to induce photobiomodulation to modulate cell function, proliferation and repair of photodamaged tissue[66,68]
ii. Unlike lasers, the effects are seen without heating of tissue through non-coherent, monochromatic light with spontaneous emission

F. No adverse side effects were noted with the use of either LED system[69–71]

XI. Intense Focused Ultrasound Therapy

A. Intense focused ultrasound is a new non-ablative modality
B. Utilized for the treatment of facial skin tightening and reduction of rhytides
C. Intense focused ultrasound system

i. Device is called the Ulthera System (Ulthera)
ii. Incorporates both ultrasound imaging capability for visualizing skin and subcutis and a therapeutic ultrasound module used to create zones of thermal coagulation[72,73]

iii. Provides the ability to visualize the deep soft tissue, which allows for precise treatment while leaving the surrounding regions unaffected[74,75]
iv. Histologic examination of intense ultrasound exposures showed coagulative necrosis induced by thermal damage to the superficial musculoaponeurotic system region[74]

D. Clinical benefits

i. One study showed that a single ultrasound treatment of the forehead produced an average of 1.7 to 1.9 mm brow elevation and was preserved 3 months post-treatment[73]

E. Benefits of ultrasound energy

i. Delivers energy to the deeper subcutaneous layers of the face, including the superficial musculoaponeurotic system
ii. There is no scatter or absorption of energy in the epidermis and dermis that may cause inadvertent cutaneous injury[73]
iii. Effective in all skin types[76]

1. The absorption of ultrasound energy is determined by the microscopic and bulk mechanical properties of tissue and is independent of the melanin content of the skin

F. Side effects: transient erythema and edema, which resolved in majority of patients by day two post-treatment

i. Pain during treatment was most commonly characterized as mild to moderate
ii. No serious adverse events have been reported[73]

XII. Non-Invasive Body Contouring

A. Laser-enhanced and traditional liposuction are the gold standard for body contouring at this time
B. As with all aesthetic procedures, patients are looking to reshape their bodies with minimal amount of recovery necessary

C. A variety of non-invasive modalities have been researched, tested and FDA-approved to be effective

   i. These include low-level laser therapy and cryolipolysis

D. Cryolipolysis

   i. New, FDA-approved, non-invasive way to selectively reduce the number of fat cells in a target area

      1. Device called the Zeltiq System (Zeltiq Aesthetics)

   ii. Mechanism of action[16,77]

      1. A target area is subjected to advanced controlled, localized cooling resulting in adipocyte apoptosis
      2. Adipocyte apoptosis induces an inflammatory process that results in phagocytic digestion of their remnants
      3. Resorption process occurs over the course of 90 days

   iii. Clinical benefits

      1. One study demonstrated that ultrasound measurements of a 10-subject subset showed fat layer reduction in 100% of the subjects with an average reduction of 22.4% at four months post-treatment[58]

   iv. Side effects including mild discomfort, erythema, bruising and dyaesthesia were minor and temporary[77]

      1. No significant adverse events have been associated with treatment

   v. Clinical trials to assess for adverse events

      1. To test for permanent neurological damage[78]:

         a. In one study, although six of the nine subjects experienced transient reduction in sensation of the treated area, sensation returned within 7 weeks post-treatment with a mean of 3.6 weeks
         b. Biopsies confirmed that no long-term change in nerve fiber structure occurred

2. To test for changes in lipid profiles and liver function tests[79]:
   a. A study showed that over the 90-day follow-up periods, there were no significant changes in lipid profiles or liver function tests

E. Low Level Laser Therapy (LLLT)

i. LLLT involves treatment with low-level diode laser
   1. The device is called the Zerona (Erchonia)
   2. The device consists of 5-independent-diode laser heads each with a scanner, each emitting 635 nm with an intensity of 17 mW

ii. LLLT has been proven a safe and effective therapeutic option for multiple non-cosmetic applications including:
   1. Acute pain associated with rheumatoid arthritis,[80] osteoarthritis,[81] and neck pain[82]
   2. Increasing the speed of wound healing[83,84] and of healing infections around dental implants[85]

iii. LLLT is a viable non-invasive option for adipose tissue reduction[86]
   1. It has been approved by the FDA for circumferential reduction of the waist, hips and thighs

iv. Mechanism of action[87,88]:
   1. Application of laser therapy at 635 nm to cultured adipocytes creates a transitory pore within the bi-lipid membrane resulting in the release of fat cell contents into the extracellular space
   2. Multiple studies have shown the collapse of adipose cells subsequent to laser irradiation of 635 nm with scanning and transmission electron microscopy (SEM and TEM) images

v. Clinical benefits
   1. In one study, subjects assigned to the test group demonstrated a statistically significant mean reduction in total circumference of 3.521 inches from baseline to endpoint while those in the control group showed only a 0.684 inch reduction

vi. No adverse events or side effects have been reported[89,90]

1. One study conducted showed that fat released from LLLT did not adversely affect the lipid profile[91]

vii. Advantages of LLLT[89,90]:

1. LLLT is painless
2. No adverse side effects
3. Does not require any anesthesia or downtime

XIII. Combination Therapy

A. A combination of the minimally-invasive procedures can and should be performed in order to obtain the maximum aesthetic benefit[92]

B. Non-ablative lasers and lights

i. Used to improve many characteristics of photodamage (pigmentation changes and vascular abnormalities)

C. Fractionated modalities

i. Lessen the appearance of rhytides and scars

D. Ultrasound and radiofrequency

i. Shown to tighten tissue and further reduce the appearance of fine wrinkles

E. Cryolypolosis and LLLT

i. Useful for body contouring purposes

F. Minimally-invasive procedures are not limited to devices

i. Dermal fillers — counter volume loss and simultaneously fill lines and folds

ii. Chemical peels — effectively target photodamaged skin, pigmentary disorders, superficial scarring and acne[93,94]

iii. Botulinum toxin

1. Number one minimally-invasive procedure performed in 2010[7]
2. Decreases static and dynamic rhytides
3. Prophylactically prevents their formation

iv. Topical prescription creams and cosmeceuticals[95,96]

1. Help maintain the aesthetic improvements achieved

XIV. Conclusion

A. Minimally invasive procedure benefits

i. Effective at reversing the intrinsic and extrinsic signs of aging
ii. Offer dramatic benefits to the cosmetic patient with minimal downtime, side effects and risks

B. Minimally-invasive procedures limitations and patient satisfaction

i. Patients' goals must be realistic
ii. The limitations of the treatment(s) must be thoroughly explained
iii. Drastic improvement may not be feasible without more invasive procedures
iv. Physicians must evaluate the needs, desires and expectations of the aesthetic patient in order to ensure patient satisfaction

C. Lasers and their future

i. Unimaginable strides have been made in the advancement of lasers and aesthetic technology within the last two decades

1. Lasers have revolutionized cosmetic dermatology

ii. Refinements to current technology continuously occur

1. Lasers and aesthetic devices have become safer, less invasive and more effective

iii. Cutaneous conditions currently treated with lasers include: rosacea, acne, melasma, psoriasis, benign pigmented and vascular lesions, skin neoplasias, hypertrophic scars, keloids, hypertrichosis, warts and photodamage

1. As technology evolves and research progresses, lasers may be a safe and effective treatment modality in a variety of other conditions

References

1. Gold MH, Goldman MP, Biron J. (2007) Efficacy of novel skin cream containing mixture of human growth factors and cytokines for skin rejuvenation. *J Drugs Dermatol* **6**(2): 197–201.
2. Sarifakioglu N, Terzioglu A, Ates L, Aslan G. (2004) A new phenomenon: "sleep lines" on the face. *Scand J Plast Reconstr Surg Hand Surg* **38**(4): 244–247.
3. Knize DM. (2000) Muscles that act on glabellar skin: a closer look. *Plast Reconstr Surg* **105**(1): 350–361.
4. Berneburg M, Plettenberg H, Krutmann J. (2000) Photoaging of human skin. *Photodermatol Photoimmunol Photomed* **16**(6): 239–244.
5. Yaar M, Eller MS, Gilchrest BA. (2002) Fifty years of skin aging. *J Investig Dermatol Symp Proc* **7**(1): 51–58.
6. Fisher GJ, Varani J, Voorhees JJ. (2008) Looking older: fibroblast collapse and therapeutic implications. *Arch Dermatol* **144**(5): 666–672.
7. Surgery ASfAP. 2000/2009/2010 National Cosmetic Procedures. New York, NY, Contract.
8. Tanzi EL, Lupton JR, Alster TS. (2003) Lasers in dermatology: four decades of progress. *J Am Acad Dermatol* **49**(1): 1–31; quiz 4.
9. Anderson RR, Parrish JA. (1983) Selective photothermolysis: precise microsurgery by selective absorption of pulsed radiation. *Science* **220**(4596): 524–527.
10. Bolognia J, Jorizzo J, Rapini R. (2008) *Dermatology*. Mosby, Philadelphia, PA.
11. Anderson R. (1997) Laser-tissue interactions in dermatology. In: Anrndt K, Dover J, Olbricht S (eds.), *Lasers in Cutaneous Aesthetic Surgery*. Lippincott-Raven, Philadelphia, pp. 25–51.
12. Alster TS, Wilson F. (1994) Treatment of port-wine stains with the flash-lamp-pumped pulsed dye laser: extended clinical experience in children and adults. *Ann Plast Surg* **32**(5): 478–484.
13. Stratigos A, Dover J. (2000) Overview of lasers and their properties. *Dermatol Ther* **13**: 2–16.
14. Alster TS, Lupton JR. (2001) Lasers in dermatology. An overview of types and indications. *Am J Clin Dermatol* **2**(5): 291–303.
15. Ramsdell W. (2009) Carbon dioxide laser resurfacing. *Arch Facial Plast Surg* **11**(1): 62–63.
16. Nelson AA, Wasserman D, Avram MM. (2009) Cryolipolysis for reduction of excess adipose tissue. *Semin Cutan Med Surg* **28**(4): 244–249.

17. Alexiades-Armenakas MR, Dover JS, Arndt KA. (2008) The spectrum of laser skin resurfacing: nonablative, fractional, and ablative laser resurfacing. *J Am Acad Dermatol* **58**(5): 719–737; quiz 38–40.
18. Adrian RM. (1999) Pulsed carbon dioxide and long pulse 10-ms erbium-YAG laser resurfacing: a comparative clinical and histologic study. *J Cutan Laser Ther* **1**(4): 197–202.
19. Nestor M. (2004) Ablative laser resurfacing. In: Rigel D, Weiss R, Lim H, Dover J (eds.), *Photoaging*. Marcel Dekker Press, New York.
20. Lapidoth M, Yagima Odo ME, Odo LM. (2008) Novel use of erbium:YAG (2,940-nm) laser for fractional ablative photothermolysis in the treatment of photodamaged facial skin: a pilot study. *Dermatol Surg* **34**(8): 1048–1053.
21. Chapas AM, Brightman L, Sukal S, Hale E, Daniel D, Bernstein LJ, *et al.* (2008) Successful treatment of acneiform scarring with CO_2 ablative fractional resurfacing. *Lasers Surg Med* **40**(6): 381–386.
22. Tierney EP, Kouba DJ, Hanke CW. (2009) Review of fractional photothermolysis: treatment indications and efficacy. *Dermatol Surg* **35**(10): 1445–1461.
23. Hantash BM, Bedi VP, Kapadia B, Rahman Z, Jiang K, Tanner H, *et al.* (2007) *In vivo* histological evaluation of a novel ablative fractional resurfacing device. *Lasers Surg Med* **39**(2): 96–107.
24. Kim KH, Geronemus RG. (2004) Nonablative laser and light therapies for skin rejuvenation. *Arch Facial Plast Surg* **6**(6): 398–409.
25. Geronemus RG. (2006) Fractional photothermolysis: current and future applications. *Lasers Surg Med* **38**(3): 169–176.
26. Alster TS, Tanzi EL, Lazarus M. (2007) The use of fractional laser photothermolysis for the treatment of atrophic scars. *Dermatol Surg* **33**(3): 295–299.
27. Lee HS, Lee JH, Ahn GY, Lee DH, Shin JW, Kim DH, *et al.* (2008) Fractional photothermolysis for the treatment of acne scars: a report of 27 Korean patients. *J Dermatolog Treat* **19**(1): 45–49.
28. Rokhsar CK, Fitzpatrick RE. (2005) The treatment of melasma with fractional photothermolysis: a pilot study. *Dermatol Surg* **31**(12): 1645–1650.
29. Goldberg DJ, Berlin AL, Phelps R. (2008) Histologic and ultrastructural analysis of melasma after fractional resurfacing. *Lasers Surg Med* **40**(2): 134–138.
30. Naito SK. (2007) Fractional photothermolysis treatment for resistant melasma in Chinese females. *J Cosmet Laser Ther* **9**(3): 161–163.
31. Rahman Z, Alam M, Dover JS. (2006) Fractional laser treatment for pigmentation and texture improvement. *Skin Ther Lett* **11**(9): 7–11.

32. Manstein D, Herron GS, Sink RK, Tanner H, Anderson RR. (2004) Fractional photothermolysis: a new concept for cutaneous remodeling using microscopic patterns of thermal injury. *Lasers Surg Med* **34**(5): 426–438.
33. Dierickx CC. (2006) The role of deep heating for noninvasive skin rejuvenation. *Lasers Surg Med* **38**(9): 799–807.
34. Wanner M. (2005) Laser hair removal. *Dermatol Ther* **18**(3): 209–216.
35. Levy JL, Elbahr C, Jouve E, Mordon S. (2004) Comparison and sequential study of long pulsed Nd:YAG 1,064 nm laser and sclerotherapy in leg telangiectasias treatment. *Lasers Surg Med* **34**(3): 273–276.
36. Trelles MA, Weiss R, Moreno-Moragas J, Romero C, Velez M, Alvarez X. (2010) Treatment of leg veins with combined pulsed dye and Nd:YAG lasers: 60 patients assessed at 6 months. *Lasers Surg Med* **42**(9): 609–614.
37. Kaudewitz P, Klovekorn W, Rother W. (2002) Treatment of leg vein telangiectases: 1-year results with a new 940 nm diode laser. *Dermatol Surg* **28**(11): 1031–1034.
38. Trelles MA, Allones I, Martin-Vazquez MJ, Trelles O, Velez M, Mordon S. (2004) Long pulse Nd:YAG laser for treatment of leg veins in 40 patients with assessments at 6 and 12 months. *Lasers Surg Med* **35**(1): 68–76.
39. Kouri B. (2009) Current evaluation and treatment of lower extremity varicose veins. *Am J Med* **122**(6): 513–515.
40. Trelles MA, Martin-Vazquez M, Trelles OR, Mordon SR. (2006) Treatment effects of combined radio-frequency current and a 900 nm diode laser on leg blood vessels. *Lasers Surg Med* **38**(3): 185–195.
41. Eremia S, Li C, Umar SH. (2002) A side-by-side comparative study of 1064 nm Nd:YAG, 810 nm diode and 755 nm alexandrite lasers for treatment of 0.3–3 mm leg veins. *Dermatol Surg* **28**(3): 224–230.
42. Fiskerstrand EJ, Svaasand LO, Volden G. (1998) Pigmentary changes after pulsed dye laser treatment in 125 northern European patients with port wine stains. *Br J Dermatol* **138**(3): 477–479.
43. Gaston DA, Clark DP. (1998) Facial hypertrophic scarring from pulsed dye laser. *Dermatol Surg* **24**(5): 523–525.
44. Babilas P, Schreml S, Szeimies RM, Landthaler M. (2010) Intense pulsed light (IPL): a review. *Lasers Surg Med* **42**(2): 93–104.
45. Nestor M, Goldberg D, Goldman M, Weis R, Rigel D. (1999) Photorejuvenation: non-ablative skin rejuvenation using intense pulsed light. *Skin Aging* **7**: 3.
46. Chan HH, Kono T. (2004) The use of lasers and intense pulsed light sources for the treatment of pigmentary lesions. *Skin Ther Lett* **9**(8): 5–7.

47. Sami NA, Attia AT, Badawi AM. (2008) Phototherapy in the treatment of acne vulgaris. *J Drugs Dermatol* **7**(7): 627–632.
48. Bjerring P, Christiansen K, Troilius A. (2001) Intense pulsed light source for treatment of facial telangiectasias. *J Cosmet Laser Ther* **3**(4): 169–173.
49. Li YH, Wu Y, Chen JZ, Gao XH, Liu M, Shu CM, *et al.* (2008) Application of a new intense pulsed light device in the treatment of photoaging skin in Asian patients. *Dermatol Surg* **34**(11): 1459–1464.
50. Anderson RR, Geronemus R, Kilmer SL, Farinelli W, Fitzpatrick RE. (1993) Cosmetic tattoo ink darkening. A complication of Q-switched and pulsed-laser treatment. *Arch Dermatol* **129**(8): 1010–1014.
51. Ashinoff R, Levine VJ, Soter NA. (1995) Allergic reactions to tattoo pigment after laser treatment. *Dermatol Surg* **21**(4): 291–294.
52. Ross EV, Yashar S, Michaud N, Fitzpatrick R, Geronemus R, Tope WD, *et al.* (2001) Tattoo darkening and nonresponse after laser treatment: a possible role for titanium dioxide. *Arch Dermatol* **137**(1): 33–37.
53. Wimmershoff MB, Scherer K, Lorenz S, Landthaler M, Hohenleutner U. (2000) Hair removal using a 5-msec long-pulsed ruby laser. *Dermatol Surg* **26**(3): 205–210.
54. Touma DJ, Rohrer TE. (2004) Persistent hair loss 60 months after a single treatment with a 3-millisecond alexandrite (755 nm) laser. *J Am Acad Dermatol* **50**(2): 324–325.
55. Sadick NS, Prieto VG. (2003) The use of a new diode laser for hair removal. *Dermatol Surg* **29**(1): 30–33; discussion 3–4.
56. Ross EV, Ladin Z, Kreindel M, Dierickx C. (1999) Theoretical considerations in laser hair removal. *Dermatol Clin* **17**(2): 333–355, viii.
57. Battle EF Jr., Hobbs LM. (2004) Laser-assisted hair removal for darker skin types. *Dermatol Ther* **17**(2): 177–183.
58. Dover J, Burns J, Coleman S, Fitzpatrick R, Gradner J, Goldberg D, *et al.* (2009) A prospective clinical study of non-invasive cryolipolysis for subcutaneous fat layer reduction — interim report of available subject data. *Laser Surg Med* **S21**: 45.
59. Brightman L, Goldman MP, Taub AF. (2009) Sublative rejuvenation: experience with a new fractional radiofrequency system for skin rejuvenation and repair. *J Drugs Dermatol* **8**(11 Suppl): S9–S13.
60. Alster TS, Lupton JR. (2007) Nonablative cutaneous remodeling using radiofrequency devices. *Clin Dermatol* **25**(5): 487–491.
61. Kist D, Burns AJ, Sanner R, Counters J, Zelickson B. (2006) Ultrastructural evaluation of multiple pass low energy versus single pass high energy radiofrequency treatment. *Lasers Surg Med* **38**(2): 150–154.

62. Bogle MA, Ubelhoer N, Weiss RA, Mayoral F, Kaminer MS. (2007) Evaluation of the multiple pass, low fluence algorithm for radiofrequency tightening of the lower face. *Lasers Surg Med* **39**(3): 210–217.
63. Fitzpatrick R, Geronemus R, Goldberg D, Kaminer M, Kilmer S, Ruiz-Esparza J. (2003) Multicenter study of noninvasive radiofrequency for periorbital tissue tightening. *Lasers Surg Med* **33**(4): 232–242.
64. Dover JS, Zelickson B, Physician Multispecialty Consensus P. (2007) Results of a survey of 5,700 patient monopolar radiofrequency facial skin tightening treatments: assessment of a low-energy multiple-pass technique leading to a clinical end point algorithm. *Dermatol Surg* **33**(8): 900–907.
65. el-Domyati M, el-Ammawi TS, Medhat W, Moawad O, Brennan D, Mahoney MG, *et al.* (2011) Radiofrequency facial rejuvenation: evidence-based effect. *J Am Acad Dermatol* **64**(3): 524–535.
66. Sadick NS. (2003) Update on non-ablative light therapy for rejuvenation: a review. *Lasers Surg Med* **32**(2): 120–128.
67. Hruza G, Taub AF, Collier SL, Mulholland SR. (2009) Skin rejuvenation and wrinkle reduction using a fractional radiofrequency system. *J Drugs Dermatol* **8**(3): 259–265.
68. Baez F, Reilly LR. (2007) The use of light-emitting diode therapy in the treatment of photoaged skin. *J Cosmet Dermatol* **6**(3): 189–194.
69. Russell BA, Kellett N, Reilly LR. (2005) A study to determine the efficacy of combination LED light therapy (633 nm and 830 nm) in facial skin rejuvenation. *J Cosmet Laser Ther* **7**(3–4): 196–200.
70. Bhat J, Birch J, Whitehurst C, Lanigan SW. (2005) A single-blinded randomised controlled study to determine the efficacy of Omnilux Revive facial treatment in skin rejuvenation. *Lasers Med Sci* **20**(1): 6–10.
71. Weiss RA, Weiss MA, Geronemus RG, McDaniel DH. (2004) A novel non-thermal non-ablative full panel LED photomodulation device for reversal of photoaging: digital microscopic and clinical results in various skin types. *J Drugs Dermatol* **3**(6): 605–610.
72. Gliklich RE, White WM, Slayton MH, Barthe PG, Makin IR. (2007) Clinical pilot study of intense ultrasound therapy to deep dermal facial skin and subcutaneous tissues. *Arch Facial Plast Surg* **9**(2): 88–95.
73. Alam M, White LE, Martin N, Witherspoon J, Yoo S, West DP. (2010) Ultrasound tightening of facial and neck skin: a rater-blinded prospective cohort study. *J Am Acad Dermatol* **62**(2): 262–269.
74. White WM, Makin IR, Barthe PG, Slayton MH, Gliklich RE. (2007) Selective creation of thermal injury zones in the superficial musculoaponeurotic system

using intense ultrasound therapy: a new target for noninvasive facial rejuvenation. *Arch Facial Plast Surg* **9**(1): 22–29.
75. Kennedy JE, Ter Haar GR, Cranston D. (2003) High intensity focused ultrasound: surgery of the future? *Br J Radiol* **76**(909): 590–599.
76. Laubach HJ, Makin IR, Barthe PG, Slayton MH, Manstein D. (2008) Intense focused ultrasound: evaluation of a new treatment modality for precise microcoagulation within the skin. *Dermatol Surg* **34**(5): 727–734.
77. Avram MM, Harry RS. (2009) Cryolipolysis for subcutaneous fat layer reduction. *Lasers Surg Med* **41**(10): 703–708.
78. Coleman SR, Sachdeva K, Egbert BM, Preciado J, Allison J. (2009) Clinical efficacy of noninvasive cryolipolysis and its effects on peripheral nerves. *Aesthetic Plast Surg* **33**(4): 482–488.
79. Klein KB, Zelickson B, Riopelle JG, Okamoto E, Bachelor EP, Harry RS, *et al.* (2009) Non-invasive cryolipolysis for subcutaneous fat reduction does not affect serum lipid levels or liver function tests. *Lasers Surg Med* **41**(10): 785–790.
80. Brosseau L, Robinson V, Wells G, Debie R, Gam A, Harman K, *et al.* (2005) Low level laser therapy (Classes I, II and III) for treating rheumatoid arthritis. *Cochrane Database Syst Rev* (4): CD002049.
81. Jamtvedt G, Dahm KT, Christie A, Moe RH, Haavardsholm E, Holm I, *et al.* (2008) Physical therapy interventions for patients with osteoarthritis of the knee: an overview of systematic reviews. *Phys Ther* **88**(1): 123–136.
82. Chow RT, Johnson MI, Lopes-Martins RA, Bjordal JM. (2009) Efficacy of low-level laser therapy in the management of neck pain: a systematic review and meta-analysis of randomised placebo or active-treatment controlled trials. *Lancet* **374**(9705): 1897–1908.
83. da Silva JP, da Silva MA, Almeida AP, Lombardi Junior I, Matos AP. (2010) Laser therapy in the tissue repair process: a literature review. *Photomed Laser Surg* **28**(1): 17–21.
84. Posten W, Wrone DA, Dover JS, Arndt KA, Silapunt S, Alam M. (2005) Low-level laser therapy for wound healing: mechanism and efficacy. *Dermatol Surg* **31**(3): 334–340.
85. Sculean A, Schwarz F, Becker J. (2005) Anti-infective therapy with an Er:YAG laser: influence on peri-implant healing. *Expert Rev Med Devices* **2**(3): 267–276.
86. Jewell ML, Solish NJ, Desilets CS. (2011) Noninvasive Body Sculpting Technologies with an Emphasis on High-Intensity Focused Ultrasound. *Aesthetic Plast Surg* **35**(5): 901–912.

87. Neira R, Arroyave J, Ramirez H, Ortiz CL, Solarte E, Sequeda F, *et al.* (2002) Fat liquefaction: effect of low-level laser energy on adipose tissue. *Plast Reconstr Surg* **110**(3): 912–922; discussion 23–25.
88. Neira R, Solarte E, Isaza C, *et al.* (2001) Effects of the electric laser diode beam on *in vitro* human adipose tissue culture. Congreso Bolivariano de Cirugia Plastica Reconstructiva.
89. Jackson RF, Dedo DD, Roche GC, Turok DI, Maloney RJ. (2009) Low-level laser therapy as a non-invasive approach for body contouring: a randomized, controlled study. *Lasers Surg Med* **41**(10): 799–809.
90. Turok DI. (2009) A new non-invasive approach for body contouring: the application of low-level laser therapy. *Anti-Aging Medical News*, pp. 31–33.
91. Maloney R, Shanks S, Jenney E. (2009) The reduction in cholesterol and triglyceride serum levels following low-level laser irradiation: a non-controlled, non-randomized pilot study. *Laser Surg Med* **21S**: 66.
92. Nestor MS. (2004) Combination therapy in clinical and cosmetic dermatology: the marriage of device and drug. *J Drugs Dermatol* **3**(5 Suppl): S4–S11.
93. Clark E, Scerri L. (2008) Superficial and medium-depth chemical peels. *Clin Dermatol* **26**(2): 209–218.
94. Fitzgerald R, Vleggaar D, Burgess C. (2008) Facial dermal fillers. *Aesthet Surg J* **28**(6): 699–701; author reply.
95. Singh M, Griffiths CE. (2006) The use of retinoids in the treatment of photoaging. *Dermatol Ther* **19**(5): 297–305.
96. Draelos ZD. (2008) The cosmeceutical realm. *Clin Dermatol* **26**(6): 627–632.

PLASTIC SURGERY INVOLVING THE INTEGUMENT

CHAPTER 5

BENIGN AND MALIGNANT SKIN LESIONS

Wrood M. Kassira

Illustrative Case

Patient with a lesion on the shoulder.

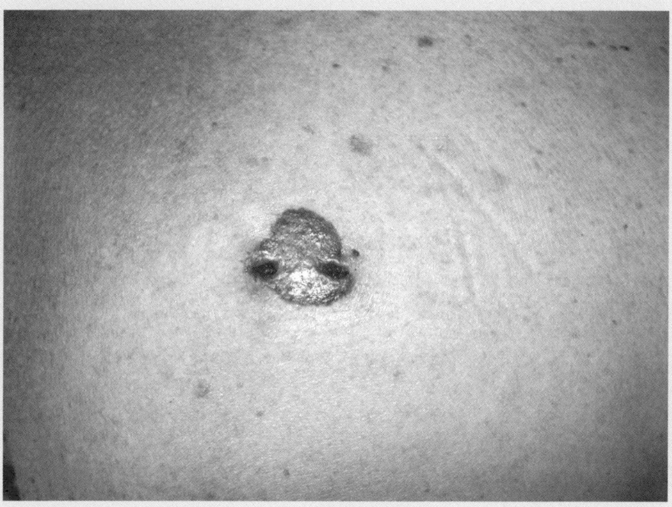

Diagnosis?

Review ABCDs
- Asymmetry
- Border irregularity
- Color variegation
- Diameter
- Enlarging

- Suspect melanoma
- Biopsy
- Thickness guides margins of resection
- Sentinel lymph node biopsy (Multidisciplinary approach)
- Closure with skin graft vs. local flap

Melanoma

Risk factor: UV light[1]

Atypical mole syndrome (B-K mole, dysplastic nevus syndrome, familial atypical multiple mole melanoma)[2,3]

- Autosomal dominant
- 10% risk of melanoma
- At least 100 melanocytic nevi
- ≥1 nevi ≥8 mm
- ≥1 nevi with atypical findings

Premalignant lesions (have atypical melanocytes)[3]

- Dysplastic nevus
- Lentigo maligna aka Hutchinson's freckle
- Melanoma *in situ*

ABCD's of melanoma [4,5]

- Asymmetry
- Border irregularity
- Color variegation
- Diameter >6 mm
- Evolving or enlarging

Other lesions:

Distinguish from pigmented BCCa with biopsy

Nevi[3,6]

- Intradermal: raised, pale papule

- Junctional: pale to dark brown, flat, smooth, round macules, appear between age 4 and 12, minimal if any growth
- Compound nevi: palpable, darker nevi, with or without hair, may appear during puberty and fades with age
- Spitz nevus: most are benign, smooth, red/pink dome-like lesion, <6 mm

Atypical moles[3]

- Nevus of Ota
- Blue nevus: blue-black lesion <5 mm
- Solar lentigo

Seborrheic keratosis: multiple, raised verrucous papules appear stuck-on, well-defined border[3,5]

Types of Melanoma:[5]

- Superficial Spreading Melanoma: most common
- Nodular Melanoma: aggressive, worst histologic type, but similar survival for match thickness
- Lentigo Maligna Melanoma: flat, large, may not be aggressive, depends on depth
- Acral Lentiginous Melanoma: soles, palms, hands, nail beds
- Amelanotic: no pigment
- Desmoplastic Melanoma: rare, high risk perineural invasion

Staging:[7]
TNM

T = Thickness (Breslow staging): Most significant prognostic predictor
T1 ≤1 mm
T2 1.01–2 mm
T3 2.01–4 mm
T4 >4 mm

Ta without ulceration
Tb with ulceration

Ulceration : worse prognosis[7]
Increased mitotic rate: worse prognosis[3]
Amelanotic: worse survival since often thicker

N: number of nodes
N1 1 node
N2 2–3 nodes
N3 4 or more nodes, or matted or satellite met

Metastasis[7]
M1a other skin, subcutaneous tissue, or nodes
M1b lung
M1c viscera or any distant mets

Clark's levels:[8]
I above basement membrane, *in situ*
II into papillary dermis
III papillary-reticular dermis
IV reticular dermis
V subcutaneous

Work-up for local melanoma

- Complete history and physical examination
- Chest X-ray
- LDH (lactate dehydrogenase)
- Sentinel lymph node biopsy

If recurrent or logoregional: CBC, CT or MRI[9]

Diagnosis

- If <1.5 cm: excisional biopsy into subcutaneous tissue, do not resect fascia, approx. 2 mm border[3,10]
- Incisional biopsy for large lesions or anatomically sensitive areas, or full thickness punch biopsy of most irregular area (needs to be full thickness into subcut.)

For nails: remove nail or create a window to perform biopsy

Margins for excision:[3,5]

- Dysplastic nevus: 0.5 cm
- Melanoma *in situ*/lentigo maligna: 0.5–1 cm
- 0–1 mm thick melanoma: 1 cm
- 1–2 mm thick: 1–2 cm
- 2–4 mm thick: 2 cm
- >4 mm thick: 2–3 cm

Subungal melanoma confined to the nail bed: amputation proximal to IP of thumb or DIP of finger

If tumor extensive: amputate[3,11]

Indications for SLNBx (sentinel lymph node biopsy):[3,12]

- 0.76 mm or greater thick melanoma
- Clark III or greater, ulcerated
- Male with <0.76 mm truncal melanoma

Adjuvant treatment:[3,5,13]

- Interferon for mets or >4 mm deep lesions
- Immunotherapy

Congenital Nevi[3,14,15]

- Precursors of melanoma, larger greater risk
- Small <1.5 cm
- Medium 1.5–2 cm
- Giant >20 cm, greater risk of malignant degeneration, treatment is excision, wait until 6 months of age; approximately 14% risk of transforming into melanoma

Basal Cell (BCCa) and Squamous Cell Cancer (SCCa)

- Often the result of accumulated actinic changes
- Less melanin, more sensitive to sun damage
- Lower Fitzpatrick skin types greater risk
- Greater lifetime burns, greater risk SCCa
- Irregular interval burns, greater risk BCCa[15]

Genetic Syndromes

1. Nevoid Basal Cell Syndrome[16,17,18]
    - Autosomal dominant
    - Chromosome 9
    - Multiple BCCa
    - Odontogenic keratocysts (jaw cysts)
    - Scoliosis
    - Bifid ribs
    - Palmar/plantar pits
    - Brachymetacarpalism
    - Broad nasal root
    - Large supraorbital ridges
    - Calcified falx cerebri
2. Porokeratosis[16]
    - Autosomal dominant
    - Abnormal keratin growth, degenerates into squamous cell cancer
    - Ringshaped plaques, sharp hornlike borders
3. Albinism[5]
    - Autosomal recessive
    - Lack melanin
    - Increased risk skin cancer
4. Xeroderma pigmentosum[5]
    - Autosomal recessive
    - Defect in DNA repair of UV damage
    - Symptoms include erythema, freckles, multiple skin cancers
    - Avoid sun exposure, protection from sun

Predisposing lesions[5,16]

1. Actinic keratoses aka solar keratoses or senile keratoses
    - Precancerous
    - May remit, stay stable or degenerate to SCCa (10–13% risk)

2. Nevus sebaceous of Jadassohn
    - Yellow plaque, present on scalp or face at birth
    - Raised, hairless, well-circumscribed
        - 10% risk BCCa
3. Cutaneous horns
    - Keratotic mass
    - Biopsy recommended to rule out SCCa or actinic keratoses

Environmental exposure[16]

1. UVB rays (290–325 nm)
    - Most carcinogenic
2. Ionizing radiation
3. Chemicals: nitrogen mustard, nitrosurea, arsenic, dimethyl benzanthracene, aromatic hyrdrocarbons[19]

Prevention[16]

- Sunscreen (Para-aminobenzoic acid), cinnamates, benzophenones absorb UV radiation
- Titanium dioxide, zinc oxide, kaolin: best protection, act as barrier to UV
- Sunprotective clothing, hats
- Avoid tanning beds (high UVA radiation)
- Regular dermatologic examinations

Diagnosis:[16]

- Shave excision or incisional biopsy
- Excisional biopsy: if small or patient with history of multiple skin cancers
- If biopsy positive but site heals clinically with no obvious tumor, still need to perform curative surgery because of microscopic residual tumor left behind

Basal Cell Cancer

Often in light skin complexion
Different histologic types include:[16,20]
Types:

- Nodular : most common, nodule flesh color with telangiestasias,
- Superficial : within epidermis, scaly, erythematous, or crusting or shallow ulcer
- Cystic
- Adenoid
- Pigmented: brown color, melanin, may appear blue-black, may confuse with melanoma
- Morpheaform or sclerosing: firm, white or yellow plaque, indurated, poorly defined borders, often positive margins post excision
- Atypical

Treatment

1. Surgical[16]

- Excision: most advocate a 3–5 mm margin for small nodular, well demarcated lesions, worse cure rate for morpheaform, infiltrative, fibrosing
- Or Mohs micrographic surgery: involves excision of tumor and mapping of the lesion using a microscope with continued resection of remaining tumor until all tumor is removed
- Advantage is high cure rate (99% for primary BCCa), tissue conservation[21]
- Disadvantage is a staged reconstruction: cost, inconvenience

Indications for Mohs:
Primary skin tumors with

- Poorly defined borders
- Originating from scar tissue
- Morpheaform or sclerosing BCCa
- Cosmetically sensitive areas, e.g. eyelid

- High recurrence areas: paranasal, nasal, periorbital, periauricular
- SCCa with perineural invasion
- Aggressive features
- Recurrent BCCa or SCCa
- Dermatofibroscarcoma protuberans
- Microcystic adnexal carcinoma

2. Destructive[16,22]

    - Cryosurgery: requires trained operator and strict guidelines, for small lesions; contraindicated in sclerosing or morphea form BCCa or cold intolerance
    - Electrodessication and curettage: most common, high cure rate, heal by secondary intention, for small (ideally <2 mm), superficial tumors in non-cosmetically sensitive area
    - Laser, CO_2 laser: for superficial BCCa, unable to examine margins, risks of hypo- or hyperpigmentation

3. Medical treatment[16]

- Injection with methotrexate, 5-FU, 5-MU, actinomycin D or interferon; for patient unable to undergo other treatment or multifocal
- Topical 5-FU not for invasive skin cancer
- Radiation: for elderly patients who cannot undergo surgery, long-term effects include fibrosis, ulceration, ectropion

Positive margin (on permanent pathology despite negative frozen section 5–16% of cases), i.e. incomplete excision: best course is re-excision (other options: observation or radiotherapy not ideal)[16,23,24]

Lesions to differentiate from Basal Cell Cancer:

Microcystic adnexal carcinoma[16,25,26]

- Histology: small cysts with basaloid cells resemble eccrine gland ducts
- Aggressive

- Perineural invasion
- Wide local excision (negative margins) or Mohs

Trichoepithelioma[16]

- Similar features to BCCa, flesh-colored papules
- Distinguished by symmetry, with smooth margins, hair structures, large horn cysts, fibrosis around basaloid cells, rare infilrative inflammatory cells

Desmoplastic Trichoepithelioma[27]

- Benign, removed to rule out malignancy, small round lesions with depressed center, confused with morpheaform BCCa, narrow strands of basaloid cells

Eccrine Epithelioma[28]

- akaBCCa with eccrine differentiation
- Aggressive, invasive, high recurrence
- Treatment is Mohs or wide local excision

Squamous Cell Cancer
Grow much faster than BCCa
Sunexposed areas, scars, sinus tracts

Precursor lesions:
Actinic Keratoses

- Scaly, rough macules or papules
- Skin colored or red or yellow
- Malignant potential
- Treatment is recommend to prevent degeneration to squamous cell cancer (SCCa)
- 5-FU, laser, chemical peel, cryotherapy, curettage, tangential excision
- Reversed with topical retinoids

Treatment of SCCa:[5,16]
Surgical excision, destructive (electrodessication and curretage or cryosurgery for superficial, small lesions), or medical treatment (radiation: for patient who cannot undergo surgery)

Excision[16,29]

- For well-differentiated <2 cm lesions: 4 mm margin
- Large tumors: 10 mm margins or more
- Or Mohs

5-FU and photodynamic therapy are not treatment for SCCa
SCCa has metastatic risk (vs. BCCa rare)[5,16]

- Perform lymph node exam
- If lymphadenopathy perform lympadenectomy
- Treatment of metastases: chemotherapy and radiation

Recurrence of SCCa increased if:[16]

- Poorly differentiated
- Depth Clark IV or V
- Perineural invasion

Marjolin's ulcer[16]

- Refers to squamous cell cancer arising from scarred tissue, burn, osteomyelitis tracts, fistula tracts
- High metastases
- Low survival
- False negative biopsies due to foci of invasive cancer
- Treatment is wide local excision

Subungal SCCa[16]

- Often misdiagnosed as infection
- Mohs surgery[30] or distal phalanx amputation (aggressive tx)

Bowen's disease[16]

- SCCa *in situ*
- Slowly growing red patch with sharp border
- Scaly, crusting
- 10% become invasive
- Treatment: surgical excision

Erythroplasia of Queyrat

- Bowens' disease of penis

Verrucous Carcinoma[16,31]

- SCCa that is well differentiated
- Palms and soles commonly affected (carcinoma cuniculatum)
- Treat with surgical excision or Mohs

Other lesions:
Keratoacanthoma[5,16]

- Characterized by rapid growth followed by resolution
- Firm raised half-moon lesion with keratin plug
- Not malignant
- Treatment: surgical excision

Bowenoid Papulosis[16,32]

- HPV related
- Anogenital area
- Flat small warts-like lesions or plaques
- Benign
- Treatment is conservative

Pseudoepitheliomatous Hyperplasia

- Benign
- Arises in bed of chronic inflammation[16]

Proliferating Epidermoid Cysts[16]

- Benign
- Begin as nodule that enlarges with central ulcer
- Most are on the scalp, more common in older women[16]

Merkel Cell Skin Tumor[16,33]

- Aggressive, arises in dermis
- Elderly pts.

- Aggressive
- Excision 3–5 mm margins
- Multidisciplinary treatment
    - +/– nodal dissection
    - Postop radiation therapy

Desmoplastic Melanoma[5,16]

- Often amelanotic
- Late diagnosis
- Higher local recurrence
- Confused with undifferentiated SCCa

Dermatofibrosarcoma Protuberans[5,16]

- Excision with 3 cm margins with fascia or Mohs
- Low rate of metastasis
- Imatinib (Gleevec®)

References

1. Fears TR, Bird CC, Guerry D 4th, *et al.* (2002) Average midrange ultraviolet radiation flux and time outdoors predict melanoma risk. *Cancer Res* **62**: 3992–3996.
2. Marghoob AA, Kopf AW, Rigel DS, *et al.* (1994) Risk of cutaneous malignant melanoma in patients with "classic" atypical mole syndrome. A case-control study. *Arch Dermatol* **130**: 993–998.
3. Anderson RG. (2004) Skin tumors II: melanoma. *Select Read Plast Surg* **10**(3): 2, 5–7, 19, 20, 22, 23, 28, 36, 38.
4. Devesa SS, *et al.* (1987) Cancer incidence and mortality trends among whites in the United States, 1947–1984. *J Natl Cancer Inst* **79**: 701–770.
5. Feig BW, Berger DH, Fuhrman GM. (2006) *The MD Anderson Surgical Oncology Handbook*. Lippincott Williams & Wilkins, Philadelphia, pp. 63, 74, 113, 114, 116, 124, 139.
6. Reed RJ, *et al.* (1975) Common and uncommon melanocytic nevi and borderline melanomas. *Semin Oncol* **2**: 119–147.
7. Balch CM, Buzaid AC, Soong SJ, *et al.* (2001) Final version of the American Joint Committee on Cancer staging system for cutaneous melanoma. *J Clin Oncol* **19**: 3635–3648.

8. McGovern VJ, *et al.* (1973) The classification of malignant melanoma and its histologic reporting. *Cancer* **32**: 1446–1457.
9. Gershenwald JE, Fischer D, Buzaid AC. (2000) Clinical classification and staging. *Clin Plast Surg* **27**(3): 361–376.
10. Ho VC, Sober AJ, Balch CM. (1998) Biopsy techniques. In: Balch CM, Houghton AN, Sober AJ, Soong S-J (eds.), *Cutaneous Melanoma*, 3rd Edn. St Louis, Quality Medicine Publishing, Ch 7.
11. Papachristou DN, Fortner JG. (1982) Melanoma arising under the nail. *J Surg Oncol* **21**: 219–222.
12. Phan GQ, Messina JL, Sondak VK, Zager JS. (2009) Sentinel lymph node biopsy for melanoma: indications and rationale. *Cancer Control* **16**(3): 234–239.
13. Kirkwood JM, Strawderman MH, Ernstoff MS, *et al.* (1996) Interferon alfa-2b adjuvant therapy of high-risk resected cutaneous melanoma: the Eastern Cooperative Oncology Group Trial EST 1684. *J Clin Oncol* **14**: 7–17.
14. Kopf AW, Bart RS, Hennessey P. (1979) Congenital nevocytic nevi and malignant melanomas. *J Am Acad Dermatol* **1**: 123–130.
15. Moss ALH, Briggs JC. (1986) Cutaneous malignant melanoma in the young. *Br J Plast Surg* **39**: 537–541.
16. Zbar RIS. (2004) Skin tumors I: basal cell and squamous cell carcinoma. *Select Read Plast Surg*. **10**(3): 1–8, 10, 17, 20–24.
17. Rayner CRW, Towers JF, Wilson JSP. (1976) What is Gorlin's syndrome? The diagnosis and management of the basal cell naevus syndrome, based on a study of thirty-seven patients. *Br J Plast Surg* **30**: 62–67.
18. Gherardini G, Bhatia N, Stal S. (1997) Congenital syndromes associated with nonmelanoma skin cancer. *Clin Plast Surg* **24**(4): 649–661.
19. DuVivier A, Vonderheid EC, Van Scott EJ, Urbach F. (1978) Mycosis fungoides, nitrogen mustard and skin cancer. *Br J Dermatol* **99**: 61–63.
20. Pollack SV, Goslen JB, Sherertz EF, Jegasothy BV. (1982) The biology of basal cell carcinoma: a review. *J Am Acad Dermatol* **7**(5): 569–577.
21. Cottel WI, Proper S. (1982) Mohs'surgery, fresh-tissue technique. Our technique with a review. *J Dermatol Surg Oncol* **8**: 576–587.
22. Vine JE. (2001) Skin cancer update. Treatment alternatives for basal-cell and squamous-cell carcinoma. *N J Med* **98**(5): 35–37.
23. Kumar P, Orton CI, McWilliam LJ, Watson S. (2000) Incidence of incomplete excision in surgically treated basal cell carcinoma: a retrospective clinical audit. *Br J Plast Surg* **53**(7): 563–566.
24. Hallock GG, Lutz DA. (2001) A prospective study of the accuracy of the surgeon's diagnosis and significance of positive margins in nonmelanoma skin cancers. *Plast Reconstr Surg* **107**(4): 942–947.

25. Dixon AY, Lee SH, McGregor DH. (1989) Factors predictive of recurrence of basal cell carcinoma. *Am J Dermatopathol* **11**: 222–232.
26. Mayer MH, *et al.* (1989) Microcystic adnexal carcinoma (sclerosing sweat duct carcinoma). *Plast Reconstr Surg* **84**: 970–975.
27. Mamelak AJ, Goldberg LH, Katz TM, Graves JJ, Arnon O, Kimyai-Asadi A. (2010) Desmoplastic trichoepithelioma. *J Am Acad Dermatol* **62**(1): 102–106.
28. Sanchez NP, Winkelmann RK. (1982) Basal cell tumor with eccrine differentiation (eccrine epithelioma). *J Am Acad Dermatol* **6**(4): 514–518.
29. Brodland DG, Zitelli JA. (1992) Surgical margins for excision of primary cutaneous squamous cell carcinoma. *J Am Acad Dermatol* **27**: 241–248.
30. Mikhail GR. (1984) Subungual epidermoid carcinoma. *J Am Acad Dermatol* **11**: 291–298.
31. Schwartz R. (1995) Verrucous carcinoma of the skin and mucosa. *J Am Acad Dermatol* **32**(1): 1–21.
32. Wade TR, Kopf AW, Ackerman AB. (1979) Bowenoid papulosis of the genitalia. *Arch Dermatol* **115**(3): 306–308.
33. Pectasides D, Pectasides M, Economopoulos T. (2006) Merkel cell cancer of the skin. *Ann Oncol* **17**(10): 1489–1495.

CHAPTER 6

INFANTILE HEMANGIOMA

Karim W. Sadik and Haaris S. Mir

Introduction

Infantile hemangiomas are a benign vascular tumor of infancy. They may result in significant physiologic, cosmetic and psychological effects. The word "hemangioma" comes from the Greek word haema- (Greek: αίμα) meaning "blood", angeio (Greek: αγγείο) meaning "vessel" and the suffix -oma (Greek: -ωμα) meaning "tumor".

Incidence

Hemangiomas are the most common tumors of infancy affecting approximately 1 in 10 children.[1] They occur in infants of all races but are most common in those who are white.[2] These lesions are more preponderant in females as compared to males with rates of 3:1 to 5:1.[2] Approximately 23% of pre-term infants <1000 g develop hemangiomas.[3]

Etiology

Presence of GLUT-1 cells of placental origin imply embolization of these cells in utero. A second theory is the alteration of the pluripotent cell to that of placentalorigin.[4] Chorionic villus sampling at 9 to 12 weeks of gestation has been associated with a 21% increased incidence of hemangiomas in infants.[2]

The origin of infantile hemangioma is likely a somatic mutation in a single endothelial cell leading to clonal expansion.[5] The possibility of a germline mutation is suggested by kindreds that show a hereditary transmission. Most hemangiomas occur sporadically without a hereditary component. However, in a few families, hemangiomas segregate as a highly penetrant, autosomal dominant trait. Gene linkage studies of familial infantile hemangiomas show evidence of linkage to chromosome 5q31–33.[2]

Pathophysiology

The life cycle of spontaneous growth to rapid involution in most patients is not fully understood.[6] Infantile capillary hemangiomas are composed of a complex mixture of clonal endothelial cells associated with pericytes, dendritic cells, and mast cells.[7] Regulators of hemangioma growth and involution are poorly understood. During the involution phase, apoptosis has been seen.[7]

Proliferation

Vascular endothelial cells rapidly divide during this phase producing vast sinusoids. During the growth phase, two major proangiogenic factors are involved: basic fibroblast growth factor (bFGF) and vascular endothelial growth factor (VEGF); histologic studies have shown that both endothelial and interstitial cells are actively dividing in this phase. [7] Certain collagenases are also noted to be present and active in remodeling the extracellular matrix, allowing for the growth of aberrant capillaries. Erythrocyte type glucose transporter protein-1 (GLUT1) is immunopositive throughout the life cycle and negative in most other vascular tumors and vascular malformations.[4]

Involution

During this phase, endothelial growth gradually decreases to the point of cellular apoptosis. There is a marked deposition of perivascular fibrous tissue. This occurs along with the arrival of fibroblasts, mast cells and macrophages. The arrival of Tissue Inhibitor of Metalloproteinase 1 (TIMP-1) heralds the inhibition of any further blood vessel growth.[8] Although mast cells are present towards the end of the proliferative phase, they are more prominent in the involuting phase suppressing further endothelial growth.[3]

Involuted

Once complete, there remains a few capillaries and veins. Some of the hallmarks of the proliferative phase can still be seen around these remaining vessels (i.e. multilayered basement membranes). The highly cellular parenchyma is now replaced with fibrofatty tissue with collagen islands.[3]

Diagnosis

Diagnosis is possible with an accurate history and physical examination. Deep anomalies (subcutaneous, intramuscular, visceral) can be difficult to diagnosis and would warrant radiological screening. If the lesion is suspicious for malignancy, biopsy may become necessary.

Radiology

During the proliferative phase ultrasonography of a hemangioma will show decreased arterial resistance and increased venous velocity. It is difficult to distinguish from arteriovenous malformation because both are fast-flow.

MRI with contrast is the gold standard, however it is typically used to delineate the extent of involvement of deep hemanigomas (i.e. abdomen or orbit) that are not well defined on physical examination. MRI usually requires sedation or general anesthesia if the child is younger than 6 years old. It shows soft tissue of intermediate intensity on T1-weighted spin-echo images and moderate hyper-intensity on T2-weighted spin-echo images. Prominent flow-voids are located around and within the tumor, indicating rapid flow in feeding arteries and dilated draining veins. At some time in the late involuting phase, the hemangioma becomes a slow-flow lesion, often with prominent fatty parenchyma.[3]

Classification

International Society for the Study of Vascular Anomalies (ISSVA)
Malformation vs Hemangiomas

Hemangioma:

Acquired

The endothelial proliferation along with involution seen in infants.

- Superficial — superficial dermis
- Deep — deep dermis/Subcutaneous tissue
- Mixed — components of both[9,10]

Congenital Hemangioma

Develops in utero and presents fully formed at birth.

- Superficial — superficial dermis
- Deep — deep dermis/Subcutaneous tissue
- Mixed — components of both[9,10]

Malformation — abnormally formed vascular channels lined with quiescent endothelial cells; congenital, may not be visible at birth; always grow; never regress.

Slow flow

Derived from capillary, venous and lymphatic vascular anomalies.[9,10] Lymphatic malformations, of which there are three types: truncal malformations, extra-truncal malformations and hemolymphatic anomalies, are the most frequent vascular malformation.[11]

Fast flow

Derived from arterial and arterio-venous anomalies.[10]

Combined

Combined anomalies are often associated with soft tissue and skeletal hypertrophy.[3]

Soft tissue and skeletal growth

Pure anomalies (fast or slow) can be associated with soft tissue and skeletal hypertrophy in rare circumstances. Capillary malformations

(Port-Wine Stains) can be associated with soft tissue growth and even skeletal hypertrophy (Klippel-Trenaunay Syndrome).[12–14] Lymphatic malformations can also be associated with soft tissue and skeletal growth.[11]

Clinical Features

80% of hemangiomas are solitary; 20% are multifocal.

Many hemangiomas are discrete, well-circumscribed masses present in the head and neck. Some hemangiomas are segmental and diffuse, often involving large areas of the extremities or the head and neck.[3] They tend to appear within 2 weeks after term birth, however deep subcutaneous and visceral hemangiomas may not become clinically apparent for months.[3] 30–40% of infantile hemangiomas are obvious at birth presenting as a pale red stain or ecchymotic area. *Congenital hemangiomas* present fully formed at birth.[3]

Proliferation

Hemangiomas grow rapidly during the first 6–8 months of life. As the growth invades the superficial dermis, the tumour becomes deep red, and raised. If the growth goes into the deep dermis or subcutis, there is minimal raising of the skin and the coloration becomes bluish. Draining veins are usually seen circum navigating the lesion in a radial pattern.[3]

Involution

Hemangiomas reach their peak before the first year of age at which point it grows in proportion to the child. The color fades to a purplish hue with a grey mantle, and the lesion becomes softer to palpation. Involution continues until 5–10 years of age. Most of the color fades by 7 years.

Regression is complete in 50% of children by age 5 years and in 70% by age 7 years, with continued improvement until age 10 to 12 years. Complete involution results in normal skin in 50%, the remained have mild discoloration, laxity, and scarring if the hemangioma became ulcerated.

Skeletal involvement is rare with hemangiomas. However when they occur, the result manifests in cartilaginous or bony overgrowth presumably secondary to increased blood flow from the hemangioma.[3]

Congenital hemangioma

These present fully formed at birth. They may be detected during routine prenatal ultrasonography. Due to the relative size proportionate to the infant in utero, it may result in cardiac overload and hydrops fetalis. They do not, however, undergo the rapid proliferation noted in infantile hemangiomas.

Two types: Rapidly Involuting Congenital Hemangiomas (RICH) and Non-Involuting Congenital hemangiomas (NICH). They are both similar in incidence, location, etc. Interestingly however, infantile hemangiomas lack the GLUT-1.[15]

RICH — pale halo, grey, involuted by 6–14 months. May be large enough to cause congestive heart failure.[15,16]

NICH — pale halo, pink/blue, continues to grow with the infant.[15,17]

Infantile hemangioma can rarely co-exist with RICH or NICH. Also, RICH can convert to a NICH.[3,16]

RICH, NICH, and common infantile hemangioma have overlapping clinical and pathologic features and may be variations of a single entity.[16]

PHACES

Facial hemangiomas can be associated with P-posterior cranial fossa malformations i.e. dandy walker or cysts, HA-large facial hemangioma, C-cardiac defects, E- eye anomalies, S- sternal cleft.[18]

Lumbosacral Anomalies

Lumbosacral hemangioma also presents in association with occult spinal dysraphism
(lipomeningocele, tethered cord, and diastematomyelia).[3]

Perineal Anomalies

Diffuse hemangioma of the perineum and lower limb is also seen with urogenital and anorectal anomalies.[3]

Natural Course

Most infantile hemangiomas result in growth in the first 5 months of life.[19]

Unlike other tumors, hemangiomas enter an involution phase, during which they usually regress over the next several months to years. Sometimes intervention is required due to proliferative growth which is complicated by ulceration, obstruction, bleeding, persistent aesthetic deformity or infection.[1,20]

Ulceration, obstruction and/or infection occurs in 10% of infantile hemangiomas. If ulceration extends to deeper tissue, it may result in loss of the associated structure i.e. the eye or ear etc.[3]

1% of hemangiomas may lead to a life threatening sequelae i.e. bleeding (GI hemangiomas) or shunting (hepatic hemangiomas) resulting in congestive heart failure.[3]

Why Actively Intervene?

There are several rationales for active intervention in treating rapidly growing and aggressive lesions as early as possible:

1. The avoidance of hemangioma growth in or near the vital and functional organs. i.e. lesions in the nose, mouth, and throat areas can affect breathing and swallowing. Bleeding in these areas can be life threatening. Lesions in the eye and ear area can affect vision and hearing. Complicated lesions in the facial area can cause permanent cosmetic damage and mental stress.
2. A shorter course of treatment. Intervening early means intervening whilst the lesion is still small and the endothelial cells more sensitive to treatment. As a result, the total chosen treatment dose may be less in the long run.
3. The mitigation of the risk of infection and associated sequelae.[21]

MANAGEMENT

Observation

The majority of infantile hemangiomas are minor and are monitored by pediatricians without the need for specialist consultation. Family anxiety is a large factor and once threshold for specialist consultation is met, time should be spent explaining the disease course in and adequate fashion with visual aids.

Corticosteroids

Corticosteroids can inhibit the proliferation of vascular endothelial cells. Oral corticosteroids are the standard of care for vascular lesions that can cause functional impairment or significant cosmetic deformity. They can also be used topically or intralesionally.[7,22]

Dose

— Intralesional injection — give if <2.5 cm hemangioma and localized. Administer Triamcinilone (25 mg/mL), give 3–5 mg/kg in 3–5 separate injections spaced over 6–8 weeks.
— Systemic injection — first line for large endangering hemangioma. i.e. obstructing airway. Administer oral prednisone at 2–3 mg/kg/day as a single morning dose for 4–6 weeks. Then slowly taper for several months and discontinue by 10–11 months.

Advantages

— Sensitive hemangiomas will respond within days to a week.
— With intralesional or systemic steroids, the hemangioma response rate is 85% (accelerated regression or stabilized growth).[8]

Disadvantages

— Inability to give live vaccines during the period of treatment.
— Pause in infant growth (length and weight) in 1/3rd of patients during the period of steroid administration. Growth resumes after stopping steroids.[23]
— Chushingoid stigmata (moon facies, etc.)
— If steroid taper is too rapid, will result in rebound of the hemangioma.

— Causes gastric irritation, H2 blocker will be protective.
— Myopathy.
— Rarely myopathy, cardiomyopathy, premature thelarche and hirsutism can result.
— Intralesional steroid injection of eyelid can result in embolic occlusion of retinal artery.[23]

Propranolol (Non-Selective Beta-Blockade)

Propranolol, a nonselective beta-blocker, has recently been introduced as a novel modality for the treatment of proliferating haemangiomas.[24] The exact mechanism of action of propranolol in the treatment of haemangiomas remains unclear. Vasoconstriction, which is immediately visible as a change in color, associated with a palpable softening of the hemangioma may occur.[25] Decreased expression of angiogenic VEGF and bFGF genes and their factors through the down-regulation of the RAF–mitogen-activated protein kinase pathway is probable.[26] Up-regulation of apoptosis of capillary endothelial cells may also be responsible for the reduction of hemangiomas.[27] Suggestions of inhibition of MMP-9 and HBMEC expression have been made.[1]

Literature in Support

Prospective Studies (in reverse chronology):

Qin *et al.* gave propranolol to 58 infants with hemangiomas at a dose of 1.0–1.5 mg per kilogram of body weight per day in Shandong and Shanghai. There were 19 males and 39 females 1 to 12 months old with a mean age of 4 months. The primary tumor size was 1.5 cm × 1.0 cm to 18.0 cm × 5.0 cm. Twenty-seven were superficial, nine deep-seated and 22 mixed. The tumors were located in head and neck (n = 41), trunk and extremities (n = 12), labium vulvae (n = 2), perianal region (n = 1), perineum (n = 1) and scrotum (n = 1). The patients were hospitalized for 7 to 10 days, continued medication at home and revisited every 2 weeks. At 24 hours post-medication, all the tumors decreased in density, color and size. The changes became conspicuous within 5 to 7 days. Seven patients had medication for 2 months, 22 for 3 months, 21 for 4 months and 8 for

5 months. The follow-up period was 5 to 9 months. The overall response was scale I (poor) in 1 patient (1.7%), scale II (moderate) in 12 patients (20.7%), scale III (good) in 35 patients (60.4%) and scale IV (excellent) in 10 patients (17.2%). Statistical analysis showed that the treatment response for deep-seated hemangiomas was significantly better than that for superficial hemangiomas ($P < 0.05$), but no significant difference was found among different primary sites ($P > 0.05$).[27]

Léauté-Labrèze *et al.* wrote in NEJM

We have observed that propranolol can inhibit the growth of these hemangiomas. Our preliminary data from 11 children are summarized. The first child had a nasal capillary hemangioma. Despite corticosteroid treatment, the lesion was stabilized but obstructive hypertrophic myocardiopathy developed, so the patient was treated with propranolol. The day after the initiation of treatment, the hemangioma changed from intense red to purple, and it softened. The corticosteroids were tapered, but the hemangioma continued to improve. When the corticosteroids were discontinued, no regrowth of the hemangioma was noted. When the child was 14 months of age, the hemangioma was completely flat. The second child had a plaque-like infantile capillary hemangioma involving the entire right upper limb and part of the face. At 1 month of age, a subcutaneous component developed, and despite corticosteroid treatment, the hemangioma continued to enlarge. Magnetic resonance imaging revealed intraconal and extraconal orbital involvement, as well as an intracervical mass causing compression and tracheal and esophageal deviation. Ultrasonography showed increased cardiac output, and treatment with propranolol, at a dose of 2 mg per kilogram of body weight per day, was initiated. Seven days later, the child was able to open his eye spontaneously, and the mass near the parotid gland was considerably reduced in size. Prednisolone was discontinued at 4 months of age, without any regrowth of the hemangioma; at 9 months of age, the eye opening was satisfactory, and no major visual impairment was noted. After written informed consent had been obtained from the parents, propranolol was given to nine additional children who had severe or disfiguring infantile capillary. In all patients, 24 hours after the initiation of treatment, we observed a change in the hemangioma from intense red to purple; this change was associated with a palpable softening of the lesion. After these initial changes, the hemangiomas continued to improve until they were nearly flat, with residual skin telangiectasias. Ultrasound examinations in five patients showed an objective regression in thickness associated with an increase in the resistive index of vascularization of the hemangioma.[24]

Retrospective Studies (in reverse chronology):

Maturo *et al.* performed a retrospective case series at Massachussettes Eye and Ear hospital. They noted two children who demonstrated significant response to oral propranolol therapy and avoided not only invasive surgical procedures, but also long-term administration of oral corticosteroids. This is the first report of treating infantile airway hemangiomas with only propranolol without additional surgical intervention or corticosteroid use.[28]

Buckmiller *et al.* performed a retrospective single institution review of children treated with propranolol for problematic hemangiomas followed by a blinded prospective analysis of serial photographs taken during the course of their therapy. Parental questionnaires were obtained to evaluate perceived therapeutic response and complications to oral propranolol. Thirty-two children with complete photo documentation were treated with oral propranolol for infantile hemangiomas between September 2008 and June 2009. Twenty-seven patients began therapy during the proliferative phase of their lesions (mean age, 4.9 months), whereas five patients began during the involutional phase (mean age, 19.4 months). Ninety-seven percent of patients displayed improvement in the quality of their hemangiomas during propranolol therapy. Patients were determined to be excellent responders (n = 16, 50%), partial responders (n = 15, 47%), or nonresponders (n = 1, 3%). Partial and nonresponders received adjuvant therapy (75%, laser therapy; 31%, steroid injections). Ten patients experienced minor but reportable side effects to propranolol, including somnolence (27.2%), gastroesophageal reflux (9.1%), respiratory syncytial virus exacerbation (4.5%), and rash (4.5%).[29]

Case Reports (in reverse chronology)

General

Massive response of severe infantile hepatic hemangioma to propranolol by Marsciani *et al.* (Abstract unavailable).[30]

Life-threatening infantile haemangioma: a dramatic response to propranolol by Theletsane *et al.* (Abstract unavailable).[31]

Orbital/Peri-Orbital Hemangioma

Propranolol for isolated orbital infantile hemangioma by Fay *et al.*[32]
Propranolol for orbital hemangioma by Taban *et al.*[33]

Subglottic / Tracheal Hemangioma

Propranolol for the treatment of a life-threatening subglottic and mediastinal infantile hemangioma by Truong *et al.*[34]

Jephson *et al.* describe the successful treatment with propranolol, of a stridulous four-month-old child with a 95% obstructing subglottic haemangioma. This was achieved without the need for tracheostomy or any other surgical intervention, and with no reported side effects. They believe the new discovery of a dramatic response to propranolol allows treatment in the acute setting and following further study may render surgical treatment of subglottic haemangioma obsolete.[35]

Buckmiller *et al.* report the successful management of tracheal hemangiomas using oral propranolol in a young patient with otherwise treatment-resistant airway lesions. Despite various endoscopic therapeutic attempts, the patient remained stridulous with airway disease that persisted into the involution phase of the average hemangioma cycle. Within 6 weeks of beginning oral propranolol (2 mg/kg/day), her airway compromise was eliminated and she had complete resolution of endoscopically visible disease. No side effects from propranolol occurred.[36]

Denoyelle *et al.* looked at the efficacy of propranolol for subglottic hemangiomas and to discuss its place among the other available therapies. They report 2 infants with subglottic hemangiomas, which were resistant to other established medical treatments. One infant presented with PHACES association, the other with widespread cutaneous congenital hemangiomas. Both were subsequently treated with systemic Propranolol. Both patients' subglottic hemangiomas responded dramatically to systemic Propranolol. No side effects of the therapy occurred, and a safety protocol previously designed for Propranolol prescribed for other indications was applied to their patients. They concluded that propranolol appears to be an effective treatment for subglottic hemangiomas and should now be used as a first-line treatment in subglottic hemangiomas when intervention is required.[37]

Mediastinal Hemangioma

Propranolol for the treatment of a life-threatening subglottic and mediastinal infantile hemangioma by Truong *et al.*[38]

Trunk Hemangioma

Mousa *et al.* discuss a premature female infant, born at 28 weeks of gestation, who presented with a large hemangioma of the right thoracic wall. Within the first few weeks, the hemangioma showed rapid horizontal and vertical growth as well as ulceration, which led them to initiate systemic therapy. They began oral propranolol treatment, in close interdisciplinary cooperation. After a few days of therapy, the tumor had stopped expanding. After 18 weeks, there has been marked regression but the therapy is still being continued. They propose that propranolol may be an effective and relatively well tolerable alternative in the management of selected cases of severe hemangiomas in infancy, providing interdisciplinary cooperation between dermatologists and pediatricians is available.[38]

Limb Hemangioma

Michel *et al.* report the case of an 8-month-old girl with a voluminous ulcerated hemangioma of the left forearm with a large, painful, central ulceration. Conventional treatment with topical and/or systemic antibiotics was unsuccessful. Flashlamp-pumped pulsed-dye laser (FPDL) could not be used because of the thickness of the lesions. They decided to use beta-blocker therapy (propanolol) for 4 months with a noteworthy efficacy.[39]

Letters to the Editor or Reviews (in reverse chronology)

Propranolol may become first-line treatment in obstructive subglottic infantile hemangiomas by Denoyelle *et al.*[40]

Propranolol therapy to treat problematic hemangiomas: a new standard therapy makes its debut by Loffler *et al.*[41]

Propranolol treatment for infantile hemangiomas by Buckmiller *et al.* A Review.[42]

In 'Pharmacologic therapy for periocular infantile hemangiomas: a review of the literature' Nguyen *et al.* review the rapidly evolving field of pharmacologic treatment of infantile hemangiomas. Various modalities, including local and systemic pharmacologic agents (propranolol), lasers, surgery and embolization, are employed to halt growth and to induce regression and are discussed in the paper.[43]

A comment in NEJM 'More on propranolol for hemangiomas of infancy' by Siegfried *et al.*[44] states: The response of infantile hemangiomas to propranolol reported in the letter by Léauté-Labrèze *et al.* (June 12 issue) catapulted the use of this treatment to first-line status among physicians managing this disease. Not included in their letter was a discussion about initiating and monitoring propranolol use, or about potential risks, which may be unique among these patients. The most common serious adverse effects are bradycardia and hypotension. Infants with very large hemangiomas or miliary hemangiomatosis are at risk for high-output cardiac compromise. Propranolol may mask the clinical signs of early cardiac failure and diminish cardiac performance. Propranolol may also blunt the clinical features of hypoglycemia. Sustained hypoglycemia in infancy has been associated with long-term neurologic sequelae. We know of two infants who had unrecognized side effects from propranolol. We developed a treatment protocol to optimize safety: baseline echocardiography and 48-hour hospitalization or home nursing visits to monitor vital signs and blood glucose levels. Medication is given every 8 hours, with an initial dose of 0.16 mg per kilogram of body weight. If the vital signs and glucose levels remain normal, the dose is incrementally doubled to a maximum of 0.67 mg per kilogram (to a maximum daily dose of 2.0 mg per kilogram). Propranolol should be gradually tapered over a period of 2 weeks.

Efficacy of beta-blockers in infantile capillary haemangiomas: the physiopathological significance and therapeutic consequences by Léauté-Labrèze *et al.*[45]

Literature Against

Studies (in reverse chronology)

Nil

Case Reports (in reverse chronology)

Lawley *et al.* at Emory comment that dramatic improvement of complicated hemangioma of infancy to propranolol was recently reported, but details for initiating therapy, monitoring, and potential risks were not included. They present two infants treated with propranolol, who suffered complications and propose a treatment protocol to minimize potential adverse events.[46]

Letters to the Editor or Reviews (in reverse chronology)

Nil

Literature (Unknown if For or Against no Abstract Available)

Propranolol as first-line treatment for infantile hemangiomas by Holmes *et al.*[47]

Propranolol for infantile hemangiomas: promise, peril, pathogenesis by Frieden *et al.*[48]

Propranolol and hemangiomas by López Gutiérrez JC.[49]

Dose: (The following are doses used in different studies. Note: no treatment protocols have been established as of yet.)

—1–1.5 mg/kg/day for 2–5 months.[27]
—2 mg/kg/day for > 6 weeks.[36]
—2–3 mg/kg/day for 5–10 months.[24]
—Before starting needs baseline echocardiogram. Start at 0.1 mg/kg every 8 hrs then gradually increase to 0.67 mg/kg to a max of 2 mg/kg/day. Hospitalization or close home nurse monitoring for first 48 hours. To stop, needs to be tapered over 2 weeks.[44]

Advantage

— Response within days if hemangioma is sensitive, 50% reduction in size in 1 week is achievable.[50]
— Does not need to be pretreated with steroids.[24]

Disadvantages

— Novel use; no treatment protocols established.[51]
— May result in significant masked hypoglycemia.[52,53]
— Undetected hypoglycemia can result in permanent neurologic sequelae.[54]
— May result in masked early symptoms and signs of cardiac failure.[44]
— Potential for bronchospasm.
— Hypotension/Bradycardia/Syncope.[55]
— Risk of overdose.[56]
— Somnolence.[29]
— Gastro-esophageal reflux.[29]
— Respiratory syncytial virus infection.[29]
— Rash.[29]
— Risk of seizures.[56]
— Risk of prolonged QRS complex.[56]

Interferon-alpha

Recombinant interferon (IFN) alpha-2a or alpha-2b is a second line agent reserved for life threatening lesions.[57,58]

Indications for use are: failure to respond to steroids, contraindication to steroids, complications of steroids, or parental refusal of steroids.[3]

Steroids and interferon should not be co-administered; the steroids should be quickly tapered prior to commencing interferon.

Dose

2–3 mU/m2 administered subcutaneously daily. It is important to titrate the dose as the infant gains weight or else rebound growth may occur.

The rate or response is 80% however 6–10 months of therapy are required.[8]

Advantages

— Response rate of 80% with full course of treatment (accelerated involution or stabilization of growth.
— Infants grow and gain weight in a normal fashion
— Effective treatment for Kasabach-Merritt phenomenon

Disadvantages

— Requires 6–10 months of continuous therapy for effect
— Fever with first 1–2 weeks of administration (pretreat with acetaminophen 1–2 hrs prior to each treatment)
— Causes transient neutropenia (due to margination and not bone marrow suppression), anemia and liver transaminase disarray (5x baseline).
— Most worrisome is spastic diplegia which slowly resolves on halting the medication.
— Require periodic neurologic and functional assessment.[3]

Vincristine

Reserved for life threatening lesions as a second line agent.[7, 57]
Same indications of use as interferon.

Advantages

— Effective treatment for hemangioendotheliomas (esp Kaposiform)
— Response rate is >80%

Disadvantages

— Must be administered through a central line (infection risk, pneumothorax, etc)
— Peripheral neuropathy, constipation, minor hair loss, sepsis

Bleomycin

Bleomycin A5 is an antineoplastic antibiotic drug with a strong antiangiogenic activity.[59]

It works by inhibiting endothelial cell migration and decreasing endothelial cell growth resulting in apoptosis.[60]

Direct intralesional injection of bleomycin A5 can specifically induce a sclerosing effect on vascular endothelium.[61]

Hemangiomas pretreated with angiographic microembolization with subsequent bleomycin A5 administration has been shown to improved outcomes.[62]

Dose

0.3–0.6 mg/kg per dose. 3–8 doses administered over 12–18 months.[63]

Advantages

— 50–90% response rate.[63]

Disadvantages

— Hyperpigmentation[63]
— Flu-like symptoms[61]
— Superficial ulceration[61]
— Cellulitis[61]
— Transient hair loss[61]
— Pulmonary fibrosis/hypertension[61]

Lasers

Various lasers have been specifically designed based on the theory of selective photothermolysis of vessels to treat cutaneous vascular lesions.

The general consensus is that the 585-nm or 595-nm Pulse Dye Laser (PDL) is particularly useful for superficial hemangiomas because of its selective penetration depth based on wavelength,[64] whereas the neodymium-doped yttrium aluminium garnet (Nd:YAG) laser (1064 nm) is more useful for hemangiomas with subcutaneous components.[65,66]

Advantage

— May improve skin discoloration
— Excellent for treatment of residual telangectasias of the involuted stage.
— May help with very superficial dermal hemangiomas.[3]

Disadvantage

— PDL penetration is only 0.75 — 1.2 mm.
— Lightens involved skin, but no evidence that it causes involution of hemangioma.
— If overused can result in ulceration, hypopigmentation, second degree skin loss and scarring.[3]

Selective Microembolization

Selective embolization rarely is used in the treatment of hemangiomas but may be required in cases of intractable bleeding, severe heart failure, large and poorly involuting hemangiomas, and as preparation for surgery.[67]

Endovascular microembolization is performed using polyvinyl alcohol (PVA-500). This is often performed to downsize the hemangioma for surgery.[68]

Embolization can also be performed prior to bleomycin A administration.[69]

Embolization should be performed only after a thorough angiographic evaluation of the pattern of the blood flow in the tumour and adjacent vessels is performed.[68]

Advantage

— Assist in downsizing the hemangioma in preparation for surgery.
— Emergently stem uncontrolled bleeding.
— May improve bleomycin treatment.[62]

Disadvantage

— Not all areas can be microembolized.

— Risk of ischemic/infracted tissues/organs.
— Difficult procedure in the younger infants.
— Requires specialized interventional radiology center.[69]

Surgery

Excess skin post involution can be handled via circular excision and pursestring closure which causes the smallest scar.[70]

Proliferating Phase

Indications for resection of a well-localized tumor in the first year are: Obstruction, deformation (i.e. periorbital tumor causing amblyopia), bleeding, ulceration unresponsive to medical treatment, inevitable scar/hair loss.[3]

Involuting Phase

Indications for removal prior to entering school are:

Resection is inevitable, for example, postulcerative scarring, unalterably expanded skin, or high probability of fibrofatty residuum; same scar length/appearance if excision were postponed; scar easily hidden in relaxed cutaneous tension lines or a border of a facial esthetic unit, necessity for staged resection or reconstruction.[3]

Involuted Phase

Resection of an involuted hemangioma is usually undertaken for:

Damaged skin, abnormal contour (fibrofatty residuum), distortion or destruction of an anatomic structure; or because staged removal or reconstruction is necessary.[3]

References

1. Zimmermann AP, Wiegand S, Werner JA, Eivazi B. (2010) Propranolol therapy for infantile hemangiomas: Review of the literature. *Int J Pediatr Otorhinolaryngol* **74**(4): 338–342.
2. Phung TL, Hochman M, Mihm MC. (2005) Current knowledge of the pathogenesis of infantile hemangiomas. *Arch Facial Plast Surg* **7**(5): 319–321.

3. Mulliken J. (2007) Vascular anomalies: infantile hemangioma. In: Thorne CH (ed.), *Grabb and Smith's Plastic Surgery*, 6th Edn. Lippincott Williams & Wilkins, pp. 191–194.
4. North PE, *et al.* (2001) A unique microvascular phenotype shared by juvenile hemangiomas and human placenta. *Arch Dermatol* **137**: 559–570.
5. Boye E, *et al.* (2001) Clonality and altered behaviour of endothelial cells from hemangiomas. *J Clin Invest* **107**: 745–752.
6. Ritter MR, Butschek RA, Friedlander M, Friedlander SF. (2007) Pathogenesis of infantile hemangioma: new molecular and cellular insights. *Exp Rev Mol Med* **9**: 1–19.
7. Frieden IJ, *et al.* (2005) Infantile hemangiomas: current knowledge, future directions. Proceedings of a research workshop on infantile hemangiomas, April 7–9, 2005, Bethesda, Maryland, USA. *Pediatr Dermatol* **22**(5): 383–406.
8. Mulliken JB, Fishman SJ, Burrows PE. (2000) Vascular anomalies. *Curr Prob Surg* **37**: 517.
9. Marler J, Mulliken JB. (2005) Current management of hemangiomas and vascular malformations. *Clin Plast Surg* **32**(1): 99–116.
10. Mulliken JB, Glowacki J. (1982) Classification of pediatric vascular lesions. *Plast Reconstr Surg* **70**(1): 120–121.
11. Salazard B, *et al.* (2006) The lymphatic malformations: clinical aspects and evolution. *Ann Chir Plast Esthet* **4–5**: 412–422.
12. Rasheed R, Durr-e-Sabih RM, Uddin N. (2009) Klippel-Trenaunay syndrome. *J Coll Physicians Surg Pak* **19**(11): 729–731.
13. Redondo P, *et al.* (2009) Foot or hand malformations related to deep venous system anomalies of the lower limb in Klippel-Trenaunay syndrome. *J Am Acad Dermatol* **4**: 621–628.
14. Gloviczki P, Driscoll D. (2007) Klippel-Trenauney Syndrome: current management. *Phlebology* **22**(6): 291–298.
15. Mulliken J, Enjolras O. (2004) Congenital hemangiomas and infantile hemangioma: missing links. *J Am Acad Dermatol* **50**(6): 875–882.
16. Berenguer B, *et al.* (2003) Rapidly involuting congenital hemangioma: clinical and histopathologic features. *Pediatr Dev Pathol* **6**(6): 495–510.
17. Enjolras O, *et al.* (2001) Non-involuting congenital hemangioma: a rare cutaneous vascular anomaly. *Plast Reconstr Surg* **107**(7): 1647–1654.
18. Metry DW, *et al.* (2006) A prospective study of PHACE syndrome in infantile hemangiomas: demographic features, clinical findings, and complications. *Am J Med Genet A* **140**(9): 975–986.
19. Chang LC, *et al.* (2008) Growth characteristics of infantile hemangiomas: implications for management. *Pediatrics* **122**(2): 360–367.

20. Pandey A, Gangopadhyay AN, Upadhyay VD. (2008) Evaluation and management of infantile hemangioma: an overview. *Ostomy Wound Manage* **54**: 22–6–28–9.
21. Yuan KH, *et al.* (2009) Successful combination therapy for severe infantile hemangiomas: case report and literature search. *Photomed Laser Surg* **27**(6): 973–977.
22. Bennett M, *et al.* (2001) Oral corticosteroid use is effective for cutaneous hemangiomas: an evidence-based evaluation. *Arch Dermatol* **137**: 1208–1213.
23. Boon L, MacDonald D, Mulliken JB. (1999) Complications of systemic corticosteroid therapy for problematic hemangioma. *Plast Reconstr Surg* **104**(6): 1616–1623.
24. Leaute-Labreze C, *et al.* (2008) Propranolol for severe hemangiomas of infancy. *N Engl J Med* **358**: 2649–2651.
25. Sommers SK, Smith DM. (2002) Beta blockade induces apoptosis in cultured capillary endothelial cells. *In Vitro Cell Dev Biol Anim* **38**: 298–304.
26. D'Angelo G, Lee H, Weiner R. (1997) cAMP-dependent protein kinase inhibits the mitogenic action of vascular endothelial growth factor and fibroblast growth factor in capillary endothelial cells by blockin Raf activation. *J Cell Biochem* **67**: 353–366.
27. Qin Z, *et al.* (2009) Treatment of infantile hemangiomas with low-dose propranolol: evaluation of short-term efficacy and safety. *Zhonghua Zheng Xing Wai Ke Za Zhi* **89**(44): 3130–3134.
28. Maturo S, Hartnick C. (2010) Initial experience using propranolol as the sole treatment for infantile airway hemangiomas. *Int J Pediatr Otorhinolaryngol* **74**(3): 323–325.
29. Buckmiller LM, *et al.* (2010) Propranolol for infantile hemangiomas: Early experience at a tertiary vascular anomalies center. *Laryngoscope* **120**: 677–681.
30. Marsciani A, *et al.* (2010) Massive response of severe infantile hepatic hemangioma to propranolol. *Pediatr Blood Cancer* **54**(1): 176.
31. Theletsane T, *et al.* (2009) Life-threatening infantile hemangioma: a dramatic response to propranolol. *J Eur Acad Dermatol Venereol* **23**(12): 1465–1466.
32. Fay A, *et al.* (2010) Propranolol for isolated orbital infantile hemangioma. *Arch Ophthalmol* **128**(2): 256–258.
33. Taban M, Goldberg R. (2010) Propranolol for orbital hemangioma. *Ophthalmology* **117**(1): 195–195e4.
34. Truong MT, *et al.* (2010) Propranolol for the treatment of a life-threatening subglottic and mediastinal infantile hemangioma. *J Pediatr* **156**(2): 335–338.

35. Jephson C, *et al.* (2009) Successful treatment of isolated subglottic haemangioma with propranolol alone. *Int J Pediatr Otorhinolaryngol* **73**(12): 1821–1823.
36. Buckmiller L, Dyamenahalli U, Richter GT. (2009) Propranolol for airway hemangiomas: case report of novel treatment. *Laryngoscope* **119**(10): 2051–2054.
37. Denoyelle F, *et al.* (2009) Role of propranolol in the therapeutic strategy of infantile laryngotracheal hemangioma. *Int J Pediatr Otorhinolaryngol* **73**(8): 1168–1172.
38. Mousa W, *et al.* (2010) Successful treatment of a large hemangioma with propranolol. *J Dtsch Dermatol Ges.* **8**(3): 184–186.
39. Michel J, Patural H. (2009) Response to oral propranolol therapy for ulcerated hemangiomas in infancy. *Arch Pediatr* **16**(12): 1565–1568.
40. Denoyelle F, Garabedian EN. (2010) Propranolol may become first-line treatment in obstructive subglottic infantile hemangiomas. *Otolaryngol Head Neck Surg* **142**(3): 463–464.
41. Loffler H, *et al.* (2009) Propranolol therapy to treat problematic hemangiomas: a new standard therapy makes its debut. *Hautarzt* **60**(12): 1013–1016.
42. Buckmiller LM. (2009) Propranolol treatment for infantile hemangiomas. *Curr Opin Otolaryngol Head Neck Surg* **17**(6): 458–459.
43. Nguyen J, Fay A. (2009) Pharmacologic therapy for periocular infantile hemangiomas: a review of the literature. *Semin Ophthalmol* **24**(3): 178–184.
44. Siegfried E, *et al.* (2008) More on propranolol for hemangiomas of infancy. *N Engl J Med* **359**: 2846–2847.
45. Leaute-Labreze C, Taieb A. (2008) Efficacy of beta-blockers in infantile capillary hemangiomas: the physiopathological significance and therapeutic consequences. *Ann Dermatol Venereol* **135**(12): 860–862.
46. Lawley LP, Siegfried E, Todd JL. (2009) Propranolol treatment for hemangioma of infancy: risks and recommendations. *Pediatr Dermatol* **26**(5): 610–614.
47. Holmes WJ, *et al.* (2010) Propranolol as first-line treatment for infantile hemangiomas. *Plast Reconstr Surg* **125**(1): 420–421.
48. Frieden IJ, Drolet BA. (2009) Propranolol for infantile hemangiomas: promise, peril, pathogenesis. *Pediatr Dermatol* **26**(5): 642–644.
49. Lopez-Gutierrez J. (2009) Propranolol and haemangiomas. *An Pediatr (Barc)* **71**(5): 461.
50. Truoung M, *et al.* (2010) Propranolol for the treatment of a life-threatening subglottic and mediastinal infantile hemangioma. *J Pediatr* **156**(2): 335–338.

51. Lawley L, Siegfried E, Todd J. (2009) Propranolol treatment for hemangioma of infancy: risks and recommendations. *Pediatr Dermatol* **26**(5): 610–614.
52. Love J, Sikka N. (2004) Are 1–2 tablets dangerous? Beta-blocker exposure in toddlers. *J Emerg Med* **26**(3): 309–314.
53. Seltzer H. (1989) Drug-induced hypoglycemia: a review of 1418 cases. *Endocrinol Metab Clin North Am* **18**(1): 163–183.
54. Burns C, *et al.* (2008) Patterns of cerebral injury and neuro developmental outcomes after symptomatic neonatal hypoglycemia. *Pediatrics* **122**: 65–74.
55. Clark D, Chan K, Gibbs J. (1989) Propranolol induced bradycardia in tetralogy of Fallot. *Br Heart J* **61**(4): 378–379.
56. Reith D, *et al.* (1996) Relative toxicity of beta blockers in overdose. *J Toxicol Clin Toxicol* **34**(3): 273–278.
57. Chan Y, Giam YC. (2005) Guidelines of care for cutaneous hemangiomas. *Ann Acad Med Singapore* **34**: 117–123.
58. Ezekowitz RA, *et al.* (1992) Interferon alpha-2a therapy for life-threatening hemangiomas of infancy. *N Engl J Med* **326**: 1456–1463.
59. Oikawa T, Hirotani K, Ogasawara H, *et al.* (1990) Inhibition of angiogenesis by bleomycin and its copper complex. *Chem Pharm Bull* **38**: 1790–1792.
60. Mabeta P, Pepper M. (2009) A comparative study on the anti-angiogenic effects of DNA-damaging and cytoskeletal-disrupting agents. *Angiogenesis* **12**(1): 81–90.
61. Muir T, Kirsten M, Fourie P, Dippenaar N, Ionescu GO. (2004) Intralesional bleomycin injection (IBI) treatment for hemangiomas and congenital vascular malformations. *Pediatr Surg Int* **19**: 766–773.
62. Liu X, Qin Z, Tai M. (2009) Angiographic classification and sclerotic therapy of maxillofacial cavernous hemangiomas: A report of 204 cases. *J Int Med Res* **37**(5): 1285–1292.
63. Pienaar C, *et al.* (2006) Intralesional bleomycin for the treatment of hemangiomas. *Plast Reconstr Surg* **117**(1): 221–226.
64. Ashinoff R, Geronemus RG. (1993) Failure of the flashlamp-pumped pulsed dye laser to prevent progression to deep hemangioma. *Pediatr Dermatol* **10**: 77–80.
65. Raulin C, Greve B. (2001) Retrospective clinical comparison of hemangioma treatment by flashlamp-pumped (585 nm) and frequency-doubled Nd:YAG (532 nm) lasers. *Lasers Surg Med* **28**: 40–43.
66. Batta K, *et al.* (2002) Randomised controlled study of early pulsed dye laser treatment of uncomplicated childhood hemangiomas: results of a 1 year analysis. *Lancet* **360**: 521–527.

67. Bava G, *et al.* (2002) Life-threatening hemorrhage from a vulvar hemangioma. *J Pediatr Surg* **37**(4): E6.
68. Korotkikh N, *et al.* (2007) Endovascular microembolization of the posterior auricular artery in comprehensive surgical management of capillary angioma of the floor of the auricle. *Angiol Sosud Khir* **13**(4): 74–76.
69. Li J, Hu X, Jiang X. (2005) Transcatheter arterial embolization in the treatment of extensive maxillofacial hemangioma in children. *World J Surg* **29**(12): 1550–1556.
70. Mulliken JB, Rogers G, Marler J. (2002) Circular excision of hemangioma and purse string closure-the smallest possible scar. *Plast Reconstr Surg* **109**: 1544–1554.

CHAPTER 7

BURN INJURY AND TREATMENT

Jessica A. Ching and C. Wayne Cruse

I. Illustrative Case

A 32 year old male presents to your service in the emergency department after sustaining flame burns in a house fire to his arms and anterior trunk. After initial assessment, consider how you would calculate his resuscitation and what you parameters would guide your resuscitation (Figs. 1 and 2).

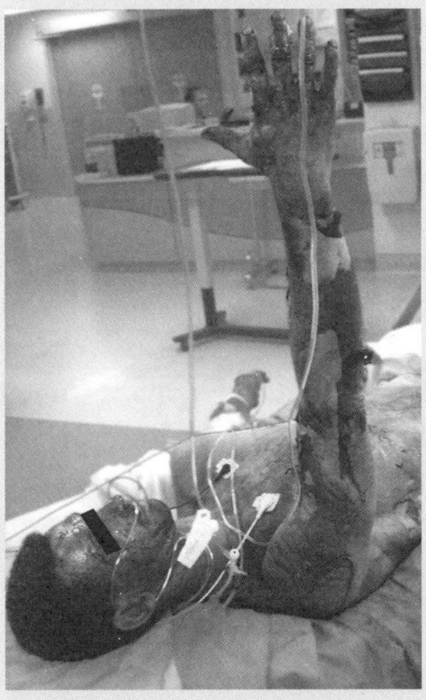

Fig. 1. Illustrative case face and upper extremity burns.

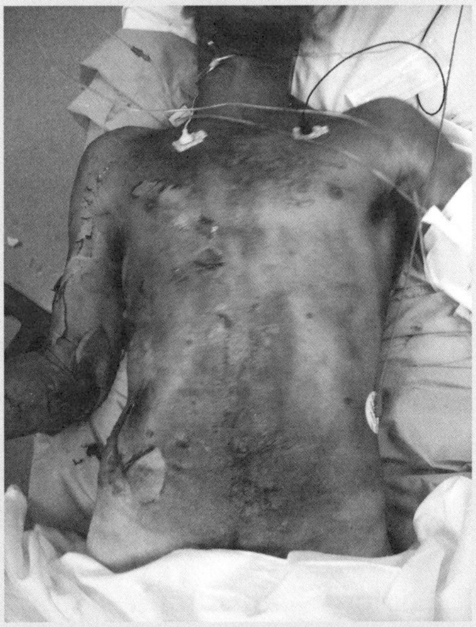

Fig. 2. Illustrative case anterior trunk burns.

II. Introduction

A. Historical Landmarks

1. Fluid resuscitation was pioneered by Frank P. Underhill, Professor of Pharmacology and Toxicology at Yale. After studying 20 people burned at Rialto Theater in 1921, he concluded loss of fluid was primarily responsible for burn mortality.[1] Prior to this, the common belief was that toxins were responsible for post burn death.
2. Lund and Browder developed diagrams to estimate burned body surface area in 1944,[2] followed by the 'rule of nines' by Knaysi *et al*;[3] both allowed for fluid resuscitation strategies based on these calculations. It was not until 1968 that the commonly referred to Parkland formula for post burn fluid resuscitation, based on burned body surface calculations, was published by Baxter and Shires.[4]
3. Infection has been a significant contributor to burn mortality, and 60–80% of patients with greater than 50% burn died of bacterial sepsis in the 1960s and 1970s.[5] More recently, the total body surface area burn estimated at 50% survival is a burn of 70% TBSA, from all causes of death not just infection.[6] Surgical techniques such as early excision and grafting along with topical treatments, such as silver nitrate, mafenide acetate, and sulfadiazine, have played key roles in decreasing burn mortality.
4. Early excision was first presented in 1954,[7] but Janzekovic in the 1960s revolutionized the burn field with tangential excision, which is now a standard of care.[8]
5. Pinch grafts were first used in the United States to cover burn wounds in the early 1900s,[9] followed by split-thickness skin grafts in the 1930s.[5] Padgett developed the adjustable dermatome in the 1940s,[10] and the meshed skin graft was introduced in 1964,[11] adding to the coverage and healing of the burn wound.

III. Etiology and Criteria

A. Etiology[6]

1. Overall in the United States: flame/flash > scald > thermal contact > electrical > chemical.

B. Criteria for transfer to a Burn Center by the American Burn Association:[12]

1. Partial-thickness and full-thickness burns greater than 10% of the total body surface area (BSA) in patients under 10 years or over 50 years of age.
2. Partial-thickness and full-thickness burns greater than 20% BSA in other age groups.
3. Partial-thickness and full-thickness burns involving the face, eyes, ears, hands, feet, genitalia, or perineum or those that involve skin overlying major joints.
4. Full-thickness burns greater than 5% BSA in any age group.
5. Electrical burns, including lightning injury.
6. Significant chemical burns.
7. Inhalation injury.
8. Burn injury in patients with pre-existing illness that could complicate management, prolong recovery, or affect mortality.
9. Any burn patient in whom concomitant trauma poses an increased risk or morbidity or mortality may be treated initially in a trauma center until stable before transfer to a burn center.
10. Children with burns seen in hospitals without qualified personnel or equipment for their care should be transferred to a burn center with these capabilities.
11. Burn injury in patients who will require special social and emotional or long-term rehabilitative support, including cases involving suspected child abuse and neglect.

C. **Intensive Care Unit Admission Indications**

1. Adults with >15–20% total body surface area (TBSA) burn injury.
2. Infants or elders.
3. Suspected inhalation injury:
   — Formal diagnosis of inhalation injury requires fiberoptic bronchoscopy.
4. Regular neurovascular checks are required, or if there is concern for developing compartment syndrome.
5. Electrical injury.

IV. Injury Assessment

A. Initial Evaluation[5,13]

1. Burn patients are trauma patients.
2. Evaluate according to Advanced Trauma Life Support (ATLS) protocol.
3. Most critical issue to address: Airway.
   a. If there are signs or symptoms of inhalation injury or circumstances surrounding the burn that raise suspicion of inhalation injury, monitor the airway closely. If there are signs of impending compromise secure an airway.
      i. Signs of inhalation injury: dyspnea, carbonaceous sputum, singed facial hair, hoarseness, dysphagia, cough, nasopharyngeal blistering.
      ii. Circumstances suggestive of inhalation injury: closed-space fire, prolonged exposure to smoke.
   b. If there is suspected exposure to cyanide or carbon monoxide, place the patient on 100% oxygen. Carbon monoxide binds to hemoglobin and impairs oxygen delivery to tissues. Inhalation injury will produce an elevated carboxyhemoglobin level (which can also be elevated in smokers). The half-life of carbon monoxide is 40 minutes on 100% oxygen. There is no indication to treat with steroids or prophylactic antibiotics for inhalation injury. Inhalation injury increases the risk of developing pneumonia and/or respiratory failure.
4. Assess for other life-threatening injuries and address appropriately.
5. Obtain a detailed history and physical, including the exact mechanism of burn injury and any past medical history.
6. If transferring a patient, prior to transport: secure an airway (err on side of intubation), IV access, Foley catheter placement, assess burn size and depth, and initiate fluid resuscitation.

B. Burn Assessment[5,13]

1. Acutely: ATLS and BLS protocols should be followed.

2. Depth.
   a. First degree (superficial thickness): only epidermis.
      i. Appears pink, no blistering, painful to touch.
      ii. Treatment: oral analgesics, topical aloe.
      iii. Ex. Sunburn.
   b. Partial thickness (second degree): involves the epidermis and a portion of the dermis, may have a superficial or deep partial thickness burn depending on depth of dermis involved.
      i. Superficial partial thickness (Fig. 3): involves epidermis to superficial portion of dermis.
      (a) Appears pink, blistering present, painful to touch, moist.
      (b) Heals in less than 3 weeks with local wound care, possible long-term pigmentation changes.
      (c) Ex: water scald.
      ii. Deep partial thickness (Fig. 4): involves epidermis to reticular dermis.

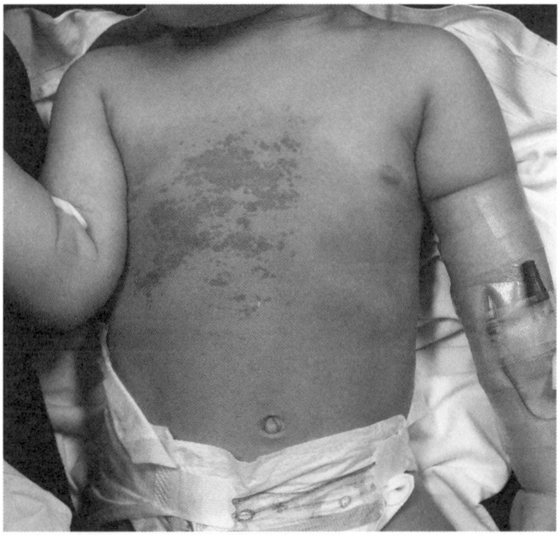

Fig. 3. Mixed superficial partial thickness and first degree burns to the anterior trunk of an infant after contact with scalding water.

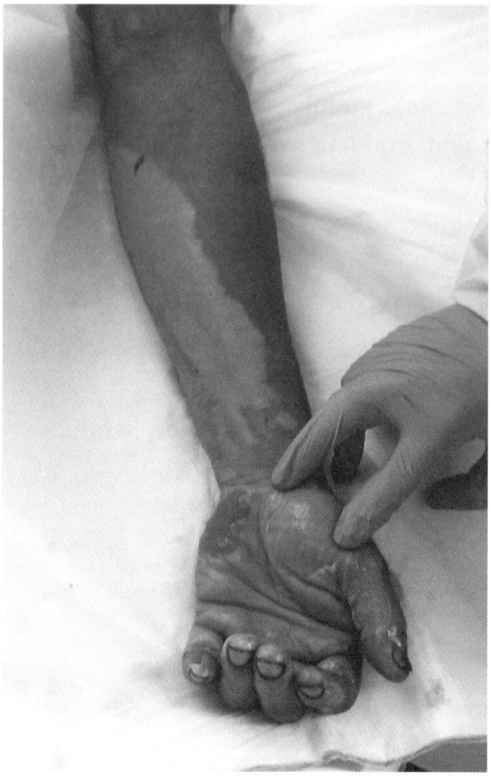

Fig. 4. Deep partial thickness upper extremity burn.

(a) Appears mottled pink to white with blistering, blunted pain sensation to touch, dry.
(b) Healing takes longer than 3 weeks without surgery and will result in significant scarring/contraction/contractures.
(c) **Goal is to obtain wound closure within 3 weeks, to improve aesthetic and functional outcomes.** Thus, surgical excision and grafting is recommended, if a burn wound will not likely heal within three weeks with wound care alone.

c. Full thickness (third degree) (Fig. 5): involves epidermis, dermis, and subcutaneous tissue.

i. Appears: brown-black, leathery, little or no sensation, non-blanching, possibly charred, thrombosed vessels may be visible under the eschar.

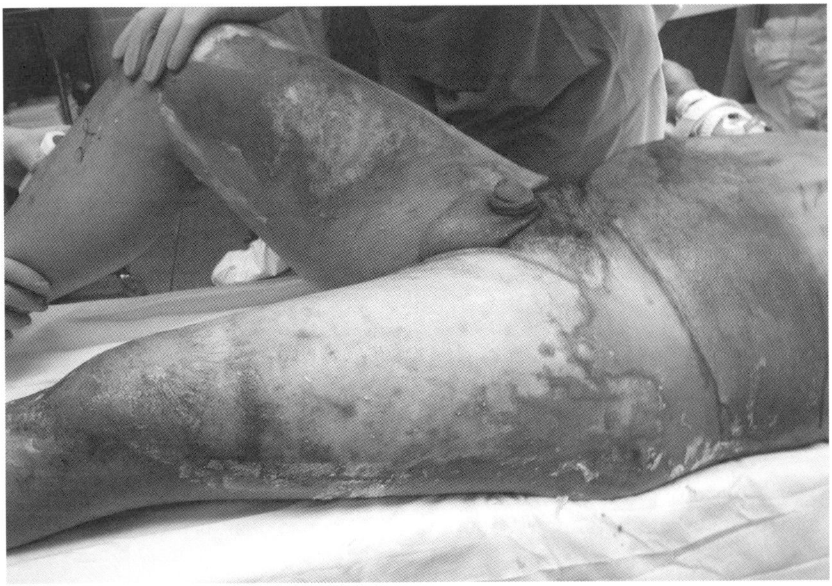

Fig. 5. Full thickness burn to anterior thighs (white and grey eschar) mixed with deep partial thickness burns (red and pink areas).

   ii. Treat with excision and grafting, unless extremely small (i.e. less than 2 cm diameter).

  d. Fourth degree (Fig. 6): involves epidermis, dermis, subcutaneous tissue and underlying structures (i.e. muscle, tendon, bone).
   i. Appears: similar to third degree but with exposed muscle or bone.
   ii. Treat with excision and grafting, like a third degree burn.

3. Estimation of total body surface area (TBSA):
  a. Surface area calculations differ between adults and children. Children have larger heads in comparison with their bodies, accounting for a larger proportion of surface area. Area of a patient's palm is about 1% TBSA, which can be used as an adjunct method of estimation.
  b. Rule of Nines: based on the following TBSA estimations.
   i. Head 9%, anterior trunk 18%, posterior trunk 18%, each upper extremity 9%, anterior lower extremity 9%, posterior lower extremity 9%, genitalia 1%.

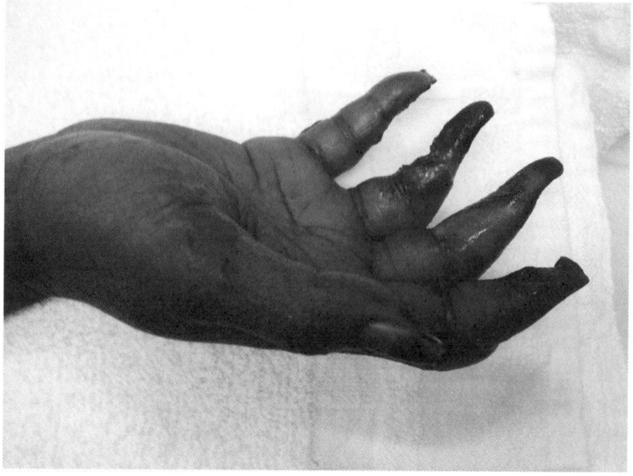

Fig. 6. Fourth degree burn to the hand showing dessication of distal digits, ultimately resulting in amputation. Patient had lost consciousness while hand was in contact with a stove burner.

   c. Lund and Browder charts: more accurate than Rule of Nines and age-based.

4. Evaluation for escharotomy.
   a. Escharotomies are generally indicated for circumferential full-thickness burns of the extremity or the chest wall if ventilation is compromised. With resuscitation, the tissue swelling and constriction effect of the circumferential burn will worsen.
   b. Often escharotomies can be performed at bedside. Release of tissues is sufficient when the eschar fully separates and the perfusion of tissue improves. This should only be through eschar, not the fascia or underlying unburned tissues.
5. Assessment in special circumstances.
   a. Tar burns
      i. The tar normally has cooled significantly prior to encountering skin, although the mother pot temperature is 400–500 degrees Fahrenheit. Burn may range from superficial to full-thickness. It is removed with petroleum-based solvents, such as mineral oil.

b. Grease scald burns

i. Grease burns tend to demarcate further over the subsequent 2–3 days. Thus, even a superficial burn on initial presentation may upon serial examination demarcate further as a full thickness burn several days after injury.

V. Acute Intervention

A. Pathophysiology[5,13]

1. After burn injury, there is a release of inflammatory mediators (histamine, prostaglandins, and cytokines) that ultimately results in increased vascular permeability, decreased cardiac output, and altered cell membrane potential. The changes are especially seen throughout the body when burn injury involves more than 15–20% TBSA; otherwise, vascular permeability tends to be localized to the area of burn injury with less effect on overall cardiac output. If inhalation injury is present, this augments the inflammatory response; subsequent vascular permeability, and decreased cardiac output as well. With these physiologic changes, there are increased fluid losses through the skin and into the interstitium (i.e. third-spacing of fluid). Resuscitation is aimed at replacing these fluid losses.

B. Resuscitation[5,13]

1. Calculated based on TBSA involved and weight in kilograms of the patient.
2. The most commonly used formula is the Parkland Formula. Intravenous fluid (IVF) should be lactated Ringer solution (LR).
3. Parkland formula: 4mL x wt x %TBSA burned = total IVF in the first 24 hours.
4. Modified Parkland formula: 3mL × wt × %TBSA burned = total IVF in the first 24 hours.
   a. Must subtract previously administered IVF from total fluid calculations, of remaining fluid: 50% within first 8 hrs, then 50% in following 16 hours. *Example*: Calculate resuscitation rate of IVF

using Parkland Formula for 70 kg male with 20% TBSA partial-thickness burns who received 1.5 L IVF en route to ER. His burn occurred 2 hours ago. 4 mL × 70 kg × 20%TBSA = 5600 mL IVF in 24 hours after injury. 2 hours have already elapsed since injury. Thus, 5600 mL – 1500 ml received en route = 4100 mL total. 4100 × 0.5 = 2050 mL in first 8 hours and 2050 mL in subsequent 16 hours after injury. 2050 mL/6 hrs since injury = 341.67 ≈ 342 mL/hr × 6 hours, then 2050 mL/16 hrs = 128.13 ≈ 128 mL/hr.

b. In children, add the maintenance fluid requirement to the calculated hourly rate of resuscitation fluids.

5. Titrate IVF rate according to urine output (UOP) of 30 cc/hr in adults, in children 1.0 cc/kg/hr.
6. **Urine output is the most accurate indicator of adequate resuscitation.**
   a. Foley catheter is needed to properly titrate fluid.
   b. Decrease IVF if UOP > 30–50 cc/hr in adults or 1.0 cc/kg/hr in children, in order to decrease risks associated with fluid overload (i.e. pulmonary edema, prolonged intubation, compartment syndrome).
   c. Inhalation injury will likely dictate higher fluid rates that calculated by resuscitation formulas, but again, titrate according to UOP.
   d. Use of pulmonary artery pressures, will lead to over resuscitation.
7. Within the first 24 hours of burn injury and high vascular permeability, colloid administered can leak to interstitial space, draw more fluid into the interstitial space with oncotic pressure, and contribute to overall interstitial fluid accumulation.
8. After the initial 24 hours of resuscitation, IVF should be continued based on the goal UOP of 30 cc/hr in adults and 1.0 cc/kg/hr in children.

C. Debridement

1. Initial non-excisional debridement should occur within 24 hours of injury.
2. Most would advocate excision and grafting to occur as soon as the patient is stabilized and the initial resuscitation has finished.

VI. Non-Surgical Management

A. Antibiotics and Wound Care[5,13]

1. Prophylactic antibiotics are not indicated.
2. Staphylococci and streptococci are the dominant colonizing bacteria in burn wounds. Topical antimicrobials are effective in decreasing colonization of wounds, such as: mafenide and silver sulfadiazine. Mafenide penetrates cartilage and burn eschar better than silver sulfadiazine. Mafenide is a carbonic anhydrase inhibitor, which can result in metabolic acidosis. The application of mafenide can also be painful, especially on partial thickness burns. Silver sulfadiazine is the most commonly used topical agent.
3. Other examples of topical wound care: silver nitrate, bacitracin, Dakin's solution, silver impregnated foam.
4. A dry gauze dressing is an acceptable covering over topical wound care antibacterial agents.

B. Nutrition[5,13]

1. Following burn injury, a patient becomes hypermetabolic and hypercatabolic. Hypermetabolism extends from the time of burn injury until the time of complete wound coverage. Feeding should be initiated immediately, and in most patients with more than 20% TBSA of burn injury, enteral feeds will be required. Ileus is common post burn, but it is minimized by starting feeds immediately upon admission. A dietician is a necessary member of a fully functional burn team.
2. Tight glycemic control is important in burn patients, whether with sliding scale insulin or an insulin drip.

C. Prophylaxis[5,13]

1. Gastric ulceration prophylaxis with histamine receptor blockers, sucralfate, and/or proton pump inhibitors is necessary to prevent stress ulcers (Curling's ulcers) in burn patients, especially if not taking an oral diet or if the patient has a history of peptic ulcer disease. Feeding the stomach soon after burn injury is also protective against gastric atony and ulcers.

2. Deep venous thrombosis is a significant risk in burn patients with prolonged bedrest, extremity injury, and indwelling venous catheters; anticoagulation with subcutaneous heparin is indicated. It is not practical in patients with extremity burns to apply sequential compression devices or antiembolism stockings in most cases. Any new onset extremity swelling after initial resuscitation should be evaluated with duplex ultrasound.

D. Infection[5,13]

1. After burn injury, the protective barrier afforded by skin is compromised, and the respiratory mucosal barrier may be injured. Cellular and humoral responses are diminished as well. All these factors contribute to an immunocompromised patient.
2. Early excision and grafting may decrease mortality from burn wound sepsis.
3. Inflammatory cytokines following burn injury commonly result in fevers and leukocytosis. Thus, in the first 72 hours of burn injury, fevers or leukocytosis do not warrant cultures to search for infection. However, after 72 hours, fevers, leukocytosis, glycemic control issues, feeding intolerance, mental status changes, and hypotension raise suspicion for infection, and urine, sputum, blood, and central lines require cultures. Antibiotics should be judiciously tailored to culture results to avoid resistant organisms among this immunocompromised population.
4. Persistent signs of infection require further investigation in the face of negative routine cultures.

E. Pain Management

1. During the hospital stay, normally non-steroidal anti-inflammatory medications are avoided due to the risk of bleeding with surgical procedures (i.e. excision and grafting). Narcotics are commonly used for pain control. With prolonged hospital stay, methadone may be considered.

VII. Surgical Management

A. Surgical Intervention[5,13,14]

1. Early excision and grafting is the standard of care for deep burns. It has resulted in decreased infection of burn wounds, decreased hospital

length of stay, and may decrease mortality. Excision should commence once the patient is stabilized after the initial resuscitation, and most would agree this occurs on approximately hospital day 3. However, some surgeons recommend complete excision within the first 24 hours.

2. The goal of treatment is to have all burn wounds closed within 3 weeks, in order to maximize both the functional and aesthetic outcomes. Excision and grafting facilitates this goal in burn wounds that are deep partial thickness to full thickness; such wounds would otherwise heal in greater than 3 weeks without excision and grafting.
3. Tangential excision is the method of choice for burn excision, which removes tissue layer by layer tangential to the wound bed until viable tissue is encountered. A Watson or Goulian knife is typically used. Pinpoint capillary bleeding is considered the marker of adequate excision and a wound bed that can support a skin graft. Hydrosurgical debridement may also be used for excision, especially over delicate areas like the fingers, hands, or face, or in concave regions like the axilla.
4. The operating room must be maintained with sufficient heat to aid the patient in maintaining body temperature. Significant energy expenditure by the patient to maintain body temperature in the operating room contributes to hypermetabolism, which uses energy stores needed for wound healing and immune function.
5. Of paramount importance is adequate hemostasis. Epinephrine solution soaked gauze, topical thrombin, and direct cauterization aid in this effort, along with topical pressure, elevation, and extremity wrapping. Fibrin sealant may also be used for hemostasis of the wound bed or aid during graft application, and it is to be placed on the wound bed shortly before graft placement.

B. Skin Grafting[5,13]

1. Fibrin secretion from recipient bed helps secure graft in place for up to 72 hours, but the graft is still vulnerable to sheering forces during this time.
2. Skin graft survival.
   a. Plasma imbibition: diffusion of nutrients from recipient bed to the skin graft, occurs from approximately days 1–3.
   b. Inosculation: the aligning of vessels in the recipient bed and the skin graft, occurs from approximately days 2–5.

c. Revascularization: re-establishment of blood flow through vessels to skin graft from recipient bed, occurs from approximately days 3–7.

3. Contraction.

   a. Primary contraction: occurs immediately after the skin graft is harvested, and increases with the thickness of the skin graft.
   b. Secondary contraction: occurs with the healing of the skin graft over weeks to months, and decreases with the thickness of the skin graft.

4. Thickness.

   a. Split thickness: (also called partial thickness), includes varying degrees of dermis but not the full dermis, from 0.008 to 0.016-inches in thickness, 0.012-inch thickness being about average. The thinner the graft, the more secondary contraction that occurs.
   b. Full thickness: includes the entire dermis. More primary contracture than partial thickness graft, but less secondary contracture than partial thickness graft.

5. Sheet and meshed grafts.

   a. Sheet graft: It is an unmeshed graft. Scarring occurs at the graft borders only. Less secondary contracture than meshed grafts, however more seroma or hematoma formation than meshed grafts.
   b. Meshed graft: It can be meshed 1:1, 2:1, 4:1, or 6:1. The more meshed holes the more scarring and contracture. Scarring occurs at the graft borders and at each meshed hole. Holes allow for fluid drainage, which may help with seroma or hematoma formation for as long as the holes remain open. Meshing grafts allows the surface area covered by a single graft to be increased because the graft can be stretched. It may also allow for easier contouring of a convex or concave area, but at the expense of increased contracture compared to sheet grafts.

6. Application.

   a. May be sutured, stapled, or glued in position. Bolsters may be sutured and tied down to aid in stabilization of grafts.

7. Dressings.

   a. Graft should be kept moist and protected from sheering forces. Greasy gauze are common for direct covering of the graft because they help with maintaining a moist environment and keep additional dressing from sticking to the graft, which could pull the graft off when the dressing is changed. Negative pressure therapy is another method for maintaining a small to moderate size skin graft in a specific position and evacuating potential seroma fluid; however, this should be left on for a full five days, if possible, to avoid prematurely disturbing the graft upon its removal. Splinting is necessary for minimizing motion of extremities, especially with skin grafts applied near joints.

b. Once the grafts show signs of healing and adequate attachment to the recipient bed (approximately 5–10 days), then treatment may be converted to moisturizing lotions and creams for long-term graft maintenance.

8. Donor sites.

a. Selection is based on availability, color match, and texture match with recipient area. If possible, a discrete location should be considered, such as the buttocks or upper thighs. Also the scalp, a less commonly considered site, is an excellent color and texture match for the face, neck, and upper clavicular areas.

b. The donor site dressing should keep the site moist, prevent infection, and decrease pain. Donor sites are often more painful than the recipient bed site. Options include silver sulfadiazine, Tegaderm (3M, Center St. Paul, MN 55144–1000), greasy gauze, Mepilex (Mölnlycke Health Care US, LLC, Norcross, GA 30092), and many others. Moisturizer is needed once initial epithelialization of the wound is complete.

C. Skin Graft Alternatives[5,13]

1. Porcine xenograft skin.

a. This is porcine derived dermis and epidermis or dermis alone.

b. Xenograft skin is most commonly applied to superficial partial thickness wounds (or donor sites).

i. It is placed on a thoroughly debrided wound either in the operating room or at bedside, and then secured in place with a dry dressing for 24 hours. After 24 hours, the dressing may be removed and the xenograft is allowed to dry completely. A heating lamp may be used to expedite the drying process; however, this may also distort the xenograft and result in rippling and loss of contour in some areas.

c. Vascular in growth will not occur with porcine xenograft.
d. It allows the wound to heal beneath it, while providing pain control.

2. Allograft.
   a. This is human cadaveric skin, including dermis and epidermis.
   b. Most often allograft is stored frozen and thawed just prior to use. It is available refrigerated as well.
   c. It is useful as coverage for a superficial partial thickness wound or over meshed skin grafts.
      i. When used to cover mesh skin grafts, allograft aids in decreasing insensible fluid losses and creates a moist wound environment to promote healing.
   d. In an immunocompromised patient, the allograft may be incorporated until a sufficient immune response is possible for rejection. In most patients, rejection occurs after 3–4 weeks, at which time the allograft becomes non-adherent to the wound bed.
3. Cultured Epidermal Autografts (CEAs).
   i. These are grown from a sample of the patients own epidermis and require 2–3 weeks to be available for application. They require no significant donor site. Therefore, CEAs are especially useful with burns of larger surface area.
   ii. CEAs are extremely sensitive to sheering forces even after areas are well-healed due to the lack of dermis. For this reason, they are often applied over a dermal substitute, such as a wound matrix.
4. Dermal substitutes.
   a. Integra (Integra Life Sciences Corporation, Plainsboro, NJ, USA).
      i. Inner layer of bovine collagen and glycoxaminoglycan chondroitin-6-sulfate, which is 2 mm thick. Pores of 70–200 μm allows for fibrovascular in growth.
      ii. Outer layer is composed of 0.23 mm thick polysiloxame polymer, and it transmits vapor similarly to epithelium.

iii. It is placed on a freshly excised burn wound and secured for 2–3 weeks to allow vascularization. After 2–3 weeks, the outer silicone layer is removed and a very thin split-thickness skin graft is applied. The skin graft is maintained in a secured position for several days to allow vascularization of the graft.

b. AlloDerm (LifeCell Corporation, The Woodlands, TX, USA).

i. It is dermis obtained from human cadavers. After being harvested as a split-thickness skin graft, epithelial particles are removed with hypertonic saline. It is then treated with detergent and freeze-dried. It is rehydrated just prior to wound application.

ii. AlloDerm creates a dermal network that is nonantigenic for vascular in growth by the host wound bed.

iii. At the time of placement, a very thin split-thickness skin graft from the patient is applied over the AlloDerm and secured.

VIII. Considerations for Non-Thermal Burns

A. Chemical Burns[13,15]

1. Injury depends on the type of agent, concentration of chemical, quantity of exposure, manner and duration of exposure, penetration, and mechanism of action of the chemical agent.
2. Typically classified as acidic, alkaline, or hydrocarbons burns.
3. The primary concern is removal of the chemical agent and all contaminated items.

   a. Adequate irrigation is confirmed by measuring skin pH.

      i. Powdered chemical substances are brushed off prior to initiating irrigation. Otherwise, an exothermic reaction may occur.

      ii. If ocular injury occurs, patient should be evaluated by ophthalmology, begin copious eye irrigation, and ocular pH measured until normalized.

4. Acidic.

   a. Coagulation necrosis: proton denatures cell proteins.

      i. Hydrolysis → protein degradation → eschar formation.

      ii. Strong acid typically has a pH < 2.0.

   b. Examples: sulfuric acid (Fig. 7), hydrochloric acid.

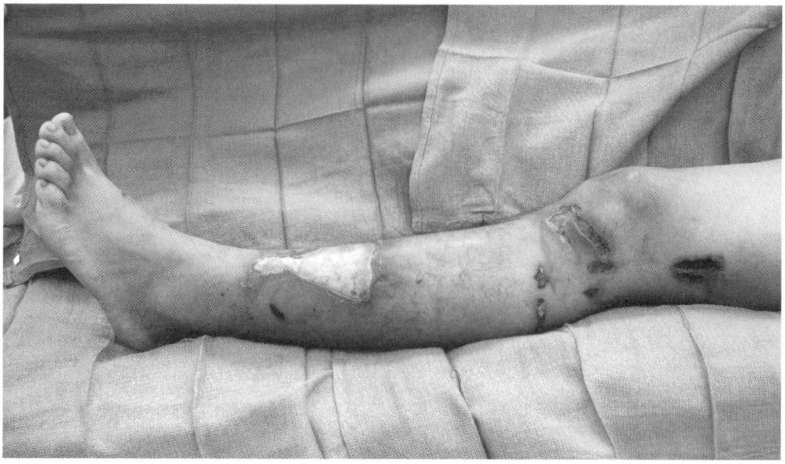

Fig. 7. Sulfuric acid burn from a car battery, occurring approximately one week prior to photo.

5. Alkaline.
    a. Tissue damage occurs by liquifactive necrosis.
        i. Alkali dissolves tissue → unites with tissue proteins → alkaline proteinates formed → more soluble ^{-}OH ions → penetrates nearby tissue.
        ii. Results in tissue dehydration and saponification of fatty tissue.
    b. For tissue injury, pH is typically > 11.5. In general alkali burns are worse than acidic burns due to the tissue penetration that occurs with liquifactive necrosis.
    c. Examples: ammonia, air bag fumes, sodium hydroxide, potassium hydroxide, and Ca carbonate.
6. Hydrocarbons.
    a. Tissue damage occurs by dissolution of cell membranes.
    b. Normally these burns are superficial.
    c. Hydrocarbons can be systemically absorbed: excretion is by lung and liver.
    d. Example: gasoline (Fig. 8).
7. Hydrofluoric.[16]
    a. Binds calcium causing severe pain locally and possible hypocalcemia systemically.

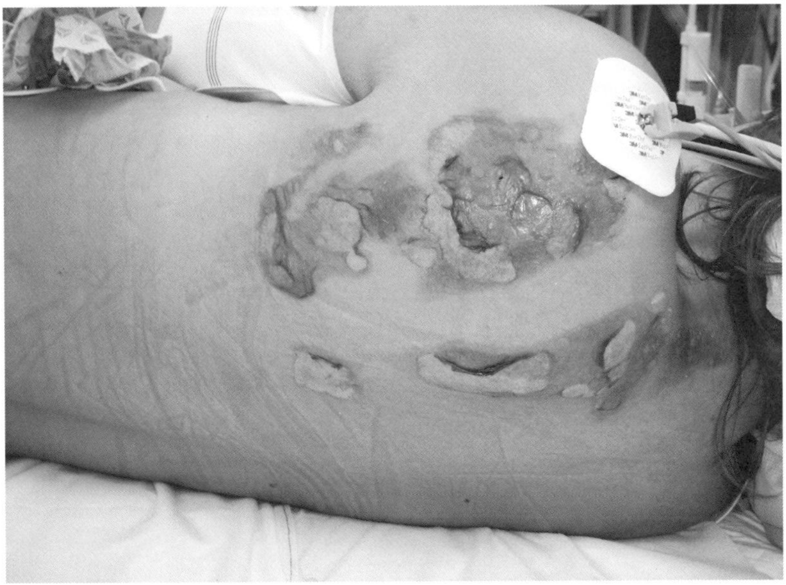

Fig. 8. Gasoline contact burn after clothing was contaminated in ATV accident and not removed for several hours.

b. Most effectively treated with calcium topical or arterial injection, and diminished pain is an indicator of adequate treatment.

B. Electrical Burns[5,13]

1. Injury types.
   a. High: > 1000 volts, deep necrosis, increased likelihood of systemic complications.
      i. Admission is indicated.
   b. Low (Fig. 9): < 1000 volts, localized tissue destruction, less likely for systemic complications.
      i. May be discharged if no loss of consciousness and no dysrhythmia. However, a child with a lip burn injury must be admitted and monitored for labial artery bleeding.
2. Mechanisms of injury.
   a. True electrical injury: current flow.

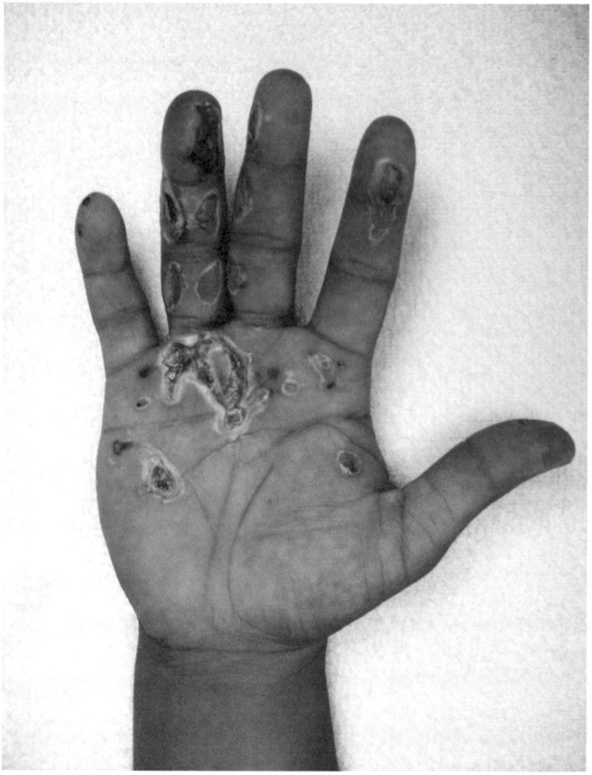

Fig. 9. Low voltage electrical burn from contact with a household electrical line during rewiring.

   b. Arc injury: electrical arc from source to object, similar to a flash burn. May arc from one body part to another. An example is an electrician working with metal objects.
   c. Flame injury: ignition of clothing/surroundings.
   d. May or may not have obvious burn contact points with any of the above mechanisms.

3. Arrhythmias.
   a. Arrhythmias are common, especially following high voltage electrical injury.
   b. An electrocardiogram (EKG) should be obtained upon arrival.

c. Cardiac monitoring on admission is indicated if there is high voltage electrical injury, significant cardiac history, elderly, observed arrhythmia since injury, or if cardiac or respiratory arrest occurred following the injury.
d. Arrhythmias are treated medically.

4. Resuscitation.
   a. Fluid resuscitation is not accurately calculated with any formula because tissue involvement is often deep and not accurately reflected by the calculated percent TBSA involved. However, a formula may give a reasonable starting point from which to begin titration according to urine output, for a goal of 30 cc/hr in an adult without myoglobinuria, 75–100 cc/hr in an adult with myoglobinuria, and 1.0 cc/kg/hr in children. LR should be used for resuscitation.
5. Myoglobinuria.
   a. Electrical current damages muscle cells and myoglobin is released into the circulation. The amount of myoglobin may overwhelm the renal filtration system, resulting in acute tubule necrosis (ATN) and acute renal failure. Serum myoglobin, urine myoglobin, and the color of the urine can be monitored for signs of significant myoglobin excretion. Pink to red urine likely indicates the presence of myoglobinuria. Treatment of myoglobinuria consists of alkanization of urine to prevent precipitation of myoglobin in renal tubules and rapid diuresis with mannitol to keep the tubules clear of potential obstruction.
6. Compartment syndrome.
   a. Keep a high index of suspicion for compartment syndrome in electrical burn patients, especially when it involves an extremity and high voltage exposure.
   b. Frequent neurovascular exams checking for: increasing pain, pallor, pulselessness (loss of arterial Doppler signal), parasthesias, poikilothermia.
   c. Increasing signs of neurovascular compromise or elevated compartment pressures (to 30 mmHg or within 20 mmHg of diastolic blood pressure) are indications for fasciotomy.
   d. Prophylactic fasciotomies are not indicated.
   e. For a fasciotomy, be sure to release all compartments fully.

7. Excisional debridement.
   a. To allow for adequate demarcation of tissue necrosis, the initial excisional debridement should wait 3–5 days post injury, unless there is persistent myoglobinuria.
8. Unique long-term sequelae.
   a. Cataracts may develop in up to 20% of high-voltage burn injury patients beginning years after the initial injury.
   b. Peripheral and central nervous system disorders that may not surface for months to years following injury.

C. Cold Injury[13]

1. Cell death results from intracellular ice crystal formation.
2. Frost bite is classified by first, second, and third degree with generally similar appearance to heat contact burns.
3. Initial treatment is by rapid rewarming of frost bitten area in water of 104 degrees Fahrenheit (40 degrees Celsius).
4. Ibuprofen may be given to decrease reperfusion injury from free radicals.
5. Non-hemorrhagic blisters are debrided, while hemorrhagic blisters are kept intact.
6. Angiography may be used for assessing the need for thrombolytic therapy.

IX. Long-Term Considerations for All Burns[5,13]

A. Hypertrophic scarring: can be painful, itch, and restrict movement.
B. Contracture: limits range of motion (Fig. 10).

   1. As long as scars are erythematous on physical exam, they are considered immature. Scars and contractures take 12 months to fully mature on average. Delaying surgery until scars are fully mature, or as long as is reasonable, will facilitate more appropriate and definitive surgical intervention.

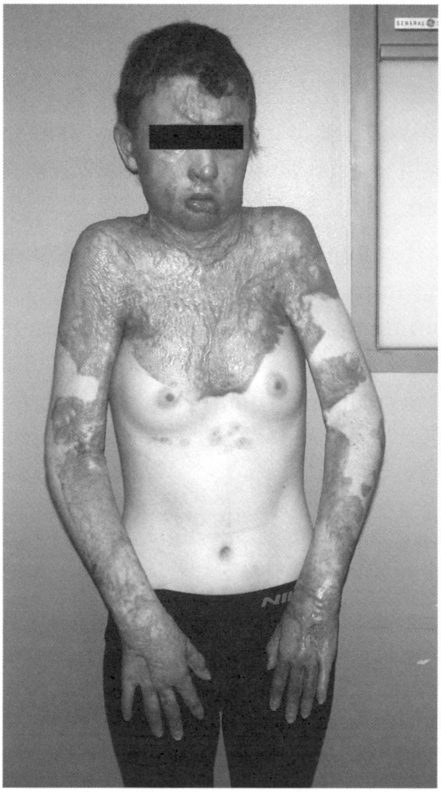

Fig. 10. Debilitating burn contractures of the neck, bilateral axilla, and bilateral upper extremities. Patient experienced flame burns about four months prior.

2. Pressure garments aid in scar maturation. The exact mechanism is controversial. Both increasing moisture within the scar tissue and relative scar tissue hypoxia have been named as potential mechanisms. Pressure garments are most effective when used as soon as grafts and open wounds are healed.
3. Splinting may be performed across joints to prevent contracture and is often begun at the time of the initial excision and grafting. Serial splinting may also be performed to increase joint range of motion by serially increased the joint angle held by the splint.

Serial splinting may begin as soon as graft and open wounds are healed.

4. Scar massage is effective at breaking up scar tissue when performed consistently, with adequate applied pressure, and using moisturizer. This can be begun as soon as wound are closed and grafts healed.

C. Heterotopic ossification: soft tissue calcium deposition around joints, which can affect joint mobility and function.

D. Need for rehabilitation: In order to regain and maintain function following burn injury, physical and occupational therapy evaluations and ongoing treatment are critical.

References

1. Underhill FP. (1930) The significance of anhydremia in extensive surface burns. *JAMA* **95**: 852.
2. Lund CC, Browder NC. (1944) The estimation of areas of burns. *Surg Gynecol Obstet* **79**: 352–358.
3. Knaysi GA, Crikelair GF, Cosman B. (1968) The role of nines: its history and accuracy. *Plast Reconstr Surg* **41**(6): 560–563.
4. Baxter CR, Shires T. (1968) Physiological response to crystalloid resuscitation of severe burns. *Ann N Y Acad Sci* **150**(3): 874–894.
5. Herndon DN. (2007) *Total Burn Care*, 3rd Edn. Saunders Elsevier, Edinburgh.
6. American Burn Association. (2009) *National Burn Report Repository of Data from 1999–2008*, version 5.0.
7. Jackson D, Topley E, Cason JS, *et al.* (1960) Primary excision and grafting of large burns. *Ann Surg* **152**: 167–189.
8. Janzekovic Z. (1970) A new concept in the early excision and immediate grafting of burns. *J Trauma* **10**(12): 1103–1108.
9. Davis J. (1914) The use of small deep skin grafts. *JAMA* **63**: 985–989.
10. Padgett EC. (1946) Indications for determination of the thickness of split skin grafts. *Am J Surg* **72**(5): 683–693.
11. Tanner JC, Vandeput J, Olley JF. (1964) The mesh skin graft. *Plast Reconstr Surg* **34**: 287–292.
12. American College of Surgeons. Committee on Trauma. (2006) Guidelines for the operations of burn units. In: *Resources for Optimal Care of the Injured Patient.* American College of Surgeons, Committee on Trauma, Chicago, Il, pp. 79–86.

13. Klein MB. (2007) Thermal, chemical, and electrical injuries. In: Thorne C, Grabb WC, Smith JW (eds.), *Grabb and Smith's Plastic Surgery*. Wolters Kluwer Health/Lippincott Williams & Wilkins, Philadelphia, pp. 132–149.
14. Heimbach DM. (1987) Early burn excision and grafting. *Surg Clin North Am* **67**(1): 93–107.
15. Sykes RA, Mani MM, Hiebert JM. (1986) Chemical burns: retrospective review. *J Burn Care Rehabil* **7**(4): 343–347.
16. Stuke LE, Arnoldo BD, Hunt JL, *et al.* (2008) Hydrofluoric acid burns: a 15-year experience. *J Burn Care Res* **29**(6): 893–896.

CHAPTER 8

CLEFT LIP AND PALATE: ANATOMY, EMBRYOLOGY, AND REPAIR

Kenneth L. Fan, Raja Mohan and Seth R. Thaller

Illustrative Case

A child is brought to your attention in the hospital after a normal vaginal delivery with a cleft lip. He is well developed and otherwise has no other problems. Family history does not reveal any other relatives with cleft lip or palate.

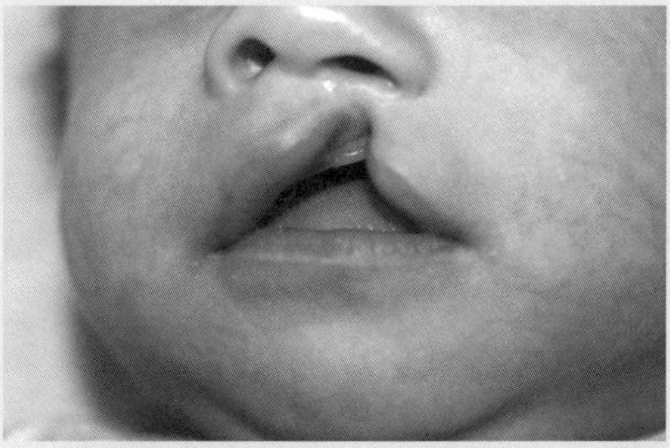

BACKGROUND INFORMATION

Regular Anatomy

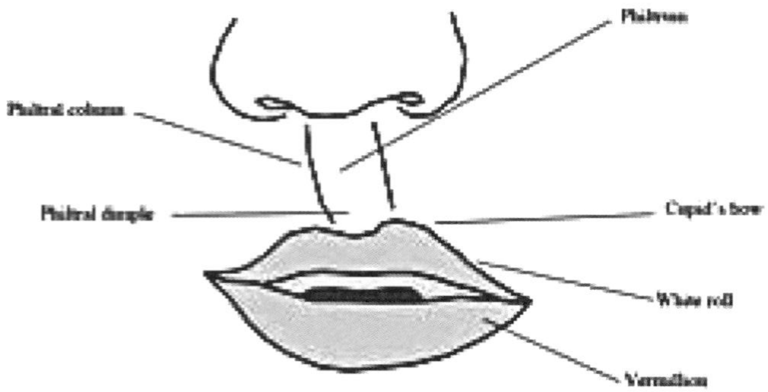

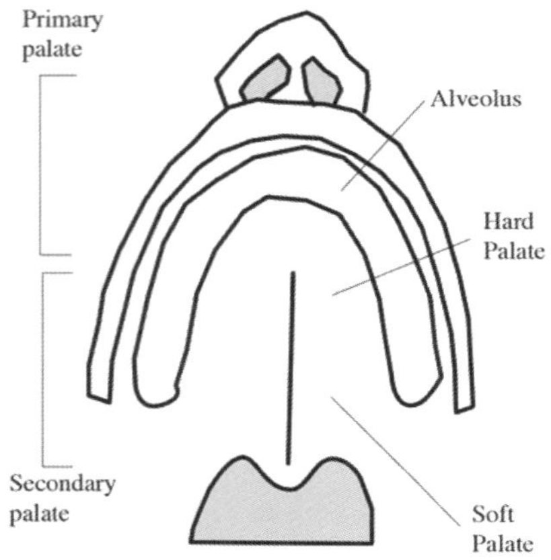

Primary palate — comprised of the upper lip, nostril sill, premaxilla, and hard palate **anterior** to the incisive foramen

Upper lip

Upper lip muscles

- **Orbicularis oris**
    - **Insertion**: interlocking orbicularis oris fibers cross over, inserting dermally to create a lift called the **philtral columns**
    - **Function**: deep portion of the oris functions as a **sphincter**
    - **Function**: superficial portion of the oris functions in **speech** and **facial expression**
- Levator labii superioris
    - **Insertion**: inferiorly on the **white roll** to contribute to peaks of **Cupid's bow**
    - **Function**: to elevate the lip

Upper lip landmarks

- Cupid's bow — two peaks formed from inferior extension of the philtral columns into the white roll
- White roll — junction between skin and vermillion
- Red roll — transition between dry/keratinized vermillion and wet/nonkeratinized mucosa
- Tubercle — portion of vermillion fullness at the central inferior apex of Cupid's bow

Upper lip blood supply and innervation

- Blood supply — bilateral superior labial arteries
- Motor innervation — facial nerve
- Sensory innervation — V2 of trigeminal

Premaxilla (anterior hard palate)

- Comprised of the anterior nasal spine and alveolar segment in the maxilla, which hold and support anterior four teeth
- Formed by the palatine process of the maxilla (median palatine process)
- Premaxilla blood supply and innervation
  - Blood supply — nasopalatine branch of the sphenopalatine artery via incisive foramen
  - Sensory innervation — **nasopalatine nerve** (V2) exits incisive foramen to innervate the anterior hard palate (premaxilla)

Important sutures

- **Incisive suture** separates the primary and secondary palate
- **Median palatine suture** divides palate in half, running form between incissors all the way to the posterior nasal spine
- The **Y shape** created by incisive sutures and posterior median palatine suture marks sites of fusion between premaxilla and the palatal shelves of the maxilla
  - Clefts of the alveolus and the hard palate typically occur here [1]

- **Transverse palatine suture**, which is perpendicular to the median palatine suture, marks joining of anterior and posterior hard palate

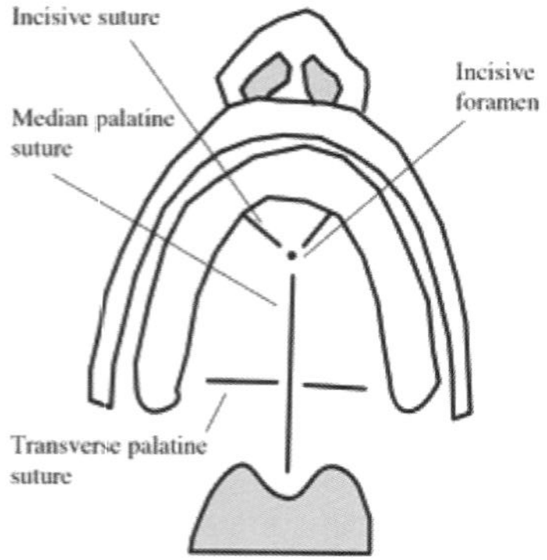

Secondary palate — comprised of the hard and soft palate **posterior** to the incisive foramen formed from the palatal shelves of the maxilla

Posterior hard palate

- **Posterior hard palate** formed by the horizontal plate of the palatine bone, which articles with the medial pterygoid plate of sphenoid bone posteriorly
- The lateral alveolar segment within the maxilla supports the canines, bicuspids, and molar teeth
- Midline/superiorly, hard palate joins with the **vomer**
    - Unilateral cleft palate — vomer is attached to the noncleftеd side
    - Complete cleft of hard palate — vomer can be seen midline
- Blood supply and innervation — **the dual blood supply** allows for hard palate viability during lifting of mucoperiosteal flaps for palate closure[1]
    - Blood supply — **greater palatine artery** (main) off the descending palatine artery through the greater palatine foramen
    - Blood supply — **nassopalatine branch**, via anastamosis, provides secondary blood supply
    - Innervation — greater palatine nerve (V2)

Soft palate comprises of the velopharyngeal muscles necessary for swallowing, breathing, and importantly speech

Upper sling attached to the soft palate

- **Levator veli palatini**
  - **Origin**: temporal bone and the Eustachian tube
  - **Insertion**: muscles interdigitate at midline behind the palatal aponeurosis
  - **Function**: raises the soft palate and pulls it posteriorly
- **Tensor veli palatini**
  - **Origin**: membranous wall of Eustachian tube
  - **Insertion**: tendon passes around the pterygoid hamulus, a projection off the medial pterygoid plate, to give rise to the palatal aponeurosis
  - **Function**: dilates the Eustachian tube by pulling the end open
  - **Function**: performs milking action on the tube when in concert with the levator veli palatini[2]

Lower sling attached to the soft palate

- **Palatoglossus**
  - **Origin**: posterior tongue
  - **Insertion**: passes through anterior tonsillar pillar to insert onto the anterior velum
  - **Function**: pulls soft palate forward and down
- **Palatopharyngeus** makes up the posterior tonsillar pillar
  - Origin: posterior pharynx
  - Insertion: passes through the posterior pillar to insert onto the velum
  - Function: depressors the palate

Uvula (the only intrinsic muscle of the palate) — pulls itself via upward

Soft palate blood supply and innervation

- Blood supply — **ascending palatine artery** (main) courses around the levator veli palatini to supply the lateral muscular structures and a large portion of the soft palate

- Blood supply — **lesser palatine artery** runs through the lesser palatine foramen
  - Both greater and lesser palatine foramen located posterolaterally on the horizontal plate of the palatine bone
- Vessels supplying the palate typically run between the periosteum and mucosa of the hard palate, and velar musculature and mucosa in the soft palate. Extensive dissection during intravelar veloplasty can place blood supplies at risk[1]
- Sensory innervation — lesser palatine nerve (V2)
- Motor innervation — muscles innervated by pharyngeal plexus containing CN IX, CN X, and CN XI, except for tensor veli palatini
  - Motor nerves reach their respective targets via lateral pharyngeal walls (avoid extensive dissection)
  - Tensor veli palatini is innervated by medial pterygoid nerve off of V3
- Sympathetic and secretory fibers — facial nerve to V2 via pterygopalatine ganglion

Embryology

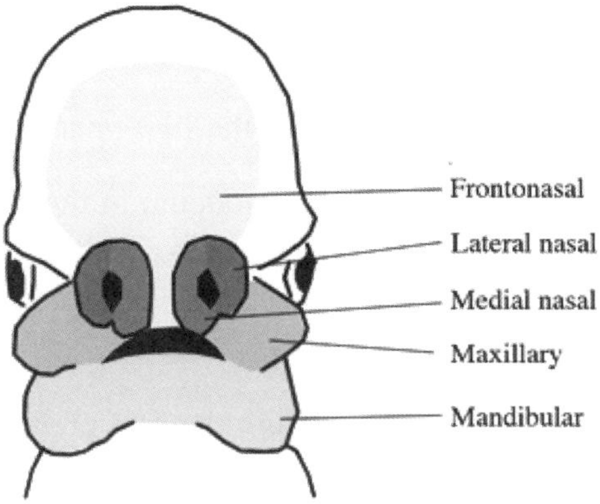

Embryonic prominences

Of the five arches, the first two are most closely associated with the development of the face and cranium. Face is derived from 5 different facial prominences, **frontonasal prominence and the bilateral maxillary prominences and mandibular process.** All surrounding the **stomadeum** (the primitive mouth) at the fourth week of development.

Muscles of mastication are derived from the **first branchial arch**, along with the mylohyoid, anterior belly of digastric, tensor tympani, and tensor veli palatini. Muscles of facial expression are derived from the **second branchial arch**. Neural crest cells from the first and second arch become the trigeminal and facial nerves respectively. Trigeminal and facial nerve innervates muscles derived from the same respective arch.

Frontonasal prominence — formed by proliferation of the mesenchyme ventral to the forebrain (not from a pharyngeal arch)

a. Forms the superior border of the stomadeum
b. Derivatives — forehead, nasal dorsum, medial and lateral nasal prominences
c. Medial nasal prominence
    i. Derivatives — nasal tip, columella/philtrum/Cupid's bow, prolabium, frenulum, primary palate (from the median palatine process), premaxilla, anterior nasal septum

d. Lateral nasal prominence

   i. Derivatives — nasal alae, lateral cartilage, lateral crus of the alar cartilage

Maxillary prominence — derived from the first pharyngeal arch

a. Forms the lateral border of the stomodeum in the fetus
b. Derivatives — upper cheek, zygoma, maxilla, orbital floor, upper lip excluding the philtrum (a frontonasal prominence structure), secondary palate (from the lateral palatine process)

Mandibular prominence — derived from the first pharyngeal arch

a. Forms the lower border of the stomodeum in the fetus
b. Derivatives — lower jaw, lower lip, lower cheek, chin regions of the face

It is important to note that cleft lip with or without cleft palate is a genetically, embryologically, and anatomically, distinct entity from isolated cleft palate.[3] Clefting can occur in with varying degrees in the primary or secondary palate ranging from incomplete to complete.

End of 6 weeks

1. **Maxillary prominence** migrate medially, fusing with the **medial nasal process** to form the upper lip and philtrum respectively for separation of the nasal pit from the stomodeum and formation of upper lip
   a. Defect in fusion of one or both side results in unilateral or bilateral cleft lip respectively
   b. May be complete or incomplete with a band of tissue at the nasal tissue (Simonart's band)
2. At this time, nasal floor is open to the oral cavity. The tongue fills the cavity, and reaches the nasal septum
   a. Nasal floor will be eventually sealed off by the **lateral palatine processes** from the medial edges of the **maxillary process** at the end of 8 weeks

End of 8 weeks

1. Closure of facial fissures affords more humanoid appearance
2. Primary and secondary palate formed by **medial nasal** and **maxillary prominence**, fusion which forms the complete palate

   a. Fusion of the **medial nasal prominences** gives rise to the **median palatine process**, which forms the premaxilla and primary palate

      i. Defects in fusion during **4–7 weeks of gestation** between the median palatine process to fuse with the lateral palatine process form **primary clefts palates**

   b. Fusion of the **maxillary prominences** give rise to the **lateral palatine processes**, which form the secondary palate behind the incisive foramen

      i. Lateral palatine process switch from vertical to horizontal (right before left, leading to increase in left sided clefts) with the mandible becoming more prognathic to allow transition without interference from tongue
      ii. Defects in fusion during **5–12 weeks of gestation** between the lateral palatine process to fuse with each other posterior to the incisive foramen are **secondary cleft palates**

   c. Upon fusion of the paired lateral and median palatine processes, the **nasal septum** grows downward from the merged medial nasal prominences
   d. Primary palate and anterior portion of secondary palate undergo **ossification** anterior to posterior

      i. An incomplete cleft will extend posterior

   e. Soft palate is derived from posterior portion of the secondary palate, which does not undergo ossification
   f. Palatal shelves undergo fusion 1 week later in females, leading to higher incidence of cleft palate in females

Statistics

1. Among all the clefts[4]

   a. Overall oral cleft incidence: 1:750 live births
   b. Cleft lip and palate 46%
   c. Isolated cleft palate 33%
   d. Isolated cleft lip 21%
   e. Bifid uvula in 2% of the population

2. Bilateral (86%) and unilateral (68%) of cleft lips are associated with cleft palate[5]
3. Left/right/bilateral cleft lip/palate 6:3:1[6]
4. Cleft lip and palate are more common in males 2:1[7]
5. Isolated cleft palate more common in females 2:1[7]
6. Racial distribution of cleft lip/palate[5]

   a. 2.1:1000 in Asian
   b. 1:1000 in Caucasians
   c. 0.4:1000 in African Americans

7. Isolated cleft palate

   a. 0.5:1000 with no racial variation[5,7]

8. Associated with increasing parental age over 30 years of age; paternal age more significant than mother's[8]

Nonsyndromic clefts appear to be multifactorial. However, a genetic component is recognized. Cleft lip with or without cleft palate is distinct genetically from isolated cleft palates.[3] The increased presence of isolated cleft palate does not increase chances of cleft lip with or without cleft palate and vice versa.

Familial incidence of cleft[7]	CL and CL/P	CP
One child affected	4%	2%
Two children affected	9%	1%
One parent affected	4%	6%
One parent, one child affected	17%	15%

Management and Preoperative Tests

Preoperative evaluation of the craniofacial patient:

1. Analysis of morphologic abnormality
2. Functional risk evaluation
3. Detection of associated malformations (i.e. cardiac or cerebral)
4. Recognition and classification of existing syndromes
5. Preoperative evaluation for surgery

Analysis of Morphologic Abnormality

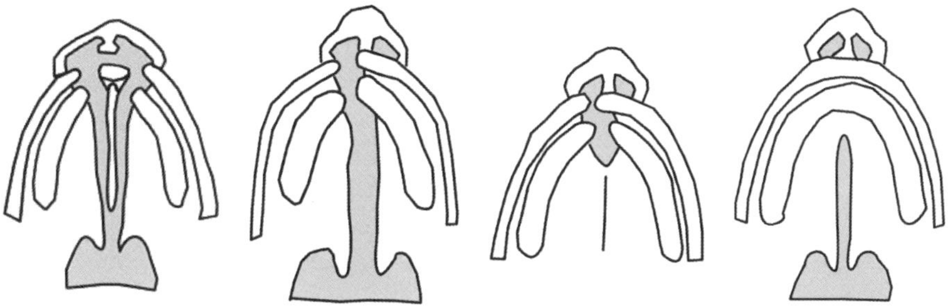

(Left) Bilateral cleft lip and palate, (2nd to left) unilateral cleft lip and palate, (2nd to right) cleft of the primary palate, (right) cleft of the secondary palate

Different Cleft Lips

Microform (forme furste) cleft lip

- Incomplete cleft characterized by a groove or scar/fibrous tissue extending from the vermillion to nasal floor with varying degrees of lip shortening, with several components[9]
    - Vermillion notch
    - Fibrous tissue from the vermillion to nasal floor
    - Ipsilateral alar deformity
    - Vertical lip shortness
- Surgery should only be performed if outcome is better than defect
    - Intraoral approach should be used if only orbicualris oris disrupted

Unilateral incomplete cleft lip

- Varying degrees of cleft in the upper lip with an intact nasal sill (Simonart band) consisting of skin, mucous membrane, and fibrous tissue, which assists in limiting the projection of the premaxilla
- Notched alveolus does not necessitate bone graft: small dimples and grooves may fill as the jaw grows
- Similar surgical technique as complete cleft required if orbicularis oris is completely disrupted, although degree of undermining can be tailored

Unilateral complete cleft lip

- Defect through the lip, **nostril sill,** and **alveolus**
- Completed clefted alveolus between the maxillary lateral incisors and canines
    - In 80–90%, the maxillary lateral incisor on cleft side is absent or smaller/dysmorphic[10]
- Nasal deformity
    - Depressed nasal base, collapsed ala, widened floor, and deviated septum
    - Lack of nostril sill causes anterolateral rotation of the premaxilla on the noncleft side
    - Abnormal attachments of the orbicularis oris leads to varying degrees of lower lateral cartilage collapse
    - Missing portions of inferior piriform aperature and hypoplasia of the lateral nasal bony platform at the maxillary wall
- For complete description on anatomy, see the cited article[11]

Bilateral cleft lip

- Soft tissues may or may not be symmetrically affected (asymmetrical)
- Simonart's band affected to varying degrees (complete/incomplete)
- In a complete cleft, the prolabium lacks muscle tissue, philtral columns, dimples, or Cupid's bow[12]

  - Lack of connections laterally and posteriorly leads to over-projection of premaxilla, excess tissue within the prolabium horizontally and a deficiency in vertical height
  - Lack of anterior premaxilla pull leads to collapse of lateral palatal shelves toward midline

- Nasal deformity

  - Flared alae, depressed nasal tip, slumped lower lateral cartilages due to failure to migrate to the nasal tip and extend the columella
  - The premaxilla is suspended from the tip of the nasal septum, while the lateral alveolar segments remain behind

Different Cleft Palates

Primary vs. secondary cleft palate

- Primary: cleft of the lip, alveolus, nostril sill, and palate anterior to the incisive foramen
- Secondary: soft palate (velum) and/or hard palate posterior to the incisive foramen

Unilateral vs. bilateral cleft palate

- Unilateral: septum contacts noncylefted palatal shelf
- Bialteral: septum does not contact any of the shelves

Complete vs. incomplete cleft palate

- Complete clefts penetrate the entire structure, while incomplete clefts do not
- Muscles of palate may be defective
  - Levator veli palatini muscle is discontinous and longitudinally oriented resulting in inability to close palate against posterior pharyngeal wall
  - Aberrant levator function influences tensor veli palatini function, which fuses to the posterior palate to open the Eustachian tube

  - 97% incidence of otitis media[13]
  - Myringotomy and PE tube required to improve hearing and speech outcomes[14]

Bifid uvula

- Most common cleft palate
- 2% of American population
- Maybe associated with palatal incompetance

Submucous cleft palate

- Intact mucous layer but with a discontinuous levator palatine muscle; triad of defects:
  - Bifid uvula
  - Palpable notch in the posterior palate
  - Muscular diastasis of the velum, creating a zona pellucida (thin mucosa) on contracture
  - Note: muscular diastasis can present without bifid uvula[15]
- Majority are asymptomatic, requiring serial speech evaluations and audiometric surveillance[16]
- Up to one third of patients can develop velopharyngeal insufficiency: short palatal length, limited mobility, and easy fatigability of the palate[17]
  - Associated with hypernasal speech and serious otitis media due to levator veli palatini dysfunction
- Furlow opposing Z-plasty can be used to correct velar diastasis

Unilateral complete cleft palate

- Direct communication is seen through entire length of the nasal passage and the oropharynx
- Feeding, speech, and impaired growth issues arise
- Repair must address all defects through the nasal mucosa, bony palate, velar musculature, oral mucosa
- Pierre Robin sequence should be looked for in those who present with isolated cleft palate

Bilateral complete cleft palate

- Premaxilla containing the central and lateral incisors are separated from the lateral alveolar segments
- As the bilateral cleft lip, presurgical techniques to reposition the premaxilla is required, especially when the lateral segments collapse together, locking out the premaxilla from the alveolar arch[16]

Typical Timing of Cleft Repair[18,19]

1. First contact: at birth or 2–4 weeks of age
2. Chelioplasty: 2 weeks – 3 months
    a. Rule of 10 for operation
        i. Ten weeks
        ii. Ten pounds
        iii. Hemoglobin of 10
    b. Presurgical orthopedics or lip adhesion may be performed before definitive lip repair in extremely wide cleft lips
3. Palatoplasty: 6 to 18 months
    a. May be delayed in children with airway obstruction or wide palatal clefts
    b. Early closure curbs speech abnormalities and hypernasal speech, but may impair facial growth
    c. Delayed repair results in improved growth, but poor speech
    d. Two stage repair is associated with less adverse effect on maxillary growth than single stage, but with worse velopharyngeal function and greater oronasal fistula[20,21]
4. Speech evaluation: started at 2 ½ years and every 6 months until normal
5. Velpharyngeal insufficiency (VPI): correction desired before starting school at the age of 5–6 years
    a. Despite closure of palate, hypernasal speech persists due to VPI
    b. Usually evident by age 2 to 3

   c. Correction entails posterior pharyngeal flap, pharyngoplasty, speech prothesis, or augmentation of posterior pharyngeal wall

6. Alveolar bone grafting: primary @ cleft lip repair, secondary 7–12 years
7. Revision of lip: age 5–6 years if necessary
   a. Ensure function and aesthetic appearance in a time of critical peer interaction
8. Surgery for maxillary retrusion correction: 14–18 years if necessary
   a. Maxillary retrusion may need to be corrected once facial growth is complete
   b. Lefort I or distraction osteogenesis

Functional Risk Evaluation

Multidisciplinary team should evaluate the cleft patient for feeding, speech, hearing abnormalities, as well as genetic counseling, presurgical orthopedics, and development of a treatment plan. The team usually consists of a:

- Plastic surgeon experienced in comprehensive cleft repair
- Pediatrician
- Pediatric otolaryngologist
- Speech pathologist
- Orthodontist
- Pediatric dentist
- Audiologist
- Geneticist
- Prosthodontist
- Psychologist
- Social worker

Airway management

- Most often a problem in Pierre Robin sequence (see section)

Feeding

- Children with clefts are underweight and require close monitoring[22]

- While normal sucking motion exists, difficulty exists in building up suction and nasal regurgitation
- Strategies include:
    - Preemie nipple with additional cross cuts
    - Lamb's nipple
    - Squeezeable bottles or bulb syringes may deliver too much milk
- Decreased body weight is associated with increase perioperative complications and higher fistula rates[22,23]

Detection of Associated Malformations

- Incidence of associated malformations in all cleft children: 21%[24]
    - 33% of abnormalities associated with malformations of the upper or lower limbs or vertebral column
    - 24% of abnormalities associated with cardiovascular system and congenital heart disease
- Incidence of isolated associated anomalies with cleft lip/palate: 7–14%[25]
- Incidence of isolated associated anomalies with cleft palate: 71% (17% with Pierre Robin)[26]

Cleft Associated Syndromes

Syndromic cleft

- Definition: more than one malformation resulting from an intrinsic error of morphogenesis resulting in defects in multiple developmental fields
- 36% of clefting has a positive family history[27]
- Incidence of syndromic cleft[27]
    - 13.8% for cleft lip and palate
    - 41.8% for isolated cleft palate

van der Woude syndrome

- Inheritance: most common autosomal dominant (variable expression) with cleft lip and palate
    - Penetrance of 70 – 100%[28]

- Mutation with IRF6 gene on 1q32–q41
- Incidence: 1:35,000–1:100,000 in Caucasians
- 1–2% of cleft patients[29]
- Features
    - Bilateral paramedian lower lip pits in 90% of patients[30]
    - Maxillary or mandibular second premolars and maxillary lateral incisors may be missing

Digeorge, conotruncal anomaly syndromes, **velocardiofacial** syndromes

- Inheritance: autosomal dominant
- Associated with 22q11 deletion
- Can occur as an isolated cleft palate
- Features
    - Cardiovascular abnormalities: VSD, tetrology of fallot, right sided aortic arch
        - Carotid may be displaced medially into the pharynx; important in planning a pharyngeal flap[1]
    - Abnormal facies: small ears, mandibular retrusion, narrow palpebral fissures, malar flattening, excessive maxillary height vertically
    - Developmental delay
    - Abnormality in palate typically a spectrum: palatal weakness, submucous to complete cleft

Pierre Robin sequence

- Inheritance: autosomal recessive and x-linked reported
- Should be screened for in those with isolated cleft palate
- Features
    - Micrognathia
    - Glossoptosis
    - U-shaped cleft palates
- Embryology
    - Theorized micrognathia and glossoptossis causes obstruction of palatal shelves, leading to horseshoe instead of V shaped palate deformities

- Management
  - Prone position to ensure airway acutely
  - Severe cases require mandibular distraction osteogenesis or tracheostomy
  - Cleft repair may be delayed for several months to ensure proper airway
    - Early repair of palate with micrognathia can narrow the area for respiration
    - Repair can be safely performed if mandible reaches normal size

Stickler syndrome

- Inheritance: autosomal dominant
- Mutation affects type II collagen on chromosome 12
- Features
  - Orofacial abnormalities
    - Cleft palate
    - Flattened facies
    - High frequency sensorineural hearing loss
    - Eye abnormalities: severe myopia, cataracts, glaucoma and/or retinal detachment
  - Early osteoarthritis
  - May present with Pierre Robin sequence[31]

Preoperative Evaluation for Surgery

- Thorough family history and genetic check list
- Evaluation of airway
  - Pierre robin sequence requires extensive airway management
  - Must ensure adequate airway will exist post-operatively
- Heart exam
  - 16 times higher prevalence of heart defects, most common being VSD[24]

- Rule of 10 for operation (last three associated with five times less complications)[32]
    - Ten weeks
    - Ten pounds
    - Hemoglobin greater than 10
    - WBC less than 10,000

Presurgical Preparations

Techniques for Bony Anatomy Reconstruction

Tessier has stressed the importance of reconstructing the bone anatomy before reconstruction of the soft tissue overlying.[33] The concept is especially applicable in the realm of cleft lip and palate surgery. Correcting underlying anatomy can simplify lip reconstruction and provide better outcome.

- **Lip adhesion**
    - Preliminary closure of lip for decreased tension during definitive repair
    - Applicability in unilateral or bilateral cleft lip with wide and poorly aligned maxillary segments
        - Can be used to retract premaxilla for lateral segment alignment[34]
    - Exact qualifying width has never been determined: depends on surgeon comfort
    - According to Loma Linda protocol, performed at 6 weeks[35]
    - Benefits
        - Affords minimal tension lip closure, especially if done young when rapid growth occurs
        - Improves maxillary arch alignment
        - May enable more predictable correction of nasal deformity due to improved alar base support
    - Disadvantages
        - Procedure is unpredictable: may not align segments ideally and can lead to alveolar collapse

    - Maxillary segments may become medially collapsed
    - Scarring created by procedure may lead to growth disturbances
  - Randall and Graham concluded lip adhesion has poor utility when the lip elements are[36]
    - Not markedly separated
    - The alveolar segment is only mildly displaced
    - Cleft lip can be approximated with little tension

- **Presurgical orthopedics**
  - Alignment of alveolar cleft prior to surgery during first few months of life
  - Requires extensive multidisciplinary approach
  - Devices can be classified into active or passive

Latham device

- Best known active device
- Technique
  - Two piece maxillary splint that overlies the palate[37]
  - Expansion screws between two pieces can be moved to adjust the lateral palatal segments
  - Elastic chain used to pull back premaxilla
  - Takes 3–5 weeks of active movement of maxillary segments to achieve approximation of alveolus
- Found that Latham device combined with gingivoperiosteoplasty disturbed facial growth, leading to an increased incidence of open bite, posterior cross bite, and a decreased length of the upper jaw[38]

Nasoalveolar molds (NAM)

- Most common passive device: gradually approximates alveolar segment by adding and removing material
- Performed before 6th week of age to take advantage of plasticity of the cartilage caused by increased estrogen

- Benefits
  - Helps avoid secondary bone graft in 60% of alveolar clefts and extensive undermining during gingivoperiosteoplasty[39]
  - Nasal stents allows correction of alar, columella, and nasal septum deformities
  - Can elongate columella and prolabium to create nasal project and upper lip length, as well as realign alveolar segments and premaxilla, in the bilateral cleft lip, all of which is difficult in the unmolded cleft
- Disadvantages
  - Labor intensive
  - Requires 3–6 months to achieve satisfactory results[40]

Operative Techniques

Surgical Closure of Alveolar Cleft

Bone grafting

- Objectives[16]
  - Closure of the fistula
  - Stabilization of the maxillary arch
  - Support of the root of teeth adjacent to the arch
  - Support of prosthesis
- Benefits
  - Results in improved nasal cosmesis
  - Grafted bone can be placed at the hypoplastic inferior piriform aperature ipsilateral to the cleft palate to support the alar base
- Primary alveolar graft
  - Placement of bone, usually rib, into alveolus at the upper buccal sulcus before 2 years of age
  - Attractive due to desire to close alveolar gap early to avoid further surgery
  - Disadvantage: graft at this time decelerates maxilla growth[41]

- Secondary alveolar graft
  - Most preferred
  - Performed between 8 to 11 years old before eruption of permanent maxillary canine for best success
  - Important to coordinate with orthodontics to ensure maxillary segment alignment presurgically
  - Iliac crest cancellous bone has a 93% success rate[42,43]
    - Other sites, as cranial bone, have been used with less pain but less success[44]
  - Advantage: not been found to have growth disturbance[45]

Gingivoperiosteoplasty

- A mucoperiosteal tunnel created between the exposed bone surfaces of the alveolar cleft via bilateral mucoperisteal flaps without dissection of the anterior face of the alveolus to encourage bone growth across the alveolar gap
- Usually performed at time of primary cleft lip repair
- Can only be performed if alveolar edges have close contact
  - 60% of the alveolar clefts did not require secondary bone graft at time of gingivoperiosteoplasty after nasoalveolar molding[39]
  - Without presurgical treatment, very wide undermining over the maxilla is required, leading to growth impairment
- Controversial operation: some surgeons report success,[46–48] while others report poorer outcomes, including higher posterior cross bite, open bite, and shorter jaw[38]

Repair of Unilateral Cleft Lip

- Rose[49]–Thompson[50] repair
  - Excision of cleft margin with primary straight line closure of the defect
  - Z-plasty's are incorporated for establishing vertical height of the upper lip
  - Used to correct smaller clefts, including the microform variant

- Randall–Tennison[51] repair
  - Z-plasty at the cleft lip edge near the vermillion border creates a lower lip triangular flap
  - Randall's modification involved applying geometric principles, tailoring flap to the cleft size[52]
  - Preserve Cupid's bow by lowering the peak on the cleft side at the expense of a lip scar across the philtral column with partial flattening of the philtral dimple and excessive vertical lip height[53]
  - Can be used for wider clefts
- Millard Rotation advancement repair
  - Based on the tenant that in the cleft lip, structures of the upper lip were intact, but merely distorted in position
  - Correction involves releasing and downwardly rotating the medial (non-cleft) segment, while advancing the lateral (cleft) flap into the upper lip defect[53]
  - Key points[34,54]
    - A back cut is made at the rotation incision of the medial lip
    - Advancement of the lateral lip is performed to correct the alar deformity and fill in the gap that the rotation cannot
    - C flap taken from the edge of the medial lip to extend the columella by placing the flap into the back cut after the rotation of medial lip, careful not to include the mucosal tissue
    - Both the incision at the columellar base and the C flap help gain length for the columella closest to cleft deformity
    - The L and M flap are taken from mucousal portion of lateral and medial lips respectively
      - Upon cleft alar base incision and advancement, L flap is sutured into the lateral nasal floor to increase the vestibular lining
      - M flap is used to fill cleft or augment gingivolabial sulcus
  - Benefits:
    - Preservation of Cupid's bow and philtral dimple

    - Tension is placed at alar bases, reducing flare and affording better molding of alveolar processes
        - Elevating slumped alar cartilage can correct nasal deformity at time of the repair
    - Scar mimics the projected philtral column on the opposite side, except for the oblique scar on the columella produced by the rotational component
- Disadvantages[11]
    - Tendency to create a constricted nostril on the repair side
    - Tension across the nostril sill
    - Need for wide undermining
    - Technically difficult in wide clefts
- Most commonly used modifications:[55] Noordhoff vermillion flap,[56] the Mohler modification,[57] and the Onizuka triangular flap[58,59]

Markings in the Rotation Advancement[60]

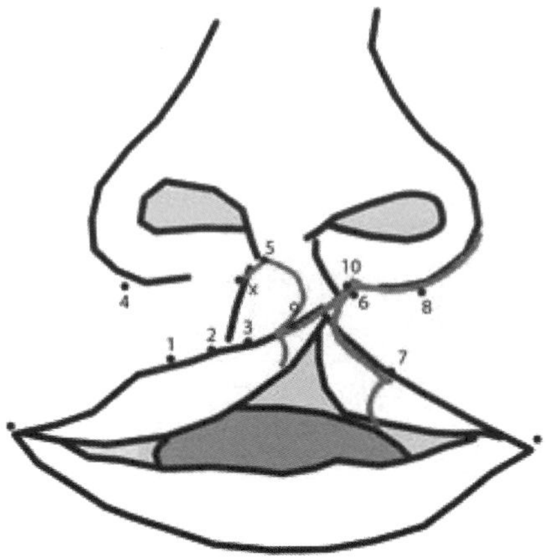

Millard's modified rotation advancement

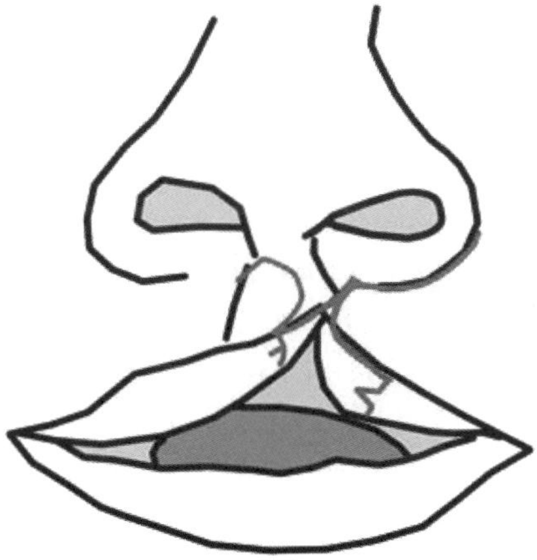

Noordhoff's vermillion flap

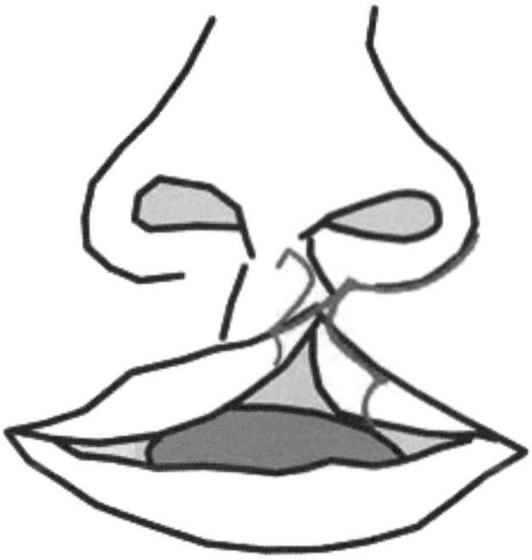

Mohler's modification

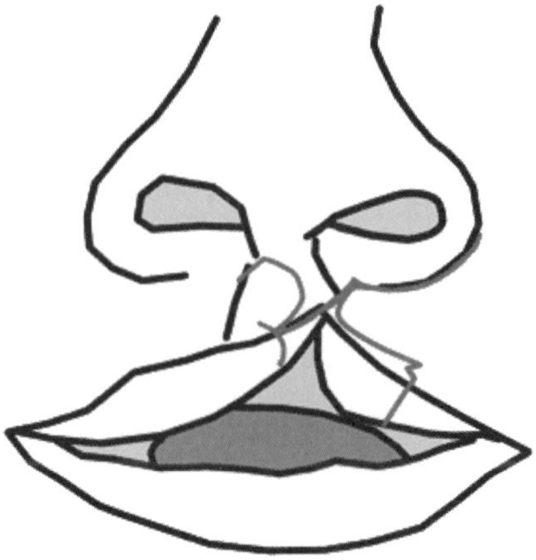

Onizuka's triangular advancement flap

Medial Lip Elements

1. Point 4: midpoint where the alar base joins with the lip on the noncclefted side
2. Point 2: mark the midpoint of Cupid's bows at the white roll
3. Point 1: mark the peak of Cupid's bow on the unclefted side of the medial lip
4. Point 3: using caliper's extrapolate the peak of Cupid's bow on the clefted side of medial lip (distance of 1 to 2 = distance of 2 to 3)
5. The columella is measured on the noncclefted philtral ridge. This measurement is transposed onto the clefted side starting at point 3, extending into the columella for creation of a philtral column
6. Point 5: the rotation incision, starting at point 3, ascending along the edge of the cleft into the base of the columella, where it curves horizontally past the midline of the columellar base into point 5. The curvilinear marking should mimic the normal philtral ridge[57]

    a. Point 5 must not cross the noncclefted philtral column. Overzealous extension of incision will cause too much vertical length of the upper lip on the normal side
    b. Point X: a back cut can be made if extra rotation is necessary to achieve symmetry of the cupid bow's element. Just before reaching

the opposite philtral column at point 5, a sharp downturn into point X can be made, usually at a 90 degree angle[61]

c. **Mohler's modification:** an extension of the rotation incision into the columella. The rotation incision does not bow toward the cleft as Millard's modified method, affording a wider C flap and a greater ability for straight line closure[57,62]

7. C flap: the C flap is mainly used to elongate the unilateral shortness of the columella on the clefted side. The arc of the rotation incision will determine the size of the C flap, as excess tissue on the medial lip not included in the rotation will be rotated into the back cut

   a. Point 9: medial edge of the C-flap
   b. Point 10: lateral edge of the C-flap

Lateral Lip Elements

1. Point 6: superior tip of the lateral advancement flap
2. Point 7: inferior tip of the lateral advancement flap located on the white roll; site of future Cupid's bow
3. Point 8: midpoint where the alar base joins with the lip on the clefted side
4. The incision marking on the lateral lip begins at point 7 to point 6 paring the cleft edge, and proceeds to curve around the alar base. The line from point to point is drawn in concavity form to eventually join the convexity of the medial lip segment

   a. Increase severity of nasal flare mandates more incision around alar base
   b. Curving of the alar base allows the use of cheek in wide clefts with small lateral lip component, and further rotation of the alar base to achieve symmetry
   c. For incomplete clefts, point 8 may be the lateral extent of the upper curved horizontal incision

5. Cleft edge of the lateral lip element (point 6 -> 7) must match the rotation incision (point 3 -> x)

   a. If extra length is required in the advancement edge to match the rotation edge, point 6 may be extended into the nasal vestibule

6. Distance of alar base to Cupid's bow on the nonclefted side (4 -> 2) must match that on the clefted side (8 -> 7)
   a. If vertical height is lacking, the lateral incision can be made to include a millimeter or more of the alar base to include it into the lateral advancement flap
7. **Noordhoff's vermillion flap:** at the vermillion edge of the lateral advancement flap, a triangular flap is created to fit into the deficient vermillion on the rotation edge. This is performed to reconstruct the cleft side Cupid's bow and provide volume to the vermillion[56]
8. **Onizuka triangular advancement flap:** three flaps are added to the unilateral cleft lip repair: 1) a small triangular flap at the vermillion border, 2) large triangular flap at the upper lip, and 3) an alar flap[58,59]

Rotation Advancement Technique[57,60,63]

1. Infiltrate local area with 1:200,000 epinephrine for hemostasis and skin turgor
2. Pare cleft mucosa edges: a vermillion flap based off the upper labial sulcus alveolar mucosa is dissected bilaterally with No. 11 scalpel. Flaps are left free for later use
   a. M flap (medial mucosal paring flap) may be used as a second layer in the closure of the alveolus and the anterior hard palate on the oral or nasal side
   b. L flap (lateral mucosa paring flap) may be used as a filler for the defect produced during incision of the lateral vestibular lining when freeing the clefted alar base from the maxilla to protect the nasal ala advancement against contracture

Freeing the medial lip segment

3. Freeing of the medial rotation flap: undermine the medial lip element from the maxilla to facilitate rotation
4. Incision, point 3 to 5: dissection begins at point 3 with a No. 11 scalpel along the marked curvilinear incision curving across midline into

point 5 at the base of the columella. More vertical height discrepancy between planned peak (point 3) vs. existing peak (point 1) requires more rotation

a. A back cut can be executed if extra rotation is required

    i. **Mulliken modification:** instead of a back cut, Mulliken devised a releasing incision,[64] which is 90 degrees perpendicular to Millard's back cut. Advantages: the rotational incision does not cross midline for better scar and the tip of the advancement flap (point 6) does not cross the philtral column. The smaller upper lip opening allows the C-flap to lengthen the hemicolumella[62]

b. Entire medial lip segment should be released upon completion of incision due to the slight tension with a skin hook. Medial lip segment is released and rotated inferiorly into its proper location

5. C flap, created by the curvilinear incision, serves to fill in the columellar defect left by the rotational incision, which can be exposed with a skin hook on the ipsilateral slumped dome

    a. Dissection: carried posteriorly in the intermembranous septum up to the tip of the nasal tip on the cleft side serves to release the C flap
    b. Scissor dissection: upward movement of the inferiorly positioned cleft crus ahead of the C-flap along the columella is facilitated by dissection between the medial crura of the bilateral alar cartilages
    c. Suture, point 9 to X: the C flap is sutured into place at this point (point 9 to x)
    d. Note: the C flap should form an abutment to keep the rotated lip segment in the desired plane. No "spring back" of the rotated segment should occur when the C flap is in place if adequate release was performed
    e. Suture point 10 to 8: tail end of the C flap is used to create part of the nasal sill

Freeing the lateral lip segment

6. Freeing of the lateral advancement flap: a releasing incision at the top of the labial sulcus can release the lateral lip from the maxilla. Wider clefts require more extensive undermining, superiorly up to the infra-orbital foramen and laterally to allow free movement of the lateral lip

   a. Cleft alar base may be freed by extending the incision into the nasal vestibule, starting laterally at the bony attachments along the piri-form opening, curving up along the intercartilaginous line
   b. Radical nasal correction: if the alar rim bends and vestibular lining kinks on advancement, the incision can be further extended along nasal rim for exposure and cartilage release to perform an alar lift is necessary[60]

7. Creation of lateral advancement flap: with a no. 11 scalpel, make an incision at at point 7 to point 6 in an effort to retain all the subcutaneous tissue, muscle, and mucosa in the lateral lip. This incision should match the rotation incision (6->7 = 3->x)

   a. Point 6 will extend into the vestibule if the lateral element is deficient length wise[61]
   b. Point 7 may also be extended more laterally along the vermillion for increased length[62]
   c. Sever the alar flare requires extension of incision around the alar base,[60] which may cause secondary nasal deformity, including scarring and narrowing of the nostril

8. Muscle dissection: with the upper half centimeter of the lateral lip intact for the key stitch, dissect the lateral lip skin and posterior mucosa off the orbicularis oris muscle

   a. The upper orbicularis on the lateral lip may be split by scissors to bring it into horizontal alignment with the medial lip. The rotation defect will be filled by the medial edge of the muscle

Closure

9. Closure of the nasal floor and nasal closure of the alveolar and anterior hard palate can be achieved with a vomerine and premaxillary mucoperisoteal free sutured onto the lateral cleft edge. The M (medial

mucosal) flap can be used as a second, oral layer in this closure. If the mucoperiosteal flaps are turned on the oral side, the M flap can be used on the nasal[53]

10. L flap is used to close the lateral nasal vestibular defect. Support for alar base can be maintained by pulling the L flap far along the line of intercartilaginous release
11. Key stitch, point 6 to X: this is the most important stitch. Using 4–0 catgut, the tip of the advancement flap at point 6 is sutured to point X
    a. Extra convexities may be removed to facilitate approximation between medial and lateral sides
    b. Mucocutaneous white roll is interdigitated to camoflauge scars at the union
12. Closure of the mucosa at the advancement incision in the upper labial sulcus is achieved with 4–0 chromic suture
13. Three layer closure
    a. With the orbicularis freed from the underlying maxilla, edges are sutured with end to end reapproximation with 4–0 Mersilene suture
    b. 6–0 silk skin suture can be placed in the lip, with 6–0 catgut in the free border of the vermillion
    c. 4–0 chromic catgut can be used to close the posterior mucosa
14. Alar base closure
    a. Epithelium off the tip of the flap is removed for several millimeter, so a 4–0 Mersilene suture can bring the tip to the area of the septum near the nasal spine under the tip of the c flap (point 9)
    b. Alar bases should be equivalent and have symmetry
    c. Once achieved, the alar base is sutured to the upper edge of the lateral advancement flap subcutaneously
15. Steristrips may be placed over the wound, and an oral airway can be placed until the airway is deemed adequate

Repair of Bilateral Cleft Lip

Repair of the bilateral cleft lip is a particularly challenging surgery. The presence of Simonart's band in incomplete bilateral cleft lip can allow the surgeon to resort to straight line closure or rotation advancement similar to those done in the unilateral cleft lip. However, in the complete bilateral cleft lip, anatomy posses a significant barrier to good cosmetic outcome. Previous techniques purely focus on the cutaneous deformity, at the expense worsening nasal shape and unstable premaxillas.[15,40] Modern approaches recognize the importance of correcting cartilage and nasal deformities for better outcome.

Skin Based Techniques

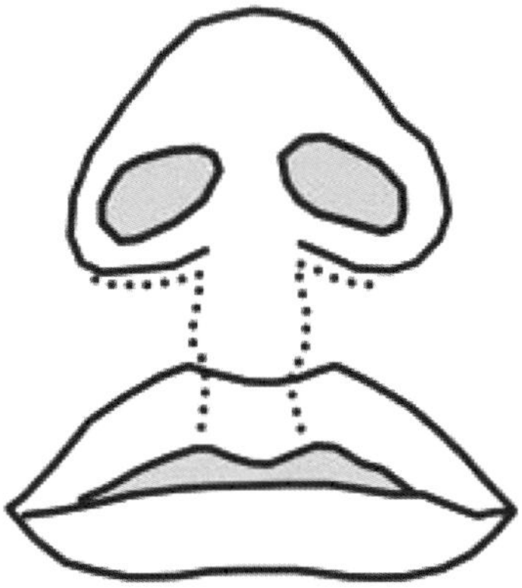

Modified Manchester repair (dotted lines = sutures)

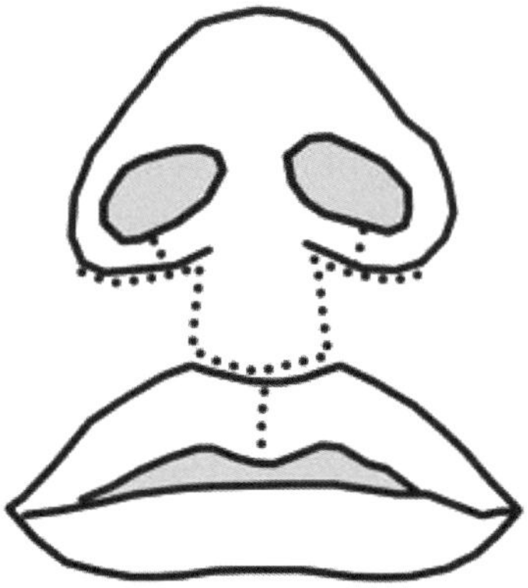

Millard bilateral cleft repair (dotted lines = sutures)

Modified Manchester by Broadbent and Wolf[65]

- Characteristics:
  - Utilizes prolabial tissue to lengthen columella[65]
  - Prolabial white roll and vermillion is retained, to construct Cupid's bow and tubercle
  - Discards lateral prolabial paring
- Technique:
  - Incision begins at the nasal floor, curves along philtral columns, and narrows at Cupid's bow
  - Philtral flap is cut to its desired width and excess tissue is discarded

  - Orbicularis muscle is be sutured to the lateral prolabial subcutaneous tissue

- Disadvantages:
  - Central vermillion to lacks bulk, due to decrease in muscle size
  - Defect in animation of the central lip
  - Two parallel scars across the central vermillion where the prolabial mucosa flap was placed
  - Skin behind prolabium becomes widened due to lateral forces pulling it apart

Millard's bilateral cleft repair (forked flap repair)

- Characteristics: two key differences versus modified Manchester[63]
  - Central prolabial white roll and vermillion is discarded with extra mucosa from prolabium used to reconstruct central gingivolabial sulcus
  - Prolabial pairings banked "whisker style" in the nasal base, instead of discarded, for future columellar lengthening if required
- Techniques:
  - Philtral flap is constructed out of the prolabium, similarly to the modified Manchester
  - After banking, orbicularis sling is constructed underneath the philtral flap via reapproximation
  - Upper lip vermillion, is reconstructed from lateral lip elements leading to a single vertical scar under Cupid's bow
  - Columellar flap is set over the lip elements
- A second stage can be incorporated:[37] V-Y advancement from the lip into the nose or flaked flaps cut from the lateral sides to be advanced into the columella for additional length of upper lip and columella
- Disadvantages:
  - Extensive amount of scarring in the lip-columella junction[40]
  - Pushing extra skin onto nasal floor for columellar length pushes footplates of medial crura into the tip, resulting in secondary nasal deformity[40]

Ultimately, the decision between using the modified Manchester or the Millard's method for bilateral cleft lip repair rests on the quality of the white roll and the vermillion. If the white roll and vermillion is of good quality, the modified Manchester method may be employed. However, with insufficient white roll and vermillion of the prolabium, it can be discarded as done in the Millard method utilizing the lateral segments instead.

Cartilage Based Techniques

Nasal repair was initially performed as late as possible. This was due to potential growth interferences before current techniques of initial nasal reconstruction.[37]

- McComb stressed the importance of correcting the displaced alar cartilages to elongate the columella and narrow nasal tip in outcome of bilateral cleft lip repair[66]
    - Described using presurgical orthopedics to reposition the premaxillary segment and to narrow soft tissue cleft
    - First stage
        - Nasal tip exposure via incisions following alar domes almost to the columellar base
        - Medial crura were suspended while sutures were placed joining alar domes
        - Prolabium was not dissected in an effort to avoid jeopardizing blood supply
        - Lips closed by lip adhesion
    - Second stage (a month later)
        - Prolabium lifted to unite the muscle below
    - At 4 and 15 year re-examination of the same patients, outcomes were satisfactory with minimal scarring[67,68]

Noordhoff and Mulliken have advocated nasal line repair at the time of primary lip repair. Noordhoff described freeing the alar cartilage via dissection from the piriform aperature upward. Cartilages were repositioned with sutures from the lower lateral cartilage to the upper lateral cartilage and the dorsal cartilage.[69] Mulliken, an initial supporter of the two stage repair with banked forked flaps, eventually began performing one stage nose/lip repair operations. Mulliken's repair differs from McComb's. It includes an extra incision in the nasal tip to approximate the crura. He closes the muscle on initial repair.[70]

Repair of Cleft Palate

Reconstruction of the cleft palate is somewhat different from the cleft lip in the outcome is not readily assessed. Operations like nasal closure and intravelar veloplasty requires years before evaluation of outcome of speech and completion of facial growth. Timing of the cleft palate repair is determined by a balance between two goals of cleft palate surgery. Normal development of speech achieved with the repair and to minimize the impaired facial growth due to transverse maxillary growth restriction. General consensus is that cleft palate repair should occur by 12 months for adequate speech development.[71] Repair should occur with phonologic development to prevent intractable compensatory maladaptive patterns of speech. However, there is no consensus regarding how early the surgery can be performed. Result of transverse maxillary growth restriction is crowding of the teeth, lateral crossbite, and open bite. Patients should be counseled on the necessary procedures, including primary palate repair with veloplasty, possible surgery on the palatopharyngeal muscle sling via sphincteroplasty or pharyngeal flap, and possible orthognathic surgery upon maturity of the skeleton.[15]

One of the most important aspects of the operation is the maintenance of the great palatine neurovascular bundle exiting the greater palatine foramen through the lateral posterior hard palate. It is important to dissect away from the pedicle to not compromise it. To obtain increased free movement of the mucoperiosteal flap for better approximation, freeing of the palatal attachments around the pedicle and stretching of the pedicle out of the greater palatine foramen is crucial.[16] By pushing back the soft palate to maintain contact with the posterior pharyngeal wall, velopharyngeal dysfunction can be avoided.

- **Two stage repair**[72]
  - 4–6 months: soft palate and veloplasty
  - 18 months: hard palate
  - Theoretically possible to achieve beneficial effect of soft palate on speech without the growth restriction early closure of the palate would incur
  - Believed the hard palate narrows as a result of the closure of the soft palate, requiring much less extensive operation
  - However, some studies have showed there is a lack of evidence of these claims, and that delaying hard palate closure has a negative impact on speech[73,74]
- **One stage repair**
  - 11–12 months: complete single stage repair
    - Pierre Robin sequence with micrognathia patients: surgery may be delayed to 14–18 months to prevent airway compromise during surgery
  - Proponents claim less speech impairment with early closure
  - Single staged **Bardach two flap** with intravelar veloplasty and the **Furlow palatoplasty** are the most popular technique, indicating a shift toward single staged repair[75]

Hard Palate Repairs

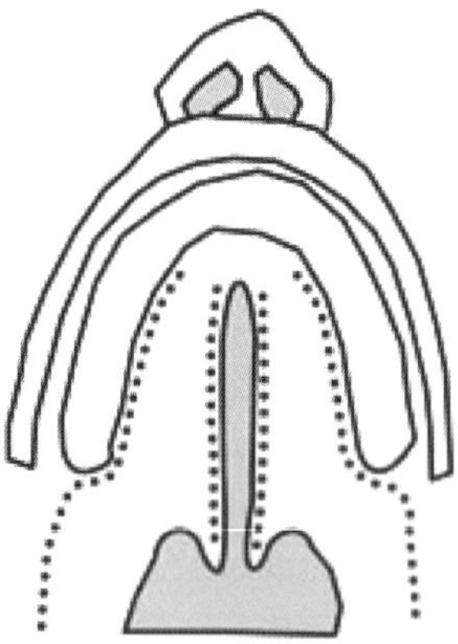

von Lagenbeck repair

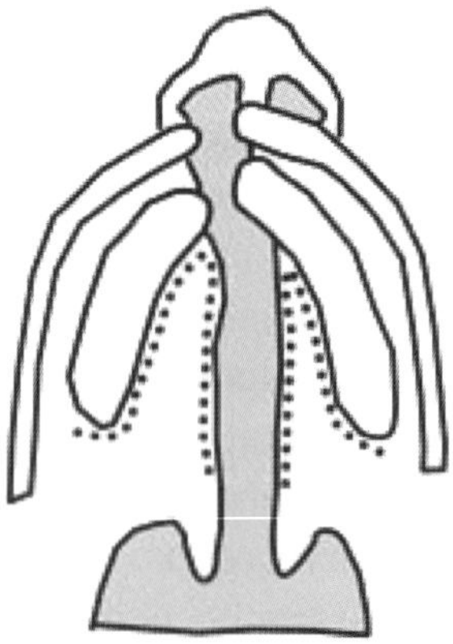

Bardach repair

- von Lagenbeck repair
  - Bilateral, bipedicled mucoperiosteal flaps
    - Incisions along the posterior alveolar and cleft margin freeing mucoperiosteum
    - Nasal and oral mucosa flaps mobilized and joined at midline
  - Often used for secondary palate repair
  - An intravelar veloplasty or levator palatini muscle can be added[16]
- Veau Wardil Kilnner pushback repair
  - Bilateral mucoperisoteal flaps based off the greater palatine arteries, which are released via osteotomy at the greater palatine foramina and dissection of periosteum behind the vessels
  - Utilizes V-Y closure to lengthen the palate
  - Hamulus fractured for better transposition of levator veli palatini
  - Vomer or buccal mucosa flaps for nasal lining (although nasal tissue was originally suggested to be left open)
    - Large open areas anteriorly of denuded palatal bone may result in decreased growth of anterior maxilla
  - Higher rate of fistula due to the nasal mucosa being the only closure of the anterior segment[76]
- Bardach repair
  - Bilateral mucoperisoteal flaps based off the greater palatine arteries
    - Essentially a modification of von Lagenbeck, with relaxing incision continuous along the alveolar edge around the cleft margins to the posterior most point
  - Wide dissection of flaps promotes mobility and allows for decreased tension on closure
  - Add intravelar veloplasty for increased success
- Vomer flaps
  - Used for hard palate closures
  - Useful in closure of wide or bilateral cleft palates

- Can be unilateral or bilateral with inferior or superior based vomer flaps
  - Inferior based flaps: incision is made high on the septum, with nasal mucosa approximated to the oral side as single layer closure
  - Superior based flaps: reflects mucosa from the septum near the cleft margin, to close the nasal mucosa
  - Inferior based flap associated with maxillary retrusion and a higher rate of fistula
- Scarring along the vomeropalatine suture is thought to influence maxillary growth[77]

Soft Palate Repairs

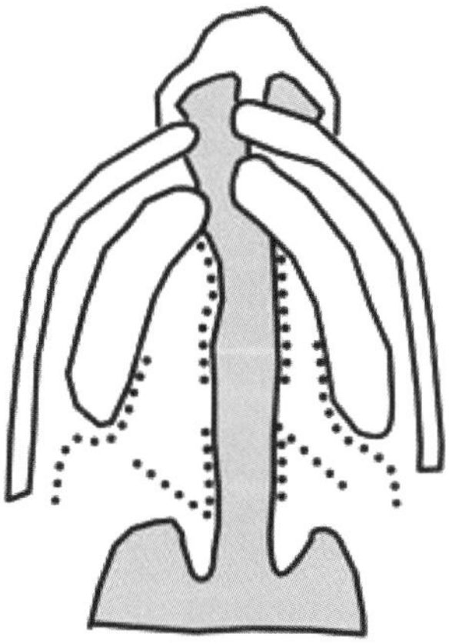

Furlow double opposing Z plasty

- Furlow's double opposing Z-plasty
  - Utilizes alternating Z-plasties on the nasal and oral mucosa to reposition the levator veli palatini
    - Central limb of Z-plasties is the cleft edge

- Anterior flaps contain only mucosa while levator muscle is maintained in the posterior flaps
  - Both flaps are based on oral and nasal mucosa but in opposite directions
  - The posteriorly based oral flap should be based on the patient's left for the right handed surgeon
- Relaxing incisions along the hard palate mucosa, vomer flaps, or both may be required to assist in closure of wide clefts
- Speech results are comparable with intravelar veloplasty if not better[78]

- Intravelar veloplasty
  - Approximates levator veli palatini at midline
  - Dissection of levator veli palatini from its abnormal insertion on the cleft margin as well as both nasal and oral mucosa is performed
  - Adherence of the thin nasal mucosa makes the dissection difficult, often times resulting in perforation
  - Levator veli palatini is closed without tension, with the oral and nasal mucosa closed in separate layers

Postoperative Care and Outpatient Rehabilitation

Lip care

- Feedings: first week, through a catheter, sryringe with soft tubing, or special feeder (e.g.: Haberman)
- Restrictions: arm splints for 2 weeks after lip repair
- Wound care: regular cleansing with half strength hydrogen peroxide, with coating bacitracin ointment
- Suture removal: 5th–7th post-operative day

Palate care

- Airway
  - Continuous pulse oximetry
  - Careful airway management required for micrognathic patients, including artificial airways

- Feedings: restrict hard foods (e.g.: pretzels, crackers)
  - 2/3 of surgeons allow immediate return to breast feeding[75]
  - 43% allow resumption of age appropriate diets once liquid is tolerated[75]
  - Liquid diet for the first 24 hours, and soft diet for one week
- Restrictions: arm splints for 2 weeks after lip repair
  - Head placed at a 30 degree angle
- Wound care:
  - Hemostasis can be achieved with fibrillar collagen
  - Apply pressure or intranasal oxymetolazone for postoperative bleeding
  - Antibiotics for 5 days

References

1. Kahn DM, Schendel SA. (2006) Anatomy and classification of alveolar and palatal clefts. In: Mathes SJ (ed.), *Plastic Surgery*. Saunders Elsevier, Philadelphia, pp. 69–89.
2. Huang MH, Lee ST, Rajendran K. (1997) A fresh cadaveric study of the paratubal muscles: implications for eustachian tube function in cleft palate. *Plast Reconstr Surg* **100**: 833–842.
3. Fogh-Anderson P, Aagesen E. (1942) *Inheritance of Harelip and Cleft Palate; Contribution to the Elucidation of the Etiology of the Congenital Clefts of the Face*. Busck, Copenhagen.
4. Fraser GR, Calnan JS. (1961) Cleft lip and palate: seasonal incidence, birth weight, birth rank, sex, site, associated malformations and parental age. A statistical survey. *Arch Dis Child* **36**: 420–423.
5. Habib Z. (1978) Genetic counselling and genetics of cleft lip and cleft palate. *Obstet Gynecol Surv* **33**: 441–447.
6. Wilson ME. (1972) A ten-year survey of cleft lip and cleft palate in the South West Region. *Br J Plast Surg* **25**: 224–228.
7. Fraser FC. (1970) The genetics of cleft lip and cleft palate. *Am J Hum Genet* **22**: 336–352.
8. Habib Z. (1978) Factors determining occurrence of cleft lip and cleft palate. *Surg Gynecol Obstet* **146**: 105–110.

9. Thomson HG, Delpero W. (1985) Clinical evaluation of microform cleft lip surgery. *Plast Reconstr Surg* **75**: 800–804.
10. Vichi M, Franchi L. (1996) Eruption anomalies of the maxillary permanent cuspids in children with cleft lip and/or palate. *J Clin Pediatr Dent* **20**: 149–153.
11. Burt JD, Byrd HS. (2000) Cleft lip: unilateral primary deformities. *Plast Reconstr Surg* **105**: 1043–1055; quiz 1056–1047.
12. Fara M, Smahel J. (1967) Postoperative follow-up of restitution procedures in the orbicularis oris muscle after operation for complete bilateral cleft of the lip. *Plast Reconstr Surg* **40**: 13–21.
13. Dhillon RS. (1988) The middle ear in cleft palate children pre and post palatal closure. *J R Soc Med* **81**: 710–713.
14. Hubbard TW, Paradise JL, McWilliams BJ, Elster BA, Taylor FH. (1985) Consequences of unremitting middle-ear disease in early life. Otologic, audiologic, and developmental findings in children with cleft palate. *N Engl J Med* **312**: 1529–1534.
15. Hopper R, Cutting C, Grayson B. (2007) Cleft lip and palate. In: Thorne CH *et al.* (eds.), *Grabb & Smith's Plastic Surgery*, 6th Edn. Wolters Kluwer, Philadelphia, pp. 201–225.
16. Hoffman WY, Mount D. (2006) Cleft palate repair. In: Mathes SJ (ed.), *Plastic Surgery*. Saunders, Philadelphia.
17. Ysunza A, Pamplona MC, Mendoza M, Molina F, Martinez P, Garcia-Velasco M, Prada N. (2001) Surgical treatment of submucous cleft palate: a comparative trial of two modalities for palatal closure. *Plast Reconstr Surg* **107**: 9–14.
18. Noordhoff MS. An integrated approach to the primary lip/nasal repair in bilateral cleft lip and palate. In: Thaller SR (ed.), *Noordhoff Craniofacial Foundation Instructional Surgical Videos*. Plastic Surgery Hyperguide.
19. Wornom IL, Will LA. (2002) Core curriculum for cleft lip/palate and other craniofacial anomalies. In: Berkowitz S (ed.), *Cleft Lip and Palate: Diagnosis and Management*. Springer, New York.
20. Liao YF, Yang IY, Wang R, Yun C, Huang CS. (2010) Two-stage palate repair with delayed hard palate closure is related to favorable maxillary growth in unilateral cleft lip and palate. *Plast Reconstr Surg* **125**: 1503–1510.
21. Noordhoff MS, Kuo J, Wang F, Huang H, Witzel MA. (1987) Development of articulation before delayed hard-palate closure in children with cleft palate: a cross-sectional study. *Plast Reconstr Surg* **80**: 518–524.
22. Lazarus DD, Hudson DA, Fleming AN, Goddard EA, Fernandes DB. (1999) Are children with clefts underweight for age at the time of primary surgery? *Plast Reconstr Surg* **103**: 1624–1629.

23. Fillies T, Homann C, Meyer U, Reich A, Joos U, Werkmeister R. (2007) Perioperative complications in infant cleft repair. *Head Face Med* **3**: 9.
24. Milerad J, Larson O, Hagberg C, Ideberg M. (1997) Associated malformations in infants with cleft lip and palate: a prospective, population-based study. *Pediatrics* **100**: 180–186.
25. Witkop C. (1979) Cleft lip with or without palate. In: Bergsma D (ed.), *Birth Defects Compendium*. Wiley & Sons, New York, p. 222.
26. Morris HL, Bardach J, Ardinger H, Jones D, Kelly KM, Olin WH, Wheeler J. (1993) Multidisciplinary treatment results for patients with isolated cleft palate. *Plast Reconstr Surg* **92**: 842–851.
27. Jones MC. (1993) Facial clefting. Etiology and developmental pathogenesis. *Clin Plast Surg* **20**: 599–606.
28. Eastman JR, Bixler D, Escobar V. (1978) Linkage studies in Van der Woude syndrome. *J Med Genet* **15**: 217–218.
29. Burdick AB. (1986) Genetic epidemiology and control of genetic expression in Van der Woude syndrome. *J Craniofac Genet Dev Biol Suppl* **2**: 99–105.
30. Janku P, Robinow M, Kelly T, Bralley R, Baynes A, Edgerton MT. (1980) The Van der Woude syndrome in a large kindred: variability, penetrance, genetic risks. *Am J Med Genet* **5**: 117–123.
31. Vander Volk CA, Menezes J. (2006) Craniofacial syndromes. In: Mathes SJ (ed.), *Plastic Surgery*. Saunders Elsevier, Philadelphia, pp. 91–112.
32. Wilhelmsen HR, Musgrave RH. (1966) Complications of cleft lip surgery. *Cleft Palate J* **3**: 223–231.
33. Tessier P, Rougier J, Mervouet F, Woillez M, Lekieffre M, Derome B. (1981) *Plastic Surgery of the Orbits and Eyelids*. Masson Publishing, New York.
34. Noordhoff MS, Chen PKT. (2006) Unilateral chelioplasty. In: Mathes SJ (ed.), *Plastic Surgery*. Saunders Elsevier, Philadelphia.
35. Witt PD, Hardesty RA. (1993) Rotation-advancement repair of the unilateral cleft lip. One center's perspective. *Clin Plast Surg* **20**: 633–645.
36. Randall P, Garham WP. (1971) Lip adhesion in the repair of bilateral cleft lip. In: Grabb WC, Rosenstein SW, Bzoch KR (eds.), *Cleft Lip and Palate*. Little Brown, Boston, p. 282.
37. Millard DR Jr, Latham RA. (1990) Improved primary surgical and dental treatment of clefts. *Plast Reconstr Surg* **86**: 856–871.
38. Henkel KO, Gundlach KK. (1997) Analysis of primary gingivoperiosteoplasty in alveolar cleft repair. Part I: facial growth. *J Craniomaxillofac Surg* **25**: 266–269.

39. Santiago PE, Grayson BH, Cutting CB, Gianoutsos MP, Brecht LE, Kwon SM. (1998) Reduced need for alveolar bone grafting by presurgical orthopedics and primary gingivoperiosteoplasty. *Cleft Palate Craniofac J* **35**: 77–80.
40. Cutting CB. (2006) Bilateral cleft lip repair. In: Mathes SJ (ed.), *Plastic Surgery*. Saunders Elsevier, Philadelphia, pp. 217–247.
41. Trotman CA, Long RE Jr., Rosenstein SW, Murphy C, Johnston LE Jr. (1996) Comparison of facial form in primary alveolar bone-grafted and non-grafted unilateral cleft lip and palate patients: intercenter retrospective study. *Cleft Palate Craniofac J* **33**: 91–95.
42. Canady JW, Zeitler DP, Thompson SA, Nicholas CD. (1993) Suitability of the iliac crest as a site for harvest of autogenous bone grafts. *Cleft Palate Craniofac J* **30**: 579–581.
43. Sadove AM, Nelson CL, Eppley BL, Nguyen B. (1990) An evaluation of calvarial and iliac donor sites in alveolar cleft grafting. *Cleft Palate J* **27**: 225–228; discussion 229.
44. LaRossa D, Buchman S, Rothkopf DM, Mayro R, Randall P. (1995) A comparison of iliac and cranial bone in secondary grafting of alveolar clefts. *Plast Reconstr Surg* **96**: 789–797; discussion 798–789.
45. Semb G. (1988) Effect of alveolar bone grafting on maxillary growth in unilateral cleft lip and palate patients. *Cleft Palate J* **25**: 288–295.
46. Millard DR, Latham R, Huifen X, Spiro S, Morovic C. (1999) Cleft lip and palate treated by presurgical orthopedics, gingivoperiosteoplasty, and lip adhesion (POPLA) compared with previous lip adhesion method: a preliminary study of serial dental casts. *Plast Reconstr Surg* **103**: 1630–1644.
47. Lukash FN, Schwartz M, Grauer S, Tuminelli F. (1998) Dynamic cleft maxillary orthopedics and periosteoplasty: benefit or detriment? *Ann Plast Surg* **40**: 321–326; discussion 326–327.
48. Sato Y, Grayson BH, Garfinkle JS, Barillas I, Maki K, Cutting CB. (2008) Success rate of gingivoperiosteoplasty with and without secondary bone grafts compared with secondary alveolar bone grafts alone. *Plast Reconstr Surg* **121**: 1356–1367; discussion 1368–1359.
49. Rose W. (1891) *Harelip and Cleft Palate.* HK Lewis, London.
50. Thompson JE. (1912) An artistic and mathematically accurate method of repairing the defect in cases of harelip. *Surg Gynecol Obstet* **14**: 498.
51. Tennison CW. (1952) The repair of the unilateral cleft lip by the stencil method. *Plast Reconstr Surg (1946)* **9**: 115–120.
52. Randall P. (1959) A triangular flap operation for the primary repair of unilateral clefts of the lip. *Plast Reconstr Surg Transplant Bull* **23**: 331–347.

53. Millard DR. (1976) *Cleft Craft: The Evolution of Its Surgery*. Little, Brown, Boston.
54. Thorne C, Grabb WC, Smith JW. (2007) *Grabb and Smith's Plastic Surgery*. Wolters Kluwer Health/Lippincott Williams & Wilkins, Philadelphia.
55. Sitzman TJ, Girotto JA, Marcus JR. (2008) Current surgical practices in cleft care: unilateral cleft lip repair. *Plast Reconstr Surg* **121**: 261e–270e.
56. Noordhoff MS. (1984) Reconstruction of vermilion in unilateral and bilateral cleft lips. *Plast Reconstr Surg* **73**: 52–61.
57. Mohler LR. (1987) Unilateral cleft lip repair. *Plast Reconstr Surg* **80**: 511–517.
58. Onizuka T. (1980) A new method for the primary repair of unilateral cleft lip. *Ann Plast Surg* **4**: 516–524.
59. Onizuka T, Ichinose M, Hosaka Y, Usui Y, Jinnai T. (1991) The contour lines of the upper lip and a revised method of cleft lip repair. *Ann Plast Surg* **27**: 238–252.
60. Millard DR. (1968) Extensions of the rotation-advancement principle for wide unilateral cleft lips. *Plast Reconstr Surg* **42**: 535–544.
61. Millard DR Jr. (1964) Refinements in rotation-advancement cleft lip technique. *Plast Reconstr Surg* **33**: 26–38.
62. Stal S, Brown RH, Higuera S, Hollier LH Jr, Byrd HS, Cutting CB, Mulliken JB. (2009) Fifty years of the Millard rotation-advancement: looking back and moving forward. *Plast Reconstr Surg* **123**: 1364–1377.
63. Millard DR Jr. (1971) Closure of bilateral cleft lip and elongation of columella by two operations in infancy. *Plast Reconstr Surg* **47**: 324–331.
64. Mulliken JB, Martinez-Perez D. (1999) The principle of rotation advancement for repair of unilateral complete cleft lip and nasal deformity: technical variations and analysis of results. *Plast Reconstr Surg* **104**: 1247–1260.
65. Broadbent TR, Woolf RM. (1974) Bilateral cleft lip: one-stage primary repair. In: Georgiade NG (ed.), *Symposium on Management of Cleft Lip and Palate and Associated Deformities*. CV Mosby, St. Louis.
66. McComb H. (1990) Primary repair of the bilateral cleft lip nose: a 15-year review and a new treatment plan. *Plast Reconstr Surg* **86**: 882–889; discussion 890–883.
67. McComb H. (1994) Primary repair of the bilateral cleft lip nose: a 4-year review. *Plast Reconstr Surg* **94**: 37–47; discussion 48–50.
68. McComb HK. (2009) Primary repair of the bilateral cleft lip nose: a long-term follow-up. *Plast Reconstr Surg* **124**: 1610–1615.
69. Noordhoff MS. (1986) Bilateral cleft lip reconstruction. *Plast Reconstr Surg* **78**: 45–54.

70. Mulliken JB. (1995) Bilateral complete cleft lip and nasal deformity: an anthropometric analysis of staged to synchronous repair. *Plast Reconstr Surg* **96**: 9–23; discussion 24–26.
71. Dorf DS, Curtin JW. (1982) Early cleft palate repair and speech outcome. *Plast Reconstr Surg* **70**: 74–81.
72. Rohrich RJ, Love EJ, Byrd HS, Johns DF. (2000) Optimal timing of cleft palate closure. *Plast Reconstr Surg* **106**: 413–421; quiz 422; discussion 423–415.
73. Witzel MA, Salyer KE, Ross RB. (1984) Delayed hard palate closure: the philosophy revisited. *Cleft Palate J* **21**: 263–269.
74. Cosman B, Falk AS. (1980) Delayed hard palate repair and speech deficiencies: a cautionary report. *Cleft Palate J* **17**: 27–33.
75. Katzel EB, Basile P, Koltz PF, Marcus JR, Girotto JA. (2009) Current surgical practices in cleft care: cleft palate repair techniques and postoperative care. *Plast Reconstr Surg* **124**: 899–906.
76. Wray C, Dann J, HoSltmann B. (1979) A comparison of three technics of palatorrhaphy: in-hospital morbidity. *Cleft Palate J* **16**: 42–45.
77. Delaire J, Precious D. (1985) Avoidance of the use of vomerine mucosa in primary surgical management of velopalatine clefts. *Oral Surg Oral Med Oral Pathol* **60**: 589–597.
78. Gunther E, Wisser JR, Cohen MA, Brown AS. (1998) Palatoplasty: Furlow's double reversing Z-plasty versus intravelar veloplasty. *Cleft Palate Craniofac J* **35**: 546–549.

CHAPTER 9

ESSENTIALS IN PLASTIC SURGERY MICROTIA CHAPTER

Kenneth L. Fan, Raja Mohan and Seth R. Thaller

Illustrative Case

Background information

Auricular Anatomy

Ear is composed of a delicate and complicated cartilaginous structure, covered by a thin, adherent, and hairless epithelial curtain. Intricate

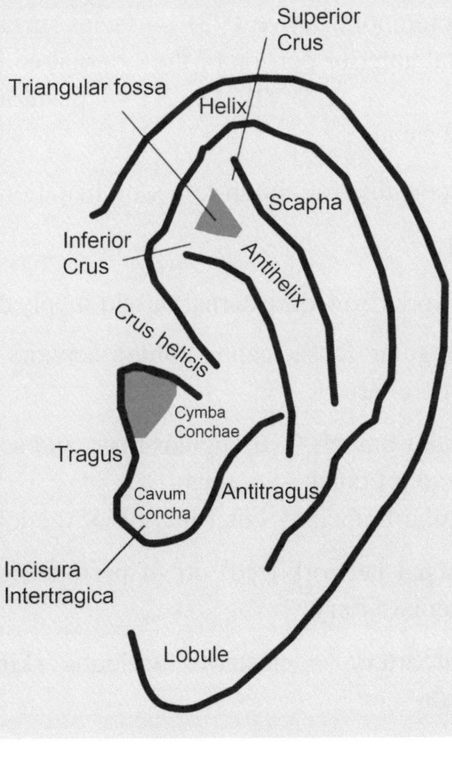

framework is composed of three primary keystones: conchal, antihelix-antitragus, and the helix-lobule complex. On a vertical axis, the auricle lies between the upper orbit and nasal spine. Horizontally, it is situated 5.5 to 7 cm posterior to the lateral orbit rim. Auricle's long axis is at 21 to 30 degrees from the cranium. It possesses a 50 to 60% width to length ratio. Less than two centimeters should lie between the helix and the skill. Inferior pole of the helix should project more than the superior counterpart. Projection from the rim to the mastoid is superiorly 10–12 mm, midear 16–18 mm, and 20–22 mm inferiorly.[1]

- Innervation[1]
    - Greater auricular nerve (C2-C3) — inferior cranial surface and lower lateral external surface innervations.
    - Lesser occipital nerve (C2-3) — superior cranial surface of the ear.
    - Auriculotemporal nerve (V3) — facial surface of the upper ear along and anterior portion of the external auditor canal.
    - Arnold's nerve (CN VII, IX, X) — posterior, inferior external auditory canal.
        - Responsible for cough reflex on irritation.
- Blood supply[1,2]
    - Two networks from the external carotid supply the majority of the ear
        - Triangular fossa-scapha (blue) network off the superficial temporal artery
- Upper auricular branch — triangular fossa and scapha
- Middle auricular branch — tragus
- Lower auricular branch — outer margin of the lobule
        - Conchal network (red) off of perforators from the posterior auricular artery
    - Occipital artery — posterior auricular skin in a minority of population

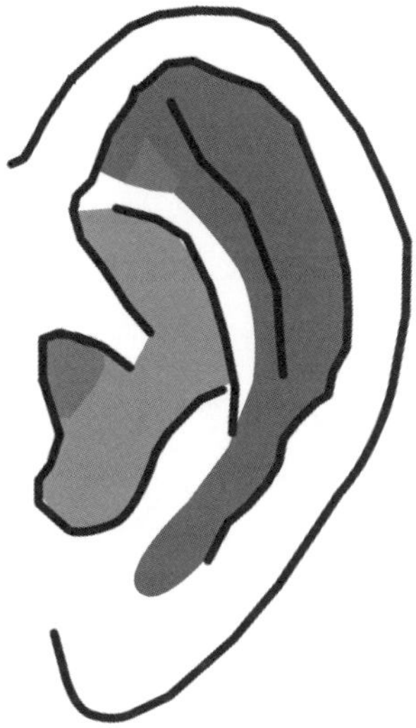

- Communication between STA and PAA allows either network to support the ear

- Venous drainage[1,2]
  - Posterior auricular veins draining into the jugular vein — posterior aspect
  - Superficial temporal and retromandibular veins — anterior and superior regions of the ear

- Lymphatic drainage
  - Follows embryological development
  - Tragus, root of the helix, superior helix (first branchial arch) — parotid and infraclavicular nodes
  - Antihelix, antitragus, lobule (second branchial arch) — mastoid and superior cervical nodes
  - Important in cutaneous carcinoma, but not always predictible

- Muscles
  - Extrinsic muscles — anterior, superior, and posterior auricularis muscles

- Intrinsic muscles — largely vestigial remanents
  - Helicis major and minor, tragicus, antitragicus
  - Intrinsic transverse and oblique muscles are found on the cranial surface

- Three tiers of cartilage

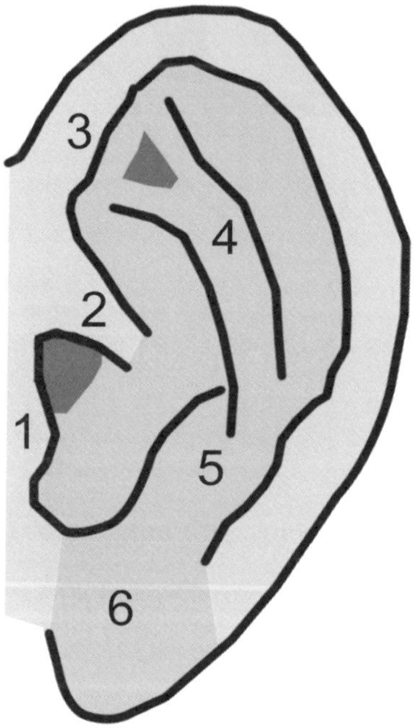

- Helical-lobular complex
- Antihelical-antitragal complex
- Conchal complex

Embryology[2,3]

- Commences development in the 3rd to 6th week of life, completed by 12 weeks
- External ear

- 6 hillocks from the 1st (mandibular) and 2nd (hyoid) pharyngeal arches
  - 1st arch (Figure, green) gives rise to anterior three hillocks to form tragus, helical root, and superior helix
  - 2nd arch (Figure, peach) gives rise to posterior three hillocks to form the antihelix, antitragus, and lobule
- Microtia arises from suppression or failure of hillock development
  - Accessory tags arise from accessory hillocks

- External auditory meatus/eardrum/middle ear
  - External auditory meatus derives from the first pharyngeal groove between the first and second pharyngeal arches during the 6th week
  - Eardrum forms from the thin membrane separating the first pharyngeal groove and arch
  - Middle ear forms from the first pharyngeal arch beginning at 4 weeks, completed by 30 weeks
    - Malleus and incus develop from the cartilage of the first pharyngeal arch beginning at 8 weeks, ossified by 4 months
    - Stapes forms from the second pharyngeal arch in a similar time line, except for the medial lamina of the footplate of the stapes, which is developed from the otic capsule

- Inner ear
  - Inner ear developed from the otic placode, a small patch of ectodermal cells stimulated through interactions from adjacent hindbrain and underlying mesenchyme
    - Otic placode appears at the level of the hindbrain and eventually develops into the inner ear during the 4th and 7th weeks of development
    - Because of separate embryologic origins, the inner ear is almost always intact during microtia, with conductive hearing loss being the major sensory defect
  - Mastoid air cells develop after birth

Epidemiology and Genetics[2–4]

- Prevalence of microtia — 0.8–4.2 per 10,000
  - Most often found in men at a ratio of 1.5
  - Higher incidence of Hispanics and Asians than African or Caucasian
- Unilateral microtia occurs 79–93% of the time, more often in the right ear
  - Hearing in contralateral ear is maintained, but children have higher risk of language delay and attention deficit disorder
- 55–93% have atresia or stenosis of the ear canal
  - Aural atresia leads to conductive hearing loss, usually reduced 40–65 dB, seen in 80–90% of cases
- Sensory loss is found in 10–15% of patients[4]
- Anotia and microtia associated with certain congenital deformities to variable degrees[2]
  - 30% — facial cleft and cardiac defects
  - 14% — anopthalmia/micropthamlia
  - 11% — limb reductions of renal malformations
  - 7% — holoprosencephaly
- Familial inheritance occurs in 3–34% of cases
  - Many modes of inheritance proposed: autosomal recessive or dominant with variable expression and incomplete penetrance
  - Possible each represents different processes leading to similar phenotypic outcome
  - Both single gene and chromosomal abberations reported in different microtia associated syndromes
- Syndromes associated with microtia
  - Oculoauriculovertebral dysplasia
    - Spectrum ranging from isolated microtia to full blown Goldenhar's syndrome

    - Defects in first and second branchial arch derivatives, leading to hemifacial microsomia, ocular malformations, and vertebral defects

  - Goldenhar's syndrome
  - Treacher Collins syndrome — associated with bilateral microtia
  - CHARGE
  - Klippel-Feil syndrome
  - Walker-Warburg syndrome
  - Meir Gorlin syndrome

- Significantly associated with hemifacial microsomia

  - Findings include asymmetry of the lower face leading to aural, oral, and mandibular development malformation
  - Tanzer found 50% of his patients with microtia had evidence of hemifacial microsomia[5,6]

    - Defects as hypoplasia of the adjacent malar and maxillary bones, poor mandibular development, facial hemiatrophy, asymmetry of the skull, and facial nerve paresis[7]

  - Many shared characteristics exist between microtia and hemifacial microsomia, including asymmetrical nature, right sided associaton, facial nerve pariesis, and male prediliction

    - Some propose microtia is in a spectrum along with hemifacial microsomia, both of which is localized to pathology in the first and second branchial arch[8]

Management and Preoperative Tests

Evaluation

- Usually evaluation by both plastic surgeon and otologist occurs within 12 months of age
- Initial assessment includes family history of syndromic disease and/or microtia
- Complete physical examination should document structure of ear and facial symmetry is necessary

- Presence of tragus has been associated as an indication of a functional middle ear
  - However, middle ear abnormality does not correlate well to the degree of external malformation probably because the middle ear is formed later embryologically than the external ear
- In the case of the atretic external ear, the presence of middle ear and cholesteatoma, squamous epithelium trapped in the middle ear, must be evaluated

- Audiologic studies can identify conductive and sensorineural hearing loss
- High resolution CT scan of the temporal bone can evaluate the middle ear ossicle and identify middle ear cleft — axial and coronal planes are necessary to assess middle ear development
- MRI can be used to determine the course of the facial nerve, often displaced in middle ear abnormalities

Classification Systems

- Marx/Meurman classification[8–10]
  - Devised by Marx[11] and later modified by Meurman[9]
  - Described microtia according to the vestigial remnants present and observation
  - **Grade I microtia** — retained all structures but with variable degrees of hypoplasia of the auricle with cupping and external auditory stenosis
  - **Grade II microtia** — missing anatomic subunits
    - Variable hypoplasia of the concha, often accompanied with the absence of the external auditory canal
  - **Grade III microtia** — classic "peanut" ear
    - Auricle is absent, with abnormal shaped and malpositioned lobule
  - **Grade IV microtia** — anotia, most severe; complete absence of outer ear

- Nagata classification[10]
  - Devised based on the type of surgical correction needed for each deformity
  - **Anotia type** — most severe, complete absence of the external ear
  - **Lobule type** — sausage-shaped remnant ear and lobule with no acoustic meatus, conchus, or tragus
  - **Concha type** — lobule, concha with or without the acoustic meatus, tragus, and intertragal notch are all present but with varying degrees of deformity
  - **Small concha type** — small indentation instead of the concha; lobule and remnant ear present
  - **Atypical type** — those that do not fit in any other category

Presurgical Preparations

Surgical Planning[2]

- Timing
  - Contralateral ear continues to grow until 10 years old, but 85% of ear development will be attained by 3 years old
  - Rib cartilage is not sufficient for necessary carving until 5–6 years old
  - Brent recommends repair at 4–6 year old, before first grade, to save patient for peer ridicule, but allow sufficient time for costal cartilage to develop and for psychological maturation[12]
- Some surgeons found the psychological stresses of few extra years until 9–10 are handled without difficulty, with added benefit of patient cooperation[13]
  - Nagata delayed repair until 10 years old, or at least 60 cm chest secondary to the large amount of cartilage needed for the procedure[10]
- Construct size

- Autologous cartilage construct grows at a rate comparable to the contralateral ear, except in the youngest patient
- Tanzer recommends making reconstructed ear 2 mm larger than normal ear in children less than 8 years old. Found cartilage constructs in 50% of patients 6 to 7 years old lagged behind in growth[6]
- Brent recommends creating construct to match the opposite ear, except in the youngest patient where costal cartilage growth is expected to accelerate faster than auricular cartilage based on findings that young children on follow up: 48.1% of ears grow at the same rate, 41.6% grew several millimeters larger, and 10.3% lagged behind the normal side[12]
  - A few mm for the skin envelope must be taken into account

- Preoperative molding
  - Must predesign framework X-ray film of the contralateral ear
  - Consider thickness of skin envelope by substracting a few mm off the framework
  - Tolleth described ideal auricle proportions[14]
- Middle ear surgery
  - Auricular reconstruction is ideally performed before middle ear surgery to ensure good skin covering over cartilaginous construct
  - Done to restore binaural hearing for improved speech and sound localization
  - Results are less than satisfactory, due to reliance on the nondefected ear and lack of binaural circuitry development,[2] although some results indicate possibility of plasticity affording middle ear hearing[15]
  - Despite experience, high stenosis rate of the external auditory canal[16]
  - Coordination with otologist in middle ear surgery is necessary

Operative Techniques

While ear reconstruction has been attempted for ages, Tanzer is credited with developing modern autologous ear reconstruction. His procedure, published in 1959, utilized autologous costal cartilage for microtia reconstruction in a 4-staged procedure as follows[5–7]:

- Rotation of the lobule horizontally into a transverse position
- Fabrication and insertion of new cartilage framework
- Elevation of the ear away from the head, and superior, posterior, and inferior conchal wall construction
- Forming of the tragus and conchal floor

Brent Reconstruction[12]

Building on the principles set forth by Tanzer, many surgeons perfected the art of ear reconstruction. Brent devised a 4 staged procedure spaced over 3 months. In his two decade experience on microtia, he reported excellent results with constructed ears growing at the same pace as the natural ear, able to with stand trauma, and a greater than 80% satisfaction rate among 621 reconstructed ears, with a low complication rate.[12] Main criticisms are the number of stages, lack of definition, difficulty achieving perfect contours, and poor tragus outcome.[17] Composite cartilage and skin graft comprising the tragus may contract, diminishing the tragus and occasionally causing eversion.[16] Scarring and contraction of the skin graft covering the auriculocephalic junction can cause decreased projection.[18] Although, this issue can be partially mitigated with coverage of thicker skin grafts.

Stage 1 — Framework construction and placement

- Placement[12,19]
  - Determined by mimicking the contralateral ear. It's relationship to the lateral canthus and nose along with lobule position
  - In the case of hemifacial microsomia, use the superior pole of the contralateral ear instead of the lateral canthus as a landmark
  - Constructed ear can be placed halfway between vestige and contralateral helical root's location
  - Do not sacrafice position of the ear to avoid the hairline on the apex of the ear

        - Brent uses electrolysis or skin grafting if extensive hair coverage exits

- Donor site
    - Cartilage for the framework base obtained from the contralateral synchondrotic region of ribs 6 and 7 for its inherent tapering shape
    - Helix harvested from floating eight rib
    - Superficial perichondrium is harvested along with graft to promote survival and adherence to the graft site
    - Posterior perichondroium is left at donor site to help cartilaginous regeneration at the donor site

- Pocket
    - Thin cutaneous pocket created via undermining posterior inferior border of the vestige incision
    - Borders of undermining need to be wide to recruit skin for tension free closure, but does not disrupt the subdermal vascular plexus
        - Blanching of the skin coverage signifies excess skin tension
        - Brent describes using intraoperative expansion to stretch the skin in such situations

Stage 2 — Lobule reconstruction

- Several months after the first stage, the lobule is reconstructed by mobilizing the lobule remnant, often times as an inferiorly based flap into the inferior pole of the previously placed auricular framework
- Done as a secondary procedure, distinct from Tanzer's steps
- Framework construction and placement is done before lobule reconstruction to reduce the risk of vascular compromise

Stage 3 — Framework elevation and creation of auricular cephalic sulcus

- In this stage, the ear is separated from the head
- Split thickness graft is added to define the ear's posterosuperior margin, after retroauricular scalp is advanced and fixed

- Banked rib cartilage can be used to achieve greater projection of the auricle. Occipitalis fascia is used to cover the graft.[19]
  - Cartilage may be banked underneath the chest incision or underneath the scalp, posterior to the site of the framework

Stage 4 — Tragus reconstruction and conchal excavation

- Tragus is constructed from a conchal composite graft in the contralateral ear, if a deep concha exists
  - If ears are symmetrical or the concha are not prominent, donor cartilage can be grafted elsewhere
- Cartilage is inserted via a J-shaped incision along the posterior tragal margin
- Excess tissue in the conchal floor removed to simulate the auditory meatus
- Brent also described methods in which tragus was added to the original framework{{219 Brent,B. 1999; }}
  - Beneficial in bilateral microtia patients were concha grafts are unavailable

Nagata Reconstruction[10,20–23]

Nagata's procedure is more complicated. It consists of less steps than Brent's technique. It is based on an original framework based on the helix, crura, antihelix, conchal elements, incisura intertargica, and tragus. One of the benefits is the simultaneous rotation of the lobule and emphasis on definition of the incisura intertragica, crus helices, and antitragus.[10] His technique creates a more natural conchal bowl and tragus. The deep, dramatic framework, creates a more natural appearing tragus. Conchal excavation is not required. Depth is created by removing the remnant ear cartilage and forming a high wall with the surrounding structures. In follow up of 7 years with 36 patients, showed excellent results on follow-up. There was no infection, no deformities, no cartilage exposures or wire penetration/extrusion.[10]

Criticisms include the significant amount of cartilage required. This leads to anterior chest deformities. Leaving the perichondrium intact and creating 2–3 mm blocks with left over cartilage to fill dead space leads to histologically sufficient regeneration of cartilage and decreased chest wall deformity.[24] Combined first stage lobular translocation and framework placement can lead to compromised flap circulation and necrosis. This is especially the case in the posterior lobular flap. A high extrusion rate is seen due to the use of wire sutures. Although, this can be avoided by burying the loop of the wire. Other authors advocate a less natural tragus versus Brent's technique sacrifices the posterior lobule skin to line the concha and the underside of the tragus.[13] Finally, the use of the temporoparietal fascia to cover the semilunar cartilage graft in the second stage can lead to scalp scarring and hair thinning.[16] More experience is required for this challenging technique.[17]

Stage 1 — Framework construction with tragus, placement, and lobule transposition

- Framework/donor site
  - Ipsilateral costal cartilage graft vs contralateral in Brent technique
  - Helix and crus helics are generated from ipsilateral ninth costal cartilage
  - Baseframe, antihelix, and tragus/incisura intertragica are generated from seventh and eighth costal cartilage
  - In concha type microtia, with lobule, tragus, and concha retained, inferior and tragal portions of framework are left out
  - Pieces fixed on the base frame with 38 gauge wire at intervals of 3 mm
- Pocket creation/framework placement
  - Nagata utilizes a W-shaped incision for maximum width and surface area to increase amount of skin coverage for the framework, avoiding skin grafting versus Tanzer's V-shaped incision[6]

        - Three flaps are created: posterior and anterior skin flaps of the lobule, anterior skin flap of the tragus
    - A "closure cone", a 2 mm circular portion of skin, is created at the anterior terminus of the incision, near the inferior portion of the tragus to facilitate the shape of the incisura intertragica[16]
        - The area is undermined 1.5–2.0 mm to maintain the subdermal vascular plexus for incertion of the framework
    - Remnant cartilage is removed according to the Nagata classification (see next section)
    - The middle peak of the W is the approximate location of the subcutaneous pedicle, left attached for blood supply, this area forming the incisura intertragica. Flanking regions are sutured forming a cone protecting the pedicle.
    - Undermining proceeds 1 cm beyond outline area of the auricle
    - Concha simulated by removal of the remnant ear cartilage, and constructing high walls in the surrounding structures
    - With the tragal end of the framework facing posteriorly, hook the subcutaneous pedicle and rotate framework into place.
    - Suture line should extend from the anterior portion of the crus helices, into the tragus's outer edge, incisura intertragica, antitragus, and caudal end of the helix
- Nuances of technique exists for each Nagata microtia classification[20–23]
    - Smaller W is used in the concha type microtia due to smaller surface area requirement
        - Only upper framework needs to be inserted
    - Small concha and lobular type, cartilage is removed completely to allow for the depth of conchal depression and skin draping over the framework

Stage 2 — Framework elevation and creation of auricular cephalic sulcus

- Performed 6 months after implantation of the three-dimensional frame

- Framework is freed using a 5 mm incision posterior and superior to the helical rim[13]
- Nagata introduced use of semilunar cartilage graft, 1 cm wide created from the 6th cartilage using previous incision, placed into the sulcus mimicking a posterior conchal wall
    - Cartilage prevents collapse of elevated ear
- Pedicled temporoparietal fascial flap is created to cover semilunar cartilage graft via a subcutaneous tunnel
    - Fascial flap strengthens circulation of the posterior ear, preventing necrosis, resorption of frame, and contraction of the grafted skin
- Defect created by elevation is covered by a a full thickness skin graft

Nonautologous frameworks

- Advantage of elimination of donor site morbidity, as visible deformities in the anterior chest wall with cartilage
- Silastic (combination plastic/silicone)
    - Initially advocated due to positive initial aesthetic result.
    - Long term result indicated spontaneous exposure and failure of implant
    - Brent noticed loss of silicone ear even after mild trauma 12 years after implantation[12]
    - Abaondoned by many surgeons[2]
- Porous polyethylene framework
    - 7% exposure rate on 12 year follow up[25]
    - yet to be widely adopted

Postoperative Care

- Suction drainage is utilized to reduce dead space, avoid hematoma and secondary fibrosis. It also improves overlying skin coaptation and anatomical contours[12,17]

- Tube change every few hours during the first day, then 4–6 there after or when 1/3 full[12,16]
- Drains to be left in for 5 days or until discharge cease

- Careful monitoring of the skin flap is necssary
- Bandages should comprise of Vaseline gauze and noncompressive
    - Compressive garments can cause ischemia and is contraindicated
    - Parents should not be allowed to change ear dressings due to possibility of overly tight reapplication and cartilaginous exposure[12]
    - Dressing removal after 12 days
- Sports and running restricted for 4–5 weeks[12]
- Brent allows patients to participate in sports without conspicuous headgear[12]

Summary

Microtia repair represents one of the most challenging plastic surgery procedures. Difficulty in coordinating age, donor site morbidity, delicate framework sculpting while balancing soft tissue forces make microtia repair a difficult science and art. The highly complex nature demands experience and expertise. This can only be achieved through dedicated practice and adequate caseload. Inexperienced surgeon should not attempt to perform such reconstruction without appropriate experienced guidance.

References

1. Mohan R, Fan K, Iyer R, Thaller S. (2010) *Microtia*. http://www.plasticsurgery.hyperguides.com/tutorial.asp?tid=41470. Accessed February 21, 2010.
2. Beahm EK, Walton RL. (2002) Auricular reconstruction for microtia: part I. Anatomy, embryology, and clinical evaluation. *Plast Reconstr Surg* **109**(7): 2473–2482; quiz following 2482.
3. Alasti F, Van Camp G. (2009) Genetics of microtia and associated syndromes. *J Med Genet* **46**(6): 361–369.

4. Carvalho GJ, Song CS, Vargervik K, Lalwani AK. (1999) Auditory and facial nerve dysfunction in patients with hemifacial microsomia. *Arch Otolaryngol Head Neck Surg* **125**(2): 209–212.
5. Tanzer RC. (1978) Microtia. *Clin Plast Surg* **5**(3): 317–336.
6. Tanzer RC. (1978) Microtia — a long-term follow-up of 44 reconstructed auricles. *Plast Reconstr Surg* **61**(2): 161–166.
7. Tanzer RC. (1959) Total reconstruction of the external ear. *Plast Reconstr Surg Transplant Bull* **23**(1): 1–15.
8. Bennun RD, Mulliken JB, Kaban LB, Murray JE. (1985) Microtia: a microform of hemifacial microsomia. *Plast Reconstr Surg* **76**(6): 859–865.
9. Meurman Y. (1957) Congenital microtia and meatal atresia; observations and aspects of treatment. *AMA Arch Otolaryngol* **66**(4): 443–463.
10. Nagata S. (1993) A new method of total reconstruction of the auricle for microtia. *Plast Reconstr Surg* **92**(2): 187–201.
11. Marx H. (1926) Die missbildungen des ohres: sekundare ohrmissbildugen. In: Springer-Verlag (ed.), *Handbuch des Speziellen Pathologischen Anatomie und Histologie.* Springer-Verlag, Berlin, Vol. 12, p. 697.
12. Brent B. (1992) Auricular repair with autogenous rib cartilage grafts: two decades of experience with 600 cases. *Plast Reconstr Surg* **90**(3): 355–374; discussion 375–356.
13. Bauer BS. (2009) Reconstruction of microtia. *Plast Reconstr Surg* **124** (1 Suppl): 14e–26e.
14. Tolleth H. (1978) Artistic anatomy, dimensions, and proportions of the external ear. *Clin Plast Surg* **5**: 337.
15. Wilmington D, Gray L, Jahrsdoerfer R. (1994) Binaural processing after corrected congenital unilateral conductive hearing loss. *Hear Res* **74**(1–2): 99–114.
16. Walton RL, Beahm EK. (2002) Auricular reconstruction for microtia: part II. Surgical techniques. *Plast Reconstr Surg* **110**(1): 234–249; quiz 250–231, 387.
17. Firmin F. (1998) Ear reconstruction in cases of typical microtia. Personal experience based on 352 microtic ear corrections. *Scand J Plast Reconstr Surg Hand Surg* **32**(1): 35–47.
18. Kizhner V, Barak A. (2008) Framework changes using costal cartilage for microtia reconstruction. *Arch Otolaryngol Head Neck Surg* **134**(7): 768–770.
19. Brent B. (1999) Technical advances in ear reconstruction with autogenous rib cartilage grafts: personal experience with 1200 cases. *Plast Reconstr Surg* **104**(2): 319–334; discussion 335–318.

20. Nagata S. (1994) Modification of the stages in total reconstruction of the auricle: part IV. Ear elevation for the constructed auricle. *Plast Reconstr Surg* **93**(2): 254–266; discussion 267–258.
21. Nagata S. (1994) Modification of the stages in total reconstruction of the auricle: part III. Grafting the three-dimensional costal cartilage framework for small concha-type microtia. *Plast Reconstr Surg* **93**(2): 243–253; discussion 267–248.
22. Nagata S. (1994) Modification of the stages in total reconstruction of the auricle: part II. Grafting the three-dimensional costal cartilage framework for concha-type microtia. *Plast Reconstr Surg* **93**(2): 231–242; discussion 267–238.
23. Nagata S. (1994) Modification of the stages in total reconstruction of the auricle: part I. Grafting the three-dimensional costal cartilage framework for lobule-type microtia. *Plast Reconstr Surg* **93**(2): 221–230; discussion 267–228.
24. Kawanabe Y, Nagata S. (2007) A new method of costal cartilage harvest for total auricular reconstruction: part II. Evaluation and analysis of the regenerated costal cartilage. *Plast Reconstr Surg* **119**(1): 308–315.
25. Reinisch JF, Lewin S. (2009) Ear reconstruction using a porous polyethylene framework and temporoparietal fascia flap. *Facial Plast Surg* **25**(3): 181–189.

CHAPTER 10

HEAD AND NECK MALIGNANCY

David Nesky and Donald Weed

Illustrative Case

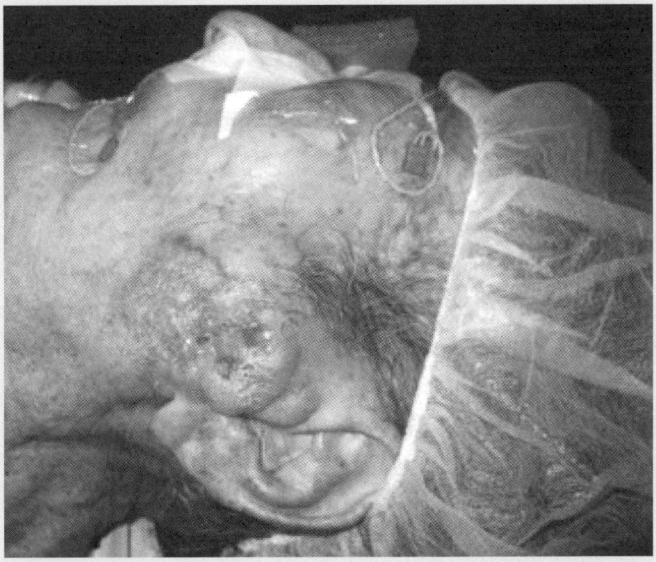

Fig. 1. Preoperative image of left temporal squamous cell carcinoma (previously excised and not pictured) with metastasis to left parotid gland.

History of Present Illness: 82 year old male with history of Mohs' excision of left forehead squamous cell carcinoma approximately six months ago presents with a firm preauricular mass measuring approximately 6×7 cm in diameter (Fig. 1).

Past Medical History: Diabetes mellitus, hypertension, cerebral vascular accident in 2004.

Past Surgical History: Several cutaneous excisions including right medial brow and right nasal ala. Coronary bypass surgery in 1967.

Social: Former smoker quit over 30 years ago.

Physical Exam:
Cranial Nerves: II–XII grossly intact, symmetric facial nerve function.
Skin: Significant solar damage with numerous actinic kerotoses. Well healed incision of left temporal region.
Face and Neck: Firm mass in preauricular region overlying the region of the facial nerve trunk measuring 6 × 7 cm. Palpable left level II lymph node measuring 3 cm in greatest diameter.
Oral Cavity and Oropharynx: Edentulous otherwise unremarkable.
Flexible Endoscopy: Oropharynx, larynx, and hypopharynx unremarkable.

Evaluation and Management

Initial evaluation of any cutaneous head and neck malignancy begins with a thorough history and examination including a fiberoptic exam of nasopharynx, oropharynx, hyopopharynx and larynx. A history of previous cutaneous surgeries must be obtained since between 50–60% of patients with regional disease from cutaneous malignancy have already had the primary lesion treated.[1] During the examination attention should be focused on identifying other synchronous cutaneous lesions and on bilateral parotid and cervical lymph node basins. If a parotid mass is identified, an assessment should be made not only of fixation to the external auditory canal but also of facial nerve function.

The majority of cutaneous squamous cell carcinoma (SCC) of the head and neck are low risk with less than 5% developing metastases to regional lymph nodes.[1] Although the overall incidence of regional metastases is low for cutaneous SCC, patients at higher risk for parotid involvement can be identified based on several clinicopathologic factors (Table 1).[2,3] In addition to identifying higher risk patients, it is essential to understand the lymphatic drainage pattern of the head and neck in order to effectively manage the regional lymph node basins (Fig. 2).

Table 1. High-risk Clinicopathologic Factors of Cutaneous SCC Associated with Increased Incidence of Regional Metastases.

Unfavorable Primary Lesion	Patient Factors
Tumor thickness >4–5 mm	Immunosuppression
Large size >1.5–2 cm	Advanced age
Local recurrence	
Perineural invasion	
Lymphovascular invasion	
Overexpression of EGFR	

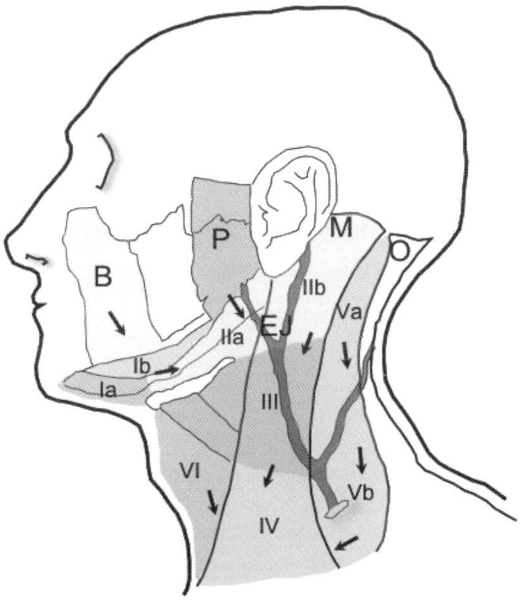

Fig. 2. Lymphatic drainage pattern of the face and scalp. B: Buccal, P: Parotid, M: Mastoid, O: Occipital, EJ: External jugular. Cutaneous lesions anterior to the auricle typically drain via main lymphatic pathway, starting within the parotid or buccal lymph nodes and progressing to level IIA. Once the upper jugular nodes are reached, lymph progresses to level III and IV.[11] Lymph associated with cutaneous lesions posterior to the auricle including the posterior scalp typically drain via the occipital and mastoid nodes. These first tier lymph nodes can drain via the deep posterior cervical, level V, or deep lateral cervical lymph nodes, level IIA, respectively.[1,11] Alternatively the lymph from the mastoid and occipital nodes can progress to external jugular chain and subsequently enter the middle and lower deep lateral cervical nodes, levels III–IV.[11]

Once a high-risk patient for regional metastasis has been indentified appropriate pre-operative testing must be completed. Computed topography imaging with contrast of face and neck is the study of choice to assess the parotid and surrounding structures including the parapharyngeal space and cervical lymph nodes. Bone windows can be used to assess mandibular or skull base invasion. If a parotid mass with fixation to external auditory canal or facial nerve paresis is present, a dedicated CT scan of the temporal bone should be obtained to assess involvement of the osseous external auditory canal, the middle and inner ear, and the mastoid.[4]

Magnetic resonance imaging can be used as an adjunct or alternative to CT and is particularly useful for extensive tumors involving the parapharyngeal space, skull base, or dura. Due to the poor cortical bone definition and equivalent assessment of cervical lymph nodes, MRI is reserved for selected patients with obvious nerve deficits or extensive disease.[4]

Audiologic testing evaluates the functional status of both the middle and inner ear. Conductive hearing loss may be due to tumor within the external auditory canal or middle ear space while sensorineural hearing loss, tinnitus, or vertigo may be attributed to inner ear involvement.

Since the incidence of distance metastases in non-melanoma cutaneous malignancies is low even in the presence of cervical lymph node disease, the role of positron emission tomography (PET) is limited. In contrast PET scan is more established in evaluation of melanoma where distant disease is more likely. For the detection of distant metastases or recurrent disease, the sensitivity and specificity of PET ranges from 70–100%.[5]

Operative Technique

The surgical intervention required to manage regionally metastatic non-melanoma cutaneous malignancies can be classified into ablative and reconstructive procedures. When addressing basal cell carcinoma, primary lesions less than 2 cm in diameter can be adequately treated with four millimeter margins achieving greater than a 95% cure rate.[6] For basal cell carcinoma lesions larger than 2 cm in diameter a 10 millimeter is recommended.[7] Alternatively for cutaneous squamous cell carcinoma the minimal recommended margin of excision is 4 mm for low risk lesions while a 6 mm margins is recommended for high risk lesions (Table 2).[8] In all cases of cutaneous basal or squamous cell carcinomas the resection margin is ultimately guided by frozen section analysis as well as pathologic features of the primary tumor, if available. If perineural disease is identified on frozen section analysis of the primary specimen a wider surgical margin is advisable to incorporate possible skip lesions. These considerations are always tempered by the proximity to critical structures such as the eye or ear, particularly if these are not clinically involved. Careful attention must be paid to the deep margin, as primary tumors in the cheek may invade to the level of the parotid fascia. Involvement of the parotid fascia typically requires a superficial parotidectomy with facial nerve preservation be performed as a satisfactory deep margin. The parotidectomy specimen will also contain regional nodes at risk of involvement. Regional node dissection, including both parotidectomy and cervical lymph node groups, should be considered for large tumors with aggressive pathologic features, for tumors with involvement of associated structures such as the ear canal, parotid gland or temporal bone, and for any tumor with clinically or radiographically positive adenopathy in any nodal station.

Cutaneous squamous cell carcinomas that have high risk features or obvious regional disease need more extensive surgical interventions. The extent of the ablative procedure correlates with the extent of the disease (Table 3, Figs. 3 to 5). The need to address the temporal bone as part of the surgical resection is based on the following 4 criteria:

- Preoperative involvement of temporal bone by direct extension
- Tumor extension to stylolmastoid foramen
- Tumor fixed to external auditory canal
- Need for intratemporal facial nerve identification

Similar to the ablative resection, the extent of the otologic resection correlates to the extent of the disease and includes the following spectrum of surgical procedures:

- Limited mastoidectomy (mastoid tip resection)
- Mastoidectomy with facial nerve mobilization and rerouting
- Lateral temporal bone resection
- Subtotal temporal bone resection
- Total temporal bone resection
- Extended infratemporal fossa

Table 2. Minimal Recommended Margins for Cutaneous Malignancies.

Primary	Margins
Basal cell carcinoma	
< 2 cm	4 mm
> 2 cm	10 mm
Squamous cell carcinoma	
Low risk	4 mm
High risk	6 mm

Table 3. Ablative Surgery for Cutaneous Malignancy Metastatic to the Parotid or Cervical Lymph Nodes.

Parotidectomy

Limited parotidectomy
Superficial parotidectomy
Total parotidectomy with nerve preservation
Radical parotidectomy[a]
Extended parotidectomy
Skin
Mandibulectomy
Lateral Temporal Bone

Neck Dissection

Selective
Modified radical[b]
Radical[c]
Extended[d]

[a] Radical parotidectomy involved complete resection of parotid tissue including the facial nerve. [b] Modified radical neck dissection is defined as removal of cervical lymph nodes from levels I–V with preservation of one or more non lympathatic structures: i.e, the spinal accessory nerve, internal jugular vein, and sternocleinomastoid muscle [c] Radical neck dissection is defined as removal of cervical lymph nodes from levels I–V including the spinal accessory nerve, internal jugular vein, and sternocleinomastoid muscle. [d] Extended radical neck dissection can be any of the above mentioned lymphadenoctomies but includes additional structures ie: carotid artery, occipital, mastoid, or external jugular lymph nodes.

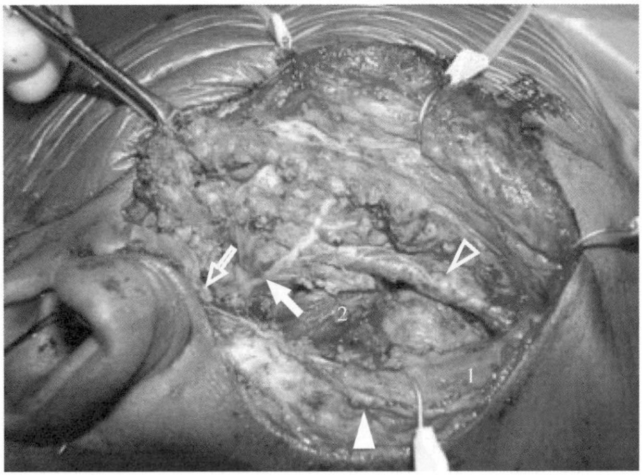

Fig. 3. Key landmarks involved in a superficial parotidectomy. 1: Sternocleinomastoid muscle. 2: Posterior belly of the digastric. Clamp shows superficial lobe of the parotid gland (reflected anteriorly and superiorly). Open arrow head: External jugular vein. White arrow head: Greater auricular nerve. Open arrow: Tragal pointer. White arrow: Main trunk of facial nerve.

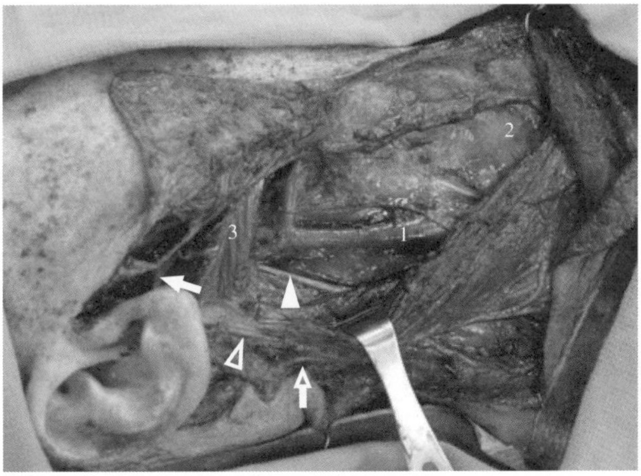

Fig. 4. Key landmarks in a total parotidectomy with facial nerve preservation and selective neck dissection level II–IV. 1: Internal jugular vein. 2: Anterior belly of omohyoid. 3: Posterior belly of digastric. Open arrow head: External jugular vein. White arrow head: Spinal accessory nerve. Open arrow: Greater auricular nerve. White arrow: Main trunk of facial nerve.

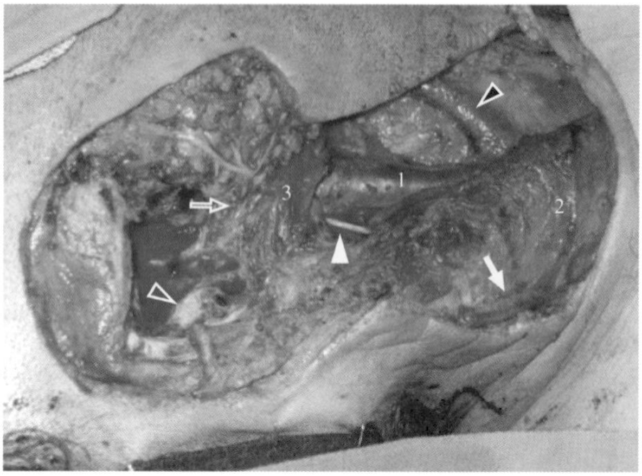

Fig. 5. Wide local excision of auricular squamous cell carcinoma primary with parotidectomy including temporal bone resection and selective neck dissection levels II–IV. 1: Internal jugular vein. 2: Sternocleinomastoid muscle. 3: Posterior belly of digastric. Open arrow head: Sigmoid sinus. White arrow head: Spinal accessory nerve. Hatched arrow head: Facial vein. Open arrow: Main trunk of facial nerve leaving stylomastoid foramen. White arrow: External jugular vein.

Reconstructive considerations for cutaneous defects depends on:

- Size and components of surgical defect
- Previous local treatment
- Need for postoperative radiation
- Medical co-morbidities
- Available reconstructive option

In order to address to various patient and tumor related factors, multiple reconstructive options have been created including:

- Primary closure
- Minor local tissue rearrangement
- Non vascualrized tissue grafts
- Locoregional axial pedicled flaps
- Microvascular free tissue transfer
- Facial nerve reconstruction
- Auricular reconstruction

Since the majority of surgical defects due to advanced cutaneous squamous cell carcinomas cannot be managed with primary closure or minor local tissue rearrangement, the focus of reconstructive options will be on local, regional, and free tissue flaps. Additionally many of these patients have been or will need radiation, therefore nonvacscularized tissue grafts are generally not recommended. Facial reanimation and auricular recinstruction are important components to the managed of lateral skull base defects but are beyond the scope of this topic.

The locoregional flaps and their blood supply (Table 4) that are emphasized will be:

- Cervicofacial advancement flap (Fig. 6)
- Pectoralis major myocutaneous flap (Fig. 7)

The free tissue transfers and their vascular supply (Table 4) that are emphasized will be:

- Radial forearm (Fig. 8)
- Anterolateral thigh (Fig. 9)

Table 4. Local, Regional, and Free Tissue Flaps with their Vascular Supply.

Local and Regional Flaps		**Free Tissue Transfers**	
Location	**Vascular Supply**	**Location**	**Vascular Supply**
Cervicofacial[a]	Random	Radial forearm	Radial artery
Temporoparietal fascia with or without skin	Superficial temporal artery	Lateral arm	Posterior radial collateral artery
Pectoralis major	Thoracoacromial artery	Anterolateral thigh	Perforators of lateral circumflex femoral branch of profunda femoris
Latissimus dorsi	Thoracodorsal artery	Rectus abdominus	Deep inferior epigastric vessels
Occipital flap	Occipital artery		

[a] Cervicofacial flaps receive their blood supply from a random distribution with the distal portion being the most unreliable. The remaining local and regional flaps are axial flaps.

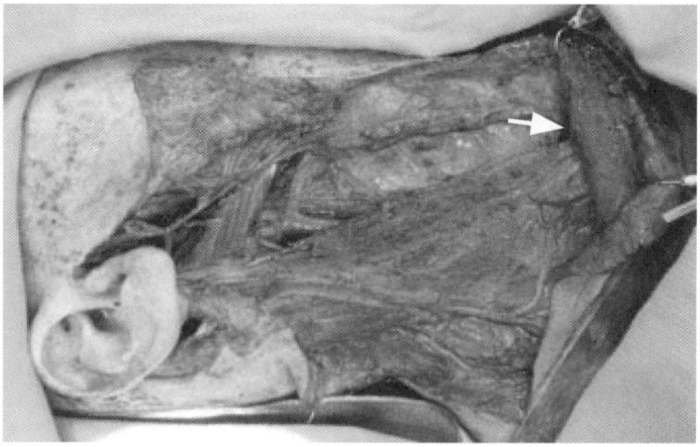

(a)

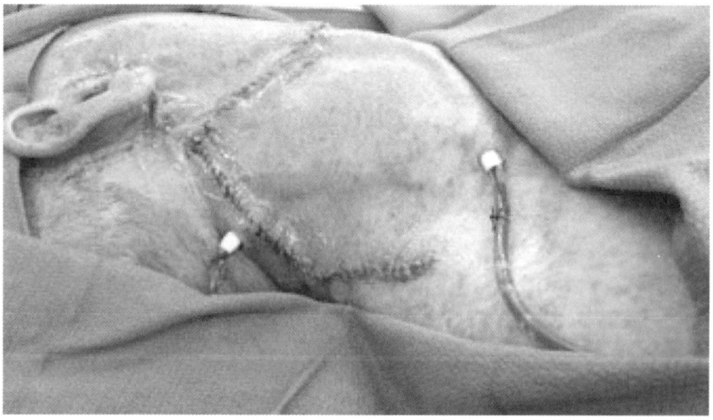

(b)

Fig. 6. Cervicofacial advancement flap. (a) Defect following total parotidectomy with facial nerve preservation and selective neck dissection level II–IV with cervicofascial flap elevated (White arrow). (b) Cervicofascial flap inset.

Post Operative Management

The post operative care of patients after a wide local excision of cutaneous malignancies is dictated by the function of the facial nerve and the reconstructive technique used to address the surgical defect. If the facial nerve is not functioning the key management points include:

1. Eye protection
   a. Artificial tears every 2 hours or as needed for dryness

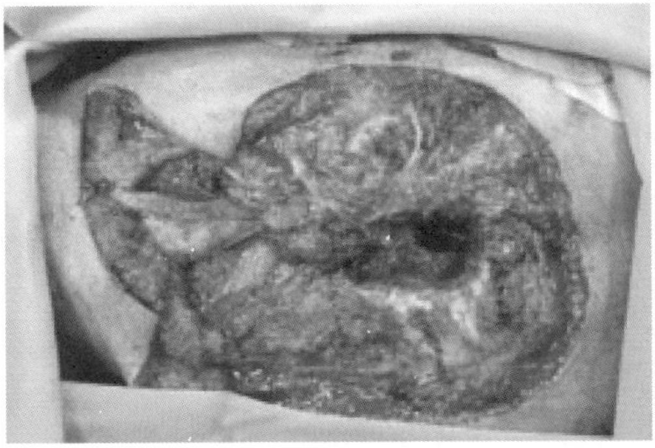

(a)

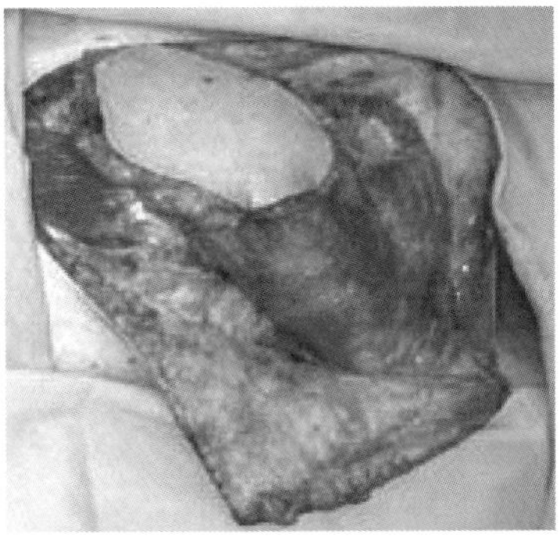

(b)

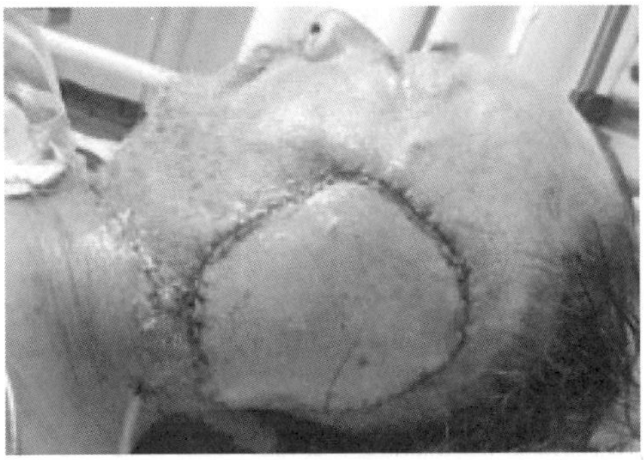

(c)

Fig. 7. (a) Defect following wide local excision, superficial parotidectomy with facial nerve preservation and lateral temporal bone resection for advanced basal cell carcinoma. (b) Elevated left pectoralis myocutaneous muscle flap. (c) Inset pectoralis myocutaneous muscle flap.

   b. Lubrication at bedtime
   c. Eye chamber or taping eye closed at bedtime
   d. Tarsorraphy

2. Oral incompetence:

   a. Diet

      i. Soft
      ii. Liquid and pureed diet are often not well tolerated

   b. Secretions, frequently suctioning of oral cavity is often required

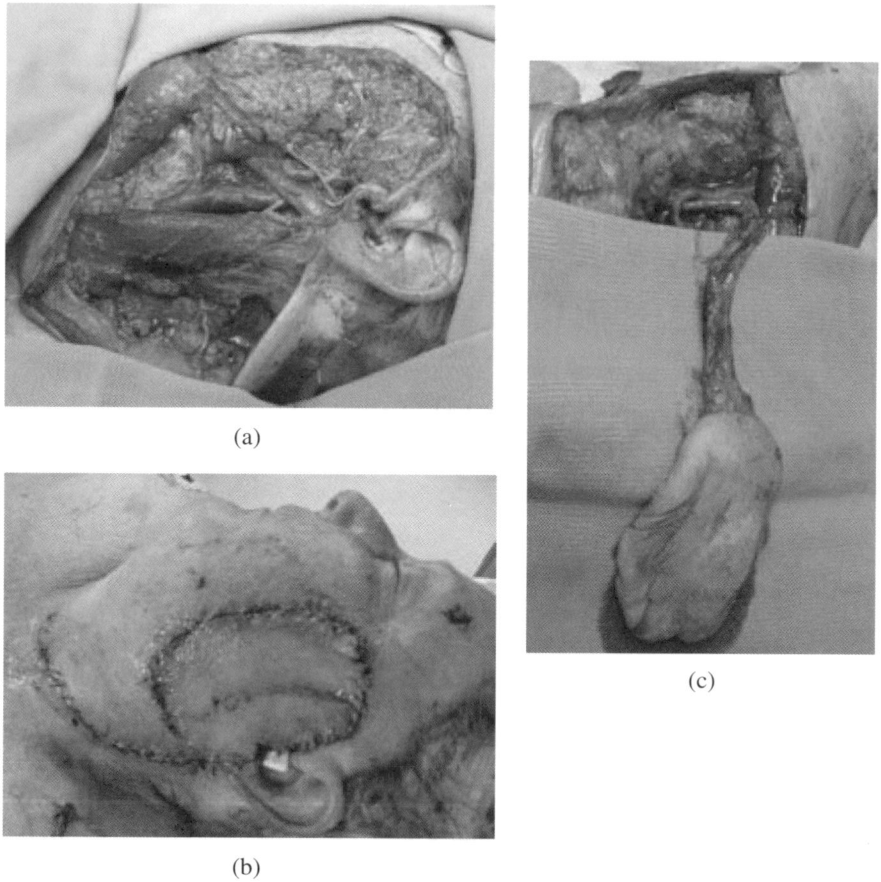

Fig. 8. (a) Defect from total parotidectomy with facial nerve preservation and left modified radical neck dissection for invasive cutaneous squamous cell carcinoma. (b) Raised radial forearm flap with dissection radial artery vascular pedicle. (c) Inset radial forearm free flap.

Regardless of the reconstructive technique it is important to closely follow the wound edges and drain outputs as the parotid or lateral skull base provides a large potential space for fluid or purulent collection. The post operative care for regional and distal flaps focuses on assessing the perfusion of the distal flap. This is primarily achieved by the detection of changes in flap:

- Color

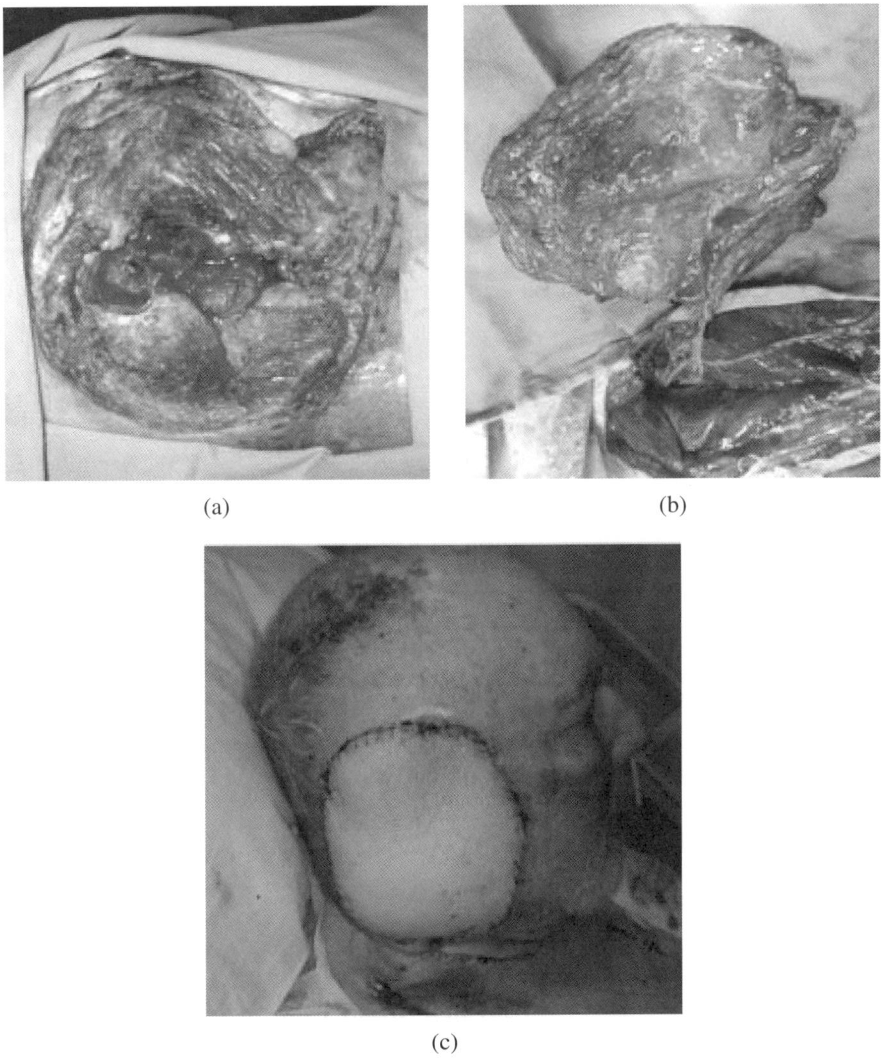

Fig. 9. (a) Defect following radical parotidectomy and lateral temporal bone resection with selective neck dissection. (b) Anterolateral thigh elevated with perforators of lateral circumflex femoral branch of profunda femoris visible. (c) Anterolateral thigh free tissue transfer inset.

- Capillary refill
- Temperature

If there is concern about flap viability, perfusion can further assessed by:

- Pin prick of skin surface
    - Assessing rate of bleeding
    - Assessing color of blood return
- Doppler of:
    - Pedicle
    - Distal flap
- Two dimension color Doppler assesses both:
    - Arterial system
    - Venous system

Specifically for free tissue transfer reconstructions is the role of post operative anti thrombotic prophylaxis.

- Low molecular weight dextran:
    - Used frequently
    - Mechanism reducing thrombus unknown
        - Impairs platelet function
        - Prolongs bleeding time
        - Destabilizes fibrin polymerization
    - Benefit in preventing thrombosis unknown
    - Increased risk of systemic (cardiac/pulmonary) complications.[9]
- Aspirin
    - Mechanism inhibits cyclooxygenase blocking formation of thromboxane A2 and therefore impairing platelet function
    - Benefit in preventing thrombosis well established both the cardiac and vascular literature
    - Low complication rate

- Low molecular weight heparin[10]
  - Mechanism inactivates thrombin factor Xa
  - Decreased rate of thromboembolic events is high risk post operative patients
  - Low rate of post operative bleeding

References

1. Veness MJ, Palme CE, Morgan GJ. (2006) High-risk cutaneous squamous cell carcinoma of the head and neck: results from 266 treated patients with metastatic lymph node disease. *Cancer* **106**(11): 2389–2396.
2. Veness MJ, Porceddu S, Palme CE, Morgan GJ. (2007) Cutaneous head and neck squamous cell carcinoma metastatic to parotid and cervical lymph nodes. *Head Neck* **29**(7): 621–631.
3. Ching S, Low I, Ng D, *et al.* (2008) Epidermal growth factor receptor: a novel biomarker for aggressive head and neck cutaneous squamous cell carcinoma. *Hum Pathol* **39**(3): 344–349.
4. Clark J, Sneddon L, O'Brien C. (2007) Management of cancer metastatic to the parotid gland. In: Myers EN, Ferris RL (eds.), *Salivary Gland Disorders*. Springer, New York, pp. 377–392.
5. Essner R. (2003) Surgical treatment of malignant melanoma. *Surg Clin North Am* **83**(1): 109–156.
6. Wolf DJ, Zitelli JA.(1987) Surgical margins for basal cell carcinoma. *Arch Dermatol* **123**(3): 340–344.
7. Albright SD, 3rd. (1982) Treatment of skin cancer using multiple modalities. *J Am Acad Dermatol* **7**(2): 143–171.
8. Brodland DG, Zitelli JA. (1992) Surgical margins for excision of primary cutaneous squamous cell carcinoma. *J Am Acad Dermatol* **27**(2 Pt 1): 241–248.
9. Disa JJ, Polvora VP, Pusic AL, Singh B, Cordeiro PG. (2003) Dextran-related complications in head and neck microsurgery: do the benefits outweigh the risks? A prospective randomized analysis. *Plast Reconstr Surg* **112**(6): 1534–1539.
10. Hirsh J, Warkentin TE, Shaughnessy SG, *et al.* (2001) Heparin and low-molecular-weight heparin: mechanisms of action, pharmacokinetics, dosing, monitoring, efficacy, and safety. *Chest* **119**(1 Suppl): 64S–94S.
11. Lengele B, Hamoir M, Scalliet P, Gregoire V. (2007) Anatomical bases for the radiological delineation of lymph node areas. Major collecting trunks, head and neck. *Radiother Oncol* **85**(1): 146–155.

CHAPTER 11

PRINCIPLES IN FACIAL INJURY MANAGEMENT

Patrick Cole and Larry Hollier, Jr.

Illustrative Case

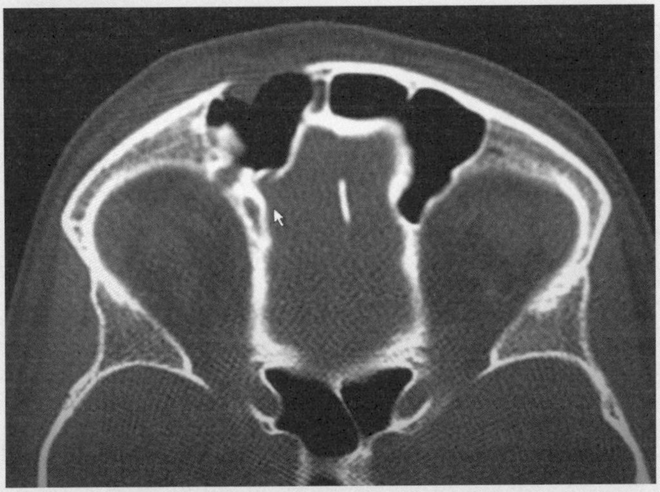

A 22-year-old male sustained a right anterior table frontal sinus fracture involving the nasofrontal duct in a motorcycle collision. Following the completion of advanced trauma live support (ATLS) protocols and cervical spine injury clearance, maxillofacial CT imaging revealed the fracture without posterior table involvement or intracranial injury (Fig. 1). Under general anesthesia, a bicoronal incision was utilized to access the injury site. Following burr destruction of all frontal sinus mucosa, a paracranial flap was inset to fully obliterate the nasofrontal duct outflow tract. Taking care not to devascularize the pericranial flap, bone fragments were reduced and permanently plate fixated. The galea was resuspended and approximated followed by skin closure.

Introduction

Injury to the face may result in complex defects involving multiple tissues types, anatomic structures, and functionalities. Perhaps most importantly, facial injury may significantly impede one's ability to both sense, as well as communicate with one's surrounding environment. With these factors in mind, current principles of facial trauma management include[1]: restoring and preserving function, and[2,3] achieving an optimal cosmetic result. It is imperative that the plastic surgeon be thoroughly familiar with proper steps in wound evaluation, initial management steps, and definitive treatment of the facial wound.

Steps in the Initial Evaluation

- Emergency trauma care must always prioritize airway maintenance, control of breathing, and circulation.
- Evaluating craniomaxillofacial soft tissue injuries should commence coincidentally with stabilization of the patient.
- Photographic documentation should be accomplished during initial presentation.
- Significant facial injuries warrant a brain CT, thus giving the opportunity to obtain a concurrent maxillofacial CT scan for clear definition of osseous injuries.
- Prior to wound cleansing and comprehensive inspection, local anesthesia with a vasoconstrictor should be administered via a 25-gauge needle.

Initial Management of the Facial Soft Tissue Wound

- While many facial wound may eventually require scar revision, complications following acute injury will be predictably better if acute care was properly performed.
- After inspection, it is helpful to thoroughly irrigate with 2% xylocaine with epinephrine 1:100,000 followed by placing a saturated gauze compress in the wound.
- All embedded foreign bodies, hematomas or fractures must be evacuated.

- If there is any suspicion of eye injury, early ophthalmologic consultation is imperative.
- Facial debridement must be conservative, with optimism for questionable tissue survival more readily expressed than in other bodily sites.
- Muscular tissues, fascial layers and others subcutaneous tissues are best approximated with monocryl or PDS.
- While in adults, one may use nylon or prolene for skin closure, the use of nonabsorbable suture for skin closure in children is best avoided. In this case, fast-absorbing gut with mastisol and steristrips is preferred.

Animal Bites

- Dog bites represent the vast majority of animal bites, may result in infection rates as high as 29%, and are often associated with *Pasteurella multocida.*[4]
- Augmentin (penicillin and clavulanic acid) usually provides adequate coverage.
- Human bites have more significant rates of infection, usually due to anaerobic streptococcus or *Eikenella corrodens*.[4]
- Bite wounds must be copiously irrigated prior to any attempt at loose closure. However, puncture wounds from teeth should not be closed. If the wound cannot be closed primarily, it is best to place a dressing and plan reconstruction at another time when the risk of infection is lower.[4]

Injuries Specific to Facial Structures

Eyelid Injuries

- Avulsion of the eyelid is a true surgical emergency. Immediate coverage is required for the prevention of further corneal damage, decreased visual acuity, and exposure keratopathy.[5,6]
- Acute care consists of an ophthalmologic consultation, placement of an antibiotic patch on the cornea, and covering of the eye with a nonpermeable occlusive eye shield. Trapping of moisture within the orbit

should prevent dryness and further desiccation of the superficial corneal layers.

- Any injury to the lower lid presents an increased risk of increased scleral show and ectropion formation.

Scalp Injuries

- Due to the extensive vascular supply to the scalp, wounds to this are may produce impressive blood loss. Ligation of identifiable bleeding vessels, and application of a compression Kerlix bandage will facilitate adequate hemostasis.[7]
- Associated skull fractures must always be suspected, and thorough palpation and inspection should be undertaken via any full-thickness scalp wound.
- Layers of the scalp are skin, connective tissue, galea aponeurosis, loose areolar tissue, and periosteum.[7] It is imperative to close scalp injuries in layers, paying particular attention to the galea.

Cheek Injuries

- Cheek wounds should be carefully irrigated, and if extension through the oral mucosa is identified, this should also be closed with vicryl or chromic sutures.[8]
- A thorough exam of the facial nerve must be carried out prior to intervention. If the nerve is lacerated, primary anastomosis should be performed at the time of laceration repair if the two ends are readily identified.[9] Otherwise, temporary closure with planned repair in the operative suite within 72 hours is appropriate.
- If suspicion or parotid duct injury exists, the orifice of Stensen's duct should be probed.[9] This may be evaluated in the emergency center by cannulating the oral papilla with a 20 gauge periopheral intravenous catheter and injecting approximately 2–3 cc of whole milk. If a parotid duct injury is present, milk can be seen exiting the external facial injury. The proximal cut end of the duct may be located by the expression of saliva from the gland. A catheter should be positioned through the area of laceration via Stenson's duct, and the duct should be repaired over the catheter.[9]

- While a majority of cheek injuries simply require layered closure, more extensive defects can be further managed with nasolabial advancement flaps, Limberg flaps, or cervicofacial flaps.[8]

Facial Fracture Management

Management of the Frontal Sinus Fracture

- The clinician must be aware that these fractures are often associated with cervical vertebrae defects, central nervous injuries and other facial fractures.[9]
- Frontal sinus fractures are not considered a surgical emergency unless associated with ophthalmologic or neurologic injury requiring other surgery.[10]
- Initially, patients should be placed on broad-spectrum intravenous antibiotics. The status of anterior and posterior tables and the naso-frontal duct determines the operative indications and technique.[10] Non-displaced anterior table fractures may be safely observed.[11]
- Displaced anterior table injuries may be managed with simple reduction and plate fixation via a coronal incision or in rare circumstances through access granted by existing traumatic wounds.[10,11]
- Fractures involving the medial aspect of the sinus and nasalrontal duct, sinus obliteration is usually the most prudent course.[9–11] If there is a question regarding the patency of the drainage system, one may test intraoperatively by placing dye within the sinus in attempting to demonstrate its passage onto cottonoids placed within the nose at the level of the middle meatus.[11]
- In the case of displaced posterior table fractures or fractures associated with CSF leaks, the sinus should be cranialized.[9–11]
- Once the forehead bone flap is free, it should be brought to the back table and the entire posterior table removed. The inner aspect of the anterior table should be burred to remove the mucosa.[10,11] A burr is most commonly used to accomplish this. Prior to burr application, it is helpful to paint the sinus cavity with methylene blue to ensure full removal. We have also found the use of a CO_2 laser to be equally effective in mucosal destruction.

- The nasofrontal duct must be completely sealed.[12] This can be accomplished using galea frontalis flaps temporalis fascia, bone or pericranium. As with obliteration, it is helpful to use fibrin glue to help the flap seal over the communication with the nasal cavity.
- Without proper management, complications of frontal sinus injury typically occur as a result of nasofrontal duct obstruction in the setting of viable sinus material, mucosal entrapment within fracture lines, or dural tears.[13]
- Early complications include cerebrospinal fluid leaks and meningitis.[14] Delayed complications include sinusitis and mucocele formation.[14]

Management of the Orbital Fracture

- In cases with suspected optic neuropathy, steroids should be administered and surgery delayed until vision stabilizes.[15,16] Unless there is clear mechanical impingement of the nerve by fracture fragments, decompressive surgery is typically not performed.[15,16]
- Release of the entrapped extraocular muscle (EOM) tissue within 48 hours of injury results in faster recovery of EOM motility.[16] Ongoing entrapment likely results in ischemia and fibrosis, compromising the final results.
- In the absence of entrapment, a delay of seven to ten days is often beneficial in allowing the swelling associated with the injury to resolve to some degree.[16,17,18]
- With respect to the approach to the lower eyelid, subciliary incisions are unacceptable due to their more frequent association with ectropion formation.[19]
- Transconjunctival incisions are preferred when supplemented by a lateral canthotomy.
- In situations where the posterior limit of the defect is hard to define, it is helpful to stick the elevator through the defect and back to the posterior wall of the maxillary sinus. The elevator can then be moved superiorly until the undersurface of the orbital floor posteriorly is reached. The elevator is then moved anteriorly until the posterior lip of the defect is reached.

- It is also helpful to consciously dissect cephalad within the orbital cone. A common mistake is dissecting straight back into the maxillary sinus. The surgeon must consciously be aware of the superior inclination of the orbital floor as one proceeds posteriorly.
- Once the defect is identified, it may be helpful to make a template of the defect to help with shaping the ultimate implant. A suture-foil pack or plastic from a saline basin are both acceptable.
- Classically, bone grafts have been strongly advocated.[20,21] However, many alloplastic materials have been developed that have performed superbly in clinical studies. These include: Titanium mesh, high-density porous polyethylene implants, and even resorbable material.[22]
- When one accounts for the swelling associated with the surgery, the operated eye should project further anterior than the uninjured eye with the orbital floor implant in place.[22–24]

Complications of Orbital Fracture

- Following orbital fracture repair, the most common complications are lower-eyelid retraction and enophthalmos.[25] Placement of a frost suture augments lower eyelid maintenance in an elevated position for 24 hours post-operatively.
- Post-operative enophthalmos, most commonly caused by poor orbital floor reconstruction and excessive orbital volumes, is particularly resistant to secondary correction.[25–27] Although fat atrophy may lead to measurable intra-orbital volume increases, it is unlikely that such change significantly contributes to post-operative enopthalmos.[24,25,27]
- Postoperative diplopia can also be an issue. The initial concern is that the cause is mechanical entrapment secondary to the implant. It is critical that a forced duction test be performed at the end of the surgical procedure. Should there be no evidence of restrictive problems at that time, it is highly unlikely that diplopia is due to the implant.[28] More commonly, there is paresis of the nerves or contusion of the muscles causing this.[28]

Management of the Nasal Fracture

- Nasal fractures are extremely common.[29,30]

- When initially seen, the diagnosis can be made simply based on clinical exam.[30,31]
- In particularly severe cases, a CT scan may be helpful in supplementing the diagnosis, particularly in ruling out injuries to the nasoorbital ethmoid (NOE) complex.[31]
- A careful intranasal exam should also be performed to rule out septal hematoma.
- It is helpful if topical decongestants are used prior to this to facilitate resolving the mucosal edema.[32]
- There are three time periods for treatment of nasal fractures: acute, subacute, and chronic.[33]
- Should the patient be seen during this period in the emergency room, closed reduction can be attempted.[33]
- This is facilitated by placing Afrin or Cocaine-soaked pledgets intranasally after anesthetizing the nose with regional blocks of Lidocaine.[32] Transeptal injections of the underside of the nasal bones facilitate this as well.[32] Most patients also benefit from sedation intravenously during the procedure.
- It is helpful once the closed reduction has been accomplished to place a dorsal nasal splint and if any significant septal manipulation has been undertaken to place Doyle intranasal splints as well.[34,35]
- In less acute settings after significant edema has set in, most patients benefit from open rhinoplasty and substantial septal remodeling following resolution of swelling.

Complications of Nasal Bone Fracture

- Nasal fractures associated with injury to the perpendicular plate and dural tear may present with leakage of cerebrospinal (CSF) fluid.[36]
- These patients frequently complain of "post nasal drip" down the back of their throat.[36]
- Should there be confusion, a small portion of fluid can be obtained and it can be sent for a Beta transferrin test.[36]
- The most important factor in managing these is to keep the patient's head elevated. At no time should the patient be recumbent as this increases the pressure at the site of the leak and prevents its

spontaneous closure. Only rarely is a lumbar drain required and open repair of the leak incredibly uncommon.[36]

Nasoorbital Ethmoidal Fracture (NOE)

- NOE fractures are historically some of the most challenging to treat.
- With the patient sedated, a definitive diagnosis can be made by placing a hemostat within the nose and pressing outward on the section of bone to which the medial canthal tendon inserts.[37]
- CT scan is very accurate in identifying NOE fractures.[38]
- The medial canthal tendon is by definition involved in the fractured segment and adequate reduction typically requires operation.[38,39]
- The majority of these injuries will require both a coronal and a lower eyelid incision.[39] Markowitz's classification of these injuries is helpful in determining the appropriate treatment.[39]
- Class I injuries have a very large single segment i.e. that can be directly plated.
- Class II fractures have a greater degree of comminution but the medial canthal tendon is still attached to bone.[39] Plating may be sufficient; however, in the more severe cases transnasal canthopexy is required.
- In Grade III fractures, the most rare, the medial canthal tendon is avulsed and transnasal canthopexy is mandatory.[39]
- One must be careful during dissection however, not to strip off any remaining insertions of the medial canthal tendon to the bone.[40]
- In more comminuted fractures or those missing bone, bone graft may be necessary.[41] This is typically harvested through the coronal incision using split calvarial bone.[41]
- Should the medial canthal tendon be insufficiently attached, a transnasal canthopexy is important.[42]
- The medial canthal tendon should be anchored at the level of the apex of the lacrimal fossa in a slight superio-posterior orientation.[41,42]
- The tendon should be transfixed by a permanent suture or a narrow gauge steel wire (30 gauge).[42] The tendon should then be passed through the drill hole to the contralateral side and secured over a screw or plate.[42,43]

- Should dorsal nasal support should be insufficient, strong consideration should be given to performing a calvarial bone graft to this region.[37]
- Finally, attention must be given to soft tissue bolsters in the medial canthal region. This can be done with a dorsal splint or preferably with bolsters tied directly over the area with sutures emanating from deep to the coronal flap.[38]

Complications of NOE Fracture Management

- The most troubling complication of NOE fractures is persistent telecanthus.[39] This is a particularly recalcitrant problem once it has been established. Unless the bones of the region have been clearly malaligned, there is very little to do about it.[37–40]

Management of Orbitozygomatic Fractures

- Second only to nasal fractures in their frequency, the malar complex is particularly vulnerable to blunt trauma.[44] Displacement of the bone typically involves enlargement of the orbital cone and enophthalmous unless anatomic reconstruction is performed.[41,44]
- CT scans form the basis for diagnosis.[42] Any displacement of the malar complex will be manifest at the broad articulation of the zygoma with the greater wing of the sphenoid.[42]
- Physical exam should also focus on the globe itself.[43] As discussed in the section on orbital injuries, a focused ophthalmologic exam to detect any problems with optic neuropathy or extra ocular muscle function is critical.[43]
- Essentially all displaced fractures should be openly reduced and fixated.[45] Non-displaced fractures may be managed conservatively without surgery.
- All fractures should initially be approached through the gingivobuccal sulcus incision.[46] This allows visualization of the fracture and up to the orbital rim T.
- The surgeon should place an elevator beneath the zygomatic arch through this incision and bluntly reduce the fracture.[46,47]

- The lower eyelid incision should be either transconjunctival with a lateral canthotomy or subtarsal to prevent the risk of lower lid retraction.[47,48,49]
- A Carol-Gerard screw placed in the malar eminence through the lower eyelid incision can be used as a joystick to both disimpact the fragment and properly position it.[50]
- Once back in anatomic position, a 1.5 mm plate is typically placed at the inferior orbital rim superiorly rather than anteriorly to minimize palpability followed by a 2.0 mm plate at the zygomatic maxillary buttress.
- Following this the orbital floor is reconstructed.
- At the end of the procedure one must carefully assess the eye position as previously discussed in the section on orbital fractures.[51,52]

Complications of Orbitozygomatic Fractures

- The most troublesome complication when one looks at orbitozygomatic fractures is persistent enophthalmos due to non-anatomic reconstruction of the malar segment.[53] If this is recognized in the very early postoperative period, removal of the plates and repositioning of the segment is possible.[53]
- As most patients complain only of the enophthalmos, one option is simply to augment orbital volume. This is best addressed using a porous polyethylene wedge carved to appropriate size and placed posterolaterally in the orbital cone until appropriate projection is achieved.[53]

Management of the Maxillary Fracture

- The first step in corrective management of the maxillary fracture is to provide maxillomandibular fixation (MMF) via arch bar application to both upper and lower dental structures.
- If the maxilla appears both displaced and impacted, efforts must be made to mobilize the injured segment. Rowe forceps can be inserted into the nose and rocked side-to-side in a forward pulling motion.

- Le Fort I injuries may be adequately exposed via an upper gingivobuccal sulcus incision and maxillary degloving, Le Fort II fractures typically require the addition of a lower lid incision.[54]
- Very severe injuries often require a coronal incision for full exposure of the nasofrontal, medial orbital, and zygomatic regions.
- Care must be taken to avoid drilling into the roots of the maxillary dentition, particularly the canines.

Management of the Mandible Fracture

- Evaluation of the patient with a mandible fracture should focus on occlusion and to a lesser degree, mental nerve sensation.[55]
- The status of the patient's dentition must be carefully evaluated as periodontal disease, particularly in the region of the third molar and in angle fractures can influence the outcome negatively.[56–58]
- CT scanning is 100% sensitive for fractures and gives a great deal more information than the panoramic radiograph, it does not give sufficient information for the teeth.[59] If there is suspicion of a dental injury, particularly important for angle fractures, a panoramic radiograph should also be obtained.
- Unlike malar fractures, there is relatively little benefit in delaying surgery of a mandible fracture for resolution of edema.[60]
- If surgery is going to be delayed, for any substantial period of time, it is beneficial to temporarily stabilize the injury with bridal wire around the teeth adjacent to the fracture.[60]
- Perhaps the most important question that must be answered by the surgeon is the appropriate form of fixation to be utilized for a fracture. The central question is whether the fixation should be load bearing or load sharing.
- Load bearing fixation implies rigidity, with the plate and screw construct bearing all of the load for the mandible.[61]
- Load sharing fixation applies functional stability with the mandible sharing some of the load with the plate.
- As a general rule, simple fractures are adequately stabilized using load sharing techniques. Problem fractures, such as those involving comminution, segmental bone loss or multiple fractures, benefit from rigid load bearing fixation.[62]

- Plates used for trauma are typically divided into 2.0 mm screws (miniplates) and those accommodating 2.4 mm screws (reconstruction plates).
- Classically, reconstruction plates are thought to be the most appropriate way to provide rigid load bearing fixation in severe fractures.[63] The disadvantage of these plates are difficult to accurately contour to the shape of the mandible and, if not perfectly adapted, can result in pulling of the bone up to the plate, shifting the bite and causing a malocclusion.[63] This problem has been minimized to some degree by locking plate technology in which the screw actually has threads within its head which screws into the hole within the plate. The screw stops tightening when the head locks into the plate itself, preventing pulling of the bone up to a maladapted plate.[64]
- Plates accommodating 2.0 mm screws, miniplates, have classically been thought to provide load-sharing fixation.[65] These plates are preferred by many practitioners in simple fractures due to the diminished likelihood of malocclusion secondary to under contouring of the plate.[65,66]

Special Considerations in the Angle Fracture Management

- Angle fractures present perhaps the most challenging case for mandibular trauma. The posterior location minimizes the surgeon's ability to visualize and manipulate the fracture.[67,68] Additionally, the presence of a third molar not infrequently raises the concern of infection.[68]
- Regardless of plate choice, most surgeons will utilize monocortical screws.[69,70] Particularly in the region of the angle, these screws should be 8 mm in length.[70] Screws of shorter length have a much greater risk of stripping, particularly if the plate is not perfectly adapted to the bone.[69–71]
- The issue of the third molar remains a controversial one. The only absolute indication to remove the third molar is if the tooth itself is damaged or particularly diseased.[72] The risk of infection in these situations is prohibitive. Although some surgeons routinely remove third molars in the line of fracture, it must be remembered that this weakens the mandible and one should consider increasing the rigidity of the fixation in such a situation.[72]

A Note on Subcondylar Fracture Management

- Management of the condylar fracture depends heavily on occlusion. If the patient exhibits no evidence of premature contact in the molar region on the affected side, conservative treatment is acceptable.[73] The patient may just be closely followed to allow healing.
- Should there be evidence of malocclusion secondary to the injury, several other considerations are important.
- Open reduction has been shown to be a safe and effective approach,[73,74] however there is quite a steep learning curve, operative times can be substantial,[75] and facial nerve paralysis or paresis is a considerable risk.[73]
- When considering intermaxillaryfixation (IMF), one must remember that the IMF does not truly reduce the fracture.[68,71] All that this accomplishes is forcing the patient to adapt their occlusion to the malreduction. Although in principle this may be suboptimal, many patients are happy with usual end result.
- The duration and type of intermaxillary fixation also serves as a source of controversy. If a patient is reliable and capable of maintaining elastics between the arch bars, this is clearly preferable to wires.[76] Elastics allow the patient to range the jaws while the occlusion is guided into the desired orientation.[76]
- Even in the most severe cases of malocclusion, patients should not be left in intermaxillary fixation for longer than four weeks.[76]

Complications of the Mandible Fracture

- The most distressing complication from mandibular fractures is malocclusion.[72]
- The surgical reduction/fixation operation should not be terminated until it is felt that the occlusion is at its preinjury level.[72,74]
- Malocclusion recognized in the postoperative period should be returned to the operating room and the fixation removed and replaced.[74]
- Infections are perhaps the most common problem seen postoperatively, and these can be simplistically divided into early and late infections.[75]

- Early infections are typically seen in the first week postoperatively and should be treated much like a simple soft tissue infection.[75] The wound should be washed out and the hardware assessed.
- More troublesome are the late infections usually manifesting three weeks or greater postoperatively.[75] These most frequently are the result of hardware failure. The patient should have the site of infection washed out and the hardware checked. Should the hardware have failed in any way, the best approach is to remove the hardware and replace it with larger more rigid hardware.[75] The reason for the infection is bone mobility and loose hardware.
- In particularly severe infections, one may feel more comfortable removing the hardware and placing the patient in intermaxillary fixation for a period of time with the administration of antibiotics prior to replacing the hardware. In the most severe situations, an external fixator may be considered.[73,75]

Conclusion

Although often complex, optimal management of facial injuries is directly dependent upon thorough initial evaluation, correct injury assessment, and timely initiation of chosen therapy. Because the face is such an integral portion of personal presentation and expression, considerable attention must be given to this aspect of the injury, including psychological preparation of the patient for the healing process, and to the possibility of both complications as well as the potential need for future revisions. As such, the goal is the judicious prevention of immediate complications and long-term disfigurement upon initial presentation. Maximum attention must be given to primary repair, with exploration and preparation of the wound borders with meticulous closure. Necessary secondary repairs should be delayed for a minimum 6 months if not more than 1 year. With time, anticipated secondary surgery may prove unnecessary. As a rule, it is probably most preferable in the acute care setting to complete the simplest possible repair and reserve more complex procedures for secondary repair.

References

1. Manson PN, Clark N, Robertson B, *et al.* (1995) Comprehensive management of pan-facial fractures. *J Craniomaxillofac Trauma* **1**: 43–56.
2. Crawley WA, Vasconez HC. (1997) Midface, upper face, and panfacial fractures. In: Ferrero J (ed.), *Fundamentals of Maxillofacial Surgery*. Springer-Velag, New York, pp. 203–214.
3. Wenig BL. (1991) Management of panfacial fractures. *Otolaryngol Clin North Am* **24**: 93–101.
4. Lim LH, Lam LK, Moore MH, *et al.* (1993) Associated injuries in facial fractures: review of 839 patients. *Br J Plast Surg* **46**: 635–638.
5. Cruz AA, Eichenberger GC. (2004) Epidemiology and management of orbital fractures. *Curr Opin Ophthalmol* **15**(5): 416–421.
6. Hussain K, Wijetunge DB, Brubnic S, *et al.* (1994) A comprehensive analysis of craniofacial trauma. *J Trauma* **36**(1): 34–47.
7. Goldschmidt MJ, Castiglione CL, Assael LA, *et al.* (1995) Craniomaxillofacial trauma in the elderly. *J Oral Maxillofac Surg* **53**: 1145–1149.
8. David DJ. (1999) Facial fracture classification: current thoughts and applications. *J Craniomaxillofac Trauma* **5**(4): 31–36.
9. Strong EB, Pahlavan N, Saito D. (2006) Frontal sinus fractures: a 28-year retrospective review. *Otolaryngol Head Neck Surg* **135**(5): 774–779.
10. McGuire TP, Gomes PP, Clokie CM, Sandor GK. (2006) Fractures of the supraorbital rim: principles and management. *J Can Dent Assoc* **72**(6): 537–540.
11. Chen KT, Chen CT, Mardini S, Tsay PK, Chen YR. (2006) Frontal sinus fractures: a treatment algorithm and assessment of outcomes based on 78 clinical cases. *Plast Reconstr Surg* **118**(2): 457–468.
12. Gossman DG, Archer SM, Arosarena O. (2006) Management of frontal sinus fractures: a review of 96 cases. *Laryngoscope* **116**(8): 1357–1362.
13. McGraw-Wall B. (1998) Frontal sinus fractures. *Facial Plast Surg* **14**: 59–66.
14. Rohrich RJ, Hollier LH. (1992) Management of frontal sinus fractures, changing concepts. *Clin Plast Surg* **19**: 219–231.
15. Chang EL, Bernardino CR. (2004) Update on orbital trauma. *Curr Opin Ophthalmol* **5**: 411–415.
16. Enislidis G. (2004) Treatment of orbital fractures: the case for treatment with resorbable materials. *J Oral Maxillofac Surg* **62**(7): 869–872.
17. Ellis E 3rd, Messo E. (2004) Use of nonresorbable alloplastic implants for internal orbital reconstruction. *J Oral Maxillofac Surg* **62**(7): 873–881.

18. Burnstine MA. (2002) Clinical recommendations for repair of isolated orbital floor fractures: an evidence-based analysis. *Ophthalmology* **109**: 1207–1210; discussion 1210–1201; quiz 1212–1203.
19. Ellis E 3rd, Tan Y. (2003) Assessment of internal orbital reconstructions for pure blowout fractures: cranial bone grafts versus titanium mesh. *J Oral Maxillofac Surg* **61**: 442–453.
20. Girotto JA, MacKenzie E, Fowler C, Redett R, Robertson B, Manson PN. (2001) Long-term physical impairment and functional outcomes after complex facial fractures. *Plast Reconstr Surg* **108**(2): 312–327.
21. Hammer B, Prein J. (1995) Correction of post-traumatic orbital deformities: operative techniques and review of 26 patients. *J Craniomaxillofac Surg* **23**: 81–90.
22. Lahbabi M, Lockhart R, Fleuridas G, Chikhani L, Bertrand JC, Guilbert F. (1999) Post-traumatic enophthalmos. Physiopathologic considerations and current therapeutics. *Rev Stomatol Chir Maxillofac* **100**: 165–174.
23. Manson PN, Grivas A, Rosenbaum A, Vannier M, Zinreich J, Iliff N. (1986) Studies on enophthalmos: II. The measurement of orbital injuries and their treatment by quantitative computed tomography. *Plast Reconstr Surg* **77**: 203–214.
24. Marin PC, Love T, Carpenter R, Iliff NT, Manson PN. (1998) Complications of orbital reconstruction: misplacement of bone grafts within the intramuscular cone. *Plast Reconstr Surg* **101**: 1323–1327; discussion 1328–1329.
25. Meyer C, Groos N, Sabatier H, Wilk A. (1998) Long-term outcome of surgically treated orbital floor fractures. Apropos of a series of 242 patients. *Rev Stomatol Chir Maxillofac* **99**: 149–154.
26. Shere JL, Boole JR, Holtel MR, Amoroso PJ. (2004) An analysis of 3599 midfacial and 1141 orbital blowout fractures among 4426 United States Army Soldiers, 1980–2000. *Otolaryngol Head Neck Surg* **130**: 164–170.
27. Manson PN, Clifford CM, Su CT, Iliff NT, Morgan R. (1986) Mechanisms of global support and post-traumatic enophthalmos: I. The anatomy of the ligament sling and its relation to intramuscular cone orbital fat. *Plast Reconstr Surg* **77**: 193–202.
28. Haug RH, Van Sickels JE, Jenkins WS. (2002) Demographics and treatment options for orbital roof fractures. *Oral Surg Oral Med Oral Pathol Oral Radiol Endod* **93**: 238–246.
29. Gruss S, Bubak PJ, Egbert MA. (1992) Craniofacial fractures. An algorithm to optimize results. *Clin Plast Surg* **19**: 195–206.
30. Reilly MJ, Davison SP. (2007) Open vs closed approach to the nasal pyramid for fracture reduction. *Arch Facial Plast Surg* **9**(2): 82–86.

31. Hwang K, You SH, Kim SG, Lee SI. (2006) Analysis of nasal bone fractures: a six-year study of 503 patients. *J Craniofac Surg* **17**(2): 261–264.
32. Cultrara A, Turk JB, Har-El G. (2004) Midfacial degloving approach for repair of naso-orbital-ethmoid and midfacial fractures. *Arch Facial Plast Surg* **6**(2): 133–135.
33. Cruse CW, Blevins PK, Luce EA. (1980) Naso-ethmoid-orbital fractures. *J Trauma* **20**(7): 551–556.
34. Oluwasanmi AF, Pinto AL. (2000) Management of nasal trauma–widespread misuse of radiographs. *Clin Perform Qual Health Care* **8**(2): 83–85.
35. Rohrich RJ, Adams WP Jr. (2000) Nasal fracture management: minimizing secondary nasal deformities. *Plast Reconstr Surg* **106**(2): 266–273.
36. Staffel JG. (2002) Optimizing treatment of nasal fractures. *Laryngoscope* **112**: 1709–1719.
37. Gotcher JE Jr, Livesay KW. (2002) Management of complex facial fractures. *J Tenn Dent Assoc Fall* **82**(3): 69–73.
38. Moos KF. (2002) Diagnosis of facial bone fractures. *Ann R Coll Surg Engl* **84**(6): 429–431.
39. Ellis E III. (1993) Sequencing treatment for naso-orbito-ethmoid fractures. *J Oral Maxillofac Surg* **51**: 543–548.
40. Gullane PJ, Gilbert RW. (1985) Approach to naso-frontal-ethmoidal complex fractures. *J Otolaryngol* **14**: 132–135.
41. Maniglia AJ, Phillips DA. (1986) Indications and techniques of midfacial degloving. *Arch Otolaryngol Head Neck Surg* **112**: 750–752.
42. Manolidis S, Weeks BH, Kirby M, Scarlett M, Hollier L. (2002) Classification and surgical management of orbital fractures: experience with 111 orbital reconstructions. *J Craniofac Surg* **13**(6): 726–737.
43. Eski M, Sahin I, Deveci M, Turegun M, Isik S, Sengezer M. (2006) A retrospective analysis of 101 zygomatico-orbital fractures. *J Craniofac Surg* **17**(6): 1059–1064.
44. Price JC, Holliday MJ, Kennedy DW, *et al.* (1988) The versatile midface degloving approach. *Laryngoscope* **98**: 291–295.
45. Tadj A, Kimble FW. (2003) Fractured zygomas. *ANZ J Surg* **73**(1–2): 49–54.
46. Covington DS, Wainwright DJ, Teichgraeber JF, *et al.* (1994) Changing patterns in the epidemiology and treatment of zygoma fractures: 10-year review. *J Trauma* **37**: 243–248.
47. Zingg M, Laedrach K, Chen J, *et al.* (1992) Classification and treatment of zygomatic fractures: a review of 1025 cases. *J Oral Maxillofac Surg* **50**: 778–790.

48. Hollier LH, Thornton J, Pazmino P, *et al.* (2003) The management of orbitozygomatic fractures. *Plast Reconstr Surg* **111**: 2386–2392.
49. Carr RM, Mathog RH. (1997) Early and delayed repair of orbitozygomatic complex fractures. *J Oral Maxillofac Surg* **55**: 253–258.
50. Kaastad E, Freng A. (1989) Zygomatico-maxillary fractures. *J Craniomaxillofac Surg* **17**: 210.
51. Czerwinski M, Martin M, Lee C. (2005) Quantitative comparison of open reduction and internal fixation versus the Gillies method in the treatment of orbitozygomatic complex fractures. *Plast Reconstr Surg* **115**: 1848–1854.
52. Pearl RM. (1992) Treatment of enophthalmos. *Clin Plast Surg* **19**: 99–111.
53. Rohrich JR, Janis JE, Adams WP. (2003) Subciliary versus subtarsal approaches to orbitozygomatic fractures. *Plast Reconstr Surg* **111**: 1708–1714.
54. Zachariades N, Mezitis M, Mourouzis C, Papadakis D, Spanou A. (2006) Fractures of the mandibular condyle: a review of 466 cases. Literature review, reflections on treatment and proposals. *J Craniomaxillofac Surg* **34**(7): 421–432.
55. Stacey DH, Doyle JF, Mount DL, Snyder MC, Gutowski KA. (2006) Management of mandible fractures. *Plast Reconstr Surg* **117**(3): 48e–60e.
56. Van Sickels JE. (2005) A review and update of new methods for immobilization of the mandible. *Oral Surg Oral Med Oral Pathol Oral Radiol Endod* **100**(2 Suppl): S11–S16.
57. Mouton-Barrett R, Rubinstein A. (1998) Complications of mandibular fractures *Ann Plast Surg* **41**: 258–263.
58. Ellis E, Walker L. (1996) Treatment of mandibular angle fractures using one noncompression miniplate. *J Oral Maxillofac Surg* **54**: 864–871.
59. Passeri L, Ellis E, Sinn D. (1993) Complications of nonrigid fixation of mandibular angle fractures. *J Oral Maxillofac Surg* **51**: 382–384.
60. Ellis E, Karas N. (1992) Treatment of mandibular angle fractures using two mini dynamic compression plates. *J Oral Maxillofac Surg* **50**: 958–963.
61. Ellis E. (1999) Treatment methods for fractures of the mandibular angle. *Int J Oral Maxillofac Surg* **28**: 243–252.
62. Stone I, Dodson T, Bays R. (1993) Risk factors for infection following operative treatment of mandibular fractures: a multivariate analysis. *Plast Reconstr Surg* **91**: 64–68.
63. Leach J, Truelson J. (1995) Traditional methods vs rigid internal fixation of mandible fractures. *Arch Otolaryngol Head Neck Surg* **121**: 750–753.
64. Moreno J, Fernandez A, Ortiz J, *et al.* (2000) Complication rates associated with different treatments for mandibular fractures. *J Oral Maxillofac Surg* **58**: 273–280.

65. Ellis E, Sinn D. (1993) Treatment of mandibular angle fractures using 2 2.4-mm dynamic compression plates. *J Oral Maxillofac Surg* **31**: 969–973.
66. Haug R, Schwimmer A. (1994) Fibrous union of the mandible. *J Oral Maxillofac Surg* **52**: 832–839.
67. Tuovinen V, Norholt E, Sindet-Pederson S, *et al.* (1994) A retrospective analysis of 279 patients with isolated mandibular fractures treated with titanium miniplates. *J Oral Maxillofac Surg* **52**: 931–935.
68. Nakamura S, Takenoshita Y, Oka M. (1994) Complications of miniplate osteosynthesis for mandibular fractures. *J Oral Maxillofac Surg* **52**: 233–238.
69. Safdar N, Meechan J. (1995) Relationship between fractures of the mandibular angle and the presence and state of eruption of the lower third molar. *Oral Surg Oral Med Oral Path Oral Radiol Endod* **79**: 680–684.
70. Champy M, Lodde JP, Schmitt R, *et al.* (1978) Mandibular osteosynthesis by miniature screwed plates via a buccal approach. *J Maxillofac Surg* **6**: 14–21.
71. Marciani R, Anderson G, Gonty A. (1994) Treatment of mandibular angle fractures: transoral internal wire fixation. *J Oral Maxillofac Surg* **52**: 752–756.
72. Ellis E. (1998) Complications of mandibular condyle fractures. *Int J Oral Maxillofac Surg* **27**: 255–257.
73. Ellis E, McFadden D, Simon P, *et al.* (2000) Surgical complications with open treatment of mandibular condylar process fractures. *J Oral Maxillofac Surg* **58**: 950–958.
74. Mathog R, Toma V, Clayman L, *et al.* (2000) Nonunion of the mandible: an analysis of contributing factors. *J Oral Maxillofac Surg* **58**: 746–752.
75. Fanibunda K. (2000) Mandibular fracture resulting in displacement of the inferior alveolar nerve and allodynia. *J Oral Maxillofac Surg* **58**: 557–559.
76. Marchena J, Padwa B, Kaban L. (1998) Sensory abnormalities associated with mandibular fractures: incidence and natural history. *J Oral Maxillofac Surg* **56**: 822–825.

CHAPTER 12

AESTHETIC SURGERY OF THE FACE: FACE LIFT

Erick Martell and Alan Matarasso

Introduction

The indication for face lift surgery (facialplasty, rhytidectomy) is rejuvenation of the aging face that is primarily due to tissue laxity and/or volumetric changes. The goal of face lift surgery is to elevate and adjust ptotic soft tissue of the cheek, midface, face and neck area or restore volume loss in order to create a more youthful and rested appearance. Facelift surgery will not rejuvenate the eyebrow or eyes and should not alter the position of the eyelids, nose or mouth.

A thorough understanding of the multi lamellar facial anatomy and their relationships to each other and the structures that lie within them are important in order to achieve optimal aesthetic results and minimize potential complications.

Anatomy

The relevant tissue layers of the face include:

(1) skin,
(2) subcutaneous fat,
(3) superficial musculoaponeurotic system (SMAS),
(4) parotidomasseteric fascia
(5) mimetic muscles and
(6) branches of the facial nerve.

SMAS

The SMAS is the superficial fascia of the facial fat compartments and mimetic muscles and represents an attenuated fibromuscular extension of the superficial cervical fascia.[1] It continues as the platysma into the lower cheek and neck inferiorly and the parotid capsule laterally. Anteriorly, it terminates as the investing fascia of the superficial layer of the mimetic muscles. Superiorly, it continues as the superficial temporal fascia (temporoparietal fascia) and galea.[2,3]

Arterial Blood Supply

The facial artery (branch of external carotid artery) is the main blood supply to the lower and mid-face. It gives off:

- the inferior and superior labial arteries;
- lateral nasal artery and;
- the angular artery.
    - The superior labial artery supplies the upper lip and lateral nasal ala while the inferior labial artery supplies the lower lip and chin region. The lateral nasal artery branches off the facial artery to supply the nasal sidewall and ala.
    - The terminal branch of the facial artery, the angular artery, is the robust blood supply to the upper cheek, midface and medial canthal area.[4]
    - The superficial temporal artery supplies the upper and lower face via the temporal/frontal branches (temporal and frontal skin regions) and the transverse facial artery, respectively.
    - The transverse facial artery comes off the superficial temporal artery within the parotid gland and crosses inferior to the zygomatic arch to supply the cheek. The transverse facial artery is the main blood supply to the facelift skin flap after it's elevation.[5]
    - The upper face (brow, forehead) is supplied by the supraorbital and supratrochlear arteries (branch of ophthalmic artery), while the infraorbital artery supplies the midface.

SMAS

The SMAS attaches to the skin via retaining ligaments of the face and serves to support the soft tissues and resist gravitational forces over time.

- The osseocutaneous ligaments (mandibular and zygomatic) anchor the dermis to the periosteum in the mandibular and zygomatic regions.
- The fasciocutaneous ligaments (parotid and masseteric) form as fascial condensations of the parotid gland and masseter muscle to the overlying dermis.[6–8]

Attenuation of these ligaments and ptosis of soft tissues adjacent to these ligaments contribute to the stigmata of facial aging. For example, prominent jowls in the region of the mandibular cutaneous ligaments and submalar hollowness.

Malar Fat Pad

- The midface is a triangular region bordered by the infraorbital rim superiorly, the zygomaticus major laterally and the nasolabial fold medially.[9]
- The malar fat pad lies superficial to the SMAS and deep to the subcutaneous fat in the midface region.
- Descent of the malar fat pad to the inferior and medial positions is one hallmark of midfacial aging and elevation and repositioning of this compartment is a goal of midfacial rejuvenation.
- Additionally, lower lid fat herniation along with malar fat pad descent accentuates a hollowed out look of the midface-lower lid region (lid-cheek junction). Therefore, some surgeons prefer to perform lower lid blepharoplasty in combination with a midface lift or variations in those operations in order to address this specific problem.

Facial Nerve

- The facial nerve exits the stylomastoid foramen at a point that corresponds to approximately 0.5 cm below the tragus.

- There can be many anatomic variations; however it commonly divides into the temporofacial and facial-cervical branches within the parotid gland prior to exiting the parotid gland as the temporal, zygomatic, buccal, mandibular and cervical branches.
    - The temporal (frontal) branch of the facial nerve innervates the frontalis, corrugator, procerus and a portion of the orbicularis oculi muscles. It lies within layer of the superficial temporal fascia (mesotemporalis). It crosses the zygomatic arch and courses toward the temporal region lying approximately 1.5 cm above the lateral brow (Pitanguy's line.) [10]
    - The buccal branch innervates the buccinator (cheek tensor), orbicularis oculi (sphinteric) and levator labii superioris, levator anguli oris and both the zygomaticus major and minor (lip elevators.)
    - The zygomatic and buccal branches have extensive collateral innervations to the mimetic muscles of the face (zygomaticus muscles, levator angularis, and orbicularis oculi).
    - The marginal mandibular nerve innervates the lip depressors (depressor anguli oris and mentalis.) Studies have shown the marginal mandibular nerve to be located in an area from the superior border of the mandible to approximately 2 cm below the inferior border of the mandible.[11,12] Eighty percent of the time it is below the mandible when it is lateral to the facial artery and above the mandible when it is anterior to the artery.
    - The cervical branch innervates the platysma, which is also a lip depressor. A cervical branch injury can mimic the appearance of a marginal mandibular branch injury.
    - All muscles of the face are innervated from their deep surface except for the levator anguli oris, buccinators, and mentalis.

Techniques

Subcutaneous Facelift

- The subcutaneous (skin-only) facelift involves elevation of the skin flaps with division of the mandibular, zygomatic and masseteric retaining ligaments and leaving the SMAS and deeper facial structures undisturbed.

- A "C" shaped incision is made in the temporal hair bearing skin and continues inferiorly onto the pre or post tragal skin and continues underneath the earlobe into the postauricular crease and then angles into the hair bearing skin of the mastoid region.
- In this area, the skin flap is densely adherent to the sternocleidomastoid fascia and meticulous dissection is necessary to avoid injury to the great auricular nerve.[14]
- Following release of the osseocutaneous retaining ligaments, the skin flaps are advanced in a cephaloposterior direction followed by excision of redundant skin and then flap closure.
- The blood supply to the skin flap is the musculocutaneous branches of the facial, superficial temporal, and ophthalmic arteries.[13]
- In the male patient, some authors prefer to avoid a post tragal incision, which can result in tragal distortion and positioning of hair bearing facial skin onto the tragus.
- An inherent issue with this technique is that the skin flap is not a structural support for the deep facial structures and therefore does not reposition the deep tissues of the face.
- If the skin is excessively tightened, it can result in an unnatural stretched appearance rather than a youthful rejuvenated appearance.

SMAS Facelift

- The SMAS is an inelastic layer that provides a meaningful and sustained support of the soft tissues of the face.
- Repositioning of the SMAS translates clinically into redistribution and enhancement of the natural facial contours (opposed to flattening), which is more characteristic of a youthful face.
- This allows the skin to be re-draped with minimal tension and thus reduces the post procedure stigmata.
- The skin incisions are essentially the same as described in the subcutaneous technique. However, a mesotemporalis layer must be developed at the transition zone just above the ear between the deep temporalis fascia of the subcutaneous skin flap dissection below. The frontal branch of the facial nerve runs within this mesotemporalis. Many variations of dissection and suspension of the SMAS alone or in continuity with the lateral platysmal muscle have been described.

- The skin vector of pull and the SMAS-platysma vector can be adjusted independent of each other to enhance the cosmetic outcome according to the needs of the patient.
- The typical SMAS dissection involves a vertical SMAS incision in the preauricular area and continued inferiorly to the angle of the mandible and neck, creating a SMAS-platysmal flap.
- A transverse SMAS incision is made inferior to the zygomatic arch, avoiding the frontal branch of the facial nerve.
- The SMAS is dissected and elevated anteriorly over the parotid fascia to a level which depends on the desired degree of re-suspension to the jowls and neck.
- The upper mobile SMAS flap is advanced and sutured to the immobile SMAS at the original incision and the SMAS-platysmal flap is sutured to the sternocleidomastoid fascia. Extension of the SMAS can accentuate the nasolabial fold.
- Recently surgeons have recognized the need for volumization in conjunction with surgical rejuvenation. Fat grafting can be done in numerous areas of the face including: tear trough, eyelid-cheek junction, nasolabial crease, mandibular angle, lips, etc.

The High SMAS Facelift

- The High SMAS facelift differs from the traditional SMAS facelift in that the superior SMAS incision and elevation is above the zygomatic arch while protecting the frontal branch of the facial nerve.[15,16]
- The superior SMAS flap is then fixated to the deep temporal fascia superior to the auricular attachment.
- The vertical lift of the malar fat pad and upper SMAS translates into greater recruitment and redistribution to the midface and upper malar regions.[17]

Extended SMAS Technique

- The Extended SMAS technique also involves incision and elevation of the SMAS above the zygomatic arch to enhance midface and upper malar rejuvenation.

- The anterior dissection is taken further anterior and superficial to the zygomaticus major muscle, which exerts a greater effect on the mid-cheek and perioral areas.[18]
- This procedure requires longer operative time and a more meticulous dissection in order to avoid nerve injury.

SMAS Plication Technique

- In the SMAS plication technique, imbrication and fixation of the SMAS at multiple sites and along different vectors results in elevation of the jowls and perioral region in patients with deformities amenable to this procedure.
- The benefits of SMAS plication are that it is less invasive, is faster to perform, with potentially less complications. The drawbacks can be that there is less effect on the midface and malar regions and can result in contour irregularities in thin-faced patients.

Lateral SMASectomy

- The lateral SMASectomy procedure, first described by Straith usually involves excising 1–2cm of SMAS anterior to the parotid gland in an oblique fashion from the angle of the mandible to the malar region.
- The mobile SMAS is then sutured to the fixed SMAS as an anchoring point. The vector of soft tissue elevation can be varied according to the obliquity in which the SMASectomy is designed.
- This technique avoids the risks inherent in a full SMAS dissection; the drawback is that it results in tightening of the deep tissues in only one vector.

Deep Plane Facelift

Skoog developed the technique of elevating the SMAS, subcutaneous fat and skin as a single unit for facial rejuvenation.[19]
The advantages are that

- it allows wide undermining and
- repositioning of the SMAS while maintaining excellent blood supply to the overlying skin.

The main disadvantage is that the SMAS and the skin are repositioned in the same vector and to the same degree, which may not meet the aesthetic goals of the patient. Furthermore, the midface and periorbital areas remain unaddressed. Hamra's composite facelift was a modification of the Deep Plane facelift to address these issues, and has evolved over the years.

Composite Facelift

The goal of the Composite facelift technique is to address

1. jowling caused by ptosis of the platysma muscle,
2. deepening of the nasolabial folds and midcheek depressions caused by descent of cheek fat.

Procedure Steps:

- This requires the patient to consent to undergoing lower lid blepharoplasty along with a facelift. This procedure allows repositioning of these three elements en bloc with the skin and without disruption of their normal relationships to each other.[20]
- The SMAS elevation is performed in the usual fashion along with elevation of the malar fat pad off of the zygomatic major and minor muscles.
- The orbicularis oculi is undermined via a lower blepharoplasty incision and joined with the facelift incision.[21]
- After the pre-platysmal dissection, the medial edges of the paired platysma muscles are advanced anteriorly via the submental incision, and sutured in the midline.
- Rejuvenation of the jowl and cheek areas is in the superiolateral vector and, for the midface, in the superiomedial vector.
- Excellent aesthetic results of the periorbital, lower, and midface regions have been obtained in selected patients using this technique.
- It requires, however, a thorough knowledge of the anatomy and experience.

Short Scar Facelift with Barbed Suture SMAS-Platysma Imbrication and Tissue Sealant

The senior author's preferred facelift technique has evolved to this method.

The procedure begins with liposuction of the neck, jowls, and face as indicated. Any fat grafting that is necessary is then performed.

A submental incision is made and the medial (anterior) edges of the platysma muscles are identified. When indicated a triangular wedge at the level of the hyoid is excised and the platysma muscle edges are approximated with 3-0 Mersilene sutures yielding an Eiffel tower design appearance of the medial platysma muscle closure. Alternatively, the edges of the redundant platysma are incised every one centimeter from hyoid to mandible, breaking up the continuity of the medial platysma bands that appear as telltale muscle cords in the neck.

The incision is made in continuity beginning with a sideburn cut, pre- or post-tragally (this is designed as a vest-over-pants tragoplasty) ending in the post-auricular sulcus at the first skin crease approximately at the edge of the mastoid bone. A subcutaneous skin flap is widely undermined as indicated.

Redundant SMAS and lateral platysma muscle laxity are identified. The excess SMAS is elevated and sutured to the junction of the zygoma in front of the ear with a di-directional barbed suture. One suture progresses anteriorly along the zygoma, imbricating redundant SMAS. The second suture imbricates the SMAS in front of the ear and then in continuity with the lateral platysma down the upper neck and sewn to the sternocleidomastoid fascia.

The anterior skin flap is elevated in a cephalo-vertical fashion and the posterior flap cephaloposteriorly. The excess skin is trimmed where it meets the edges of the ear without tension. Tissue sealant is sprayed on the dissected area and the wound edges are then closed in one layer with different material depending on location. Drains are not used.

Subperiosteal Facelift

- The subperiosteal facelift allows tissue repositioning at the level of its bony origins.
- It is aimed at rejuvenation of the upper two thirds of the face; however it can be combined with other traditional techniques in a biplanar manner in order to address the lower third of the face.

- It is typically performed via a temporal and intraoral approach but it can also be performed endoscopically.
- The combination of a brow lift, midface lift with malar augmentation as well as SMAS and platysma repositioning represents a comprehensive approach in patients with advanced facial aging.[22,23]
- A relative contraindication to the subperiosteal technique is previous extensive facial fractures, which the resultant bony irregularities make the dissection more perilous.
- A disadvantage is prolonged swelling and a higher incidence of facial nerve injury.
- A comparative 10-year study on two sets of identical twins done by four different surgeons reported the results in four of the techniques.[33]

Minimal Access Cranial Suspension

- In the MACS face lift the SMAS and its attached structures are suspended in a pure vertical vector with the excess skin being excised above the temporal hairline.
- A preauricular incision is made with the dissection limited to the lateral canthus, nasolabial fold and the angle of the mandible in the subcutaneous plane with the SMAS left undisturbed.
- The SMAS is then secured to the deep temporal fascia using multiple purse string sutures. The laterally placed suture is directed from the temporal fascia towards the angle of the mandible, which affects the cervicomental area.
- A medially placed suture is directed towards the jowls, which exerts action on the jowls and marionette groves.
- The extended MACS procedure involves a third purse string suture directed to suspend the malar fat pad which affects the nasolabial folds and midface.[24,25]
- The major disadvantage is that a relatively large area of deep tissues are suspended by a static suture, which can lead to suture palpability, facial creasing, dimpling and contour irregularities with facial animation.

Neck Lift

When indicated, the region from the jowl to the collar area can be addressed in isolation by a neck lift that will not affect the midface area. A submental incision is used to enable access to any submental platysma bands. The skin incision begins on the pre-auricular crease approximately one centimeter above the earlobe. It extends on the post-auricular sulcus for three to five centimeters and then transverses into the mastoid-post-auricular scalp area obliquely at a sixty degree angle for five to six centimeters.

Complications

Hematoma

- Hematomas are the most common complication following facelift procedures and most often occur within the first 24 hours postoperatively.
- Often the etiology is not determined and rarely is a definitive isolated bleeding vessel found to be the culprit, but rather generalized oozing is usually identified.
- Causes include failure of operative hemostasis, poor control of perioperative hypertension, unrecognized use of medication affecting coagulation, underlying coagulation disorders, or sudden increases in intrathoracic pressures (e.g. emesis, valsalva, etc.)[26]
- Expanding hematomas can result in airway compromise and should be treated as a surgical emergency.
- The incidence of hematomas requiring surgical interventions ranges from 2–4%. Symptoms include localized and increasing pain to the affected side of the face or neck. Since significant pain following a facelift is unusual, sudden unilateral pain should be treated as a hematoma until proven otherwise.[37]
- Protocols for non-expanding hematomas have been reported in order to clean them in a sterile, non-operating room area.[38]
- Smaller hematomas, less than 20 cc's, usually present when facial edema begins to subside and can be managed with needle aspiration and close follow up.

Nerve Injury

- The overall incidence of permanent nerve injury following rhytidectomy is less than 1%.[27]
- Most postoperative paralysis and neuropraxias are transient and recover within the first year. Intervention is rarely needed. If a nerve injury is recognized intraoperatively, or the level of injury recalled in the immediate post-operative period, it should be repaired. If not they are managed expectantly.
- Patient education, monitoring, close follow up and support is beneficial in this time period.
- In the immediate postoperative period, up to 12 hours or so, it is common to observe abnormal forms of sensation that mimic nerve injury but are due to the lingering effects of the local anesthetic agents or surgery.

The most commonly injured motor nerve following rhytidectomy is the buccal branch of the facial nerve.[28] The zygomatic and buccal branches have extensive collateral innervations to the mimetic muscles of the face and therefore injury to one branch usually results in a transient defect and full recovery is expected.

Injury to the temporal branch of the facial nerve

Injury to the temporal branch of the facial nerve can occur when dissecting in the superficial temporal fascial (temporoparietal) plane and can result in the inability to raise the eyebrow on the affected side.

Therefore, in a subcutaneous facelift, the nerve is within the mesotemporalis and dissection can be done in a blunt fashion using a gauze covered index finger in order to avoid transecting the nerve.

Injury to the marginal mandibular branch of the facial nerve

Injury to the marginal mandibular branch of the facial nerve can occur during the dissection of the lateral border of the platysmal below the angle of the mandible, potentially resulting in the inability to depress the lower lip on the affected side. As in the mesotemporalis, the lateral border of the platysma can be bluntly finger-tip dissected. Unlike the zygomatic and buccal branches, which have overlapping innervation, the mandibular and temporal branches are terminal branches to their respective regions and therefore are less likely to recover in the event of an injury. Pseudo-paralysis of the marginal mandibular nerve can occur from injury to the cervical branch, most commonly when performing a submental dissection. It manifests itself by weakness of the lower lip due to lack of platysmal innervation.[29]

Approximately 15% of injuries to the marginal mandibular and frontal branch nerves are permanent.

Sensory Nerve Injuries

- The most commonly injured sensory nerve is the great auricular nerve.
- It is located approximately 8 cm inferior to the external auditory meatus, or 6 cm from the lobule, and 1cm posterior to the external jugular vein.[30]
- Overall, the most commonly injured nerve; it is prone to injury during skin flap dissection over the sternocleidomastoid fascia in the postauricular area where there are dense deep dermal attachments to the underlying fascia. If an injury is recognized intraoperatively, the nerve should be repaired
- Although most patients will experience transient numbness following a rhytidectomy, greater auricular nerve injury can result in long-term sensory loss or pain of the lower portion of the ear lobe.

Skin Flap Ischemia and Necrosis

The incidence of skin flap ischemia or necrosis is variable and the etiology is often multifactorial. Soon after surgery the skin can appear mottled or irregularly discolored form the effects of the injections and surgery, albeit with appropriate capillary refill. Ischemic skin can progress to necrosis. The clinical presentation ranges from superficial skin sloughing to full thickness necrosis. Causes include:

1. vascular compromise from a large expanding hematoma;
2. excessive tension with skin closure leading to vascular compromise;
3. improper plane of dissection, or damaging the flap during dissection;

4. dermal injury secondary to thermal burns (a common occurrence of this can be seen as small areas of punctate skin necrosis ranging from a few millimeters to more than one centimeter from electrocautery burns to the underside of the skin flap);
5. tobacco exposure and;
6. tight pressure dressings or improper head positioning postoperatively.

- In general: superficial tissue injuries can be treated conservatively and allowed to re-epithelialize and heal by secondary intention.[31]
- Debridement and subsequent skin advancement should be delayed until the wound demarcates and non-viable tissue is observed.
- The late sequelae of skin necrosis can include hypertrophic scarring, hypopigmentation, and textural changes in the skin.[32] Untoward sequelae of facialplasty include, but are not limited to, skin irregularities, small fluid collections, paresthesias, discoloration, and variations in the appearance of the scar that tend to resolve spontaneously or with minimal intervention.

References

1. Mitz V, Peyronie M. (1976) The superficial musculo-aponeurotic system (SMAS) in the parotid and cheek area. *Plast Reconstr Surg*. **58**(1): 80–8.
2. Wassef M. (1987) Superficial fascial and muscular layers in the face and neck: a histological study. *Aesthetic Plast Surg.* **11**: 171–176.
3. Barton Jr FE. (1992) The SMAS and the nasolabial fold. *Plast Reconstr Surg.* **89**: 1054–1057.
4. Netter F. (2006) Atlas of Human Anatomy 4th Ed. Saunders, Philadelphia.
5. Whetzel, Thomas P. M.D; Mathes, Stephen J. M.D. (1997) The Arterial Supply of the Face Lift Flap The Arterial Supply of the Face Lift Flap. *Plast Reconstr Surg.* **100**: 480–486.
6. Furnas DW. (1989) The retaining ligaments of the cheek. *Plast Reconstr Surg.* **83**: 11–16.
7. Stuzin JM, Baker TJ, Gordon HL. (1992) The relationship of the superficial and deep facial fascias: relevance to rhytidectomy and aging. *Plast Reconstr Surg.* **89**: 441–449.
8. Pessa JE, Desvigne LD, Lyons AE. (1999) An early description of the superficial musculoaponeurotic system by Sir Charles Bell. *Plast Reconstr Surg.* **103**: 1071–1072.

9. Mendelson BC, Muzzafar AR, Adams Jr WP. (2002) Surgical anatomy of the midcheek and malar mounds. *Plast Reconstr Surg*. **110**: 885–896.
10. Pitanguy I, Ramos AS. (1966) The frontal branch of the facial nerve: the importance of its variations in face lifting. *Plast Reconstr Surg*. **38**: 352–356.
11. Dingman RO, Grabb WC. (1962) Surgical anatomy of the mandibular ramus of the facial nerve based on the dissection of 100 facial halves. *Plast Reconstr Surg*. **29**: 266–272.
12. Nelson DW, Gingrass RP. (1979) Anatomy of the mandibular branches of the facial nerve. *Plast Reconstr Surg*. **64**(4): 479–82.
13. Whetzel TP, Mathes SJ. (1992) Arterial anatomy of the face: an analysis of vascular territories and perforating cutaneous vessels. *Plast Reconstr Surg*. **89**(4): 591–603; discussion 604–5.
14. McKinney P, Katrana DJ. (1980) Prevention of injury to the great auricular nerve during rhytidectomy. *Plast Reconstr Surg*. **66**(5): 675–9.
15. Stuzin JM, Wangstrom L, Kawamoto HK, *et al*. (1989) Anatomy of the frontal branch of the facial nerve: the significance of the temporal fat pad. *Plast Reconstr Surg*. **83**(2): 265–71.
16. Trussler AP *et al*. (2010) The frontal branch of the facial nerve across the zygomatic arch: anatomical relevance of the High-SMAS technique. *Plast Reconstr Surg*. **125**(4): 1221–1229.
17. Barton Jr FE. (2002) The "High SMAS" Face Lift Technique. *Aesthetic Surg J*. **22**: 481–486.
18. Stuzin JM, Baker, TJ, Gordon, HL and Baker, TM. (1995) Extended SMAS dissection as an approach to midface rejuvenation. *Clin Plast Surg*. **22**: 295
19. Skoog (1974) T. Plastic Surgery: New Methods and Refinements. Philadelphia: Saunders.
20. Hamra, ST. (1992) Composite rhytidectomy. *Plast Reconstr Surg*. **90**(1): 1–13.
21. Hamra, ST. (1992) Composite rhytidectomy. *Plast Reconstr Surg*. **90**(1): 14–22.
22. Ramirez OM. (1996) Classification of facial rejuvenation techniques based on the subperiosteal approach and ancillary procedures. *Plast Reconstr Surg*. **97**(1): 45–55.
23. Ramirez, O.M. (1995) The subperiosteal approach for the correction of the deep nasolabial fold and the central third of the face. *Clin. Plast. Surg*. **22**: 341.
24. Aesthetic Surgery of the Facial Mosaic The MACS Lift: Minimal Access Cranial Suspension Lift; Heidelberg Springer 2007.
25. Tonnard P, Verpaele A. (2004) The MACS-Lift: Short-Scar Rhytidectomy Philadelphia QMP.

26. Grover R, Jones M, Waterhouse N. (2001) The prevention of haematoma following rhytidectomy: a review of 1078 consecutive facelifts. *Br J Plast Surg.* **54**: 481–6.
27. DC, Conley J. (1979) Avoiding facial nerve injuries in rhytidectomy. *Plast Reconstr Surg.* **64**: 781–95.
28. Baker DC and Conley, J. (1979) Avoiding facial nerve injuries in rhytidectomy: Anatomic variations and pitfalls. *Plast Reconstr Surg.* **64**: 781.
29. Ellenbogen R. (1979) Pseudo-paralysis of the marginal mandibular nerve after plastysmaa face-lift operation. *Plast Reconstr Surg*. 364–368.
30. McKinney P, Katrana DJ. (1980) Prevention of injury to the great auricular nerve during rhytidectomy. *Plast Reconstr Surg*. **66**(5): 675–9.
31. Baker TJ, Gordon HL, Mosienko P. (1977) Rhytidectomy: a statistical analysis. *Plast Reconstr Surg.* **59**(1): 24–30.
32. Stuzin JM. (2008) MOC-PS CME article: face lifting. *Plast Reconstr Surg.* **121**(1): 1–19.

Further Reading

Alpert BS, Baker DC, Hamra ST, Owsley JQ, Ramirez O. (2009) Identical twin face lifts with differing techniques: a 10-year follow-up. *Plast Reconstr Surg*. **123**(3): 1025–1033; 1034–1036.

Baker DC, Chiu ES. (2005) Bedside treatment of early acute rhytidectomy hematomas. *Plast Reconstr Surg*. **115**(7): 2119–2122; discussion 2123.

Matarasso A, Elkwood A, Rankin M, Elkowitz M. (2000) National plastic surgery survey: face lift techniques and complications. *Plast Reconstr Surg*. **106**(5): 1185–1195.

Pitanguy I, Machado B. (2012) Facial rejuvenation surgery. A retrospective study of 8788 cases. *Aesthetic Surg J*. **32**: 393–412.

Rees TD, Barone CM, Valauri FA, Ginsberg GD, Nolan WB. (1994) 3rd. Hematomas requiring surgical evacuation following face lift surgery. *Plast Reconstr Surg*. **93**(6): 1185–1190.

Warren RJ, Aston SJ, Mendelson BC. (2001) Face lift. *Plast Reconstr Surg.* **128**(6): 747e–64e.

CHAPTER 13

EYELID, CHEEK, LIP, NASAL, SCALP, EAR RECONSTRUCTION

Anuja K. Antony, Victor J. Hassid and Mimis N. Cohen

EYELID RECONSTRUCTION

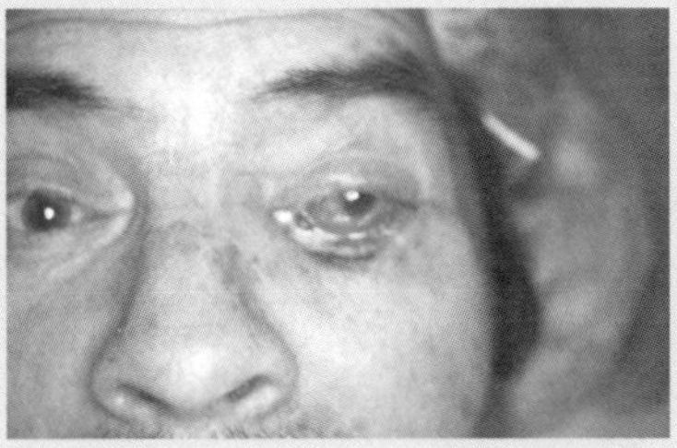

A.

Illustrative Case 1: 54 year old male with basal cell carcinoma of left lower eyelid present for Moh's resection with anticipated total loss of lower lid.

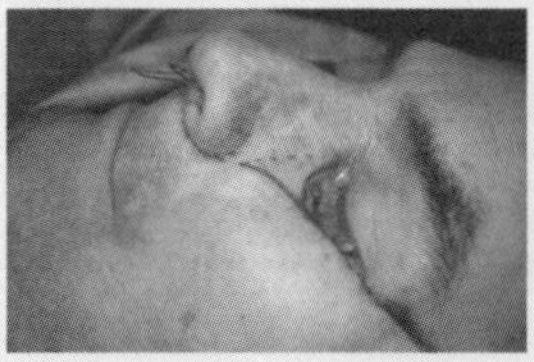

B.

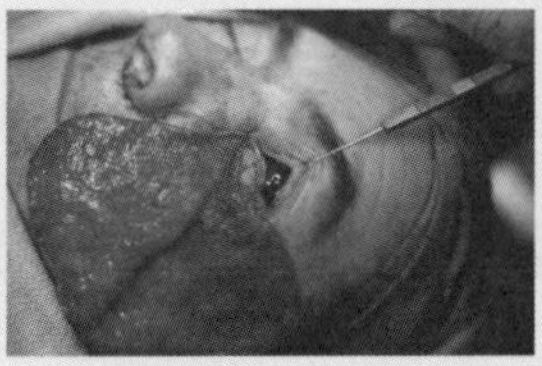

C.

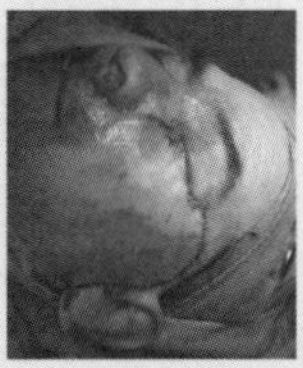

D.

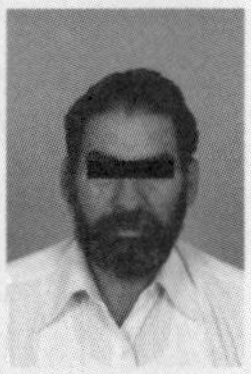

E.

1B. Proposed cheek flap. Note that nose is packed with cocaine packs prior to harvesting chondromucosal flap for conjunctival and mucosal reconstruction.
1C. Chondromucosal flap harvested with lateral canthotomy in place. Elevated cheek flap shown. (Tarsorraphy stitch recommended — not shown.)
1D and E. Immediate result and results 12 months after reconstruction.

Management, Preoperative Tests

- Important to evaluate visual acuity and orbital status; may require ophthalmology consultation
- Detailed analysis of structures involved and estimation of percent of missing eyelid tissue
- Determine if Partial or Full-thickness injury
- Lid tissue best reconstructed like-for-like with lid tissue, for improved aesthetic outcome (caution when borrowing from upper eyelid, because it contributes to a great degree to orbit protection and lid function)

Operative Techniques List

PRIMARY CLOSURE

- Primary closure for defects up to 1/3 of the lid
- 33–50% defects can be repaired primarily, along with canthotomy and cantholysis
- 50–75% defects repaired with myocutaneous advancement flaps
- >75% borrow tissue from the opposite lid or adjacent regions, such as cheek, temporal area, forehead

PARTIAL THICKNESS LOSS

- Anterior Skin Coverage: primary repair or FTSG, preferably from contralateral lid
- Tarsus: repair primarily or reconstruct with cartilage/palatal mucosal grafts, or allografts (e.g. Alloderm®)
- Conjunctiva: either advancement of adjacent conjunctiva or use buccal/nasal mucosa

FULL THICKNESS LOSS

- Full-thickness: either primary repair or will require grafts and local flap for repair of anterior skin coverage, tarsus and conjunctiva

FLAPS

Upper eyelid

- Cutler-Beard flap (bridge flap)
- Temporal forehead flap
- Paramedian forehead flap

Lower eyelid

- Tenzel semicircular flap
- Hughes tarsoconjunctival flap
- Mustarde cheek advancement flap

Operative Techniques Description — Order of Repair and Steps

— PRIMARY REPAIR:

- Full-thickness incisions should be made perpendicular to the eyelid margin and extend to the superior tarsal margin to prevent notching
- Lateral cantholysis may be needed to reduce tension of closure
- Repair completed in layers; sutures passed through anterior two-thirds of tarsal plate to avoid corneal irritation

— SKIN GRAFT:

- FTSG can adequately reconstruct small superficial anterior lamellar defects
- Excess skin from contralateral upper lid can be used (if not available: supraclavicular skin, preauricular, lateral cervical skin); medial eyelid skin is avoided to prevent lagophthalmos)
- 50–70% overcorrection should be planned to allow for secondary contraction
- Separate grafts in pretarsal area and orbital sulcus

Upper Lid Flaps

— CUTLER-BEARD FLAP:

- Full thickness lower lid bridge flap for defects up to 100%
- Incision made 5 mm inferior to lower eyelid margin to preserve lid margin vascularity
- Flap advanced under the intact lower lid margin (bridge) and inset into upper lid
- Width = defect
  - — Vertical incisions inferiorly to fornix and inferior orbital rim; relaxing incisions in capsulopalpebral fascia to allow passage of the flap
- Can be modified by adding posterior lamella spacer (ear cartilage or hard palate mucoperichondrium placed anterior to conjunctiva (biplanar flap) and sutured to levator aponeurosis to maintain lid function and stability
- Division traditionally at 6 weeks

— TEMPORAL FOREHEAD FLAP:

- Tissue is thicker and less ideal; used when other options not feasible
- Design appropriately based on size of defect
- Right angle-resembling shape starting lateral to the orbit with orientation towards midline of forehead
- Raise thin cutaneous flap and transpose it to upper eyelid region
- Defect closed in layers

— PARAMEDIAN FOREHEAD FLAP/GLABELLAR-TYPE FLAPS:

- Design appropriately based on size of defect; tissue thicker
- See section on Nasal Reconstruction for operative details
- Division of pedicle in 3 weeks and inset of flap

Lower Lid Flaps

— TENZEL FLAP:

- Defects 40–60%
- Superiorly based musculocutaneous (orbicularis) flap starting at the lateral canthus and extending in a semicircle (diameter ≥3 cm)

- Lateral canthotomy is required to rotate the flap and lateral remaining lid margin

— HUGHES TARSOCONJUNCTIVAL FLAP:

- Upper lid retracted with Desmarres retractor and a 3-sided flap is designed consisting of conjunctiva and tarsus; horizontal border should be at least 4 mm superior to lid margin
- Composite flap is advanced into lower eyelid defect, so that upper border of tarsus contained within flap is in alignment with remaining lower eyelid margin
- Anterior lamella is reconstructed with advancement of cutaneous or musculocutaneous (if orbicularis present) flap, which originates from the area caudal to lower eyelid.
- Divide pedicle in 4–6 weeks

— MUSTARDE FLAP:

- Carry the incision beyond the lateral canthus in a curvilinear fashion and extend it higher than the lateral palpebral fissure (almost at the level of the eyebrow), since height will be lost during rotation, and this will also allow the incision to be hidden in the crow's feet wrinkles
- Need the temporal skin for reconstruction
- Incision curves inferiorly to the preauricular crease
- Once it reaches the ear lobule, the incision may be carried inferiorly and medially into the neck, or extend behind the ear in the posterior auricular sulcus and alond the hairline
- The flap is raised in the subcutaneous plane and rotated to cover the eyelid defect
- A back-cut or equalizing Burow's triangle excision at the base of the flap may be useful to decrease wound closure tension
- The lateral canthus is formed by suturing the deep layer of the dermis of the rotational graft to superior and inner aspect of the lateral orbital rim
- Suspend flap to the lateral rim periosteum to add additional upward traction at apex of the flap
- The eyelids may be sutured together with a tarsorrhaphy stitch to provide additional upward tension on the flap and removed after a week

Postoperative Care

- Possibly outpatient procedure
- Local wound care
- Bolster dressing if skin graft used
- Drains as needed
- Antibiotics × 1 week
- Monitor for complications, such as eyelid retraction, notching of eyelid margin, bleeding, infection, etc.

Outpatient Rehabilitation

- Wound care
- Scar massaging

CHEEK RECONSTRUCTION

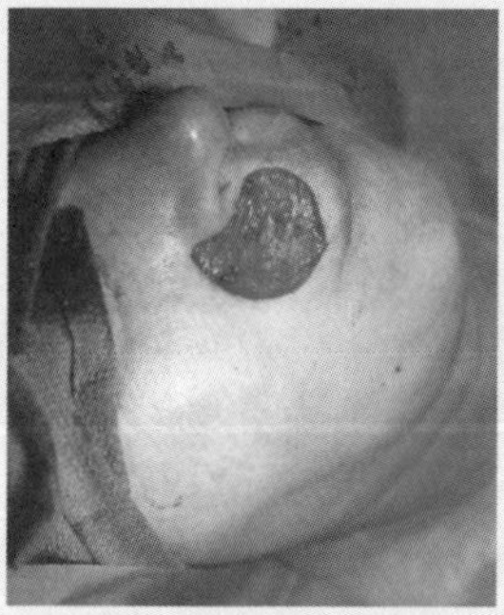

A.

Illustrative Case 2: 65 year old diagnosed with cheek/upper lip defect after excision of superficial spreading melanoma.

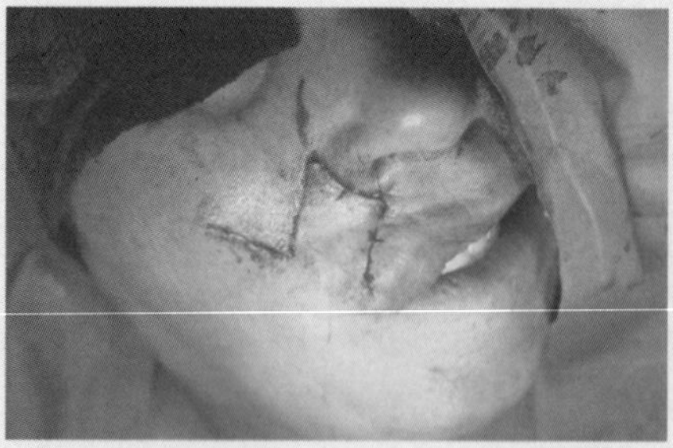

B.

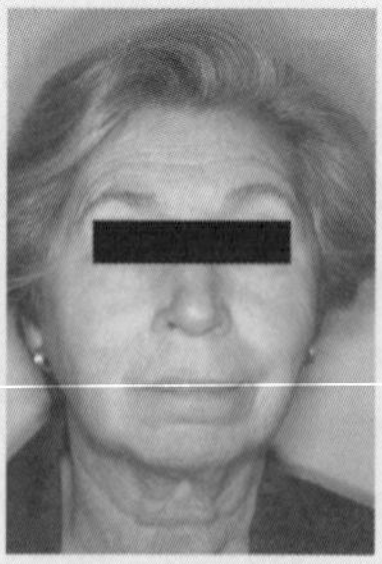

C.

2B. A rhomboid flap was used to reconstruct the defect.
2C. Final result 2 years postop.

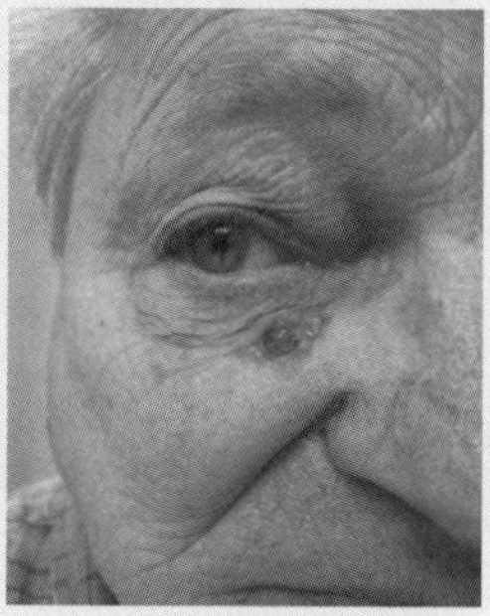

A.

Illustrative Case 3: 72 year old male with recurrent BCC of medial cheek/canthal region scheduled for Moh's resection.
3B. Defect of medial cheek/canthal region after resection.

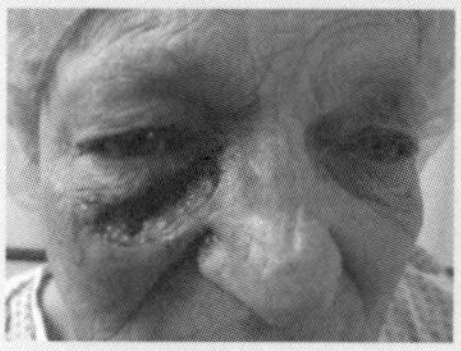

B.

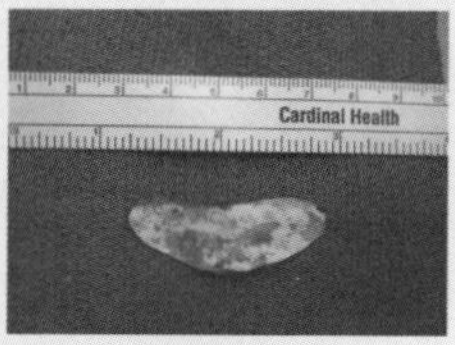

C.

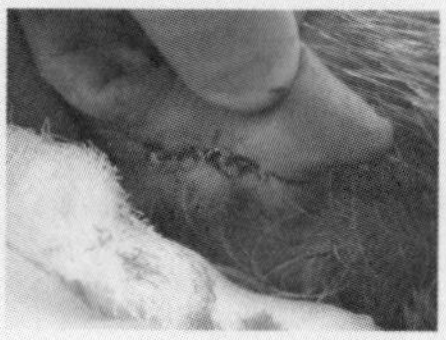

D.

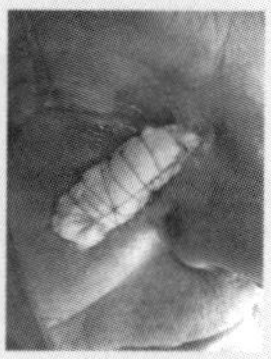

E.

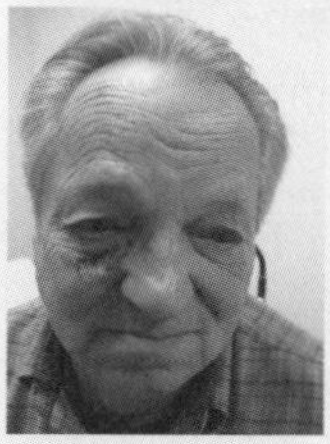

F.

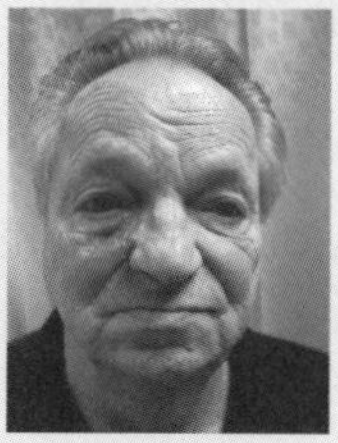

G.

3C. Template of defect for FTSG.
3D. Postauricular FTSG harvested. Defect closed primarily.
3E. Tie-over bolster placed on skin graft. Note lateral tarsorraphy stitch.
3F and G. 2 weeks and 1 month postoperative result.

Management, Preoperative Tests

- Assess mobility and laxity of skin surrounding the defect
- Assess convexity / concavity of defect
- Determine which facial structures may be distorted by secondary tissue movement (important: nasal ala, lip, lower eyelid)
- Outline borders of the cheek and adjacent facial aesthetic units; scars should be placed at borders of units for better aesthetic outcome
- Reconstructive options may differ based on the underlying etiology, e.g. defect following excision of melanoma with high risk of recurrence, which can be reconstructed either with primary closure, or healing by secondary intention, or with the use of skin graft, reserving a local flap at a second stage after appropriate time interval to ensure the recurrence is unlikely
- Freshen the edges of the defect, e.g. if the defect has been created by Mohs surgery, it typically has 45 degrees beveled edges.
- If greater than 50% of the unit is missing, consider reconstructing entire cheek unit

Operative Techniques List

- Primary closure
- Full-thickness skin graft
- Local skin flaps for lesions < 4 cm (rhomboid flap, bilobed flap)
- Local flaps for lesions > 4 cm (cheek rotation-advancement flaps)
- Tissue expansion
- Free flaps for defects usually >10 cm or full thickness; fasciocutaneous flaps are preferred, because they are relatively thin and do not atrophy (e.g. radial forearm flap, anteriolateral thigh flap)

Operative Techniques Description — Order of Repair and Steps

— PRIMARY REPAIR:

- Smaller lesions in direction of relaxed skin tension lines (RSTL)
- Repair in layers

— RHOMBOID FLAP:

- Standard design, so that final donor site scar in direction of RSTL
- Raise in a subcutaneous plane
- Remember that maximal tension at the area of donor site closure
- Rhombus designed with 60- and 120-degree angles and flap fashioned to transfer redundant skin to defect with primary closure of donor site

— BILOBED FLAP:

- See Nasal Reconstruction section for operative details

— CHEEK ROTATION-ADVANCEMENT FLAP:

- Random pattern subcutaneous flap, typically V-Y advancement with excision of Burrow's triangles
- Near eyelid margin or nasal base, anchor flap to perisoteum to prevent ectropion or nostril flare
- Defects best excised as rectangle or square to prevent trap door deformity and 1:1 base-to-lenth width safe to avoid tip necrosis
- "Cervicofacial hike" described based off of SMAS and similar to deep plane rhytidectomy advances cheek superiorly

Postoperative Care

- Local wound care; Bolster dressing if skin graft used
- Drains — surgeon preference
- Monitor for complications, such as infection, bleeding, seroma/hematoma formation

Outpatient Rehabilitation

- Wound care
- Scar massage

LIP RECONSTRUCTION

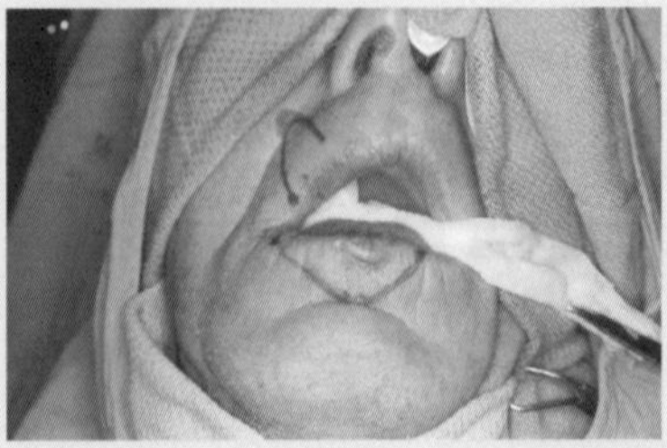

A.

Illustrative Case 4: 74 year old with large BCC of lower lip. Proposed excision of approximately ¾ of the lip with markings for planned commisure-sparing Estlander flap based on the upper lip.

4B. Ten days post resection and staged reconstruction prior to flap division.

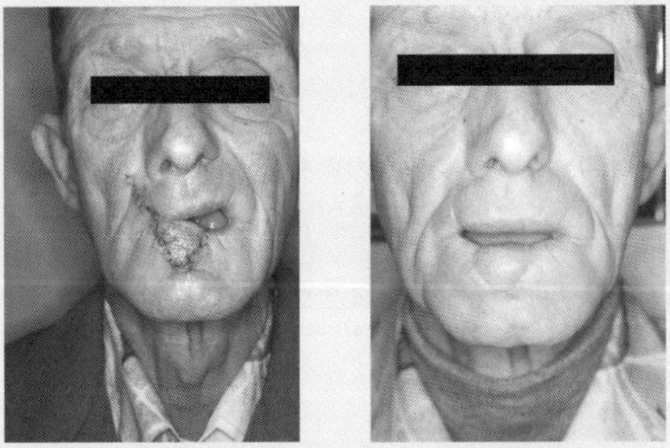

B. C.

4C. Final result 17 months after division and inset.

Management, Preoperative Tests

- Analysis of the defect (size, partial/full thickness, commissure involvement)
- Primary closure is an option for defects up to one third of lip
- Different options depending on type of defect (see operative techniques)

Operative Techniques List

- Vermilion volume deficiency
  - Axial musculovermilion advancement flap
  - Musculomucosal or mucosal labial V-Y advancement flap
  - Mucosal cross-lip flap
  - Tongue flap
- Full-thickness lip reconstruction
  - Abbé flap
  - Estlander flap
  - Karapandzic technique
- Total lip reconstruction
  - Radial forearm with palmaris longus composite free flap (the palmaris longus can be used as sling to maintain lip height)

Operative Techniques Description — Order of Repair and Steps

— PRIMARY REPAIR:

- Optimal primary repair requires approximation of mucosa, orbicularis oris, deep dermis and epidermis
- Anterior vermilion line is the principal landmark of the lip, followed by the red line (border between dry and wet vermilion)

— AXIAL MUSCULOVERMILION ADVANCEMENT FLAP:

- Full-thickness incision made along anterior vermilion line inferior to the labial artery
- The flap will include the vermilion part of the orbicularis oris muscle
- The incision should be long enough to allow for adequate stretch
- Forward advancement of the flap to cover the defect
- Careful wound closure in order to optimize final scar

— MUSCULOMUCOSAL OR MUCOSAL V-Y ADVANCEMENT FLAP:

- A simple advancement flap can be created by undermining beneath the labial mucosa in a plane that is deep to the minor salivary glands and superficial to the orbicularis oris

- If a V-Y flap is being designed a V-shaped incision is created with the apex of the incision positioned toward the gingivolabial sulcus
- The triangular-shaped island is advanced in a vertical or near-vertical orientation into the defect, maintaining adequate attachments to the deep tissues.
- The donor site is closed in a Y configuration

— MUCOSAL CROSS-LIP FLAP:

- Single pedicle flap for small defects or bipedicle flap ("bucket handle") for wider defects (it extends horizontally across the lip)
- Design a linear mucosal band at the region immediately posterior to the posterior vermilion line of the donor lip
- Width of the band based on the width of the defect, and on the ability to close the donor defect
- Elevate flap in plane superficial to orbicularis oris; include portion of the muscle if bulk needed; Labial artery usually not included, but if it is there is greater likelihood of flap viability
- Transfer flap to the vermilion defect and inset it; donor site closed primarily with advancement of labial mucosa
- Division of pedicle in 3 weeks

— TONGUE FLAP:

- Design the flap on the dorsal aspect of the tongue for upper lip defects, and on the ventral for lower lip defects
- Design pedicle at or near the free margin of the tongue
- Suture the leading edge of the flap to the anterior border of the vermilion defect (meticulous suturing because of tongue movement postoperative)
- Attachment to the posterior edge of the defect at a second stage, during the division of the pedicle, after 3 weeks
- The donor site is closed primarily or allowed to granulate while the pedicle is connected to the flap

— ABBÉ FLAP:

- The flap is pedicled on the lateral side of the donor lip (depends on the labial artery) and its width should be half of that of the defect
- Choose the pivoting point on the donor lip, and maintain the continuity of the labial artery at that point
- Make a full thickness incision on the donor lip away from the pivot point and control the bleeding from the labial artery
- Rotate the lip tissue into the defect and secure it in place in layers, including muscle
- Maintain an adequate cuff of orbicularis oris in the pedicle to safely incorporate the labial artery
- Division and inset of flap in 3 weeks
- For the upper lip, the Abbé flap is preferred to the others, because it permits preservation of cupid's bow

— ESTLANDER FLAP:

- Performed as a one-stage reconstruction or staged modification (commisure-sparing)
- Same as Abbé, but the defect is located at the lateral portion of either lip
- If the donor lip is the upper lip, design the apex of the flap in a rounded fashion, in order for donor site scar to lie in nasololabial crease

— KARAPANDZIC TECHNIQUE:

- This flap represents a circumoral composite rotation flap and involves the creation of bilateral opposing flaps which may be of different lengths, but of uniform width
- When reconstructing the lower lip, incise the skin along the course of the mental crease, parallel to the free margin of the lip; similarly design your incision for an upper lip reconstruction

- Dissect being careful to preserve as many neural and vascular structures as possible; the labial arteries and buccal nerve branches should be identified and preserved bilaterally
- Separate subcutaneous tissue and muscle bluntly with the use of scissors, by gentle spreading the orbicularis longitudinally, before division
- Dissect neural and vascular structures sufficiently to allow for stretching during rotation of the flaps
- Once adequate mobilization achieved, rotate and close in three layers (mucosa, muscle, skin)

Postoperative Care

- Nutritional education is necessary (blenderized diet, small pieces of food)
- If oral competence present, oral hygiene with swish and spit oral solution; if not, hygiene can be accomplished with swabs and chlorhexidine oral solution or a mixture of hydrogen peroxide and saline

Outpatient Rehabilitation

- Oral continence can be a long term problem for patients who have undergone lip reconstruction (esp if continuity of muscle not reconstructed)

NASAL RECONSTRUCTION

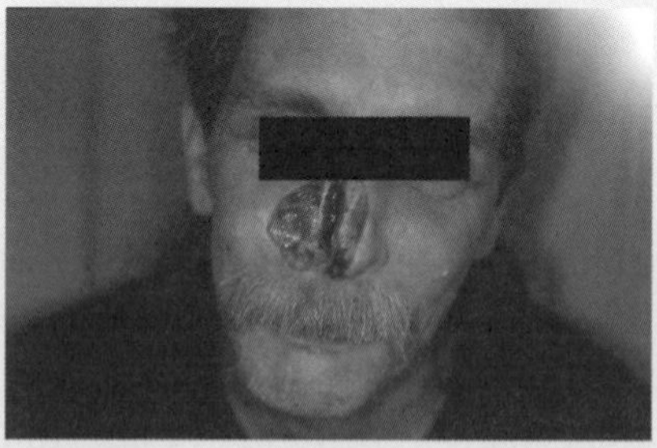

A.

Illustrative Case 5: Large nasal and cheek defect after Moh's excision of BCC.

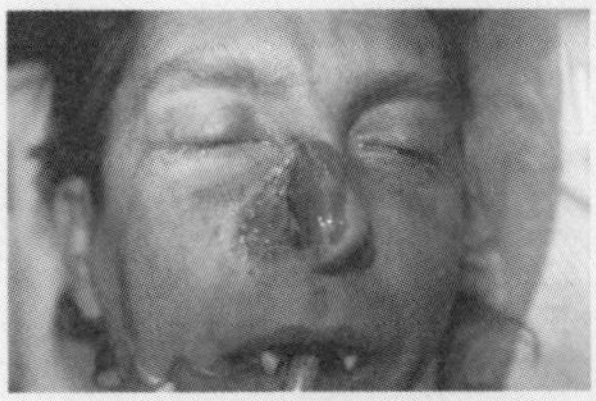

B.

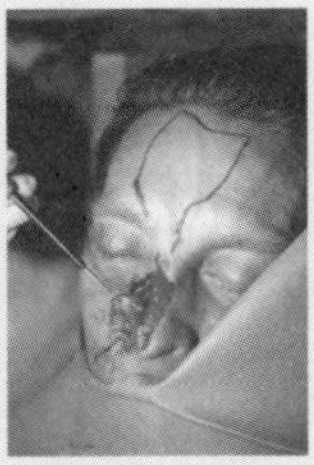

C.

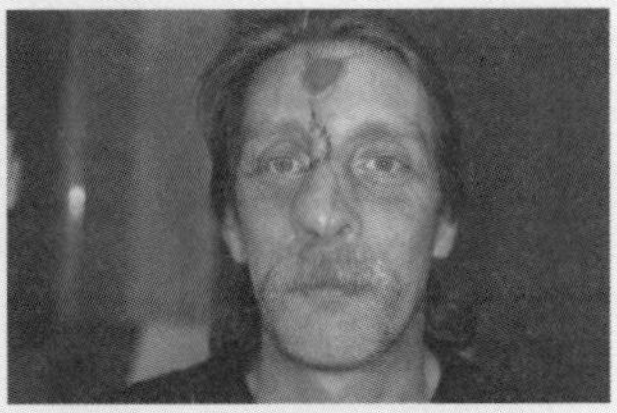

D.

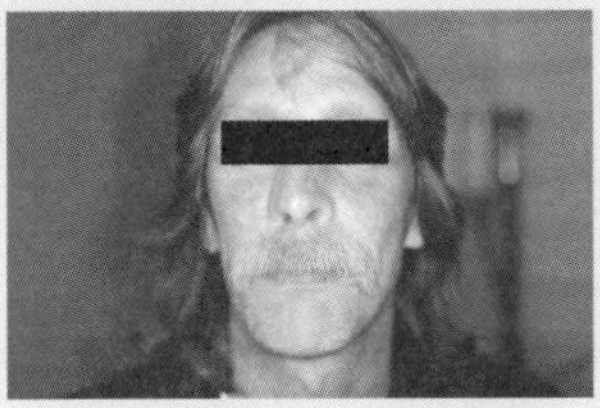

E.

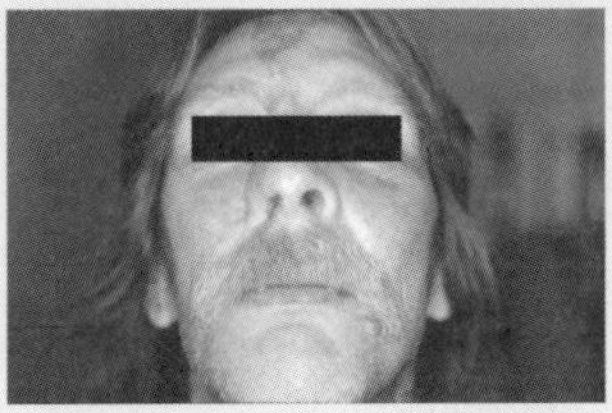

F.

5B. Close up of the defect prior to reconstruction.
5C. Reconstruction of the lining and support with septal chondromucosal pedicled flap and pattern of forehead flap using template from defect. Cheek was undermined and advanced to appropriate position prior to nasal reconstruction.
5D. Initial result with cheek advancement with reconstruction of nose with a forehead flap. Donor site to heal by secondary intention.
5E and F. Final result 7 months post reconstruction.

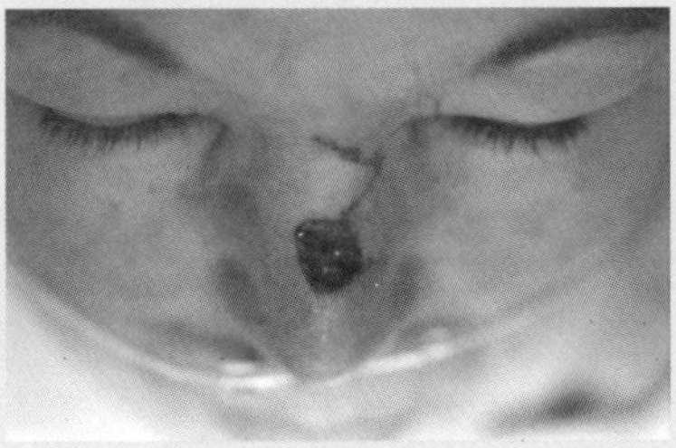

A.

Illustrative Case 6: 32 year old female with 1.5 cm full thickness defect on dorsum of nose after excision of BCC.

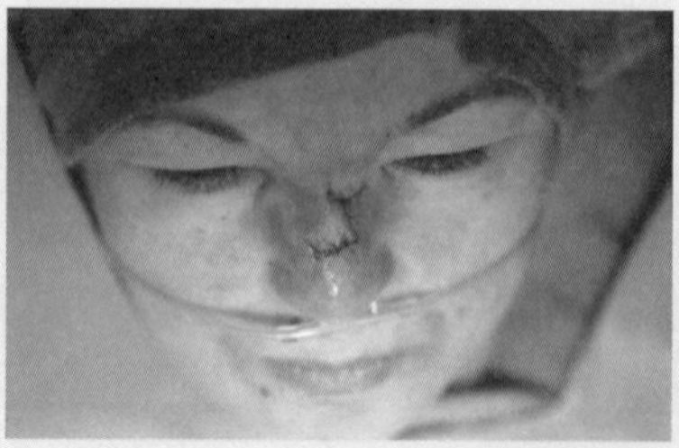

B.

6B. Immediate reconstruction was achieved with a rhomboid flap.

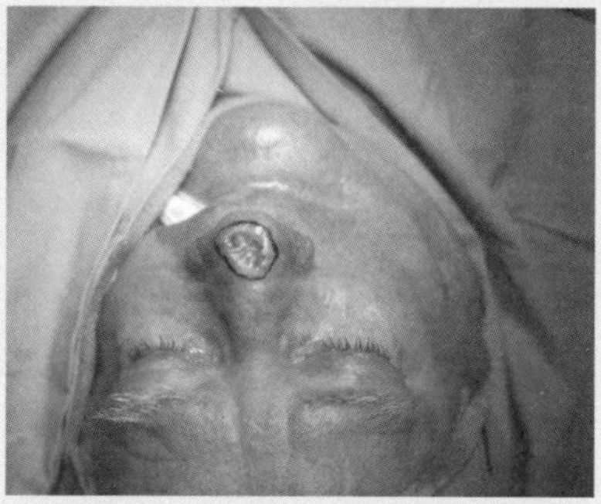

A.

Illustrative Case 7: 56 year old male with recurrent BCC on tip of nose to undergo Moh's excision of lesion.

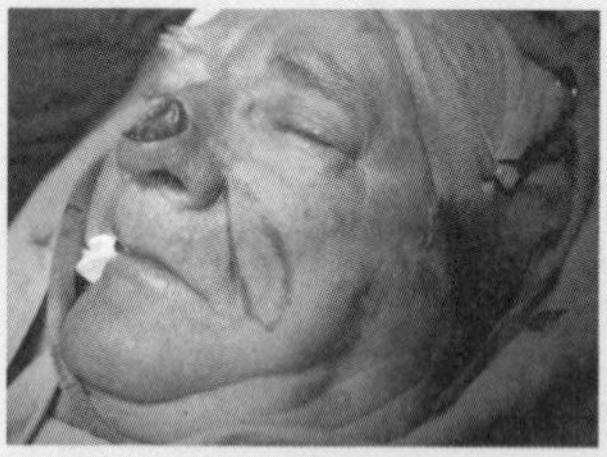

B.

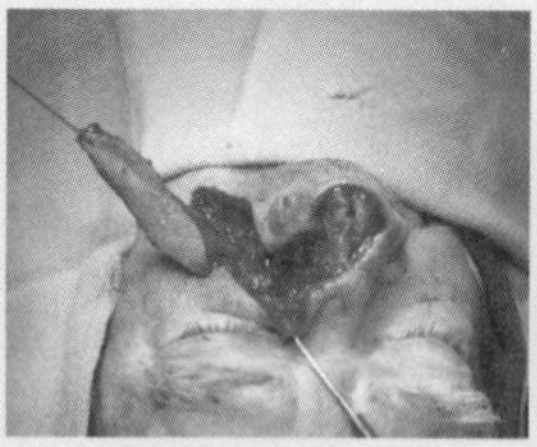

C.

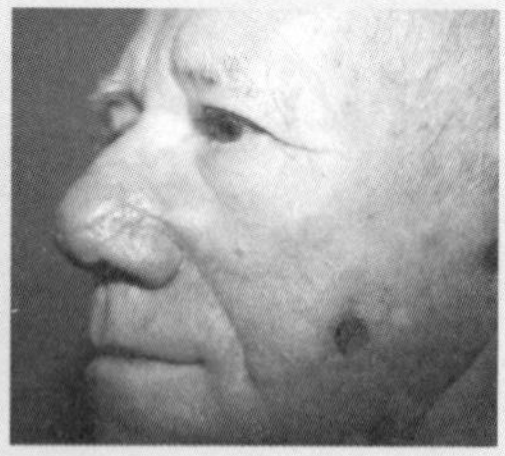

D.

7B. 2 cm defect with exposed cartilage. Proposed reconstruction with island nasolabial fold.

7C. Flap mobilized on broad subcutaneous pedicle.

7D. Final result with good contour and linear donor site scar.

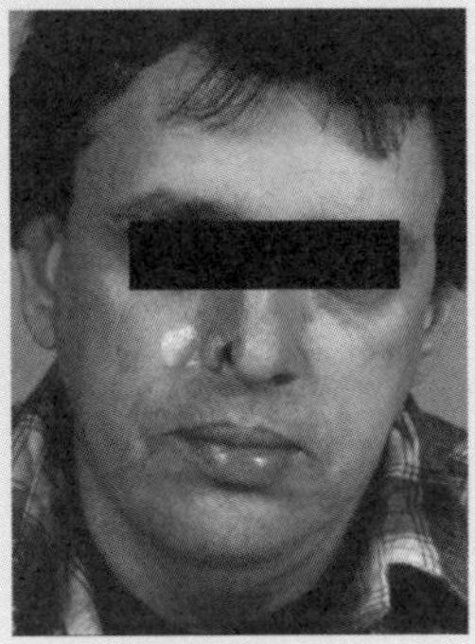

A.

Illustrative Case 8: 48 year old male with 1.5 cm defect of the left nostril after excision of BCC.

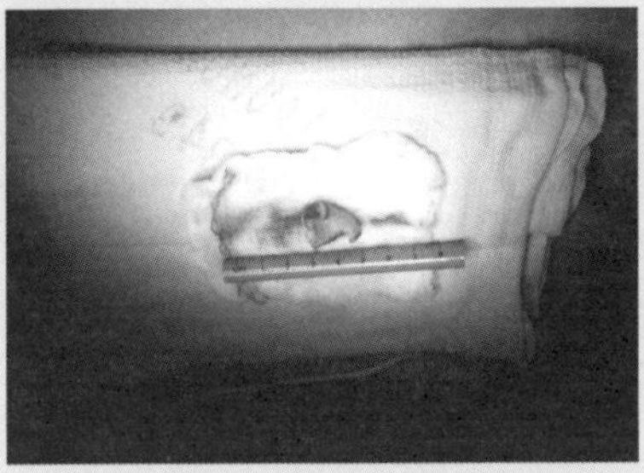

B.

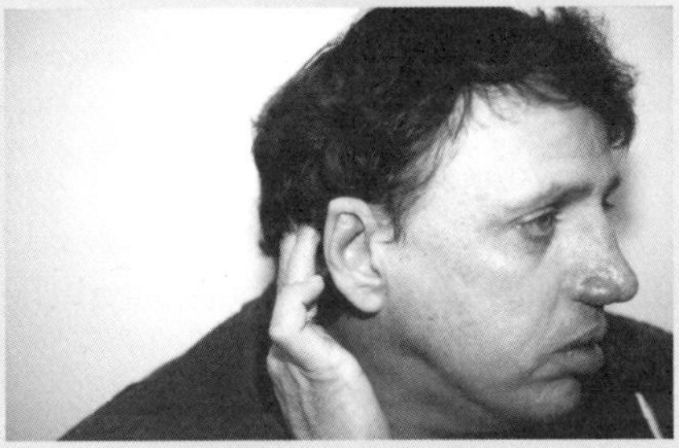

C.

8B. Reconstruction with composite graft from the ear.

8C. Early postoperative result.

Management, Preoperative Tests

- Detailed analysis of the defect: location, subunits, size of defect
- Assess tissue missing: coverage, support, lining
- If >50% defect of a subunit, enlarge defect to include the entire subunit and reconstruct it
- Different techniques based on tissue missing (see list below)

Operative Techniques List

- Coverage (skin/Soft tissue):
  - — Bilobed flap
  - — Rhomboid flap
  - — Nasolabial flap
  - — Paramedian forehead flap
- Support (cartilage/bone):
  - — Cartilage/bone from nasal septum
  - — Auricular concha
  - — Rib cartilage graft
  - — Outer table of cranium
  - — Nonanatomic alar support (alar batten graft, lateral crural strut graft, alar spreader graft, alar contour graft)
  - — Alloplasts (porous polyethylene, vitallium or titanium mesh)
- Lining (mucosa):
  - — Split/full-thickness skin graft (cannot use support grafts simultaneously, but in delayed fashion)
  - — Unipedicle caudally based septal mucoperichondrial hinge flap
  - — Contralateral dorsally based hinge flap
  - — Turbinate mucoperiosteal flap
- Total nasal reconstruction:
  - — Paramedian forehead flap (nose may be prefabricated using lining and cartilage under forehead flap prior to transfer)
  - — Free flaps (e.g. radial forearm free flap); only when forehead flap is not available
  - — Prosthetic nose (use of osseointegrated implants)

Operative Techniques Description — Order of Repair and Steps

— RHOMBOID FLAP:

- Standard design, so that final donor site scar is in the direction of RSTL
- Raise in a subcutaneous plane

- Remember that site of maximal tension is at the area of donor site closure
- Circular modification: extend the diameter of the circular defect by two-thirds towards any direction, that will lead to an optimal scar; the angle should be 60 degrees

— BILOBED FLAP:

- Pivot point is set at a distance equal to radius of defect measured from edge of defect
- Two arcs are drawn with centers the pivot point; one passes through the center and the other tangential to the defect
- Bases of both lobes of flap originate from smaller arc
- Height of first lobe extends to second arc
- Width of first lobe equals width of defect; width of second one is equal to or slightly smaller than that of first one
- Height of second lobe is double that of the first one
- Axis of defect and two lobes are approximately 45 degrees apart
- Donor site of second lobe closed first; first lobe is transposed into the defect; second lobe transposed and trimmed
- Skin closure

— PARAMEDIAN FOREHEAD FLAP:

- Design appropriately based on size of defect; do not include scalp hair if possible
- The length is determined by measurement
- The base of the pedicle is placed in the glabellar region centered over the supratrochlear artery on the same side as the majority of the nasal defect
- Raise flap in the subfascial plane, just superficial to the periosteum of the frontal bone and once adequate length has been obtained inset the flap (supratrochlear artery exits orbit approximately 2 cm lateral to midline, passing under orbicularis oculi and over corrugator supercilii; at level of eybrow it passes through orbicularis and frontalis muscles and continues superiorly in superficial subcutaneous tissue plane)

- Frontalis muscle can be trimmed along the distal three-fourths of the flap (all but 1mm of fat beneath the dermis may be removed, since the pedicle runs superficial to frontalis superior to the level of the eyebrow)
- Incisions may be extended below the eyebrow level if needed in order to obtain adequate length
- Adequate flap mobilization may require complete division of corrugator supercilii muscle
- Donor site either primarily closed or healing by secondary intention
- Division of pedicle in 3 weeks and inset of flap

— NASOLABIAL FLAP:

- Design appropriately based on size of defect
- Width of the cutaneous pedicle is approximately the width of the template, except if the template is >2 cm
- Elevate flap in the subcutaneous plane, maintaining a 3 mm of fat on the undersurface of the cutaneous pedicle
- The flap pivots 90 degrees toward the midline and is sutured to the defect
- The distal half of the flap may be thinned to match thickness of recipient site; the proximal portion bridging between nose and cheek cannot be thinned
- Cheek wound is closed primarily
- Division of the pedicle and inset of flap in 3 weeks
- The proximal portion is inset after division in the cheek by opening the superior portion of the donor site scar 1–2cm, and spreading the edges to accommodate the proximal pedicle
- One significant disadvantage of this type of flap in males is the transfer of hair-bearing skin to the nose

— IPSILATERAL SEPTAL MUCOPERICHONDRIAL HINGE FLAP:

- In general it should be designed as large as possible; flaps measuring approximately 4 (length) × 3 cm (width) are large enough to line the entire lower nasal vault and portions of the caudal aspect of the middle vault

- Lidocaine with epinephrine injected in the subperichondrial plane along the entire length of the septum
- 2 horizontal incisions extending from anterior to posterior are made with a scalpel
- The dorsal incision begins 0.75 cm posterior to anterior septal angle and continues in a line parallel to the septal plane 0.5 to 1 cm below the roof of the middle vault
- Should extend 1–2cm posterior to bony cartilaginous junction of the septum
- Inferior incision starts 1cm posterior to anterior nasal spine and extends along the junction of the nasal crest and nasal floor up to the level of the dorsal incision; the two incisions are then connected in a vertical fashion
- Raise the septal mucoperichondrial flap from above downward toward the nasal floor and anteriorly to posteriorly
- Deliver the flap out of nasal passage (bone and septal cartilage exposed and sometimes removed to be used as grafts; if not they eventually become covered by a thin epithelium during healing by secondary intention)
- The mucoperichondrial flap is turned laterally as a hinge flap, with the mucosal surface facing downward
- Flap positioning is adjusted for maximal mucosal coverage; the margins of the hinge flap are sutured to the margins of the mucosal defect

— TURBINATE MUCOPERIOSTEAL FLAP:

- Local anesthetic solution with epinephrine in injected along the turbinate, floor of the nose, and middle or inferior meatus, depending on which turbinate is used
- Turbinate medialized with a blunt elevator
- Cottle elevator or 2 mm osteotome is placed in the meatus below the turbinate and pushed superiorly to perforate the bony attachment to the lateral nasal wall (multiple perforations are made along the length of the turbinate

- Pedicled anteriorly, the posterior aspect of the mobilized turbinate is pivoted toward the nasal defect, with the use of forceps
- The bone of the delivered turbinate is removed, and the remaining mucosal flap is transferred to the recipient site and sutured in place
- If the location of the defect is at the nasal tip, the pedicle will have to be divided in 3 weeks, because it will be obstructing the airway

Postoperative Care

- Standard instructions for wound care
- Scar massaging
- Drain care based on procedure performed
- Antibiotics

Outpatient Rehabilitation

- Scar therapy

SCALP RECONSTRUCTION

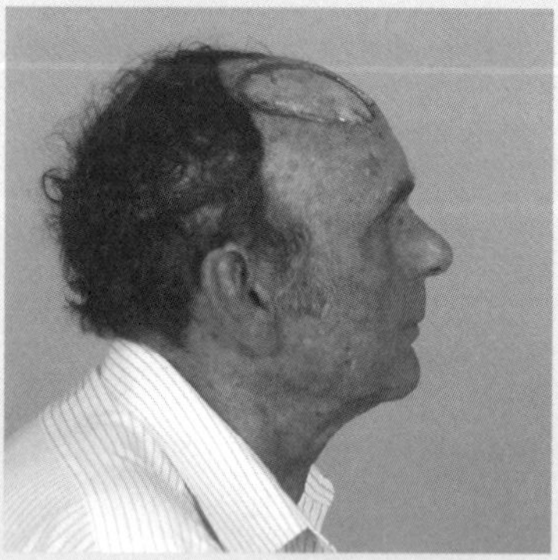

A.

Case 9: 69 year old male kidney transplant recipient with large scalp defect after excision of a squamous cell carcinoma.

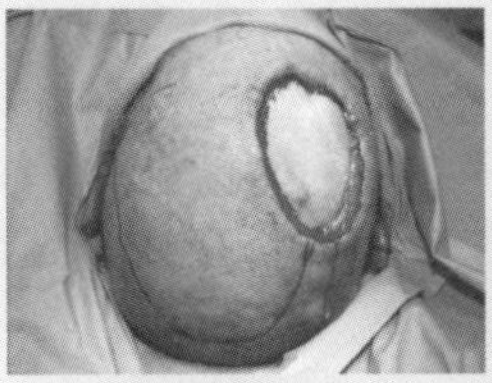

B.

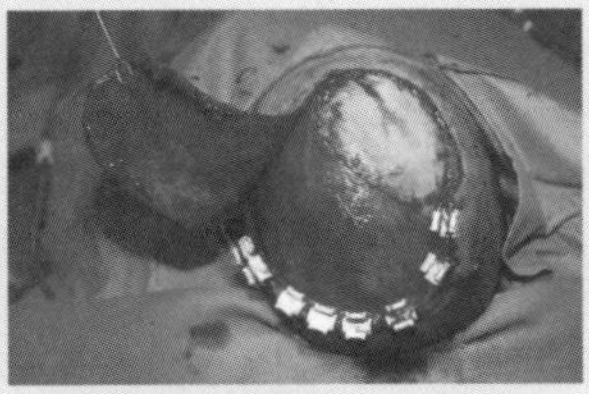

C.

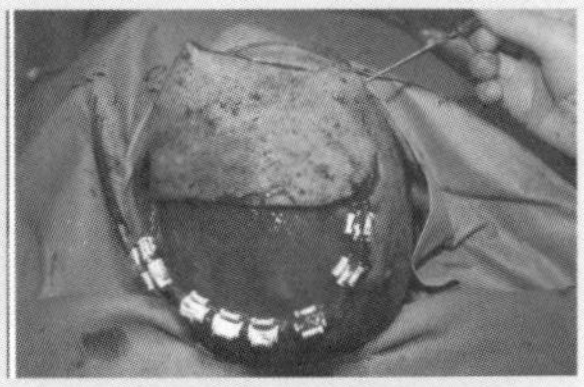

D.

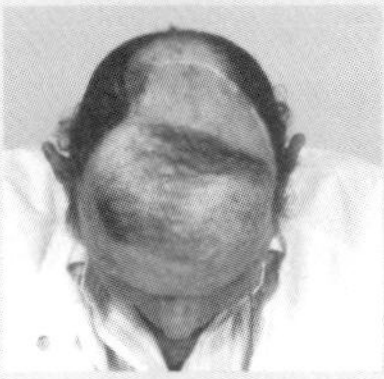

E.

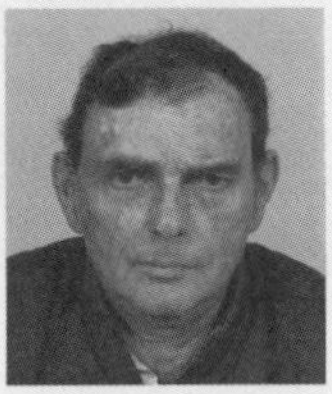

F.

9B. Proposed scalp flap for reconstruction. Negative margins determined.
9C. Flap elevated over periosteum.
9D. Flap rotated anteriorly to provide coverage and STSG was placed in the donor site.
9E and F. Early (3 months) and late (19 months) results with complete healing and improvement of anterior hair line.

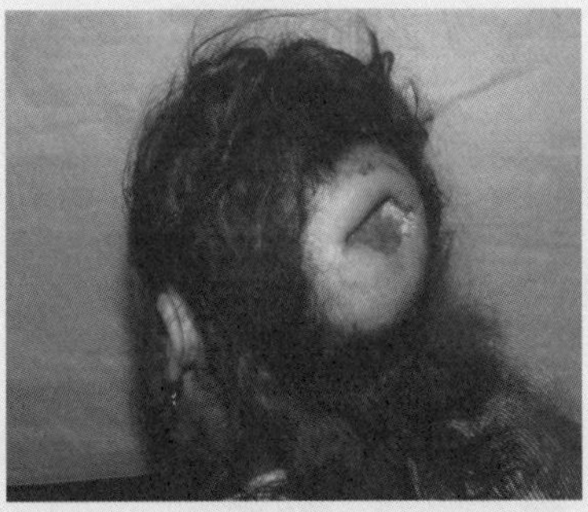

A.

Case 10: 55 year old female with large scalp defect (pressure necrosis) after trauma.

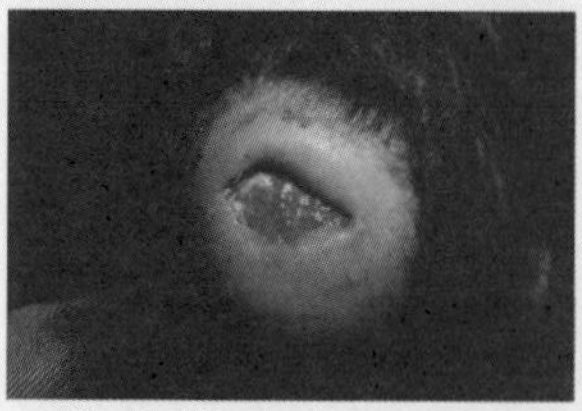

B.

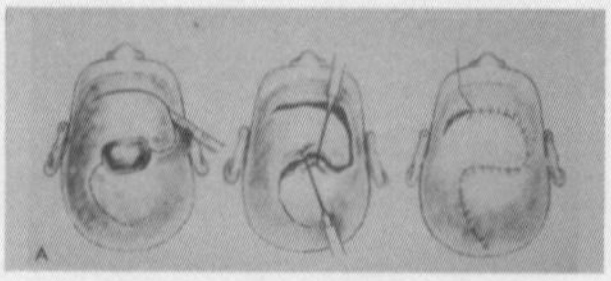

C.

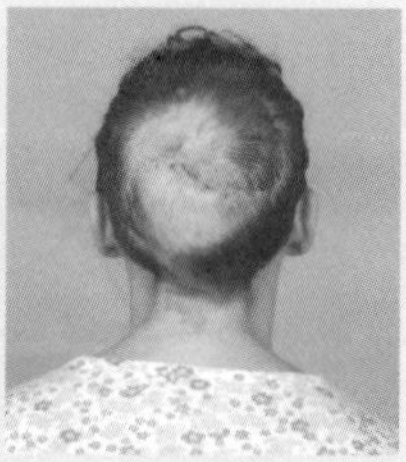

D.

10B. Close up of the defect

10C. Complete coverage with rotation of 2 (S design — see drawing) scalp flaps

10D. Postoperative result

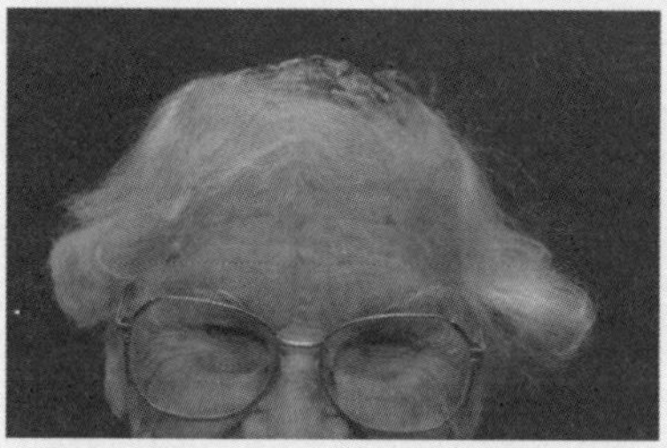

A.

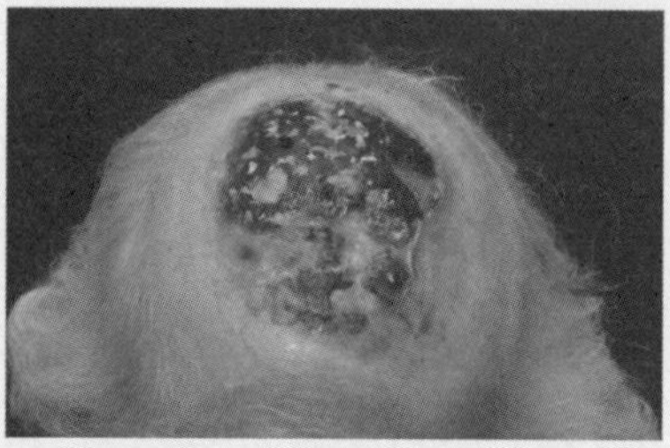

B.

Case 11: 83 year old female with recurrent invasive SCCA of scalp.

11C. Post en bloc resection of SCCA with cranial (inner and outer table) resection and placement of mesh plate.

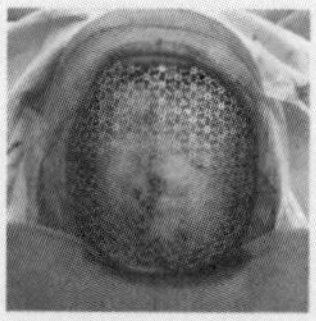

C.

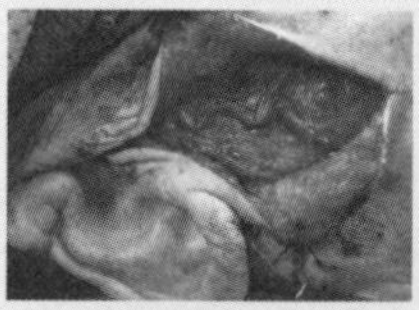

D.

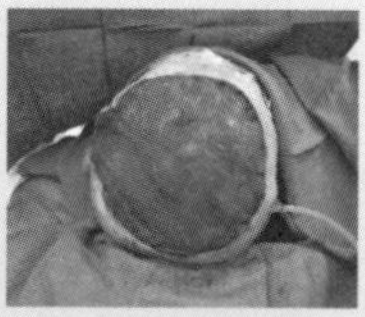

E.

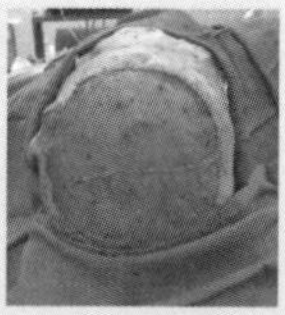

F.

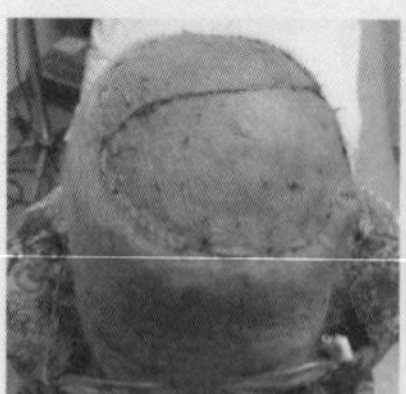

G.

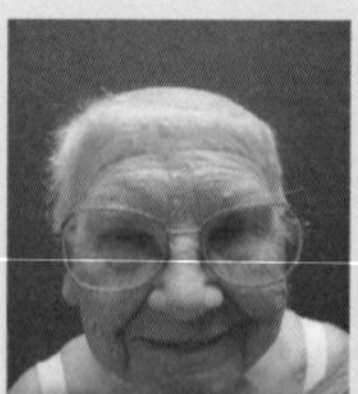

H.

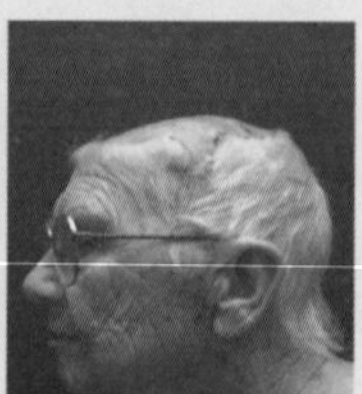

I.

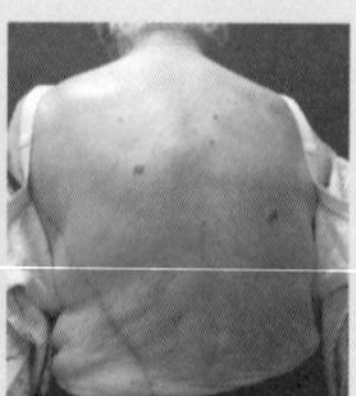

J.

11D. Exposure of recipient vessels (STA/V).

11E. Inset of free latissimus flap after anastomosis.

11F. STSG over latissimus flap.

11G to J. Early and late postoperative result.

Management, Preoperative Tests

- Replace tissue with like tissue; use adjacent scalp; include at least one named vessel into the scalp flap
- Scalp mobility is greatest at the parietal region
- Tissue expansion may be needed if there is inadequate or traumatized local tissue available, not acceptable reaarangement of hair orientation, or distortion of hairline
- Exposed bone can be covered temporarily with split thickness skin grafts, during the expansion process, either by burring the outer table or by covering the area with pericranial flaps
- Half of the scalp can be reconstructed with tissue expansion
- Hair micrografting may be needed to improve incision lines and alopecia
- Limit the use of hemostatic clips and electrocautery on scalp cut edges in order to avoid follicular damage
- Score the galea perpendicular to the direction of desired tissue gain
- Approximate galea during closure, because that's the strength layer

Operative Techniques List

- Healing by secondary intention
    - — Base of viable tissue, such as pericranium, must be present
    - — Formation of granulation tissue may be enhanced by removing the outer table of the cranium to the level of the diploic space
    - — Scalp wounds will minimally contract due to the stiff galeal layer
    - — Laborious wound care

- Primary wound closure
  - Defects up to 3 cm in diameter can generally be repaired primarily, with wide undermining of the galea
  - Galeal relaxing incisions may be needed with caution not to injure vessels superficial to the galea
  - Galeal layer should bear the majority of closure tension
- Skin grafting
  - Reliable, but suboptimal reconstruction
  - Skin graft lacks hair follicles and is thinner than normal scalp, therefore leads to contour irregularities
  - Reasonable for patients who are not candidates for extensive procedures and in whom the aesthetic outcome is of less concern
  - Useful for temporary coverage, or for coverage of secondary defects, located in less visible areas (e.g. occiput)
  - May be indicated when there is high recurrence risk after removal of scalp malignancy (other means of reconstruction can be used after reasonable time has elapsed)
  - High failure rates if need for postoperative radiation
- Local flaps
  - Advancement, pivotal flaps; advancement flaps may be difficult to use secondary to the lack of scalp elasticity
  - Incisions should be positioned to optimize vascular supply
  - Principal anatomic landmark is the anterior hairline
- Regional flaps
  - Limited to defects of inferior occipital and temporal regions of the scalp (because of limited reach of the pedicles)
  - Reported success with trapezius and latissimus dorsi musculocutaneous flaps
  - They do not provide hair-bearing tissue
- Temporoparietal fascia flap
  - Supplied by branches of superficial temporal artery and vein
  - Can be raised as a pedicled flap measuring 14 × 17 cm

- Microsurgical tissue transfer
  - — Latissimus dorsi flap has been the most commonly used free flap
  - — The muscle component of the flap atrophies over time
  - — Greatest disadvantage is the lack of hair replacement
- Tissue expansion
  - — Place the expander in the subgaleal plane
  - — Cranium provides a smooth and firm base
  - — A crescent-shaped or oval expander are frequently the most appropriate shapes
  - — Inflation starts usually 2 weeks post placement

Operative Techniques Description — Order of Repair and Steps

— ADVANCEMENT FLAP:

- Usually used for repair of longitudinal defects
- Widely undermine the galea and score it parallel to the long axis of the defect
- Approximate the galea during closure

— ROTATIONAL FLAP:

- Design it 4–6 times as long as the width of the defect
- Bevel the incision to parallel the direction of growth of the hair follicles
- Elevate the flap in the subgalelal plane and undermine the surrounding scalp in the same plane to decrease the wound closure tension
- Perform a back-cut extending from the base of the flap if needed, being cautious not to compromise the vascularity
- Do not excise standing cutaneous deformities, because you are reducing the width of the base of the flap; these will decrease significantly over time; if necessary excise it at a later date
- Pivot the flap into the defect and suture the leading border of the flap in place
- Suture the curvilinear border next, using the halves principle
- Cover the secondary defect with a skin graft, if closure by advancement is not possible

- Employ multiple rotation flaps at the same time if needed in order to distribute wound closure tension over a larger area of the scalp
- Three-flap "pinwheel" technique: three separate rotational flaps positioned around the defect in equal distances, raised and pivoted in same direction

— ORTICOCHEA TECHNIQUE:

- Three to four transposition flaps raised on named vessels in the subgaleal plane and transposed to cover the defect
- The entire scalp needs to be undermined in the course of dissection and transfer of the flaps

Postoperative Care

- Standard wound care

Outpatient Rehabilitation

- Hair restoration grafts or flaps may be needed (multiple stages of grafting are usually required, with each stage separated form the next one with several months of healing)

EAR RECONSTRUCTION

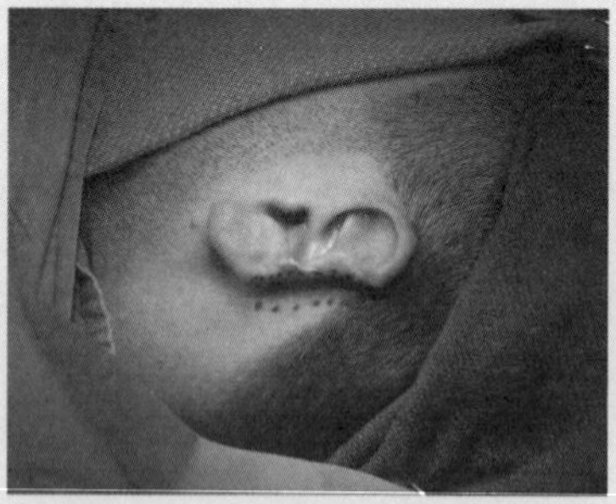

A.

Case 12: 7 year old female with dog bite to ear and resultant helical deformity.

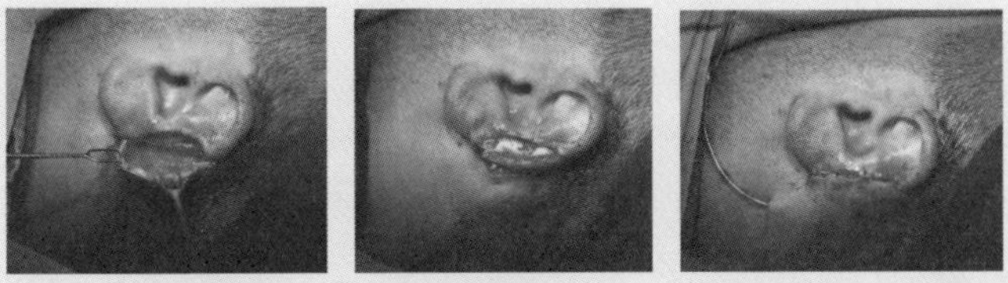

B. C. D.

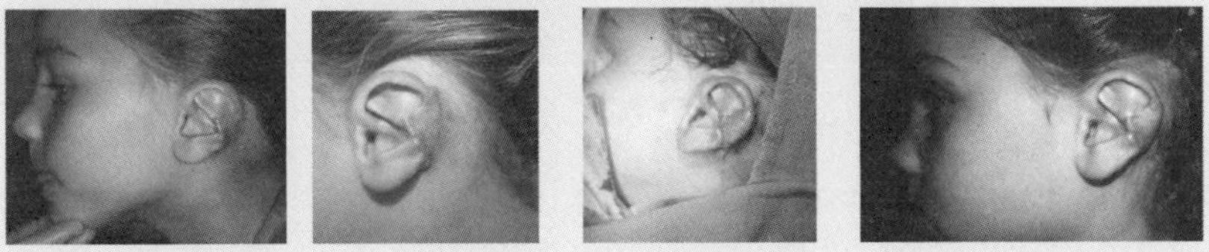

E. F. G. H.

12B to D. First stage: elevation of postauricular subcutaneous flap based on width of helical rim defect. Placement of rib cartilage graft to helical rim and subsequent inset of flap over drain. Preserve posterior auricular branches if present.

12E and F. Prior to flap division with healed first stage reconstruction.

12G and H. Second stage reconstruction with division and inset of flap with placement of STSG over posterior aspect of ear on preserved perichondrium. Early and late postoperative — note restored helical contour.

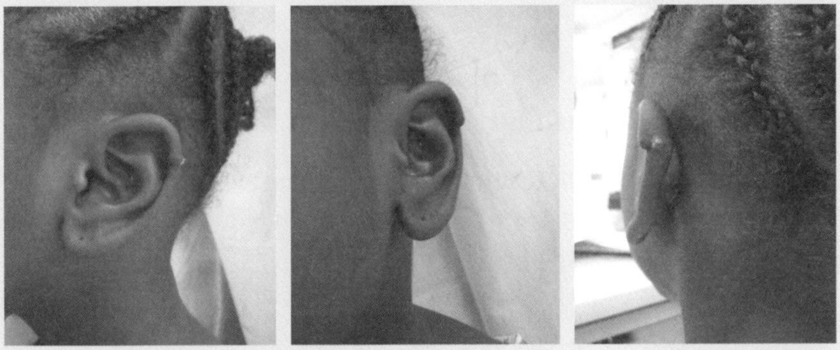

A. B. C.

Case 13: 7 year old female with h/o traumatic laceration of ear with step off deformity.

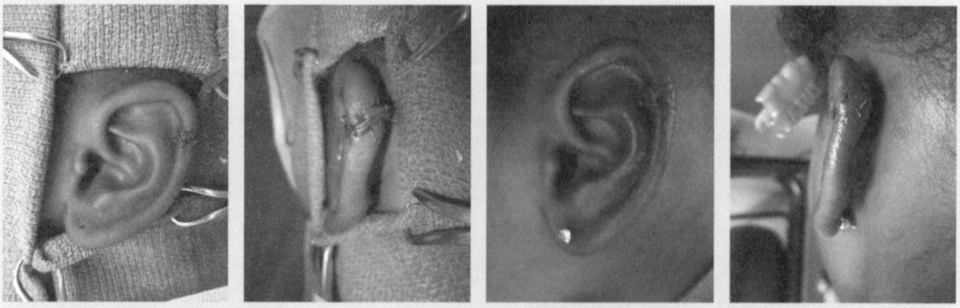

D. E. F. G.

13D and E. Excision of wound margins, reapproximation of cartilage and local tissue rearrangement using z-plasty.
13F and G. Early 2-week postoperative result.

Management, Preoperative Tests

- Assess the defect (cutaneous defect, with or without intact cartilage vs. full thickness defect)
- Additional treatment options based on the etiology (e.g. human/animal bites, lacerations, avulsions, amputations)
- Partial-thickness
- Full-thickness (helical rim, superior/middle/inferior third of the auricle, lobule)

Operative Techniques List

- Partial-thickness/intact perichondrium: advancement flaps from post-auricular or anterior-auricular skin; full thickness skin graft from contralateral postauricular skin
- Partial-thickness/perichondrium missing: Elsahy's two bipedicle flaps technique
- Primary closure for small cutaneous defects, which may occasionally require small excisions of ear cartilage or local tissue rearrangement to avoid contour irregularities

- Full-thickness:
  - Defects of conchal bowl: full-thickness skin graft (if subtotal defect), postauricular/subcutaneous tissue pedicle island advancement flap
  - Helix: Antia-Buch procedure, pre- or postauricular interpolated cutaneous tube flap, auricular cartilage grafts, Dieffenbach's flap
- Replantation and banking
- Total ear reconstruction vs. prosthetic ear (via osseointegrated implants)

Operative Techniques Description — Order of Repair and Steps

— ELSAHY'S TECHNIQUE:

- A bipedicle cutaneous flap "A" is designed on the medial surface of the auricle parallel to the defect; size of the flap and direction are determined by the size and direction of the defect
- Elevate and advance the flap around the helical rim as far as the lateral surface, and suture it in place in order to cover the lateral helical defect
- The amount of tension on the flap gives an idea about the size of the second bilobed flap "B"
- Elevate and advance the flap B in the same direction and cover the defect of flap A
- Close the defect created by the flap B primarily
- A cartilage graft can be embedded inside the flap, if needed.

— ANTIA-BUCH PROCEDURE (chondrocutaneous advancement flap):

- Make incision in helical sulcus through anterior skin and cartilage; posteromedial skin is undermined
- Advance helix into defect based on posterior skin flap
- Suture in place, in order to cover the gap
- If the defect is large enough (up to 2-cm), then perform the same technique on the root of helix and close the defect in a V-Y fashion

— DIEFFENBACH'S FLAP:

- Harvest contralateral auricular cartilage graft and suture it to the defect
- Elevate postauricular skin and advance it over cartilage graft to fill defect
- Suture the skin flap onto the wound edges
- Divide the flap 3 weeks later

— POSTAURICULAR SUBCUTANEOUS TISSUE PEDICLE ADVANCEMENT FLAP:

- Design the flap on postauricular skin, based on size and shape of the conchal defect
- Dissect the flap away from the surface of the mastoid bone in a posterior to anterior direction, in order to maintain a thick subcutaneous tissue pedicle that incorporates branches of the postauricular artery and, if present, the postauricular muscle
- Tunnel the subcutaneous tissue pedicle beneath medial auricular skin
- Bivalve the flap, by de-epithelializing a cutaneous strip, to provide skin cover of medial and lateral aspect of defect
- Suture the flap in place
- Close the postauricular defect primarily

— PRE-/ POSTAURICULAR INTERPOLATED CUTANEOUS TUBE FLAP (DEFECTS >2.5 CM):

- First stage: create tube from pre- or postauricular skin, based on the extent of helical rim defect; dissect as a bipedicled flap and tube it upon itself
- Second stage: after 3 weeks, detach one end of the cutaneous tube from its donor site and secure it to one edge of the helical rim defect
- Third stage: after 3 weeks, incise the other end of the tube and inset in the other edge of the helical defect

— EARLOBE RECONSTRUCTION:

- Up to 50% of the earlobe may be removed by wedge shaped excision followed by primary wound closure, with minimal resulting deformity
- Conchal cartilage from contralateral ear is harvested in the shape of earlobe and is embedded in a subcutaneous pocket below the auricle, in a location corresponding to the desired position of the earlobe
- After 6 weeks, the cartilage and overlying skin are elevated as a composite flap, based superiorly on the auricle
- Coverage of medial surface of reconstructed earlobe with full-thickness skin graft

— REPLANTATION AND BANKING:

- Superficial temporal artery or posterior auricular artery should be available for microvascular anastomosis
- If venous anastomosis is not available, leech therapy can be used
- Banking: skin of the amputated part is removed; the amputated portion is reattached, and exposed cartilage is covered with a postauricular skin flap
- The flap is divided after 3 months, and the defect is covered with a skin graft
- Preservation of the temporoparietal fascia for secondary reconstruction is recommended; use of the temporoparietal fascia for acute coverage of replanted cartilage is not recommended

— TOTAL EAR RECONSTRUCTION:

- An important difference between ear reconstruction in children and in adults is the fact that in children the cartilage is flexible, and the helical rim can be created by attaching a separate carved piece of rib cartilage to the framework, while in adults it is stiff, and the framework — including the helical rim — is carved en bloc
- Base the framework on a template from the contralateral ear

Postoperative Care

- Bolster dressing care in case skin graft has been used
- Avoid contact sports in order to prevent injury to the reconstructed auricle at least for 4–6 weeks

Outpatient Rehabilitation

- Revisional surgeries for contour irregularities may be needed

Suggested Readings

Eyelid Reconstruction

1. Fante RG. (2007) Reconstruction of the eyelids. In: Baker SR (ed.), *Local Flaps in Facial Reconstruction,* 2nd Edn. Mosby, Philadelphia.
2. Potter JK. (2007) Eyelid reconstruction. In: Janis JE (ed.), *Essentials of Plastic Surgery.* Quality Medical Publishing, St. Louis.
3. DiFrancesco LM, Codner MA, McCord CD. (2004) Upper eyelid reconstruction. *Plast Reconstr Surg* **114**: 98e–107e.
4. Fischer T, Noever G, Lange M, Kammer E. (2001) Experience in upper eyelid reconstruction with the Cutler-Beard technique. *Ann Plast Surg* **47**: 338–342.

Cheek Reconstruction

1. Bradley DT, Murakami CS. (2007) Reconstruction of the cheek. In: Baker SR (ed.), *Local Flaps in Facial Reconstruction,* 2nd Edn. Mosby, Philadelphia.
2. Mathes DW, Garcia CA. (2007) Cheek reconstruction. In: Janis JE (ed.), *Essentials of Plastic Surgery.* Quality Medical Publishing, St. Louis.
3. Menick FJ. (2001) Reconstruction of the cheek. *Plast Reconstr Surg* **108**(2): 496–504.
4. Mureau MAM, Hofer SQP. (2009) Maximizing results in reconstruction of cheek defects. *Clin Plast Surg* **36**: 461–476.
5. Park SS, Little S. (2007) Rhombic flaps. In: Baker SR (ed.), *Local Flaps in Facial Reconstruction,* 2nd Edn. Mosby, Philadelphia.

Lip Reconstruction

1. Renner GJ. (2007) Reconstruction of the lip. In: Baker SR (ed.), *Local Flaps in Facial Reconstruction,* 2nd Edn. Mosby, Philadelphia.
2. Mosser SW. (2007) Lip reconstruction. In: Janis JE (ed.), *Essentials of Plastic Surgery*, Quality Medical Publishing, St. Louis.
3. Anvar BA, Evans BCD, Evans GRD. (2007) Lip reconstruction. *Plast Reconstr Surg* **120**(4): 57e–64e.
4. Kawamoto HK Jr. (1979) Correction of major defects of the vermilion with a cross-lip vermilion flap. *Plast Reconstr Surg* **64**: 315.

Nasal Reconstruction

1. Baker SR. (2007) Reconstruction of the nose. In: Baker SR (ed.), *Local Flaps in Facial Reconstruction,* 2nd Edn. Mosby, Philadelphia.
2. Crosby MA. (2007) Nasal reconstruction. In: Janis JE (ed.), *Essentials of Plastic Surgery*. Quality Medical Publishing, St. Louis.
3. Menick FJ. (2004) Nasal reconstruction: forehead flap. *Plast Reconstr Surg* **113**(6): 100e–111e.
4. Zitelli JA. (1989) The bilobed flap for nasal reconstruction. *Arch Dermatol* **125**: 957–959.
5. Baker SR. (2007) Bilobe flaps. In: Baker SR (ed.), *Local Flaps in Facial Reconstruction,* 2nd Edn. Mosby, Philadelphia.
6. Park SS, Little S. (2007) Rhombic flaps. In: Baker SR (ed.), *Local Flaps in Facial Reconstruction,* 2nd Edn. Mosby, Philadelphia.
7. Baker SR. (2007) Melolabial flaps. In: Baker SR (ed.), *Local Flaps in Facial Reconstruction,* 2nd Edn. Mosby, Philadelphia.
8. Baker SR. (2007) Interpolated paramedian forehead flaps. In: Baker SR (ed.), *Local Flaps in Facial Reconstruction,* 2nd Edn. Mosby, Philadelphia.

Scalp Reconstruction

1. Hoffmann JF. (2007) Reconstruction of the scalp. In: Baker SR (ed.), *Local Flaps in Facial Reconstruction,* 2nd Edn. Mosby, Philadelphia.
2. Leedy JE. (2007) Scalp and calvarial reconstruction. In: Janis JE (ed.), *Essentials of Plastic Surgery.* Quality Medical Publishing, St. Louis.
3. Arnold PG, Rangarathnam CS. (1982) Multiple flap scalp reconstruction: orticochea revisited. *Plast Reconstr Surg* **69**: 605–613.

4. Baker SR. (2007) Rotation flaps. In: Baker SR (ed.), *Local Flaps in Facial Reconstruction,* 2nd Edn. Mosby, Philadelphia.

Ear Reconstruction

1. Cheney ML, Hadlock TA, Quatela VC. (2007) Reconstruction of the auricle. In Baker SR (ed.), *Local Flaps in Facial Reconstruction,* 2nd Edn. Mosby, Philadelphia.
2. Gosman AA, Reece EM. (2007) Ear reconstruction. In: Janis JE (ed.), *Essentials of Plastic Surgery,* Quality Medical Publishing, St. Louis.
3. Elsahy N. (2002) Reconstruction of the ear after skin and perichondrium loss. *Clin Plast Surg* **29**: 187.
4. Antia NH, Buch VI. (1967) Chondrocutaneous advancement flap for the marginal defect of the ear. *Plast Reconstr Surg* **39**: 472–477.

PLASTIC SURGERY OF THE UPPER EXTREMITY

CHAPTER 14

INFECTIOUS AND INFLAMMATORY DISORDERS OF THE UPPER EXTREMITY

Joshua M. Adkinson and Robert X. Murphy, Jr.

Illustrative Case

A 38 year old, right-hand dominant male is seen in the Emergency Department 4 days after sustaining a cat bite to his left long finger. He notes increasing swelling, pain, decreased range of motion, and subjective fevers. He has no relevant past medical or surgical history, no allergies, and takes no medications. He smokes a half pack a day of cigarettes and consumes 2–3 beers a day. An X-ray reveals soft tissue swelling, but no fracture or foreign body. His WBC is 16,000 and his temperature is 101.8. He is noted to have pain with passive extension of the digit and a flexed resting posture.

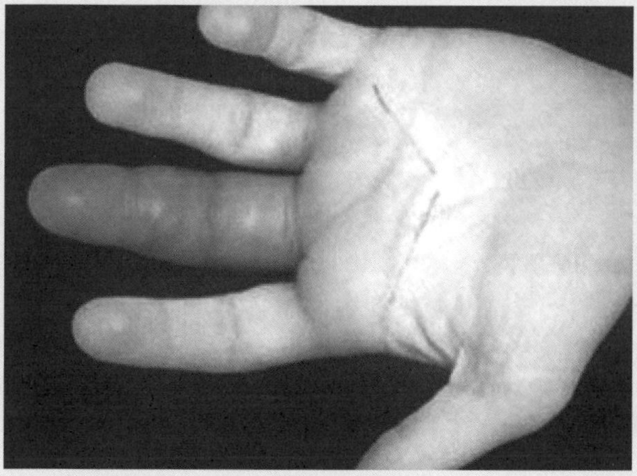

Infectious Disorders

Infections of the hand are extremely common, comprising as many as 35% of patients admitted to hand surgery services.[1] Prompt diagnosis and treatment can lead to a rapid and full recovery, while delayed therapy can lead to permanent disability.[2–4] Most hand infections arise from relatively minor wounds for which appropriate treatment was delayed or neglected. For uncomplicated cellulitis, antibiotics are the only therapy necessary. However, for significant infections of the upper extremity, surgical drainage remains the foundation of treatment with adjunctive antibiotics as guided by cultures and sensitivities.[1,2] Outcomes are dependent on multiple factors including: location of infection, the virulence of the organisms involved, timing of treatment, adequacy of surgical drainage, antibiotic effectiveness, and local and systemic host defense factors.[3,5]

General Principles

Evaluation

- Mode of injury, timing of events, hand dominance, occupation, systemic diseases and general health
- Exposure of the upper extremity and thorough examination with a systematic approach (compare to contralateral)
- Radiographs to document retained foreign bodies, skeletal injury, osteomyelitis or gas in the soft tissues and for baseline future comparison
- Tetanus when indicated

Operative principles

- Anytime an abscess is identified, drainage should be performed
- Incisions should never cross flexion creases at right angles, and should be marked widely to allow for extension, if necessary
- Tourniquet control is helpful — an Esmarch bandage is typically avoided. As an alternative to the Esmarch, the arm can be elevated arm for 2 minutes with pressure on the brachial artery prior to tourniquet inflation

Rest, heat, and elevation

- Immobilization limits opening of tissue planes, restricting spread
- Heat enhances circulation, increases delivery of inflammatory mediators, and decreases patient discomfort
- Elevation reduces edema by improving venous and lymphatic return

Antibiotic therapy

- Based on the fact that the vast majority of hand infections are caused by *Staphylococcus* and *Streptococcus*[3]
- Initially empiric and then guided by cultures and sensitivities (ideally taken before initiation of antibiotics)[5]

Paronychia

- The most common infection in the hand
- Represents an infection of soft tissue fold around the nail — can be confused with herpetic whitlow
- Hallmarks include erythema, tenderness, and swelling adjacent to the nail. May see nail plate deformity with chronic paronychia or elevation of the nail if pus accumulates on nail bed
- Caused by minor trauma: nail biting, poor manicure technique, or foreign body[5]
- Usually *S. aureus*, occasionally anaerobes
- If chronic, caused by *C. albicans* or occasionally *Pseudomonas*

Anatomy

- Nail complex: nail bed (germinal and sterile matrices), nail plate, and perionychium (border tissue surrounding the nail)
- Eponychium: thin tissue extending from the nail wall onto the nail plate
- Hyponychium: mass of keratin just distal to the sterile matrix, below the distal nail plate

Non-operative management

- If diagnosed early, may be treated by antibiotics, rest, heat, elevation, and warm soaks

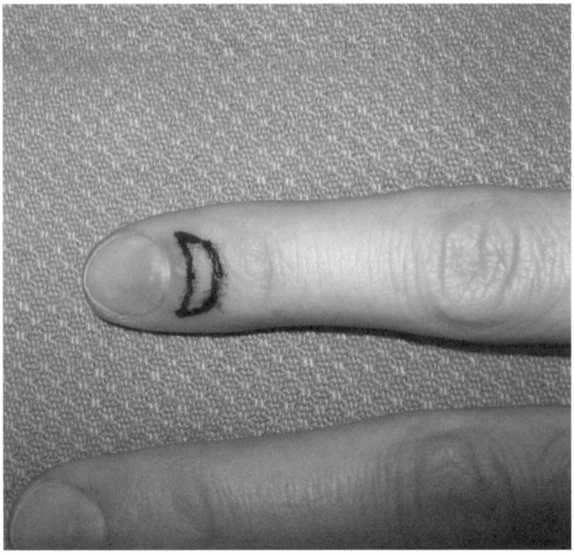

Fig. 1. Operative management of chronic paronychia with crescent-shaped excision.

Operative management of acute paronychia

- Typically, no anesthesia is necessary
- Elevate the nail fold with a small hemostat, Freer elevator, or No. 11 blade, pointing tip away from nail bed
- Abscess pocket is irrigated
- If pocket is under nail plate, a portion of plate should be removed
- Culture and place a small wick of gauze under the fold

Operative management of chronic paronychia

- Digital block anesthesia and tourniquet control are used
- A 3–5 mm wide crescent-shaped portion of skin 1 mm proximal to eponychial fold is excised not including the germinal matrix[3]
- If nail deformity, removal of the nail reported to improve cure rates and decrease risk of recurrence
- Wound is allowed to close secondarily

Postoperative care

- Remove gauze at 48 hrs and start warm soaks

- Antibiotics for 5–7 days if acute, 10–14 days if chronic
- Early ROM exercises

Felon

- An abscess of the pulp of the thumb or fingertip
- Usually present after a puncture wound with swelling, erythema, and throbbing pain made worse with dependency — can be seen in diabetics after fingersticks for blood glucose measurements[2,3]
- May progress to necrosis or infection of adjacent structures (tendon sheath, joints, bone) if delayed
- *S. aureus* most common, occasionally gram-negative organisms

Anatomy

- 15–20 longitudinal septa attach the distal phalanx to the skin and divide the pulp into separate compartments[1]
- Digital arteries run parallel to the distal phalanx, and dorsal to the digital nerves
- The highest concentration of sensory receptors in the hand is the volar aspect of the distal phalanx

Non-operative management

- Ensure appropriate tetanus management
- If diagnosed early, may be treated by antibiotics, rest, heat, elevation, and warm soaks
- Any signs of fluctuance requires surgery

Operative management

- Digital block anesthesia and tourniquet control are used
- Many incisions described — if pointing abscess, open longitudinally over the point of maximal fluctuance with a No. 11 blade scalpel avoiding injury to flexor sheath or joint capsule
- Otherwise, staying distal to DIP flexion crease and dorsal to the neurovascular bundle, a unilateral incision is made over the midaxial line (ulnar for IF/MF/RF, and radial for thumb and SF) with a No. 11 blade scalpel[3]

- Scalpel/tenotomy scissors are used to divide the fibrous septa and allow the abscess to drain
- Probe the bone to evaluate for involvement — debride any affected areas
- Culture, irrigate, and pack the wound

Postoperative care

- Start warm soaks and daily dressing changes at 24–48 hrs and stop by 5 days
- IV/PO antibiotics for 5–7 days, longer if bony involvement
- Early ROM exercises

Herpetic Whitlow

- Commonly misdiagnosed as bacterial infection, such as paronychia or felon[4]
- Distinction made from the history: prodromal phase consisting of 24–72 hrs of burning pain prior to development of skin changes
- Caused by HSV 1 and 2

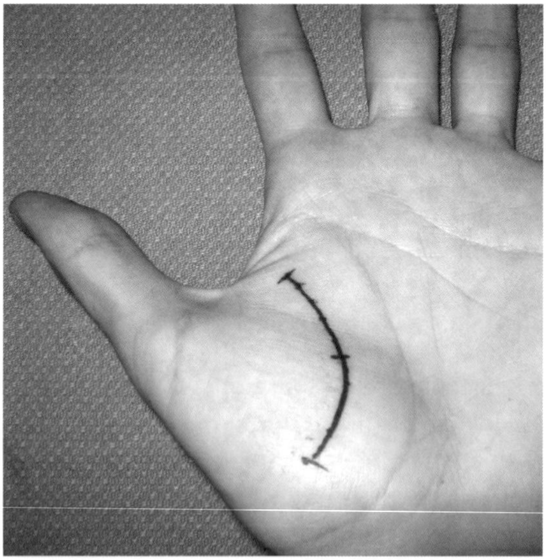

Fig. 2. Volar approach for thenar space abscess.

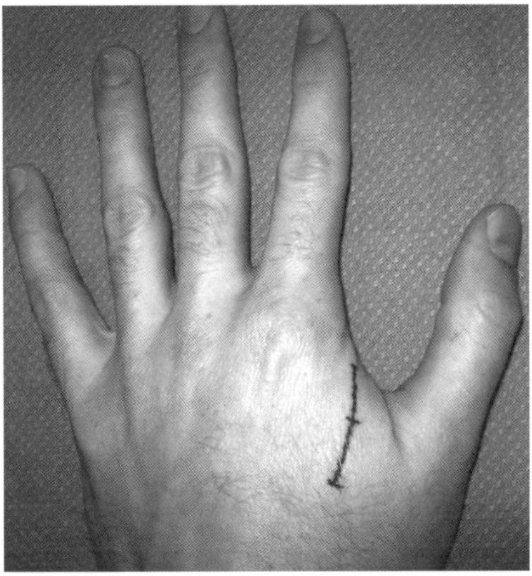

Fig. 3. Dorsal approach for thenar space abscess.

- Seen in adults (medical or dental professionals) and children (thumb or finger can become inoculated by sucking)
- Usually index finger or thumb
- Process occurs over 2 wks and then resolves over next 7–10 days
- Present with red, swollen, painful digit and subsequent clear vesicles that may coalesce or become turbid

Management

- Do NOT incise unless secondary bacterial infection, the process is self-limiting
- May unroof to obtain Tzanck smear and/or viral cultures
- Treat with rest, elevation, and anti-inflammatory agents
- Acyclovir in severe cases or with immunocompromised patients
- 20% recurrence rate

Palmar Space Abscesses

- Abscess formation within one of the potential spaces of the hand (most importantly, the thenar and midpalmar space)
- Typically occur after a penetrating wound

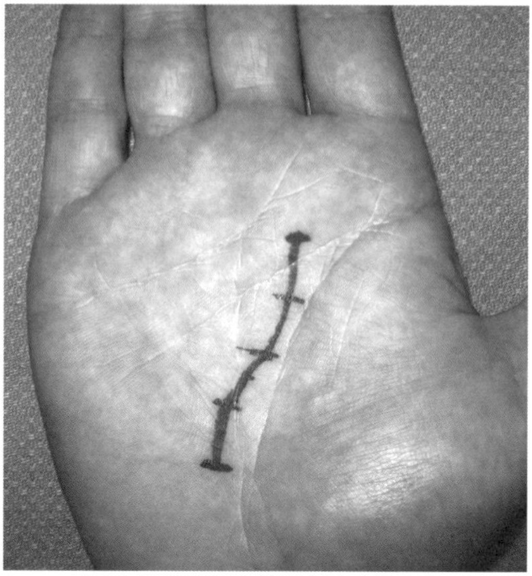

Fig. 4. Approach for mid-palmar space abscess.

- *S. aureus* is the most common organism
- Pain, swelling, and redness of the entire hand possibly with pain with flexion or opposition of thumb (thenar space) or pain on flexion of ulnar digits (midpalmar space)

Anatomy

Thenar space[3]

- Lies between the thenar eminence and the third metacarpal
- Dorsal border — fascia covering the adductor pollicis muscle
- Volar border — tendon sheath of the index finger and the palmar fascia
- Radial border — confluence of the adductor pollicis tendon and fascia as they insert on the proximal phalanx of the thumb
- Ulnar border — oblique (vertical midpalmar) septum, extending from the palmar aspect of the third metacarpal shaft obliquely and radially toward the palmar fascia

Midpalmar space[3]

- Lies between the thenar and hypothenar eminence

- Dorsal border — fascia overlying the second and third volar interosseous muscles and the periosteum of the third, fourth, and fifth metacarpals
- Volar border — flexor sheaths of the long, ring, and small fingers and the palmar aponeurosis
- Radial border — oblique (vertical midpalmar) septum
- Ulnar border — hypothenar septum, extending from the volar ridge of the fifth metacarpal shaft to the palmar aponeurosis.

Non-operative management ***rarely, if ever, indicated***

- Ensure appropriate tetanus management
- Antibiotics, rest, heat, elevation, and warm soaks

Operative management of Thenar Space Abscess

- Regional anesthesia, and tourniquet control are used
- Combined dorsal/volar approach: Using a No. 15 blade scalpel, a 3–4 cm incision is made on the palmar surface of the hand just adjacent and parallel to the thenar crease 1 cm proximal to the web space and continued proximally for 3 to 4 cm
- Protecting the motor and palmar cutaneous branches of the median nerve, dissection performed through palmar fascia toward the adductor pollicis muscle until abscess encountered
- After drainage, dissection is extended over the distal adductor to decompress the first dorsal interosseous space
- Next, a slightly curved longitudinal incision is made in the dorsal first web space, starting proximal to the web and extending perpendicularly, between the first and second metacarpals
- The dissection is continued deeper into the interval between the first dorsal interosseous and the adductor pollicis, at which point pus should be encountered
- Culture and irrigate wounds
- Drain each wound individually and splint the hand

Operative management of midpalmar space abscess

- Regional anesthesia, and tourniquet control are used

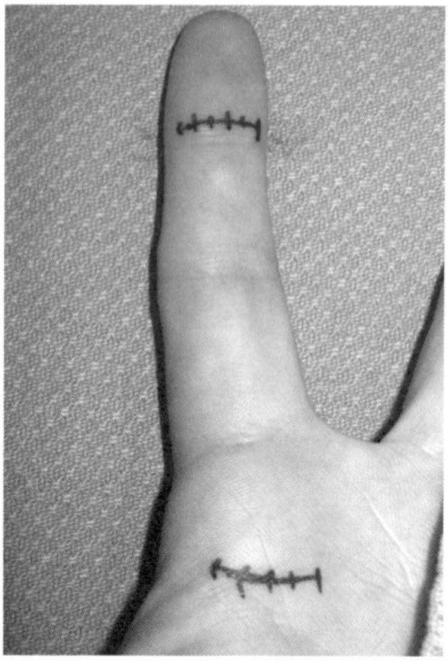

Fig. 5. Limited-incision technique for suppurative tenosynovitis.

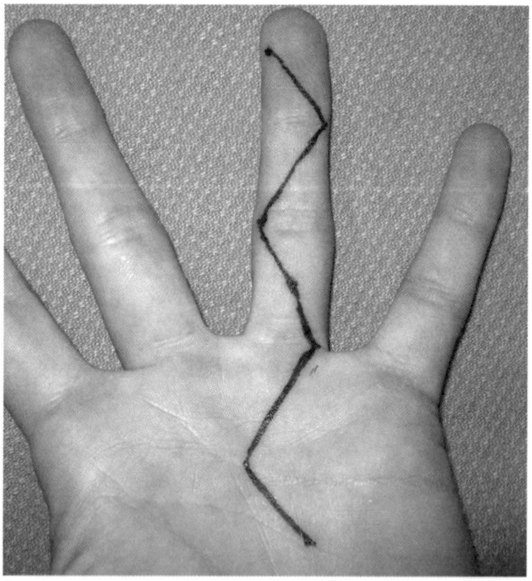

Fig. 6. Bruner incision technique for suppurative tenosynovitis.

- Using a No. 15 blade scalpel a slightly curved incision is made in the mid palm, beginning just proximal to the distal palmar crease in line with the third ray

- This extends proximally and slightly ulnarly, parallel to the thenar crease
- The palmar fascia is split, and the superficial palmar arch and the digital arteries and nerves are identified and protected
- The midpalmar space is entered by dissecting on either side of the ring finger flexor tendons
- Culture, irrigate, and pack the wound, followed by splinting of the hand

Postoperative care

- Start warm soaks and daily dressing changes at 24 hrs
- Repeat debridement in 48 hrs if not improving
- IV antibiotics for 5–7 days

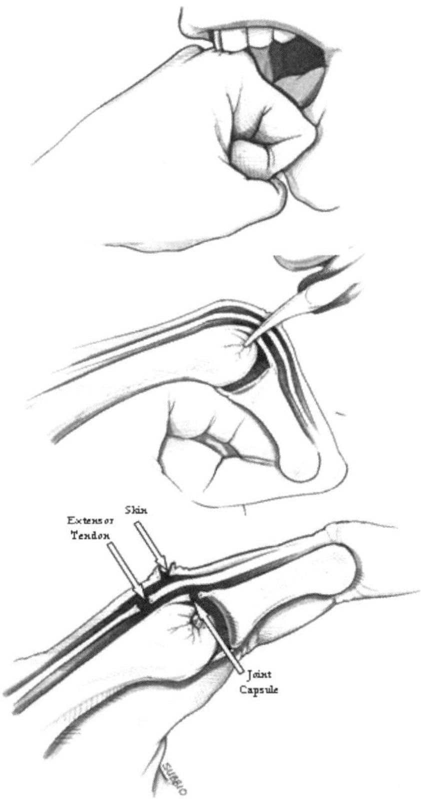

Fig. 7. Fight bite.

- Wounds are left to heal by secondary intention
- Early ROM

Suppurative Tenosynovitis

- Represents an abscess in the flexor tendon sheath usually after penetrating trauma
- Left untreated can lead to destruction of synovial gliding surfaces with adhesions, necrosis of tendons, osteomyelitis, and even amputation
- *S. aureus* is the most common pathogen, rarely gonococcus from hematogenous spread
- Consider *P. multocida* with animal bite wounds
- X-ray used to evaluate for foreign bodies, pyarthrosis, osteomyelitis, or unrecognized trauma, such as fracture

Kanavel's Signs

Pain on passive extension
Fusiform swelling of the digit
Partially flexed posture of the digit
Tenderness over the entire flexor tendon sheath

Anatomy

- Flexor tendon sheath is a double-walled structure with visceral (epitenon) and parietal (adjacent to pulleys) layers that create a hollow tubular structure, creating a closed system
- The sheaths begin in the palm at the level of the metacarpal neck and end distally just proximal to the DIP joint
- The space of Parona, which lies between the fascia of the pronator quadratus muscle and FDP conjoined tendon sheath, is a potential space of communication of the radial and ulnar bursae (horseshoe abscess)
- Nutrient supply to tendons are from vincula and diffusion from the synovial fluid
- When bacteria inoculate the flexor sheath, the synovial fluid becomes the nutritional source for the bacteria
- Bacterial proliferation leads to increased volume and pressure within the tendon sheath

- This high pressure obstructs the blood supply of the flexor tendons via the vincular system and can result in tendon necrosis and subsequent rupture[1–5]

Non-operative management

- Ensure appropriate tetanus management
- If diagnosed early, may be treated by antibiotics, rest, heat, elevation, and warm soaks (it is rare that patients present early enough for non-operative management)
- If unclear diagnosis or suspicion of non-septic tenosynovitis, diagnostic aspiration of the tendon sheath may be performed with a 20–22 g needle
- Re-evaluate at 24 hrs and operate if failure to improve

Operative management — limited-incision technique

- Tourniquet control is used
- Using a No. 15 blade scalpel, an incision is made near and parallel to the DIP flexion crease
- The tendon sheath is visualized by retracting both neurovascular bundles to their respective sides and opened through a transverse incision to allow fluid to drain (cultures are taken)

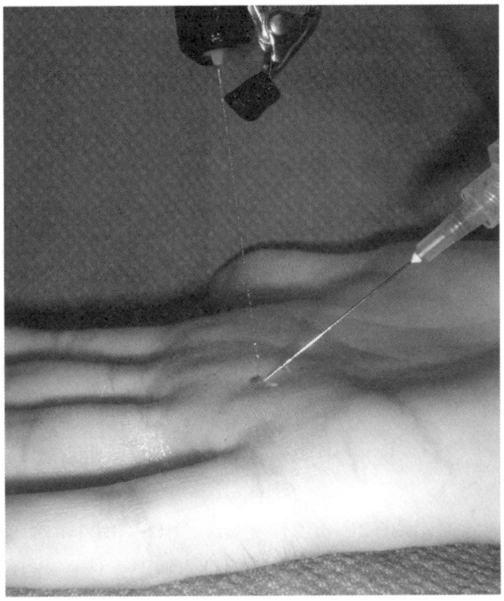

Fig. 8. Steroid injection of trigger finger.

- A second 1.5 cm transverse incision is made just proximal to the A1 pulley and the flexor tendon sheath is exposed and opened
- A polyethylene catheter with holes cut along its length is inserted into the sheath
- A syringe is attached to the catheter, and the tendon sheath is copiously irrigated from proximal to distal, noting egress of fluid from the distal incision
- The catheter is sutured in place with 3–0 or 4–0 monofilament suture so that irrigation can continue either intermittently or continuously (if severe)
- Splint the hand

Operative management — midlateral or Bruner incision technique
If pus is thick or if unable to drain adequately with limited approach
Bruner incision typically contraindicated as it leaves sheath exposed and may lead to tendon dessication

- General/regional anesthesia and tourniquet control are used
- Using a No. 15 blade, a midlateral (ulnar for IF/MF/RF, and radial for thumb and SF) is made dorsal to Cleland's ligament and extends from middle of the distal phalanx to just proximal to the web space. Alternatively, a Bruner zig-zag incision is made
- The dissection is carried out dorsal to the neurovascular bundle and down to the flexor tendon sheath
- A 5 mm incision is made in the tendon sheath distal to the A4 pulley to allow egress of fluid/pus
- Cultures are taken
- If a midlateral approach is used, a 0.5 to 2.0 cm transverse volar incision made proximal to the A1 pulley
- A 14 or 16 g intravenous catheter or a No. 5 pediatric feeding tube is introduced into the tendon sheath and advanced 1.5 to 2.0 cm into the sheath
- The sheath is then copiously irrigated
- The catheter is removed and the wounds are packed open
- Alternatives include: leaving the catheter in place as with limited-incision technique, and loosely closing the skin[3]

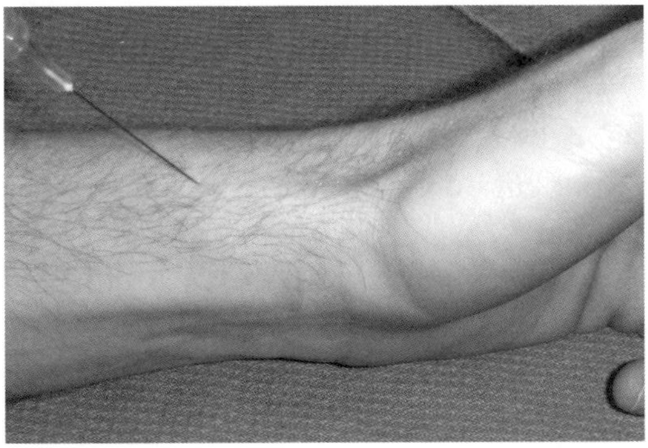

Fig. 9. Steroid injection of DeQuervains.

Preserve A2 and A4 pulleys

Be sure to debride any associated wounds at time of surgery

Postoperative care

- Pull catheter out at 24–48 hrs postoperatively if present
- If midlateral or Bruner incision used, change packing daily and remove 72 hrs postoperatively[3]
- Loosely approximate the skin edges when the infection has subsided, if not approximated previously
- IV antibiotics for 7–10 days, then postoperatively for a total of 4 wks
- Early, aggressive hand therapy

Bite Wounds (Classified according to source: Human or Animal)

Human bites

- Most commonly occur over RF/SF metacarpal head (fight bite)
- Human bites are potentially far more dangerous than animal bites owing to the mixture of gram-positive organisms (*S. viridans* and *S. aureus*) and anaerobic virulent organisms (*Eikenella corrodens* and *Bacteroides)*
- Examine hand with fingers fully flexed to reproduce position at time of injury
- X-rays are mandatory (evaluate for foreign body, fracture, or air in the joint space)[1–5]

Operative management

- Using a No. 15 blade scalpel, wide exposure around the traumatic wound is obtained
- The tendon, joint capsule, and bone are explored with the hand in a position of flexion
- If suspicion of capsule injury, open and inspect the articular surfaces
- Necrotic tissue, cartilage and bone are debrided
- Cultures are taken and the wound is copiously irrigated
- The wound is left open and injuries to the extensor tendon or extensor mechanism are NOT repaired
- A moist gauze wick is placed in the wound, and a soft bulky dressing is applied

Postoperative care

- Elevation and splinting
- Daily dressing changes
- Continue antibiotics until signs of clinical improvement
- Hand therapy at 48–72 hrs postoperatively
- Allow wound to close secondarily after 7 days of dressing changes
- If no improvement, repeat X-rays and return to operating room

Animal bites

- Dog bites most common (90%) and more likely to cause fracture, but cat bites more likely to cause an abscess
- Both require coverage for *Pasteurella*, *Staphylococcus*, *Streptococcus*, and anaerobes
- Require appropriate tetanus management and investigation for rabies
- X-rays are useful to evaluate for foreign body, fracture, or air in the joint space
- Cat bites rarely require closure[1–5]

Operative management

- Local infiltration as dictated by location and extent of the wound
- Irrigate wounds and explore joints when violated

- Large wounds should be re-approximated loosely with monofilament suture
- If wounds are substantial, splint the hand

Postoperative care

- IV/PO antibiotics based on clinical signs and symptoms
- Daily dressing changes if wounds are left open to heal by secondary intention
- High suspicion for cat-scratch fever (pustule at wound with painful lymphadenopathy) — treated with anti-inflammatory agents and antibiotics if necessary, usually self-limited

Inflammatory Disorders

The need for precision hand movements requires that tendon forces are exact with minimal friction. The direction of pull is maintained by sheaths and pulleys, while synovial lining minimizes friction. Any size discrepancy between the tendon and its sheath can increase friction, leading to inflammation and associated sequelae. Symptoms of tenosynovitis

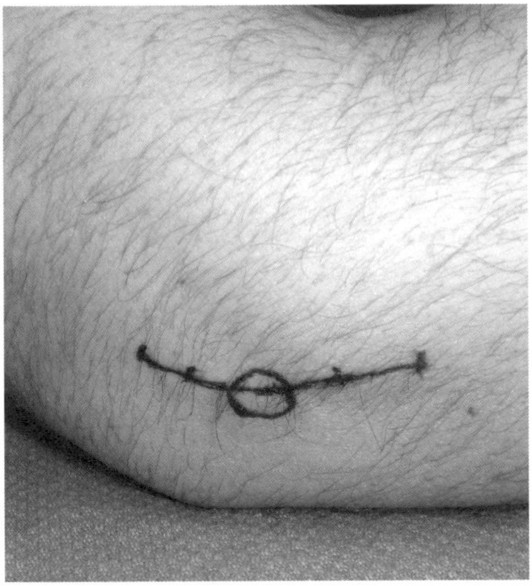

Fig. 10. Approach for lateral epicondylitis — lateral epicondyle marked with a circle.

(inflammation of tendon) worsen with edema and are more pronounced upon wakening from sleep.[6]

Any tendon can become inflamed, but the upper extremity is affected in a limited number of locations. The more common sites will be discussed individually.[2]

Digital Flexor Tenosynovitis "Trigger Finger"

- Inflammation of a tendon and its synovial lining
- Painful nodule often palpable and moves with excursion
- As process progresses, nodule enters the sheath with an abrupt motion, which causes the "triggering"
- Finger flexion may be restricted and the finger may become rigidly locked in the palm if the nodule is large enough to stop distal movement of the tendon

Non-operative management

- Ice, splinting, rest, NSAIDS
- A 3 mL syringe is loaded with 0.9 mL plain lidocaine and 0.1 mL sodium bicarbonate
- A steroid mixture (eg. triamcinolone 3–4 mg) is added to the mixture
- A 27g needle is applied to the syringe
- The hand is prepped and the digits slightly hyperextended
- The metacarpal head is palpated and the skin sprayed with ethyl chloride solution for 10 seconds
- The needle is introduced directly into the flexor tendon over the metacarpal head
- Needle placement can be confirmed, if necessary, by disengaging the syringe from the needle and asking the patient to gently bend the digit; needle motion confirms placement
- The syringe is replaced and light pressure applied to the plunger while simultaneously withdrawing the needle slowly[7]
- When the needle tip emerges from the tendon substance, dramatic relief of resistance is felt, and a fluid wave may be palpated throughout the tendon sheath proximal and distal to the injection site
- Usually relief of symptoms after 3–4 days
- If no improvement, consider surgery

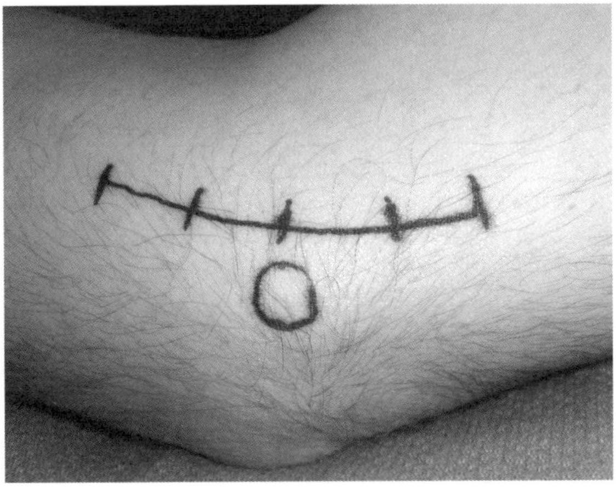

Fig. 11. Approach for medial epicondylitis — medial epicondyle marked with a circle.

Inform diabetics that this may affect blood sugar levels
Some authors advocate percutaneous needle release[8]

Operative management

- A tourniquet is applied, and 5 mL of lidocaine is injected into skin overlying the A1 pulley
- Using a No. 15 blade scalpel, a 1 to 1.5 cm transverse, oblique, or longitudinal incision is made over the involved metacarpal head
- In the thumb, the FPL tendon is approached through a 1.5 cm transverse incision in the MP flexion crease
- Blunt dissection is used to spread the subcutaneous tissues and the palmar fascia to expose the flexor sheath, ensuring protection of nerves and vessels
- The proximal edge of the thickened flexor sheath (proximal side of the A1 pulley) is identified, and a scalpel blade is used to divide the entire A1 pulley under direct vision (avoid A2 pulley to prevent bowstringing)
- If wide-awake, the patient is asked to actively move the digit to confirm complete relief of the triggering
- Hemostasis is obtained via electrocautery, and the wound is closed with two or three monofilament sutures
- A dressing is applied, with all digits left free, and motion is encouraged on the day of surgery[7]

Postoperative care

- Sutures removed 10–14 days postoperatively
- Resume full hand use within 3–4 wks of surgery

De Quervain's Tenosynovitis

- Inflammation of the APL and EPB tendons in the first extensor compartment[6]
- Hallmark is pain on the radial side of the wrist just proximal to the radial styloid
- Positive Finkelstein test — pain with adduction and flexion of thumb with ulnar deviation of the wrist[2]
- Can be seen in the postpartum period[7]

Anatomy

- APL is large with several slips, while EPB is a small single slip tendon and is occasionally absent or separated from APL by small septum

Non-operative management

- The radial styloid area is prepped with antiseptic solution
- Patient abducts and extends the thumb to palpate first extensor compartment
- While spraying ethyl chloride, a 27 g needle is introduced into the tendon sheath, and 1 mL of dexamethasone mixed with 0.5 mL of 1% plain lidocaine is injected
- The needle backed out of the tendon with pressure on plunger (a fluid wave should be palpable proximal and distal to the injection site as the abductor pollicis longus sheath fills)
- Repeat at 4–6 wks if no relief
- Surgery reserved for refractory cases[7]

Operative management

- A tourniquet is applied and the overlying skin is infiltrated with local anesthesia
- Using a No. 15 blade scalpel, a 2 cm transverse skin incision is made over the first dorsal compartment about 1 cm proximal to the tip of the

radial styloid process (be cognizant of branches of radial sensory nerve during dissection in order to prevent painful postoperative neuroma)
- The exposed annular ligament covering the compartment is incised with a scalpel (avoid excision of the entire sheath to prevent tendon subluxation)
- The tendons are mobilized out of the tunnel to ensure complete decompression from their musculotendinous junctions to a point at least 1 cm distal to the retinacular sheath
- Hemostasis is established with cautery after tourniquet release, and the skin is closed with a monofilament sutures
- A soft bulky dressing is applied[7]

Postoperative care

- Thumb motion encouraged in the immediate postoperative period
- Avoid heavy activities for 4–6 wks

Intersection Syndrome

- Tenosynovitis of the second extensor compartment, containing the ECRL and ECRB tendons[2,7]
- Pain, tenderness, and possibly swelling and crepitus of the dorsal forearm where second compartment tendons cross over first compartment tendons
- Aggravated by activities requiring wrist extension, such as weight lifting and rowing[6]

Non-operative management

- Splint wrist in 15 degrees of extension
- Steroid injection: site is located 4 cm proximal to the wrist along the distal radial forearm (see "De Quervain's Tenosynovitis" for technique)

Operative management

- A tourniquet is applied and the overlying skin is infiltrated with local anesthesia
- Using a No. 15 blade scalpel, a longitudinal incision is made along the radial wrist extending proximally to the swollen area

- After incising the deep fascia, release of the second dorsal compartment demonstrates the area of pathology
- The tendons are elevated and inspected, and no attempt is made to close the retinaculum
- Hemostasis is established with cautery after tourniquet release, and the skin is closed with a monofilament sutures[7]

Postoperative care

- Splint the wrist in extension for 2 wks to prevent bowstringing
- Patients can then use hand and wrist as tolerated

Lateral Epicondylitis "Tennis Elbow"

- Most common cause of lateral elbow pain
- Inflammation of the origin of the ECRB from the humerus
- Hallmark is tenderness over the lateral epicondyle with decreased grip strength
- Rare concomitant compression of radial nerve or posterior interosseous nerve at the arcade of Frohse
- Always attempt initial non-operative management
- Usually resolves without surgery, which is reserved for repeated courses and failed non-operative therapy[6]

Non-operative management

- Modification of activities and NSAIDs
- Splinting or use of an elastic band at the border of the proximal and middle third of the muscle (counterforce bracing)
- Steroid injection: with a 25 g needle, inject 1–2 mL of equal amounts 2% lidocaine and triamcinolone at 10 mg/mL over the area of maximal tenderness

Operative management

- After infiltration with local anesthesia, a 3–5 cm longitudinal incision is made over the lateral epicondyle and through the extensor aponeurosis using a No. 15 blade scalpel
- The ECRL muscle is retracted medially, revealing the degenerative origin of the ECRB

- The lateral epicondyle is decorticated with an osteotome or by drill holes
- The ECRB origin and associated periosteum are excised with a scalpel
- The ECRL is sewn to the extensor aponeurosis in an attempt to repair the defect
- The skin is closed with monofilament suture
- Splint or brace the elbow at 90 degrees of flexion[6,9]

Postoperative care

- Early motion in a brace may be initiated at 3–5 days after surgery
- Strengthening exercises started by 3 wks

Medial Epicondylitis "Golfer's Elbow"

- Much less common than lateral epicondylitis
- Involves the origin of the flexor-pronator mass from the medial epicondyle
- Patients may give history of multiple connective tissue inflammatory disorders
- Must differentiate from cubital tunnel syndrome (may have both)[2,6]

Non-operative management

- Modification of activities and NSAIDs
- A wrist splint is placed in neutral position to rest the flexors
- Usually resolves without surgery, which is reserved for repeated courses and failed non-operative therapy
- Steroid injection: with a 25 g needle, inject 1–2 mL of equal amounts 2% lidocaine and triamcinolone at 10 mg/mL over the area of maximal tenderness. To avoid ulnar nerve, direct patient to extend elbow as some may have ulnar nerve subluxation with flexion

Operative management

- After infiltration with local anesthesia, a 3–7 cm incision is made just anterior to the medial epicondyle
- The posterior division of the medial antebrachial cutaneous nerve must be identified and avoided during the approach
- The common flexor-pronator origin is identified, and the ulnar nerve is identified and protected

- The flexor-pronator fascia is incised and detached from the medial epicondyle with a 2 mm rim of superficial fascia to be used for later repair
- The periosteum of the medial epicondyle or the epicondyle itself is excised
- The common flexor-pronator origin is then repaired to the superficial fascia with interrupted sutures
- The subcutaneous tissue and skin are closed with monofilament suture[2, 6]

Postoperative care

- Splint or cast for 1–3 wks
- ROM exercises are started after removal of the splint or cast
- Stretching and strengthening program started 6 wks postoperatively

References

1. Chao JJ, Morrison BA. (2006) Infections of the upper limb. In: Aston SJ, Beasley RW, Thorne CHM (eds.), *Grabb and Smith's Plastic Surgery*, 6th Edn. Lippincott, Philadelphia, PA.
2. Beasley RW. (2003) *Beasley's Surgery of the Hand*. Thieme, New York, NY.
3. Stevanovic MV, Sharpe F. (2005) Acute infections in the hand. In: Green DP, Hotchkiss RN, Pederson WC (eds.), *Green's Operative Hand Surgery*, 5th Edn. Churchill Livingstone, New York, NY.
4. Ong YS, Levin LS. (2009) Hand infections. *Plast Reconstr Surg* **124**(4): 225e–233e.
5. Duncan SFM, Smith AA. (2009) Infections including tenosynovitis of the hand and forearm. In: Guyuron B, Eriksson E, Persing J (eds.), *Plastic Surgery: Indications and Practice*. Saunders, New York, NY.
6. Soltanian H. (2006) Tenosynovitis. In: Aston, SJ, Beasley RW, Thorne CHM (eds.), *Grabb and Smith's Plastic Surgery*, 6th Edn. Lippincott, Philadelphia, PA.
7. Wolfe SW. (2005) Tenosynovitis. In: Green DP, Hotchkiss RN, Pederson WC (eds.), *Green's Operative Hand Surgery*, 5th Edn. Churchill Livingstone, New York, NY.
8. Schramm JM, Nguyen M, Wongworawat MD. (2008) The safety of percutaneous trigger finger release. *Hand* **3**(1): 44–46.
9. Scher DL, Wolf JM, Owens BD. (2009) Lateral epicondylitis. *Orthopedics* **32**(4): 276–281.

CHAPTER 15

COMPRESSION NEUROPATHIES IN THE UPPER EXTREMITY

Askari Morad

Illustrative Case

A 55 year old right-hand-dominant female receptionist presents with 5-month history of transient paresthesia on the tip of her right long finger while typing or driving. Over the past month, several nights a week, she has been waking up with discomfort and paresthesia for which shaking her hand or putting it in warm water have helped. More recently, she has also noted paresthesia in her right thumb and index finger. On examination, she has decreased 2-point discrimination on her long finger. Tapping over the volar wrist crease results in paresthesia in the radial three digits. There is also evidence of early thenar atrophy.

Compression neuropathy is among the most common problems that are encountered in a hand surgery clinic. The three nerves (median, ulnar, radial) of upper extremity may be subjected to chronic compression in specific locations. The most common among these is compression of the median nerve at the wrist (i.e. carpal tunnel syndrome), followed by compression of the ulnar nerve at the elbow (i.e. cubital tunnel syndrome). It is of crucial importance that clinicians distinguish symptomatic compression neuropathy in the upper extremity from other neurologic entities (e.g radiculopathy, brachial plexopathy, CNS problems, somatoform, or factitious disorders, etc.)

Pathophysiology of Compression Neuropathy[1]

Neural changes depend on the duration and force of compression and proceed through a sequence:

1. Break down in the blood-nerve barrier.
2. Endoneural edema and increased pressure.
3. Perineural thickening.
4. Decreased microneural circulation.
5. Localized demyelination.
6. Diffuse demyelination.
7. Axonal degeneration.

Diagnosis[2]

History

Parallel to histologic changes of the compressed nerve, a continuum of symptoms starting from intermittent paresthesia or aching, to constant paresthesia and weakness, to eventual numbness and muscle loss are reported. Several conditions are thought to contribute to increased susceptibility of the nerve to compression neuropathy:

- Systemic conditions: diabetes mellitus, hyper/hypothyroidism, sarcoidosis, mucopolysacharidosis, amyloidosis.
- Alcoholism.
- Exposure to toxic metal/industrial solvents.
- Aging.
- Long-term hemodialysis.
- Hereditary motor-sensory neuropathy.
- Occupational risk (a point of controversy with limited data).

Physical Exam

— *Provocation tests*: Maneuvers that subject the nerve to increasing tension or compression to pinpoint a specific location of nerve compression. A positive test is one that elicits symptoms.

— *Nerve percussion test (Tinel's sign):* This test is positive if digital percussion over a potential site of nerve compression results in tingling sensation down the pathway of the nerve. This implies a chronically irritated nerve with evidence of neural injury.

— *Sensory evaluation:* The degree of nerve injury can be quantified through a series of sensory exams.

  — Threshold testing: Measures the minimum stimulus needed to elicit a response. Commonly, Semmes-Weinstein monofilament testing or ten test are used to assess the threshold. Changes in threshold precede changes in tactile discrimination.
  — Tactile discrimination: Indirectly measures the amount of innervated sensory receptors on the skin. This test is commonly performed by using static and moving two-point discrimination. Changes in tactile discrimination reflect a late finding in compression neuropathy.

Electrodiagnostic Studies (EDS)

EDS has two components:

1. Electromyelography (EMG):

Performed by readings from needle-recording electrodes in various muscles to assess their resting, volitional, and insertional electrical activity.

— Insertional *positive sharp wave* or electrical silence is evidence of denervation or chronic muscle degeneration.
— Fibrillation potential in resting muscle implies early muscle denervation.
— Incomplete or reduced motor unit potential (MUP) recruitment is seen with nerve injury in EMG.

2. Nerve conduction study (NCS):

Advantages: Tests conduction across large myelinated sensory and motor fibers. Increased conduction latency reflects nerve demyelination and extensive nerve injury. Additionally, velocity of conduction is recorded.

Disadvantages: Ignores small pain and temperature sensory axons which are usually the first to be affected. Normal latency may be obtained even if many nerve fibers are injured. NCS is also limited in assessing very proximal and distal sites of compression.

Double Crush Phenomenon

Compression of nerve at one level will make it susceptible to damage at another level:

- Presence of a proximal lesion may render the distal nerve trunk more vulnerable to the effects of compression (antegrade theory) or vice versa (retrograde theory). This may be due to disturbance of axonal flow kinetics and transport of enzymes and the essential components that need to reach the distal axon or disruption of the retrograde transport of byproduct and metabolic breakdown products resulting in vulnerability of a proximal portion.
- A thorough evaluation of the entire upper extremity, brachial plexus, thoracic outlet, as well as cervical spine is necessary to identify double crush.

Compression of Median Nerve[1,3]

Anatomy

— Originates from medial and lateral cord of the brachial plexus (C5–8, T1).
— Runs laterally along with the brachial artery between biceps and brachialis muscles.
— Crosses the artery medially and passes under lacertus fibrosus at antecubital fossa.

  ○ Innervates PL, FCR, FDS, PT.

— Passes between deep and superficial heads of PT.
— Gives off anterior interosseous nerve (AIN) to innervate FPL, FDP,[3,4] PQ.
— Passes under FDS and becomes more superficial in distal wrist as it goes through carpal tunnel. Palmar cutaneous branch is given off 5 cm proximal to carpal tunnel.

— In the hand, provides innervation to thenar muscles, lumbricals,[3,4] and sensation to thumb, index, long, and radial aspect of ring finger.

Sites of compression:

— Ligament of Struthers (an aberrant ligament that runs from supracondylar process to medial epicondyle).
— Between 2 heads of PT.
— Arch of FDS.
— Anomalous/accessory muscles (e.g. Ganzer's muscle).
— Carpal tunnel (most common).

Carpal Tunnel Syndrome

Most common compression neuropathy of the upper extremity.
Borders:

- Roof: transverse carpal ligament.
- Ulnar side: hamate and triquetrum.
- Radial side: scaphoid and trapezium.
- Content: Median nerve, FPL, 4 FDS, 4 FDP tendons.

Clinical Presentation

— Numbness or tingling at the tips of long (early), index fingers, and thumb.
— Exacerbated symptoms at night which results in awakening.
— Exacerbated symptoms with repetitive movement and prolonged flexed wrist postures (e.g computer work or driving).

Diagnosis

— Physical exam:

Provocation test:
— *Tinel's sign*: Digital percussion over the tunnel.
— *Phalen's test*: Wrist maintained in flexion with elbow elevated for 1 minute.
— *Pressure provocation test*: Digital pressure maintained proximal to carpal tunnel with wrist in neutral for 1 minute.

— EDS:

Increased sensory latency across the wrist are among earlier findings on NCS followed by fibrillation potential on EMG in more chronic settings.

Non-Operative Management

- *Wrist splinting:* Maintains wrist in neutral position and thus reduces pressure on the nerve.
- *Corticosteroid injection:* Can provide temporary relief therefore useful in making the right diagnosis. Those who respond to injection are more likely to have relief from surgical release.
- *Nerve gliding exercises:* Occupation therapy with focus on stretching and gliding exercises have been shown to improve function of median nerve.

Operative Management

Open carpal tunnel release (CTR)

- Anesthesia: Monitored anesthesia care (MAC) with local anesthesia is likely sufficient in most cases.
- Incision markings: Approximately 3.5 cm long, straight and longitudinal starting proximally at the wrist crease, traveling along a line parallel to the ulnar border of palmaris longus alongside the thenar crease (Fig. 1).
- The extremity is exsanguinated and the tourniquet is inflated to 250 mmHg. Incision is then made through the skin.
- Palmar fat is bluntly dissected to expose the underlying transverse carpal ligament (TCL). Crossing veins or overlying fibers of palmar fascia are divided. Distally, fibers of palmaris brevis are teased off the ligament.
- With visualization of TCL, a small full thickness cut is made with no. 15 blade in the proximal ulnar aspect of the ligament just radial to its the bony insertion.
- Through this small opening in TCL, a freer elevator is passed carefully into the tunnel. The flat part of the instrument is placed under the ligament to protect underlying structure.
- In a controlled fashion, the ligament is incised over the freer along its ulnar border from proximal to distal until yellow mid-palmar fat is visualized.

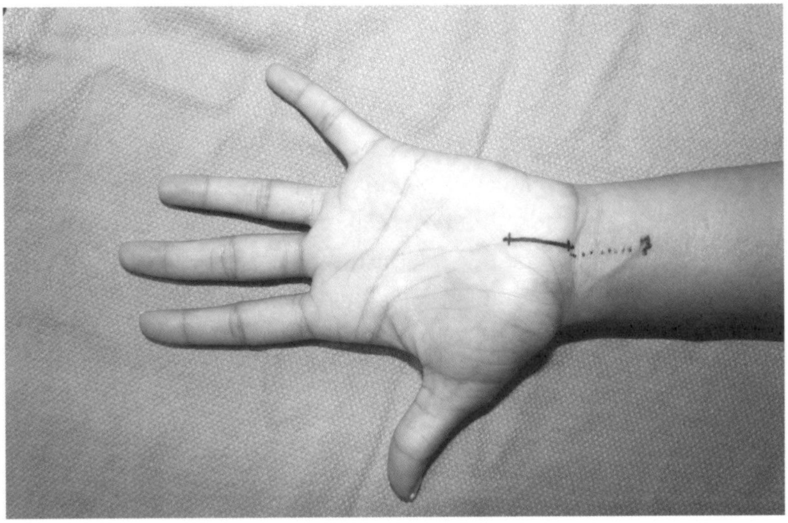

Fig. 1. Incision marking for open carpal tunnel release. An incision is made in proximal palm just ulnar to position of palmaris longus (PL) in the forearm.

— Proximal portion of TCL is then released with scissors.
— With adequate retraction of the skin, antebrachial fascia is incised proximally for about 1.5 cm with dissecting scissors with the tips of the scissors pointed ulnarly to avoid injury to the palmar cutaneous branch of the median nerve.
— One should be able to pass the tip of the small finger freely proximally and distally in tunnel to assure adequate release.
— Tourniquet is then deflated and hemostasis is attained with bipolar cautery.
— The wound is then irrigated and closed with mattress type sutures to properly evert the palmar skin edges with a 4–0 non-absorbable monofilament suture.
— A soft compressive bulky dressing is applied over the wound. Range of motion exercises are initiated 2–3 days after the surgery. Sutures are removed in 2 weeks. Strengthening exercises will be initiated in 3–4 weeks and may return to fully activity after 6 weeks.

Endoscopic carpal tunnel release
These techniques are quite variable.

One-port technique:

- Similar anesthesia and preparation to above.
- A 1.5 cm incision is made transversely over proximal wrist crease just ulnar to PL.
- A small cut is made in antebrachial fascia under the incision.
- The fascia is then lifted and increasing size obturators are carefully passed through the tunnel on the ulnar side. Finally the dissector-obturator slotted cannula is passed and camera is inserted.
- Using a dissector or a Q-tip, the deep surface of TCL is cleaned of any synovial tissue.
- Distally, the end of TCL and mid-palmar fat is identified.
- Using the fork knife, release is initiated proximal to distal under direct visualization with the camera. Release is terminated when palmar fat is visualized distally.
- Similar protocol as open CTR is followed post operatively.

Two-port technique:

In this technique after initial entrance into the tunnel, a second port incision is made at the distal aspect of the tunnel where the tip of the cannula is palpated. Here, the camera is passed from the distal port to visualize the incision of TCL through the proximal port in a distal to proximal direction.

Pronator Syndrome

- Rare form of median nerve compression neuropathy.
- Presentation: *Sensory* alteration in median nerve distribution in the hand with involvement of palmar cutaneous branch.

Diagnosis

- *Provocation test:*
    - Resisted pronation of the forearm.
    - Resisted elbow flexion with maximal supination of the forearm.
    - Resisted long finger FDS flexion.

  - o Digital pressure over the leading edge of PT with forearm in maximal supination.
- — EDS is thought to be poor predictor of surgical intervention.

Anterior Interosseous Nerve (AIN) Syndrome

- — Another rare form of median nerve compression neuropathy in proximal forearm.
- — Presentation: Weakness or loss of motor function in FPL, FDP to index and long fingers, and pronator quadratus.
- — May be associated with prior trauma.
- — NO sensory loss.
- — Parsonage-Turner syndrome (mononeuritis usually following a viral illness with associated history of pain) should be ruled out.
- — Occupational therapy and forearm flexor muscle stretching exercises can be beneficial in avoiding surgery.
- — Operative approach is the same for pronator and AIN syndrome.

Operative Management

In both pronator syndrome and anterior interosseous syndrome, the fibrous bands of the PT are commonly the source of compression.

- — Anesthesia: General or regional anesthesia is preferred.
- — Incision: Lazy "S" pattern measuring about 10 cm starting proximally at antecubital fossa and extending distally.
- — The extremity is exsanguinated, the tourniquet is inflated to 250 mmHg, and the incision is made through the skin.
- — Subcutaneous fat is dissected bluntly until lacertus fibrosus is visualized. Crossing cutaneous nerves are dissected and preserved.
- — Lacertus fibrosus is divided.
- — Tendon of superficial head of PT is identified under lacertus fibrosus.
- — A step-lengthening of PT tendon is performed distally.
- — With less tension on PT, median nerve is identified as it passes under this head of PT.
- — Median nerve is dissected proximally and distally.

— Distally where the deep head of PT and tendinous arch of FDS merge is identified.
— Tendinous portion of the arch is then divided along the path of median nerve.
— Surgeon should be able to run a small finger proximally and distally along the path of median nerve to assure complete release.
— Wound can be closed with buried absorbable sutures and a long-arm soft compression dressing is placed.
— Post operative care is otherwise similar to carpel tunnel release.

Ulnar Nerve Compression[3,4,5,6]

Anatomy

— Originates from C8 and T1 roots and continues as the terminal branch of medial cord.
— In the upper arm, the nerve travels posteromedial to brachial artery, posterior to intermuscular septum, and anterior to medial head of the triceps muscle and deep to brachialis. It remains anterior to medial antebrachial cutaneous nerve (MABCN).
— Approximately 8 cm proximal to elbow, passes through the arcade of Sruthers which is a band of fascia that connect medial head triceps to intermuscular septum.
— At the elbow, it passes posterior to medial epicondyle and medial to olecranon through epicondylar groove.
— It enters cubital tunnel in proximal elbow. Cubital tunnel is bordered by the ulnar and humeral heads of FCU and is roofed by arcuate ligament of Osborne which is a thickened transverse band between the two heads of FCU. The floor of cubital tunnel is the joint capsule and medial collateral ligament of the elbow.
— In the distal cubital tunnel, it pierces the pronator-flexor fascia and travels through the forearm superficial to FDP and deep to FDS. Distally, it passes just radial to FCU tendon.
— In distal forearm, approximately 5 cm proximal to pisiform, the dorsal sensory branch separates to innervate the ulnar dorsum of the hand.
— At the wrist, it passes through ulnar tunnel (used interchangeably with "Guyon's canal"), superficial to flexor retinaculum and divides to

superficial and deep branches. Ulnar tunnel starts at proximal edge of volar carpal ligament (the roof of the tunnel) and extends for 4–4.5 cm until the fibrous arch of hypothenar muscle. Ulnar tunnel contains both sensory and motor branches as well as ulnar artery and its accompanying veins.

- *Superficial branch*: Innervates palmaris brevis and provides sensation to small finger and ulnar ring fingers.
- *Deep branch*: Innervates hypothenar muscles, medial two lumbricals, the interossei muscles, and adductor pollicis muscle.

— 3 zones of ulnar tunnel

- Zone 1: Proximal to bifurication of nerve (contains both sensory and motor fascicles).
- Zone 2: Area deep to hypothenar arch where deep branch travels (motor only).
- Zone 3: Area around superficial branch (sensory primarily).

Cubital Tunnel Syndrome

- Most common ulnar nerve compression neuropathy and second most common compression neuropathy of upper extremity.
- Presentation: Varies from mild numbness and paresthesia in small and ring finger to pain radiating to the elbow. Patients frequently report weakness of grasp and "clumsiness" leading to dropping objects.
- Despite the name, includes various sites of compression outside of cubital tunnel.
- Known sites of compression in cubital tunnel syndrome:

    1. Arcade of Struthers.
    2. Medial intermuscular septum.
    3. Hypertrophy of medial head of triceps.
    4. Medial epicondyle (e.g. valgus deformity following trauma).
    5. Epicondylar groove.
        - Factor inside the groove (e.g. tumor, arthritic bony spurs).
        - Factor outside of the groove (e.g. anomalous anconeus epitrochlearis muscles).
        - Subluxation of the nerve.

6. Cubital tunnel/Osborne ligament (most common site).
7. Deep fascia of flexor/pronator muscle.

Diagnosis

— Physical exam:

- o Ulnar nerve is palpated along its path for any area of tenderness, masses, or other deformity implying a cause for compression.
- o Provocation test: *Elbow flexion test* (maintaining the elbow in flexion with wrist in extension for 1 minute).
- o Numbness or paresthesia at the dorso-ulnar aspect of the hand helps distinguish compression at the level of elbow from one at the wrist level.

— EDS:

- — Increased sensory latency as well as increased motor latency in ulnar nerve innervated intrinsic muscles of the hand.
- — Decrease conduction velocity of ulnar nerve across the elbow (less than 50 m/s).
- — Fibrillation in ulnar-nerve-innervated intrinsic muscle implies axonal degeneration.

Non-Operative Management

- — Avoiding postures that places elbow in full flexion.
- — Static night splinting of elbow in extension.
- — Stretching and nerve gliding exercises may be helpful in some.

Operative Management

Indication:

- — Failure of conservative treatment after 3 months or worsening symptoms.
- — Atrophy of ulnar-nerve-innnervated intrinsic muscles.
- — Subluxation of the nerve at the elbow.
- — Conduction velocity of <40 m/s across the elbow.

Techniques of cubital tunnel release

- Decompression without transposition
  - *In-situ decompression*: Nerve remains in its natural path and the fascial layer overlying is released.
  - *Decompression with medial epicondylectomy*: Same as *in-situ* decompression plus removal of about 30% of superficial medial epicondyle.
  - *Endoscopic release*: *In-situ* release of the nerve using an endoscope with a smaller incision at the elbow.
- Decompression with anterior transposition
  - *Subcutaneous transposition*: Nerve is transposed anteriorly and secured under the subcutaneous tissue in antecubital fossa.
  - *Submuscular transposition:* Pronator-flexor is divided at its origin at medial epicondyle, nerve is transposed anteriorly under the muscle belly, and the origin is repaired to medial epicondyle.
  - *Intramuscular transposition:* Nerve is transposed anteriorly and buried in a groove in pronator-flexor muscle mass.

Open *in-situ* decompression, as well as subcutaneous and submuscular transposition are among the more commonly utilized procedures by clinicians and are described in more details below.

In situ Decompression

— Anesthesia: General versus regional block.
— Positioning: Supine on the bed and a soft bump under the elbow.
— Marking: With elbow flexed, a longitudinal line is drawn from approximately 5–8 cm proximal to the medial epicondyle parallel and slightly posterior to the medial intermuscular septum. This line is passed between olecranon and medial epicondyle and brought 5 cm distally along the medial volar forearm (Fig. 2).
— A sterile tourniquet is place on the upper arm and is inflated to 250 mmHg after exsanguination. The incision is made along the marking through the skin.

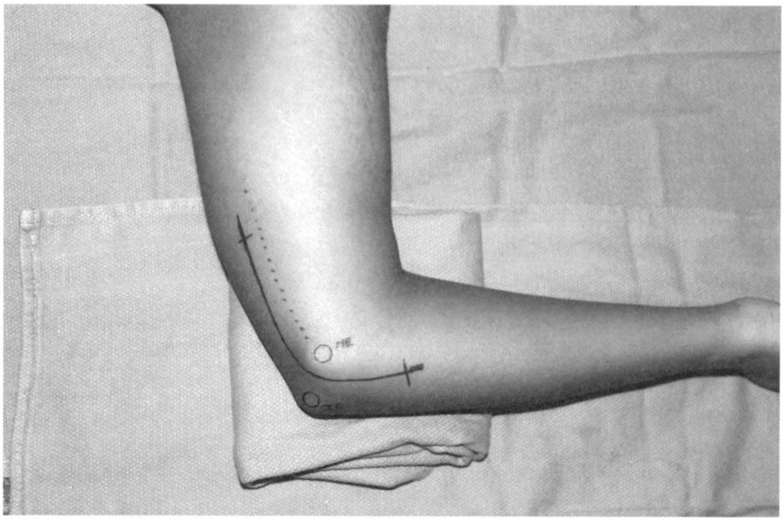

Fig. 2. Incision marking for open cubital tunnel release. Incision is made just posterior to medial intermuscular septum and passed between olecranon (OLE) and medial epicondyle (ME) before extending into the forearm.

— With blunt dissection, crossing branches of medial antebrachial cutaneous nerve are identified and preserved in subcutaneous layer until underlying fascia is visualized.
— Intermuscular septum is identified proximal to the elbow. Just posterior to the septum, ulnar nerve trunk is found.
— The nerve is kept in its bed while carefully the overlying fascia is incised. The dissection is continued about 10 cm proximal to medial epicondyle to fully release arcade of Struthers.
— The dissection is then continued distally to release the roof of epicondylar groove. Special attention is paid not to mobilize the nerve from the groove to prevent subluxation.
— Distally, the nerve is followed as it travels between two heads of FCU. The fascia between the two heads (Osborne ligament) is divided.
— With gentle spreading, the nerve is released as it travels deep in the muscle and through the deep fascia.
— Tourniquet is deflated. Hemostasis is attained with bipolar cautery.

— The wound is closed with subdermal and subcutaneous absorbable monofilament sutures and a soft long arm compression dressing is placed.

Anterior transposition

— Ulnar nerve is approached in a similar fashion as in-situ technique.
— After the nerve is visualized proximally, it is circumferentially dissected and a vessel loop is passed around it with no tension. This will allow to further mobilize the nerve proximally and distally.
— The nerve is released and elevated along the entire path of dissection as described in *in-situ* technique.
— The medial intermuscular septum is dissected from its surrounding tissue distally and a segment of 4 cm long and 1 wide is resected from the septum just proximal to the elbow
— The nerve is then transposed anteriorly without any tension. Care is taken to avoid creating a new compression sites. Capsular branches of ulnar nerve have to be divided to allow transposition.
— Subcutaneous transposition: The nerve will lie anteriorly between the fascia of pronator-flexor muscle and the overlying subcutanous fat-skin flap. Medial to the position of transposed nerve, a laterally based fascial flap is raised from the pronator-flexor muscle mass and secured carefully to the overlying dermis to keep the nerve in its new anterior position.
— Submuscular transposition: The pronator-flexor mass is further dissected laterally. Median nerve along with the vascular bundle lateral to the muscle is identified and protected. This pronator-flexor tendon is circumferentially dissected over the medial collateral ligament around its origin on medial epicondyle. The muscle is then taken off from it origin directly or through a step-cut incision. The nerve is then transposed anteriorly over the elbow joint. The divided muscle is then brought over the nerve and fixed to medial epicondyle (suture anchors versus step-cut lengthening repair).

Post Operative Care

— Soft compression dressing is removed 2–5 days after the surgery.
— Range of motion exercises are started 2–3 days following the surgery.

- Weight restriction of object lighter than 5 lbs for the first month.
- No restriction by second month.
- Cases of submuscular transposition will be immobilized in a long arm splint for 4–6 weeks.

Comparison of Various Techniques

- The results of several meta-analyses and randomized prospective studies have not shown any significant difference in outcomes among various open techniques of cubital tunnel release. Similarly, complication rate or re-operation rates have not been different. Further studies comparing endoscopic technique to various open techniques are needed to draw a reliable conclusion.

Ulnar Tunnel Syndrome

- Less common type of ulnar nerve compression.
- Compression is generally due to space-occupying mass or lesions (e.g. tumors, ganglion cysts, thrombosed vessels, pseudoaneurysms, anomalous muscles, etc) or may result from repetitive or acute trauma (e.g fracture of the hook of hamate).
- Depending on location of compression of ulnar nerve in ulnar tunnel, presentation can be a combination of motor and sensory (zone 1), motor only (zone 2), or primarily sensory (zone 3) deficits (Fig. 3).
- Presentation:
    - Weakness of ulnar-nerve-innervated intrinsic muscles of the hand and sensory changes in small finger and ulnar aspect of ring finger.
    - Dorsal ulnar aspect of the hand (dorsal sensory branch of ulnar nerve) is not affected.
- EDS is helpful in localizing the problem to the wrist.
- Management is primarily operative in light of non-resolving symptoms.

Operative Management

- Anesthesia and preparation is similar to open CTR.
- Marking: A palmar incision is designed about 1 cm ulnar and parallel to that of open CTR such that field of dissection is ulnar to the hook

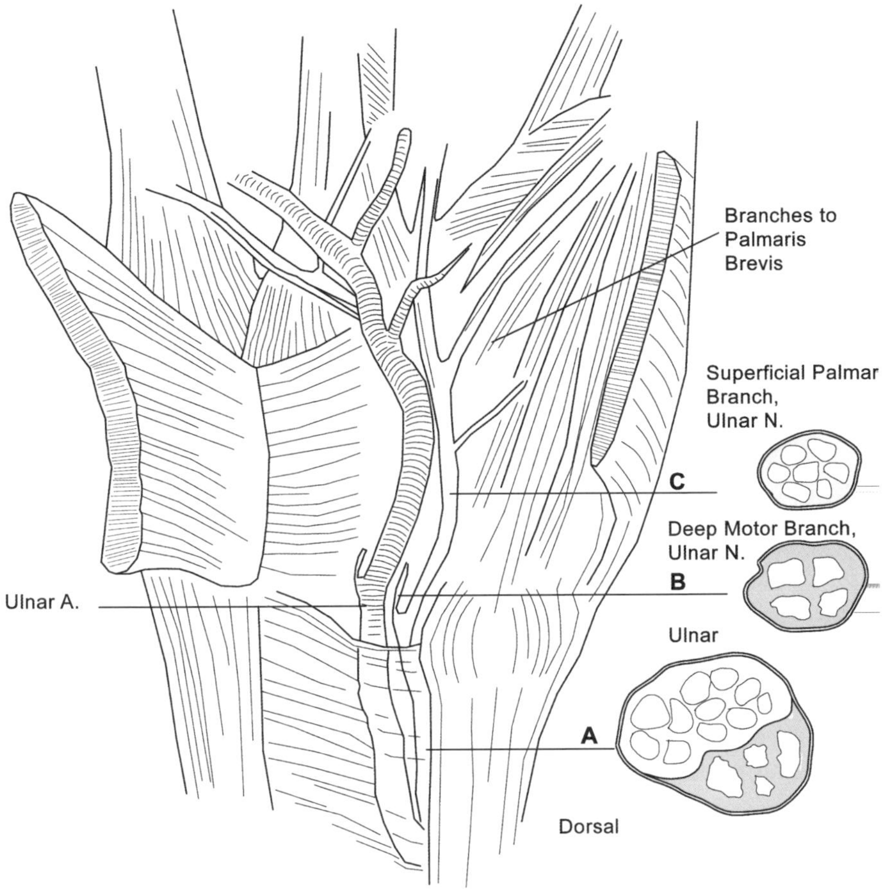

Fig. 3. Ulnar tunnel anatomy. Proximal to the distal edge of volar carpal ligament ulnar nerve contains both sensory and motor fasciles (zone 1) but beyond this point it divides into a deep motor branch (zone 2) and a superficial branch (zone 3).

of the hamate. The incision is extended more proximally in a zig-zag pattern across the wrist crease.

— After exsanguination and tourniquet inflation, the incision is made through the dermis.
— With blunt dissection, volar carpal ligament and palmaris brevis are identified and released. Guyons' canal is thus opened.
— Neurovascular bundle is more easily identified proximally and traced distally.

- Ulnar nerve is then dissected medially at the proximal edge of the hypothenar muscle to find the deep branch as it curves around the hook of the hamate. Part of the proximal edge of hypothenar muscle is divided to better decompress this branch.
- Ulnar nerve proper is then fully decompressed through Guyon's canal by releasing part of the distal antebrachial fascia. Distally, superficial branch and its branches are identified and released as it travels over hypothenar muscle.
- Hemostasis is attained after deflating the tourniquet and wound is closed with 4–0 non-absorbable monofilament sutures in a mattress pattern.
- Post operative regimen is similar to open CTR.

Radial Nerve Compression Neuropathy[1,4,7]

- Rare entity.
- 2 groups:
    - Compression in proximal forearm can result in radial tunnel syndrome or posterior interosseous (PIN) syndrome.
    - Compression of superficial branch of radial nerve (SBRN) in distal forearm can result in Wartenberg Syndrome.

Anatomy

- One of terminal branches of posterior cord.
- Splits away from axillary nerve just proximal to quadrangular space.
- Lies behind the brachial artery and anterior to long head of triceps.
- Travels posterior and lateral and becomes deep to long head and follows between the lateral and medial heads of the triceps at around the spiral groove of humerus. At this level, it innervates the triceps.
- Approximately 10 cm proximal to lateral epicondyle, it pierces the lateral intermuscular septum to assume an anterior position. Distal to this point, it sends branches to brachialis, brachioradialis (BR), anconeus, and extensor carpi radialis longus (ECRL) prior to entering the forearm.

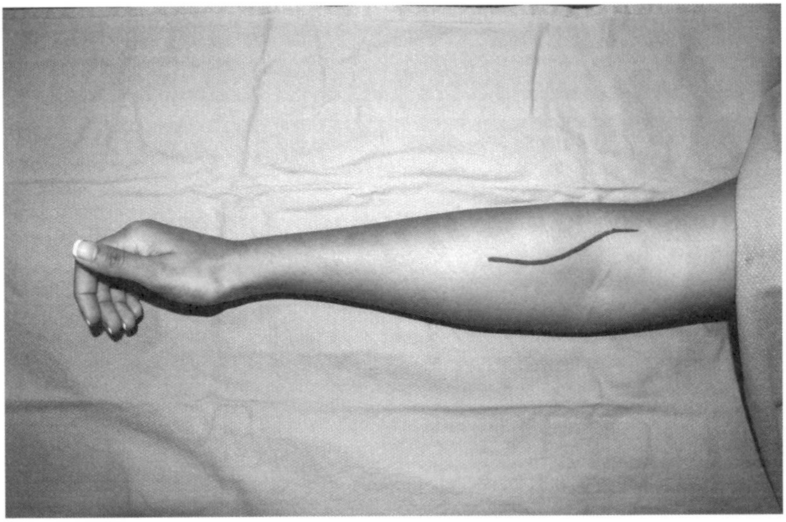

Fig. 4. Radial tunnel anatomy. Radial nerve travels between BR and brachialis to pass under arcade of Fröhse as it enters supinator muscle.

— The nerve passes anterior to the lateral epicondyle and enters the radial tunnel at the elbow. Radial tunnel is about 5 cm long and lies anterior to radiocapitellar joint capsule, medial to BR and ECRL, lateral to biceps tendon. The tunnel is roofed by BR as it passes anteromedially over the nerve in the forearm (Fig. 4).

— Upon entering the tunnel, the nerve is crossed by several prominent vessels forming the leash of Henry (radial recurrent artery/veins).

— At the level of lateral epicondyle, radial nerve then divides to PIN and SBRN. Extensor carpi radialis brevis (ECRB) is innervated distal to the elbow usually by PIN and at times by SBRN.

— SBRN travels deep to BR and enters subcutaneous tissue between the tendons of BR and ECRL or in some cases by piercing BR tendon. At about 5 cm proximal to radial styloid, SBRN divided to a palmar and dorsal branches that will distally provide sensation to dorsum of the thumb, index, long finger, and half of ring finger.

— PIN passes under the arcade of Fröhse which is a fibrous proximal border of the supinator muscle as it enters the interval between the two heads of supinator.

— After exiting the supinator muscle, the nerve branches into a deep and superficial branch providing innervation to the muscles of the forearm (deep branch: APL, EPL, EPB, EIP; superficial branch: ECU, EDC, EDQ).

Radial Tunnel Syndrome and Posterior Interosseous Syndromes

— Uncommon syndromes resulting from compression of radial nerve in the region of proximal elbow.

Sites of compression (Fig. 4):

— Fibrous opening of radial tunnel.
— Leash of Henry.
— ECRB tendinous edge.
— Arcade of Fröhse (most common site).
— Distal edge of supinator fascia.

Radial Tunnel Syndrome

— An unusual pain syndrome.
— Presentation: Pain and weakness upon resisted elbow extension or rotation with pain localizing to lateral proximal forearm (radial tunnel) and weakness usually secondary to pain.

— *Diagnosis*

- Tenderness over radial tunnel.
- Provocation test: Pain over edge of proximal ECRB with resisted long finger extension; pain with resisted supination.
- EDS not helpful.
- Radial nerve block maybe helpful in establishing diagnosis.
- May be mistaken or occur simultaneously with lateral epicondylitis.
- Nerve gliding exercise may be helpful but generally non-operative management is of limited benefit.
- Overall, a controversial diagnosis due to presentation (a pain syndrome vs. a true compression neuropathy).

Posterior Interosseous Syndrome

— Compression of PIN usually with an onset after a traumatic event, iatrogenic causes, or due to mass effect.
— Presentation: Weakness of ECRB, supinator, ECU, EIP, EDC, EDQ, EPL/B, and APL with no sensory symptoms.

— *Diagnosis*

- Radial deviation of the hand with forceful wrist flexion (ECRL intact but ECRB affected).
- Weakness on extension of index finger.
- Provocation test: Digital pressure over PIN in the interval between BR and ECRB may elicit symptoms (inconsistent).
- EDS may be helpful.

Operative Management

Anterior Approach: Radial nerve is approached volarly between BR and brachialis.
Posterior Approach: Radial nerve is approached dorsally between EDC and ECRB.
Muscle–Splitting Approach: BR muscle is split to expose the nerve.

Anterior (Henry's) Approach:
— Anesthesia: General versus regional block.
— Marking: Incision is marked starting proximal and lateral to the antecubital fossa, continued on the anteromedial edge of BR and extended about 10 cm distal to the elbow (Fig. 5).
— After inflation of tourniquet, the incision is made through the dermis and subcutaneous fat to expose the underlying the muscular fascia. Cutaneous nerves are dissected and protected.
— Carefully, the interval between BR and brachialis is identified. Within in this interval, radial nerve paper is visualized and carefully dissected.
— Medial to brachialis (lateral to biceps tendon), lateral antebrachial nerve is identified and protected.
— The vessels (leash of Henry) crossing over radial nerve are dissected and ligated.

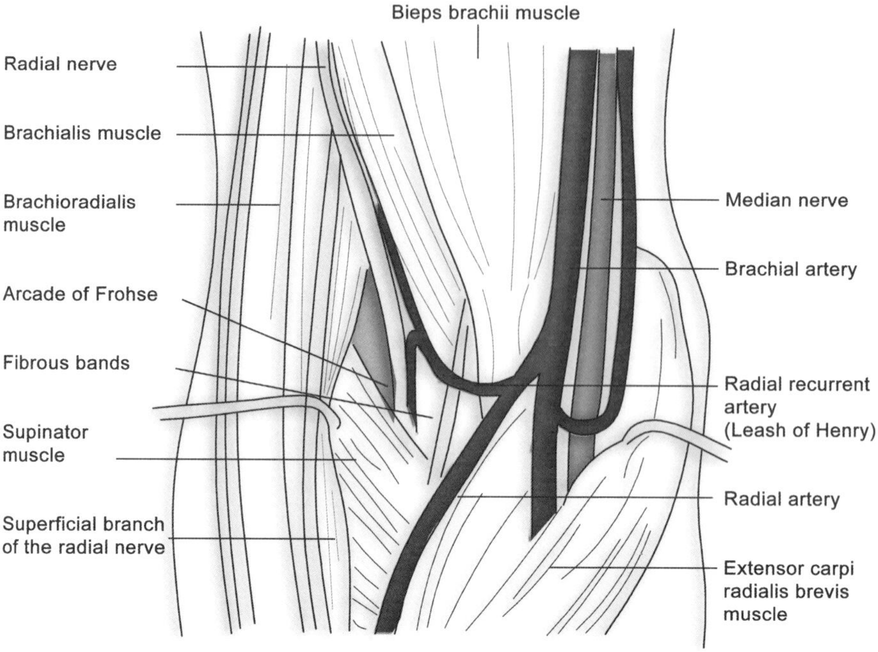

Fig. 5. Incision marking for anterior (Henry's) approach to radial tunnel release. Incision is initiated lateral to antecubital fossa in distal arm and extended distally along the medial border of BR.

— The nerve is traced distally to where it branches to SBRN and PIN.
— The leading edge of supinator is exposed as PIN passes deep to it. This fibrous edge (arcade of Fröhse) is released.
— PIN is then traced and released through its path in the supinator. The distal edge of the supinator fascia is divided.
— The wound is then irrigated and closed with subdermal and subcuticular absorbable mono-filament sutures and soft compression dressing is applied from the hand up to mid arm. Range of motion exercises are started 1 week after the surgery and strengthening exercises are initiated about 3–4 weeks after the surgery.

Posterior (Thompson's) Approach:

— Marking: Incision is marked on proximal dorsal forearm along a line drawn from lateral epicondyle to radial styloid.

— Under tourniquet control, incision is made through the skin and subcutaneous fat to expose underlying muscular fascia. Subcutaneous nerves are identified and protected.
— The interval between EDC and ECRB is identified and entered. PIN is visualized as it exits deep to supinator muscle. Branches to ECRB are protected. The distal edge of supinator is then released.
— The nerve is released proximally through its path in supinator. The leading edge of ECRB tendon and the proximal tendinous edge of supinator muscle are released and vessels of leash of Henry are divided and ligated.
— Post operative care will be similar to anterior approach.

Muscle-Splitting Approach:
— A lazy-S incision is marked starting proximal to radial head and 2–3 cm lateral to biceps tendon on the lateral proximal forearm.
— With tourniquet inflated, incision is made through skin and subcutaneous layer. Subcutaneous nerves are identified and protected.
— Fascia overlying the BR is identified and split. The muscle fibers over the radial head are bluntly split with dissecting scissors until the fat overlying the radial head is visualized. PIN is then identified.
— The split in the muscles is then lengthened through the radial tunnel to access proximal and distal part of the nerve. Releases will be done at the same places as described in anterior and posterior approaches.

Wartenberg's Syndrome

— Compression of sensory branch of radial nerve in its superficial location in distal forearm.
— Presentation:
 — Numbness and paresthesia in dorsum of thumb, index, and long finger as well as dorsoradial aspect of the hand.
 — May be related to a history of work-related repetitive activity, tight wrist watch bands, or handcuffs.
— *Diagnosis:*
 — Tinel's sign over area of entrapment.
 — EDS may be helpful.

Non-Operative Management

— Corticosteroid injection.
— Activity modification.

Operative Management

— Marking: Longitudinal incision of approximately 5 cm is made on the volar edge of BR in distal 1/3 of the forearm.
— Under tourniquet control, the skin is incised toward the volar aspect of BR. Dorsally, the sensory branch of radial nerve is identified.
— The nerve is released proximally as it enters the interval between BR and ECRL. The interval is opened by release BR fascia and nerve is further released proximally.
— Portion of the tendon of the BR is excised to better release the nerve.
— Surgical site is closed similar to approaches for radial tunnel syndrome. Post operative dressing is removed by day 2 or 3, range of motion exercises are initiated when dressing is removed, and strengthening exercises are started after 4 weeks.

Recurrent Compression Neuropathy Following Decompression[1]

Etiologies of recurrence or persistence of symptoms following decompression can be placed in three groups:

— *Inadequate release of all sites of compression:* Patients report the same symptoms as those prior to surgery without any resolution.
— *Formation of a new compression site*: Patients report resolution of symptoms for a time period followed by recurrence of the same symptoms as those prior to surgery (compression on medial intermuscular septum after ulnar nerve transposition).
— *Iatrogenic injury to the nerve*: Patients report entirely new symptoms (e.g. neuroma formation).

Management is will require exploration of prior surgical areas with attention to complete release of any residual compression sites or addressing any injury to the nerve (e.g. resection of neuroma).

Acknowledgments

Author would like to thank Ceren Dayicioglu for illustrations.

References

1. Mackinnon SE, Novak CB. (2005) Compression neuropathies. In: Green, DP Hotchkiss RN, Pederson WC, Wolfe SW (eds.), *Green's Operative Surgery*, 5th Edn. Elsevier, Philadelphia, pp. 999–1045.
2. Effron CR, Beasley RW. (2007) Compression neuropathies in the upper limb and electrophysiologic studies. In: Thorne CH, *et al.* (eds.), *Grabb and Smith's Plastic Surgery,* 6th Edn. Lippincott Williams & Wilkins, Philadelphia.
3. Means KR Jr, Segalman KA. (2007) Carpal tunnel syndrome. In: Tumble TE, Budoff JE (eds.), *Hand Surgery Update IV*. American Society for Surgery of the Hand, Rosemont, pp. 399–408.
4. Goldfarb CA. (2007) Cubital tunnel syndrome and radial tunnel syndrome. In: Tumble TE, Budoff JE (eds.), *Hand Surgery Update IV*. American Society for Surgery of the Hand, Rosemont.
5. Posner MA. (1998) Compressive ulnar neuropathies at the elbow. I. Etiology and diagnosis. *J Am Acad Orthop Surg* **6**: 282–288.
6. Posner MA. (1998) Compressive ulnar neuropathies at the elbow. II. Treatment. *J Am Acad Orthop Surg* **6**: 289–297.
7. Means KR Jr, Segalman KA. (2010) Compressive neuropathies. In: Trumble TE, Rayan GM, Budoff JE, Baratz ME (eds.), *Principles of Hand Surgery and Therapy,* 2nd Edn. Saunders, Philadelphia.

CHAPTER 16

BENIGN AND MALIGNANT TUMORS OF THE UPPER EXTREMITY

Sara Yegiyants, Yash Avasha and Zubin J. Panthaki

Overview:

1. SKIN TUMORS
   - Benign
   - Premalignant
   - Malignant
   - Sweat gland tumors
2. SOFT TISSUE TUMORS
   - Benign
   - Malignant
     - Low grade
     - High grade
3. BONE TUMORS
   - Benign
   - Malignant
4. VASCULAR TUMORS

1. SKIN TUMORS[1]

A. Benign

1. Sebaceous Cyst
   - Arise from obstructed apocrine glands in the skin
   - Contain sebum
   - Found on dorsum of hand only (no sebaceous glands on palmar aspect)
   - Excise if problematic

2. Cutaneous Horn (Fig. 1)
   - Protrusion of keratotic material from the skin
   - Sun-exposed areas
   - Associated with benign, premalignant, and malignant lesions
   - Smaller lesions — excisional biopsy
   - Large lesions — punch biopsy
3. Verruca Vulgaris (common warts)
   - Caused by HPV 1,4,7,10
   - Most commonly found at sites of trauma
   - Spontaneous resolution within 1 to 2 years
   - Lesions that are persistent, interfere with function, or are cosmetically unacceptable should be treated
   - Therapy
     - Topical agents — cure rates of 70% to 80% can be achieved with minimal side effects
     - Salicylic acid which is both keratolytic and a local irritant

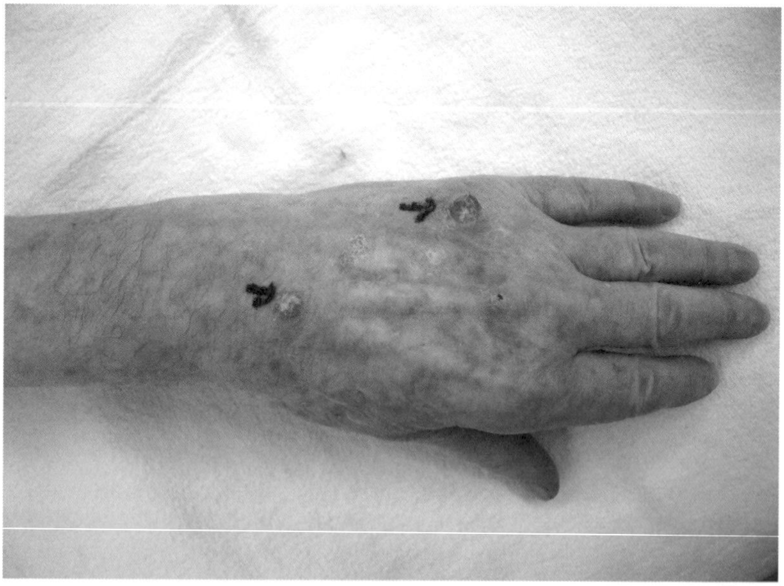

Fig. 1. Cutaneous horn (ulnar lesion).

- Other topical remedies contain glutaraldehyde and occasionally formaldehyde
- Cryotherapy — cure rates approach 60% to 80%
- Immunomodulatory agents, carbon dioxide lasers, pulsed-dye lasers, and photodynamic therapy

4. Pyogenic Granuloma (Fig. 2)

- Solitary reddish nodular tumor of the skin or mucosa
- Etiology is unknown
- Chronic vascular lesion that eventually becomes inflamed and generates localized granulation tissue
- Spontaneous resolution is unusual
- In the subungual location — may be the result of a nail plate puncture wound, whether traumatic or iatrogenic
- Treatment — excision, curettage, radiation therapy, cauterization, pulsed-dye laser, or silver nitrate
- Excision of the lesion with a 1-mm margin — most effective

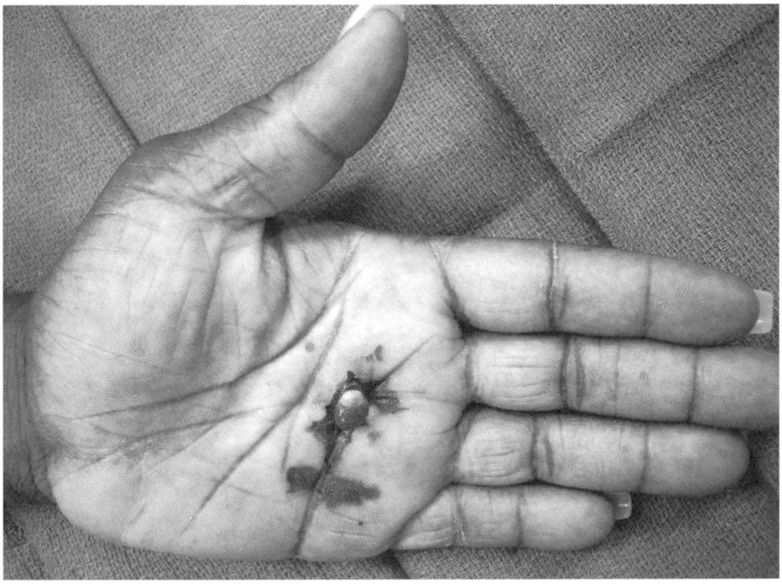

Fig. 2. Pyogenic granuloma.

5. Keratoacanthoma (Fig. 3)

- Rapidly growing skin tumor
- Resembles squamous cell carcinoma
- Occurs on sun-exposed, hair-bearing skin, beginning as a small red papule and enlarging rapidly over 1 to 2 months to become a firm, rounded tumor as large as 2.0 cm in diameter
- Central keratin plug
- Thought to arise from the epithelium of hair follicles
- Natural history is spontaneous regression
- Excise for accurate diagnosis

6. Distal Digital Keratoacanthoma

- Rare, destructive variant of keratoacanthoma involves the distal subungual tissue or the proximal nail fold
- Painful tumor that usually arises in the nail bed, causing separation of the nail plate from the bed

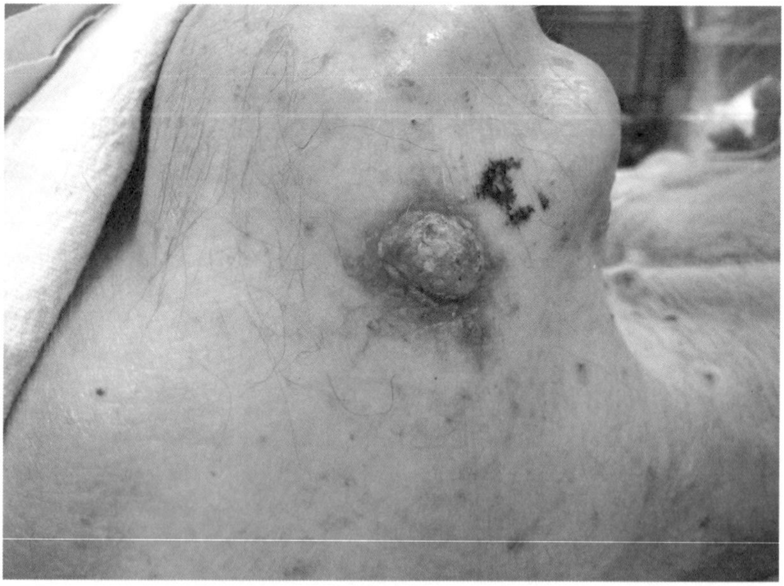

Fig. 3. Keratocanthoma.

- In the subungual location, this rapid growth can result in early bone destruction
- Treatment
  - Incisional biopsy to rule out SCC, then excision and curettage
  - In cases in which the diagnosis is unclear, bony destruction is extensive, or the lesion is recurrent, amputation or partial amputation of the digit is warranted

7. Dermatofibroma (Histiocytoma)

- Fibrous tissue tumors that involve the dermis
- Composed of fibroblasts, collagen, and histiocytes
- Solitary, firm, dome-shaped masses that exhibit varying degrees of coloring
- Excisional biopsy

8. Lentigines

- Benign pigmented macules result from increased activity of epidermal melanocytes
- Two major types: simple lentigo and solar lentigo
- May closely resemble melanoma, especially lentigo maligna, and a biopsy may be indicated to establish the nature of the lesion

9. Seborrheic Keratosis

- Benign neoplasms of keratinocytes
- Common in middle-aged and older adults
- If malignancy is not suspected remove with curettage, laser treatment, and cryotherapy

10. Melanocytic Nevi (Mole)

    a. Common acquired nevi

    - Appear after 6 months of life
    - Increase in size and number during childhood and adolescence
    - Acral nevi are located on the palmar and plantar surfaces
    - Biopsy is probably indicated in mottled or large (>7 mm) lesions

b. Longitudinal melanonychia

- Tan, brown, or black streaking of the nail caused by increased melanin deposition in the nail plate

c. Congenital nevi

- Classified by size into three categories: small (<1.5 cm), medium (1.5 cm to <20 cm), and large or giant (>20 cm)
  Malignant potential of large congenital nevi estimated the incidence of melanoma to range from 0% to 9%
  Treatment — excision

d. Blue nevi (Fig. 4)

- Dermal melanocytes that actively produce melanin
- Dermal melanin preferentially scatters the shorter wavelengths of light, giving these nevi a blue color
- Often arises in adolescence or early adult-hood

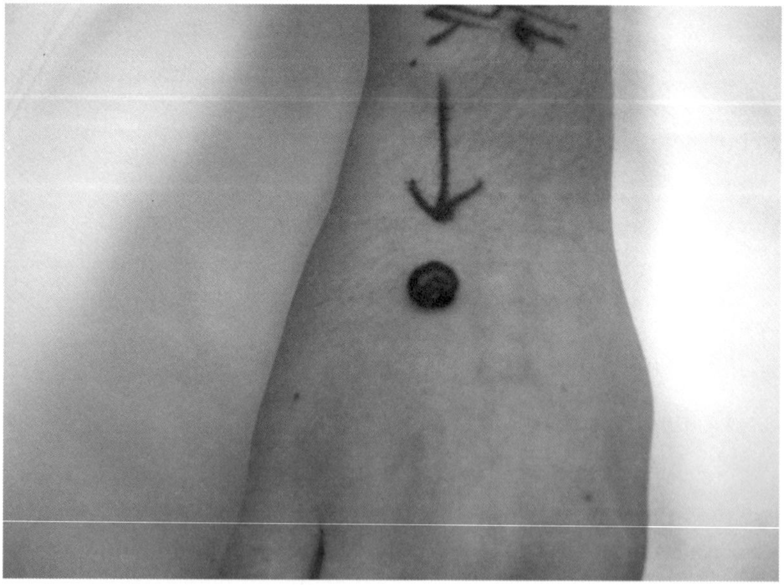

Fig. 4. Blue nevus.

  - Usually presents as a solitary lesion, 1 to 10 mm in diameter, and is often found on the dorsal surface of the hands or feet
  - Presence of multiple blue nevi is associated with — the Carney complex (multiple blue nevi, cardiac myxomas, and endocrine overactivity)
  - Treatment — observation

11. Acquired Digital Fibrokeratoma (Acral Fibrokeratoma)

- Benign tumors of fibrous tissue usually occur on the acral surfaces
- A flesh-colored, hornlike projection with a raised collar of skin at the base
- Variant of acquired digital fibrokeratoma — Koenen tumor
- Treatment — excision

B. Premalignant Tumors

1. Keratoses

- Cutaneous damage secondary to sun exposure

2. Actinic Keratosis

- Hyperkeratotic lesion with densely adherent scales attached to a pink base
- Abnormal proliferations of epidermal keratinocytes
- Related to long term sun damage
- Common in fair-skinned persons with a history of significant sun exposure
- Estimates of the conversion rate to invasive cancer range from 0.1% to 10%
- Treatment
  - Solitary lesions — cryotherapy or electrodesiccation with curettage
  - Multiple lesions — topical 5-fluorouracil, dermabrasion, and cutaneous peels (i.e., trichloroacetic acid peel), photodynamic therapy

3. Bowen's Disease (intraepidermal SCC or SCC in situ)

- Confined to epidermis, but may extend deeply into hair follicles and sebaceous glands
- Keratinocyte is the neoplastic cell
- Erythematous slow growing plaques, present in any location of hand
- Treatment — no single optimal treatment
  - 5-FU, cryotherapy, radiotherapy, photodynamic therapy
  - Simple excision — five year recurrence rate of 5% to 19%

4. Atypical Nevus (Atypical Mole)

- Characteristics of ABCD mneumonic
- Excise with a 1 to 2 mm margin, full thickness

C. Malignant Tumors

1. Melanoma

a. Melanoma in-situ — early form of melanoma confined to epithelial layer

- Lentigo maligna (Hutchinson's freckle)
- Associated with long term sun exposure
- Most commonly on extensor forearm
- Tan, flat macule, has prolonged radial growth phase that may last 1 or 2 decades
- Treatment — excise with 5 mm margins

b. Superficial spreading

- Most common type, 70% of all melanomas
- Arises within a melanocytic nevus
- Begins as a pigmented plaque and has a radial growth phase (months to years) before vertical growth begins
- Metastatic spread correlated with vertical invasion

c. Nodular melanoma (Fig. 5)

- 15% of all melanomas
- Little or no radial growth phase, increased metastatic potential
- Fast growing, arises de novo

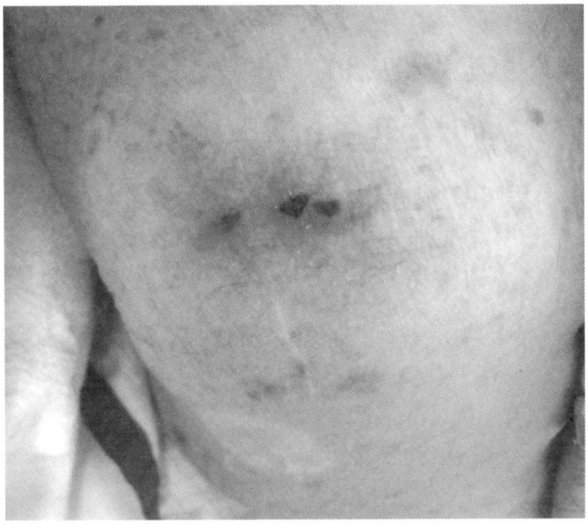

Fig. 5. Nodular melanoma.

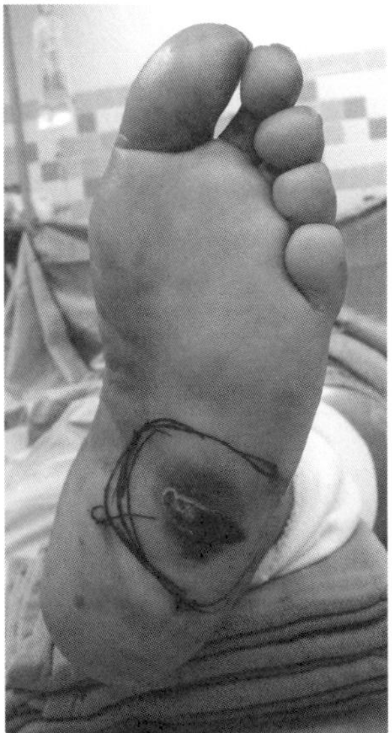

Fig. 6. Acral lentiginous melanoma.

d. Acral lentiginous melanoma (Fig. 6)

- 2% to 8% of all melanomas, found on palmar and plantar surfaces, nail, mucous membranes

- Not associated with sun exposure
- Slow growing, with long radial growth phase before vertical growth

e. Subungual melanoma

- Arises in nail matrix, usually affects thumb or great toe
- Pigmented nail lesions present over 2 months should be biopsied
- Amputation at one joint proximal to the joint closest to the subungual melanoma

Treatment

- Excision based on Breslow's classification of tumor thickness
- Sentinel lymph node biopsy and elective lymph node dissection for intermediate thickness (0.76 to 4 mm) melanoma

Tumor thickness	Margins	5 year survival
In-situ	2 to 5 mm	95% to 100%
<1 mm	1 cm	95% to 100%
1 to 2 mm	2 cm	80% to 96%
2 to 4 mm	2 to 3 cm	60% to 75%
>4 mm	3 cm	50%

2. Squamous Cell Carcinoma (SCC) (Fig. 7)

- Most frequent malignant tumor of hand
- UV radiation is most common risk factor
- Ranges from slow growing lesion to large ulcerated tumors, locally invasive but may metastasize
- Dorsum of hand and forearm are commonly involved areas in the upper extremity
- Treatment — excision, depth to include subcutaneous fat

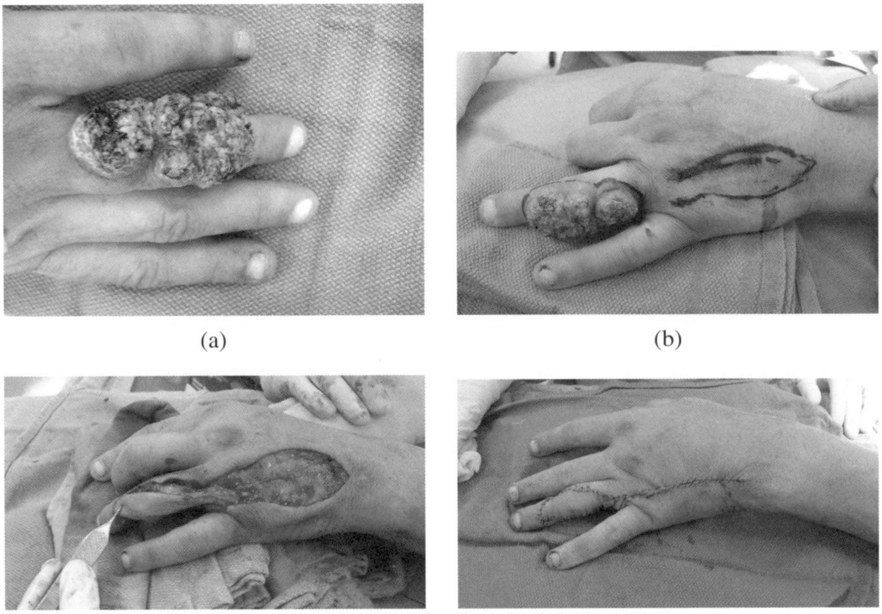

(a) (b) (c) (d)

Fig. 7. Verrucous carcinoma, an uncommon variant of SCC. Resected and reconstructed with reverse fourth dorsal metacarpal artery flap.

- 2% to 5% of SCCs metastasize to axillary nodes

Tumor size	Margin of excision
<2 cm in diameter	4 mm margin
>2 cm in diameter	6 mm margin

3. Basal Cell Carcinoma (BCC) (Fig. 8)

- Most common form of skin cancer, related to sun exposure
- Slow growing tumors, present as areas of skin atrophy, pink to reddish discoloration, telangiectatic changes, ulceration, "pearly" borders
- Invade locally, rarely metastasize, mid subcutaneous level

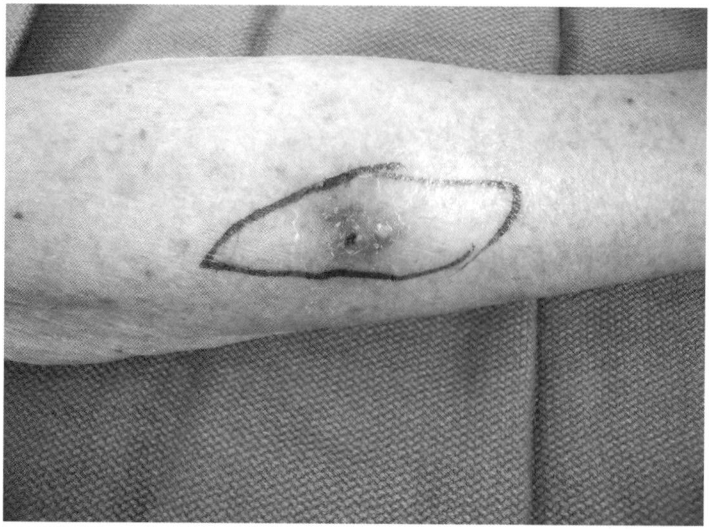

Fig. 8. BCC.

- Treatment — excision
  - <2 cm — 4 mm margin
  - >2 cm — Moh's

4. Lymphangiosarcoma (Stewart-Treves Syndrome)

- Occurs in the setting of chronic lymphedema
- Treatment — amputation of involved extremity

5. Merkel Cell Carcinoma

- Located in basal layer of epidermis, pressure — receptor,
- Treatment — wide surgical excision with lymphadenectomy
- Adjuvant chemoradiation
- High incidence of distant metastasis and recurrence

D. Sweat Gland Tumors

1. Eccrine Poroma (Fig. 9)

- Benign tumor, presents as an asymptomatic, solitary, soft, raised tumor, usually in the palm
- Treatment — excision

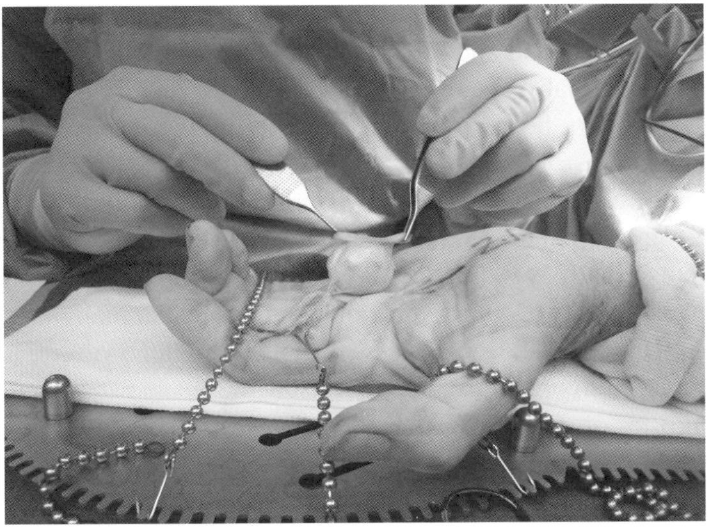

Fig. 9. Eccrine poroma.

2. Chondroid Syringoma

   - Benign, can grow very large

3. Eccrine Spiradenoma

   - Single mass or multiple nodules

4. Malignant Sweat Gland Tumors

   - Clear cell carcinoma
   - Digital papillary adenocarcinoma
   - Eccrine adenocarcinoma
   - Treatment — excision with regional node dissection

2. SOFT TISSUE TUMORS

A. Benign[2–5]

1. Ganglion Cysts

- Most common
- These mucin-filled cysts are usually attached to the adjacent underlying joint capsule, tendon, or tendon sheath

- Ganglions are most prevalent in women and generally occur (70%) between the second and fourth decades of life
- Ganglions usually occur singly and in very specific locations; however, they have been reported to arise from almost every joint of the hand and wrist
- Ganglion cysts have also been reported to cause clinically symptomatic pressure on the median and ulnar nerves of the hand
- Patients usually seek medical attention due to cosmetic appearance of the mass, pain, weakness, and concern of potential malignancy
- Malignant degeneration has never been reported; however, malignant soft tissue tumors are frequently misdiagnosed as ganglion cysts
- Ganglions may appear quite suddenly or develop over several months
- They may subside with rest, enlarge with activity, and rupture or disappear spontaneously
- Over 50% may recur if incompletely excised
- Communication between the wrist joint and cyst has been demonstrated with arthrograms but not with cystograms. A one-way valvular mechanism has therefore been postulated to connect the wrist joint to the cyst
- The main cyst may be single or multiloculated and appears smooth, white, and translucent
- The wall is made up of compressed collagen fibers and is sparsely lined with flattened cells without evidence of an epithelial or synovial lining
- The contents of the cyst are characterized by a highly viscous, clear, sticky, jelly-like mucin made up of glucosamine, albumin, globulin, and high concentrations of hyaluronic acid
- The etiology and pathogenesis of ganglions remain obscure
- Treatment
    - Non-operative
    - Observation has been advocated in the pediatric population owing to the high likelihood of spontaneous resolution
    - digital pressure, injections of hyaluronidase or sclerosing solutions, subcutaneous tenotome dissection, and cross-fixation with a heavy suture

- Aspiration of the ganglion, puncture of the cyst wall, and instillation of lidocaine, (Xylocaine) and betamethasone (Celestone) into the capsule or tendon sheath attachments reduces the mass and may alleviate symptoms for varying periods of time
- Aspiration may provide long-term relief and has been reported to be effective in 20% to 30% of patients with wrist ganglia
- Injection and aspiration of volar wrist ganglions must be approached with caution due to the proximity of the radial artery

- Operative
  - Excision
  - Open
  - Arthroscopic
  - No comparative outcome studies available
  - Technique

a. Dorsal wrist ganglion

- Transverse incision over scapholunate ligament
- Main cyst pedicle mobilized to underlying joint capsule
- Scapholunate attachements are excised

b. Volar wrist ganglion

- Longitudinal incision
- Cyst pedicle mobilized, capsular attachments excised
- Often intimately associated with the radial artery

2. Mucous Cyst

- Ganglion of the DIP joint
- Earliest sign — longitudinal grooving of nail without mass, caused by pressure on the nail matrix
- Associated with osteoarthritic changes in the joint, osteophytes need to be excised

3. Epidermal Inclusion Cysts

- Epidermal inclusion cysts are thought to result from traumatic implantation of epithelial cells into the underlying soft tissue or bone
- The cells grow over an interval of months to years to produce a painless swelling, most commonly in the fingertip
- Occur most commonly in the distal phalanx of the left long finger and thumb in men in the third and fourth decades of life
- Differential diagnosis may be more difficult when the cyst involves bone, in which case radiographs generally show a well-demarcated lytic lesion
- Occasionally, cortical penetration can be seen, and the lesion may mimic a malignant or infectious process
- Epidermal inclusion cysts are readily treated with marginal excision or with curettage and bone grafting for those lesions involving bone
- Recurrence is uncommon, and malignant transformation has not been reported

4. Lipomas (Fig. 10)

- Benign fat tumors that occur typically in several locations in the hand, most commonly subcutaneously or intramuscularly

5. Foreign Body Lesion

    - Traumatic, reactive masses in response to implanted foreign material
    - Treatment — excisional biopsy

6. Lipofibromatous Hamartomas

- Unusual tumors of the peripheral nerves most commonly involving the median nerve when seen in the upper extremity

7. Giant Cell Tumors (Figs. 11 and 12)

- Benign soft tissue tumor that is the second most common tumor seen in the hand (after ganglions)
- Localized nodular synovitis, fibrous xanthoma, and pigmented villonodular tenosynovitis

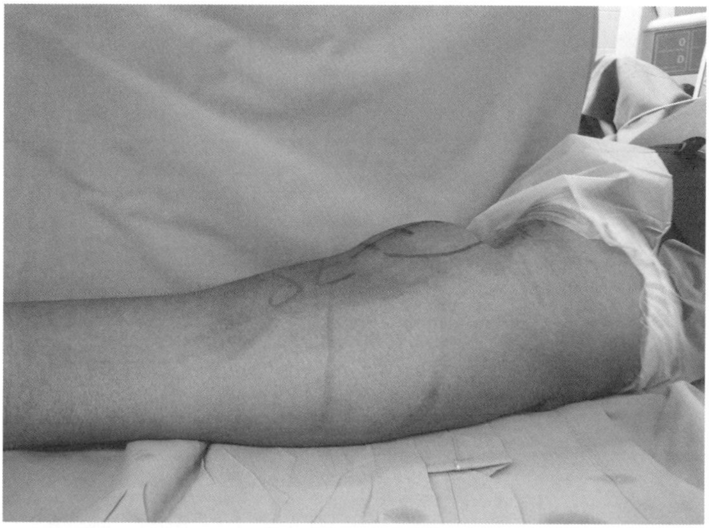

(a)

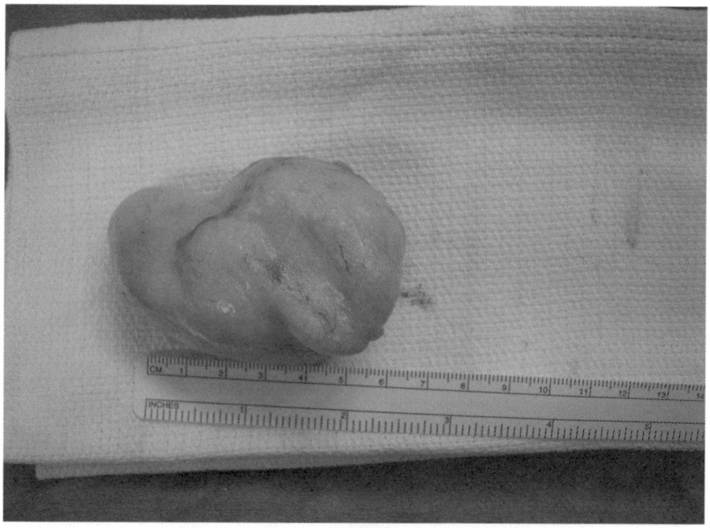

(b)

Fig. 10. Lipoma.

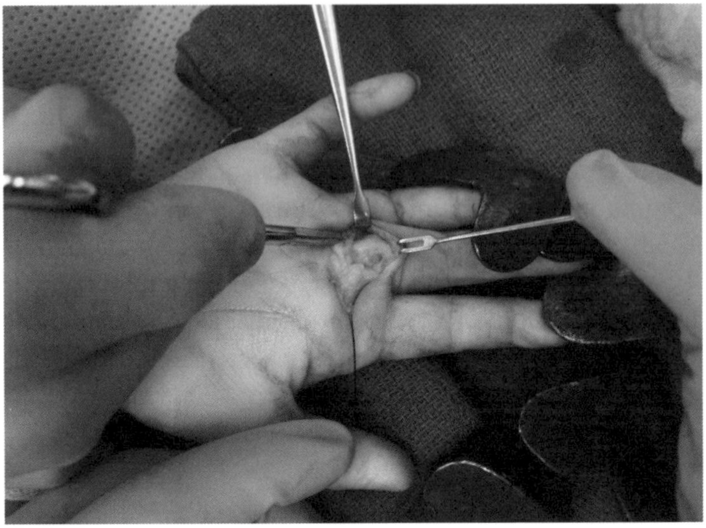

(a)

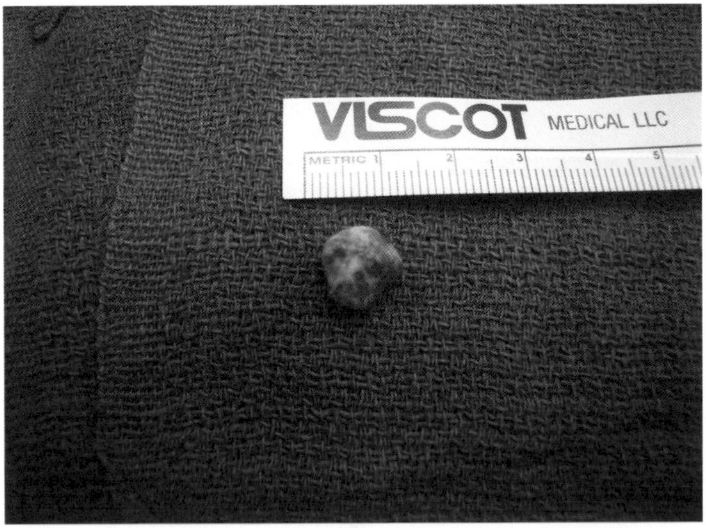

(b)

Fig. 11 Tendon sheath giant cell tumor.

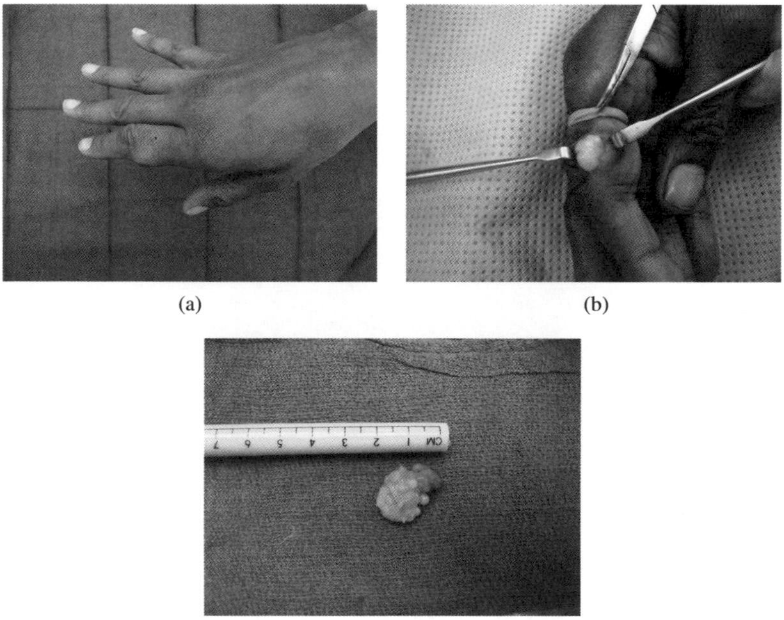

(a) (b)

(c)

Fig. 12. Volar plate giant cell tumor.

- The tumor usually occurs on the volar surface of the fingers or hand, although dorsal involvement is not uncommon. There is a propensity for involvement of the radial three digits and the DIP joint region
- Clinically, the tumor is most often firm, nodular, and non-tender
- Marginal excision is the recommended treatment, although the reported risk of recurrence is from 5% to 50%
- Malignant transformation of GCT of tendon sheath in the hand has not been reported

8. Schwannomas (Fig. 13)

- The most common benign nerve tumor occurring in the upper extremity
- This lesion arises from the Schwann cell and produces a slowly growing, well-circumscribed, eccentric lesion in the peripheral nerve
- Patients most frequently notice a painless mass, but less commonly there may be a neurologic deficit. Palpation or compression of the lesion may produce radiating pain in a specific nerve distribution

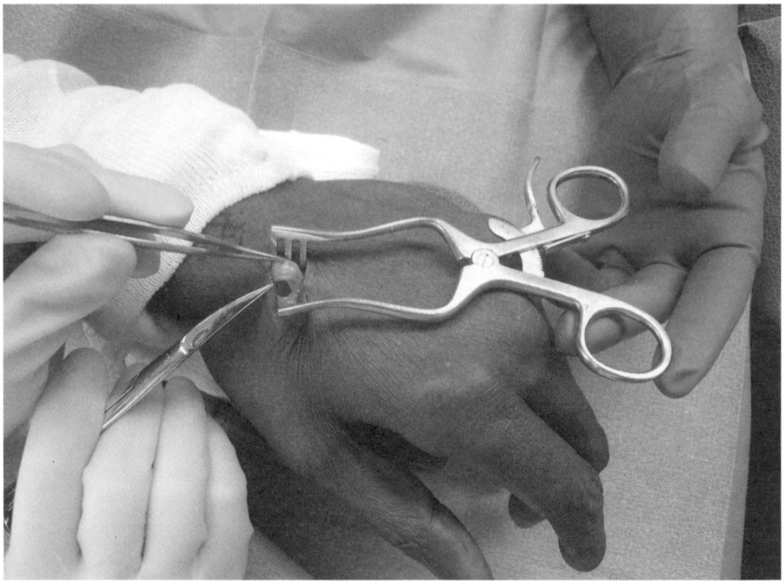

Fig. 13. Dorsal radial sensory nerve Schwannoma.

9. Neurofibromas

- Benign, arise from nerve fasciculi

10. Fibromatosis

a. Digital fibroma of infancy

- Aggressive fibrous lesion exclusively in the fingers and toes, 80% arising before age one
- Usually involved IP joint of fingers
- Treatment — observation, marginal excision, wide excision, amputation

b. Nodular fasciitis (Fig. 14)

- Rare tumor, volar surface of forearm
- Rapidly growing nodule, mimics sarcoma

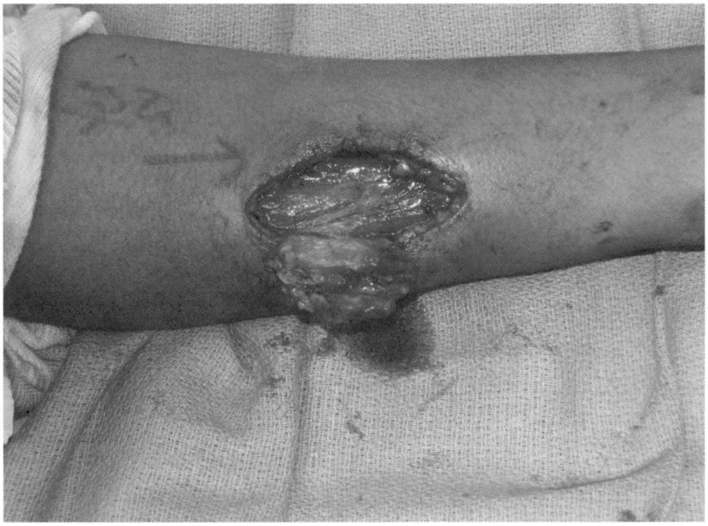

(a)

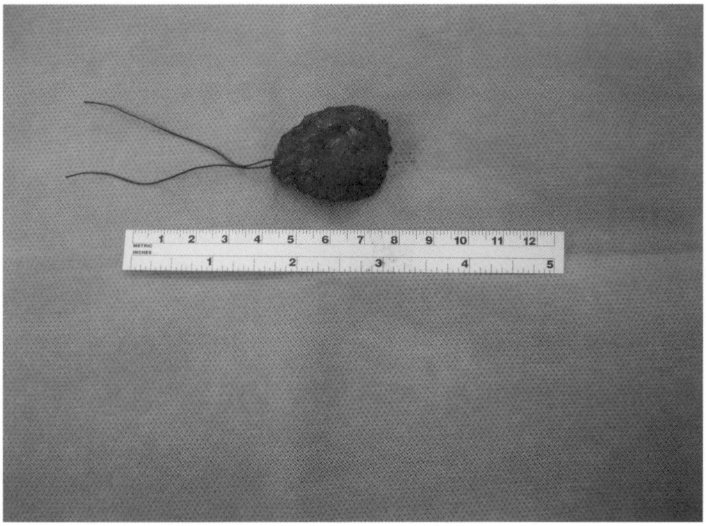

(b)

Fig. 14. Nodular fascitis.

B. Malignant[6–8]

Classification and staging of tumors

- Histologic Grade and Surgical Staging
- The histologic grade (G) of a neoplasm is determined by the malignant characteristics of tissue obtained with a biopsy
- G0: Benign
- G1: Low grade — few cells, much stroma, little necrosis, mature cells, fewer than five mitoses per high-power field
    - Low likelihood of metastasis and frequent local recurrence
- G2: High grade — many cells, little stroma, much necrosis, immature cells, more than 10 mitoses per high-power field
    - Frequent metastasis

AJCC STAGING SYSTEM FOR SOFT TISSUE SARCOMAS

Stage I	
IA	Low grade, small (<5 cm), superficial or deep to fascia
IB	Low grade, large (>5 cm), superficial to fascia
Stage II	
IIA	Low grade, large, deep to fascia
IIB	High grade, small, superficial or deep to fascia
IIC	High grade, large, superficial to fascia
Stage III	High grade, large (>5 cm), deep to fascia
Stage IV	Any metastasis to lymph nodes or distant sites

Evaluation

Clinical history and physical examination

↓

Laboratory work up

ESR, BMP, CBC, Ca, Phos, Alk phos, LDH

↓

Imaging examination

Radiographs
Ultrasound — distinguish cystic versus solid masses
CT scan — evaluate extent of bone involvement
MRI — soft tissue extension, relation to neurovascular structures
Bone scan — detection of metastasis

↓

Tissue biopsy
FNA
Core
Incisional
Excisional

1. Sarcoma (Fig. 15)

a. Epithelioid

- Most common soft tissue sarcoma occurring in the forearm and hand
- Commonly presents as a painless nodule on the volar surface of palm or digits, may ulcerate
- Characterized by tendency to spread proximally
- Treatment — wide excision, regional lymphadenectomy, adjuvant radiation, adjuvant chemotherapy with lymph node involvement

b. Synovial

- High grade sarcoma, arises in proximity to joints, tendons and bursae
- Presents as painless mass in the hand present for many years
- Lymphatic metastases in 25% of cases

c. Liposarcoma

- Rare in hand
- Clinically may resemble a lipoma
- Treatment — wide excision and adjuvant radiation

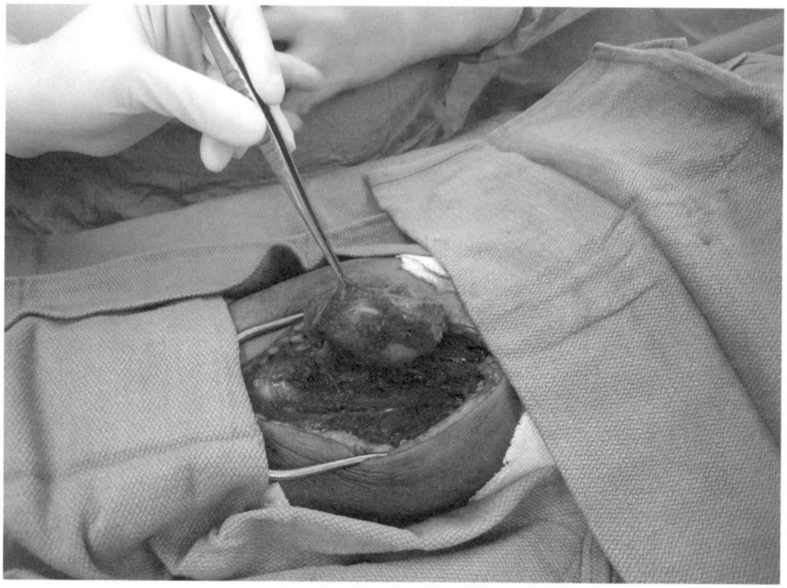

(a)

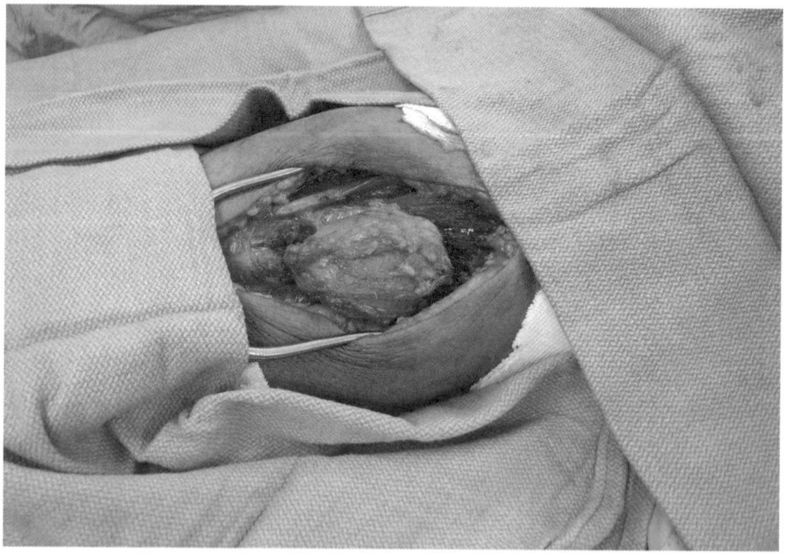

(b)

Fig. 15 High grade sarcoma arising from flexor digitorum superficialis.

d. Fibrosarcoma

- 30% occur in the upper extremity, rare in the hand

e. Dermatofibrosarcoma protuberans

- Low grade, rare in hand, arises in the dermis
- High local recurrence rate, low rate of metastasis
- Treatment — excision with 3 cm margins
- Malignant fibrous histiocytoma
    - 19% of lesions arise in the upper extremity
    - Treatment — wide excision with adjuvant radiation therapy

f. Malignant peripheral nerve sheath tumor (neurofibrosarcoma/malignant schwannoma)

- 30% occur in upper extremity, 50% are associated with neurofibromatosis
- Treatment — wide local excision or amputation
- 5 year survival of 40%

g. Rhabdomyosarcoma

- Rare in hand
- Treatment — wide local excision with adjuvant radiation therapy

h. Leiomyosarcoma

- Arises in the smooth muscle, seen in the veins in the hand

i. Clear cell sarcoma

- Rare tumor, occurs in close association with tendons
- High risk of local recurrence and regional metastasis

3. BONE TUMORS

A. Benign[6,9]

1. Enchondroma

- Benign cartilaginous lesions that are the most common primary bone tumors arising from the bones in the hand
- Approximately 35% of all enchondromas arise in the hand, and enchondromas account for as many as 90% of bone tumors seen in the hand
- The proximal phalanx is the most common site of involvement, followed by the metacarpal and middle phalanx.
- Small asymptomatic lesions with a typical radiographic appearance may simply be observed
- Large or symptomatic enchondromas, or those lesions that do not demonstrate a characteristic radiographic appearance, should be treated with biopsy and curettage
- Iliac crest bone graft has been most commonly used to fill the defect left after curettage, although fresh-frozen or freeze-dried irradiated allograft has been used with similar excellent results reported
- The risk of local recurrence after curettage is 4.5%

2. Multiple Enchondromatosis (Ollier's Disease)

- Uncommon, non-hereditary skeletal disorder characterized by the presence of multiple enchondromas or cartilaginous masses in the metaphysis and diaphysis of long bones or short tubular bones of the hands and feet
- Unilateral or predominant on one side
- May be large and produce significant cosmetic and functional deformity in the hand, as well as brachydactyly
- The risk of malignant transformation to chondrosarcoma or osteosarcoma in patients with Ollier's disease is approximately 30%
- Patients with Ollier's disease require periodic surveillance with physical and radiographic examination

3. Maffucci's Syndrome

- Extremely rare disease that affects the hands in the majority of cases
- Radiographic findings in bone are identical to those seen in Ollier's disease
- Have multiple hemangiomas
- High risk for developing both bone and soft tissue sarcomas

4. Periosteal Chondroma

- Uncommon benign cartilaginous lesion that may occur in the phalanges and be confused radiographically with enchondroma and histologically with chondrosarcoma
- Radiographs typically reveal a subperiosteal lytic lesion with erosion of the underlying cortex, buttressing at the proximal and distal extent, and occasionally an overlying rim of sclerosis
- Important to attempt to make the diagnosis of periosteal chondroma preoperatively based on plain radiographs to treat the lesion appropriately and to avoid unnecessary amputation
- Marginal excision is usually curative, with local recurrence rates of less than 4%

5. Osteochondroma

- Rare in the hand, except in patients with multiple hereditary exostoses
- Osseous growths with a hyaline cartilage cap thought to originate from the physis or regions of tendon insertion
- In the hand are most commonly seen at the distal aspect of the proximal phalanx
- The prominence caused by an osteochondroma may result in cosmetic deformity and impaired function by producing a mechanical block to motion
- Osteochondromas with a characteristic radiographic appearance that are asymptomatic and do not impair function may be observed
- Lesions that produce progressive deformity, pain, or impairment of function should be excised
- malignant transformation of an osteochondroma in the hand has not been reported

6. Chondromyxoid Fibroma

- Rare, benign cartilaginous lesion
- Long history of mild pain or swelling
- Plain radiographs most often reveal a lytic lesion in the metaphyseal region of the bone
- Curettage and bone grafting have been successful in controlling hand lesions with recurrence rates of 7% to 25%

7. Osteoid Osteoma

- 5% to 15% of osteoid osteomas occur in the hand and wrist, most commonly in the proximal phalanx and carpus
- Radiographs most commonly demonstrate a lytic lesion rather than the classic appearance of reactive sclerosis surrounding a central lucent nidus
- Physical examination usually demonstrates well-delineated tenderness and swelling
- Treatment — excision with either curettage of the nidus or en bloc excision
- Prolonged use of NSAIDs may be an alternative to surgical treatment

8. Osteoblastoma

- Rare benign tumor that is usually larger than 2 cm in diameter and is characterized by osteoid and woven bone production

9. Unicameral Bone Cyst

- Benign, cystic lesions of uncertain etiology that are extremely rare in the bones of the hand and forearm
- Usually asymptomatic until there has been a pathologic fracture
- Treatment of unicameral bone cysts has included observation, curettage and bone grafting, drilling, corticosteroid injection, and en bloc excision

10. Aneurysmal Bone Cyst

- Only 3% to 5% of all aneurysmal bone cysts occur in the hand
- Metacarpal involvement is more common
- Curettage and bone grafting
- Recurrence high

11. Giant Cell Tumor of Bone

- 5% of benign bone tumors, only 2% of giant cell tumors occur in the hand
- Local recurrence rates of greater than 80% may be seen after intralesional treatment with curettage
- Benign lesions, based on their histology, but they may behave in a locally aggressive fashion, metastasize, and ultimately result in death
- Cases of pulmonary metastases from benign giant cell tumors of bone arising in the hand

- Treatment — preoperative staging with CT of chest or total body scan, amputation for majority of non-distal distal radius lesions, wide excision for distal radius lesions with perforation of more than one cortex

B. Malignant[6,10]

A classification scheme based on a modified staging system for bone sarcoma surgical stages

1. Chondrosarcoma

- Most common primary malignant bone tumor that occurs in the hand
- May arise primarily or may develop in a preexistent benign lesion such as an enchondroma or osteochondroma

Stage	Grade	Site
IA	Low (G1)	Intracompartmental (T1)
IB	Low (G1)	Extracompartmental (T2)
IIA	High (G2)	Intracompartmental (T1)
IIB	High (G2)	Extracompartmental (T2)
III	Any (G)	Any T
	Regional or distant metastasis (M)	Regional or distant metastasis (M)

- The proximal phalanges and metacarpals are most commonly affected
- Presents as a slowly growing, firm, and often painful mass
- Extreme cortical expansion, perforation, or extension into the surrounding soft tissues helps to differentiate this lesion from enchondroma
- Majority of chondrosarcomas are slow-growing lesions that do not metastasize
- A well-planned incisional biopsy should be done for suspicious lesions
- Patients suspected of having chondrosarcoma must have their disease locally and systemically staged
- Treated surgically with wide en bloc excision or digit or ray amputation
- No role for chemoradiation therapy

2. Osteogenic Sarcoma

- Rare in the hand
- Treatment — wide en bloc excision or finger or ray amputation, adjuvant or neoadjuvant chemotherapy
- No role for radiation therapy

3. Ewing's Sarcoma

- Rare in the hand
- Commonly in the first or second decade of life
- Presents with pain, swelling and erythema
- Arises in the metacarpals or phalanges with extensive soft tissue involvement
- Radiographs with large, lytic lesion with soft tissue involvement
- Treatment — ablative surgery with adjuvant or neoadjuvant chemoradiation therapy

4. Metastatic Tumors

- Rare
- Fewer than 0.3% of patients with cancer develop acrometastases
- In 50% of patients with acrometastasis, the lesion can mimic a benign condition or can be the first presentation of malignancy or metastatic disease
- Distal phalanx is the most common site of metastasis to the hand
- Most common metastatic lesion — bronchogenic carcinoma of the lung Other reported primary malignancies include renal, esophageal, breast, colon, prostate, thyroid, and bone cancer
- Clinical findings include the typical signs of inflammation-pain, swelling, and erythema-which may lead to an initial clinical diagnosis of infection
- Radiographs usually reveal a lytic destructive lesion,
- Amputation and ray resection are effective in providing palliation and local control of disease

4. VASCULAR TUMORS[11]

A. Congenital AV Malformations (Fig. 16)

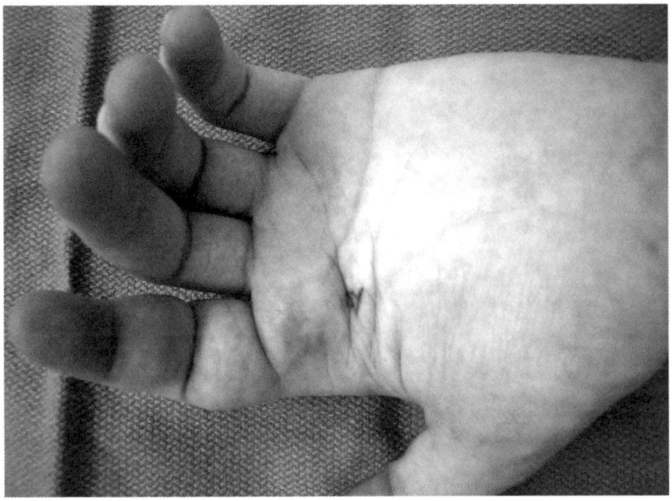

(a)

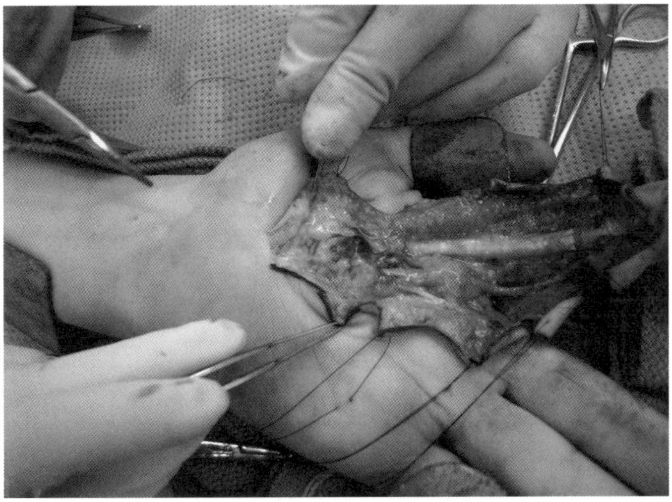

(b)

Fig. 16. Venous malformation.

- Involve the upper extremity in 30 to 60% of patients
- Common initial symptoms: (1) pain 40%, (2) swelling 50%, (3) noticable mass 30%
- Lesions are arterial, venous, capillary or a combinationin 50% of extremitites, soft tissue masses in 65%
- Diagnostic tests — plain radiographs with pahtognomonic phleboliths, MRA, CT
- Treatment — dependent on symptoms, location, and predominant vessels involved
    - Non-operative
- Selective embolization
    - Operative — last resort
- Excision of malformation including ligation of the feeding artery and draining vein
- En-bloc resection with arterial reconstruction

B. Hemangiomas

- Tumors with characteristic growth cycle
    - 1st phase — rapid, endothelial cell proliferation, lasts 10 to 12 months
    - 2nd phase — growth rate proportional to child's growth, color fades from bright red to dull red
    - 3rd phase — involutional. By age 5, 50% of the lesions have regressed, by age 7, 70% of the lesions have involuted
    - Diagnosis — radiographs with calcifications, US, CT, MRI
    - Treatment — conservative and directed toward associated complications of bleeding, ulceration, and infection
- Kasabach-Merritt syndrome — diffuse coagulopathy secondary to platelet trapping within the hemangioma

C. Glomus Tumor

- Benign vascular hematomas containing all of the cells of normal glomus apparatus, 75% in the hand, 65% at fingertips

- Normal glomus lies in the reticular layer as an arteriovenous anastomosis in the dermis and functions as a thermoregulatory control mechanism.
- Characterized by painful subcutaneous nodules usually located in the subungual region of the digits. Triad of symptoms (1) cold hypersensitivity, (2) paroxysmal pain, (3) pinpoint pain
- MRI — T1 appear as dark, well delineated lesion, T2 bright lesion
- Classified into 3 groups: (1) solitary, (2) multiple painful lesions, (3) multiple painless lesions
- Treatment — excision for symptomatic lesions

References

1. Haase H, Chung K. (2011) Skin tumors. In: Wolfe SW, Hotchkiss RN, Pederson WC, Kozin (eds.), *Green's Operative Hand Surgery*, 6th Edn. Elsevier, Philadelphia.
2. Payne TW, Merrell G. (2010) Benign bony and soft tissue tumors of the hand. *Hand Surg* **35**(11): 1901–1910.
3. Williams J, Hodari A, Janevski P, Siddiqu A. (2010) Recurrence of giant cell tumors in the hand: a prospective study. *Hand Surg* **35**(3): 451–456.
4. Rankin G, Kuschner SH, Gellman H. (1991) Nodular fasciitis: a rapidly growing tumor of the hand. *Hand Surg* **16**(5): 791–795.
5. Rockwell GM, Thoma A, Salam S. (2003) Schwannoma of the hand and wrist. *Plast Reconstr Surg* **111**(3): 1227–1232.
6. Athanesian E. (2011) Bone and soft tissue tumors. In: Wolfe SW, Hotchkiss RN, Pederson WC, Kozin SH (eds.), *Green's Operative Hand Surgery*, 6th Edn. Elsevier, Philadelphia, pp. 2141–2195.
7. Popov P, Tukiainen E, Asko-Seljavaara S, Huuhtanen R, Virolainen M, *et al.* (2002) Soft-tissue sarcomas of the upper extremity: surgical treatment and outcome. *Plast Reconstr Surg* **13**(1): 222–230.
8. Labow BI, Rosen H, Greene AK, Lee WPA, Upton J. (2008) Soft tissue sarcomas of the hand: functional reconstuction and outcome analysis. *Hand* **3**(3): 229–236.
9. Foucher G, Viet D, Lanieri L. (1997) Osteoid osteoma in the hand and wrist. *Eur J Orthop Surg Traumatol* **7**(3): 165–168.
10. Puhaindran ME, Athanasian EA. (2010) Mailgnant and metastatic tumors of the hand. *Hand Surg* **35**(11): 1895–1900.
11. Koman AL, Smith BP, Smith TL, Ruch DS, Li Z. Vascular tumors In: Wolfe SW, Hotchkiss RN, Pederson WC, Kozin SH (eds.), *Green's Operative Hand Surgery,* 6th Edn. Elsevier, Philadelphia.

CHAPTER 17

RHEUMATOID ARTHRITIS OF THE HAND

Haaris S. Mir and Stacy R. Henderson

History

- The cause of rheumatoid arthritis (RA) remains poorly understood to date. Three competing theories of RA origin exist
  1. RA is a disease of the modern era and its pathogenesis is the result of an environmental or a genetic stimulus that did not exist in ancient times
  2. RA existed among our ancient ancestors but had never been definitively characterized
  3. Hybrid theory, which suggests RA developed from indigenous populations in North America and spread to the populations in Europe through the travel of persons and/or goods[1]
- The first modern description of rheumatoid arthritis was by Augustin Jacob Landré-Beauvais in 1800. He first described symptoms and signs that resemble rheumatoid arthritis today[2]
- Paleopathologic studies done in the last century have uncovered bone samples from around the world that demonstrate skeletal damage suggesting RA in the specimen. This suggests RA existed several hundred years prior to the initial description by Landré-Beauvais[3]

Pathogenesis

I. Genetic predisposition
   - The HLA-DR4 allele has been found to be associated with RA[4–7]
   - The PTPN2 gene has also been associated with RA. The gene encodes a protein tyrosine phosphatase involved in activation and control of inflammatory cells[8]

- RA is more common in women 30–50 years of age, with a 3:1 female to male ratio[2,9,10]

II. Environmental inciting event

- There are many arthritogens postulated to incite the inflammatory response, but none have yet been proven
- These include the Epstein-Barr virus, retroviruses, parvoviruses, mycobacteria, *Borrelia*, *Proteus mirabilis*, and *Mycoplasma*[5–7,11,12]
- Citrullinated proteins, proteins modified by the enzymatic conversion of arginine to citrulline, have been strongly linked to RA. These proteins are commonly found in smokers and may explain the higher incidence of RA in that population[8,13]

III. Autoimmune inflammatory response

- Once an inciting event has taken place in a genetically susceptible individual, an inflammatory synovitis is initiated by B and T cells
- Synovial cells release an antigen that triggers B cell production of rheumatoid factor (RF), an IgM antibody specific for the Fc portion of IgG
- RF and IgG combine to form immune complexes that activate the complement system and attract inflammatory cells to the joint space causing chronic synovitis
- Chronic synovitis leads to pannus, granulation tissue within synovial tissue, formation
- The pannus releases cytokines that cause articular cartilage destruction and joint fusion[14]

Diagnosis[15–17]

I. Clinical findings

A. Skin

1. Rheumatoid nodules

- Occur in 25% of the patient population

- — Subcutaneous inflammatory masses (at ulna near elbow)
  - Correlated with worse prognosis

B. Joints

1. "Z deformities"
   - — Loss of joint tissue support
   - — Ulnar deviation of metacarpophalangeal (MCP) joints caused by radial deviation of metacarpals
2. Arthritis mutilans
   - — Osteolysis with profound destruction of joint cartilage and bony surfaces

C. Tendons

1. Tenosynovitis: 50% overall incidence in rheumatoid arthritis
2. Wrist tendon ruptures
   - — Most common ruptures (in order from most frequent)
     (1) Extensor Digiti Minimi (EDM)
     (2) Extensor Digitorum Communis (EDC) # 5
     (3) EDC # 4
     (4) Extensor Pollicis Longus (EPL)
     (5) EDC # 3
3. Flexor tendon triggering: (trigger finger) sometimes leads to rupture
   - — Flexor pollicis longus (FPL)
     - Mannerfelt syndrome[18,19]
       - ○ Attrition flexor tendon ruptures in rheumatoid arthritis caused by bony spurs in the carpal tunnel
       - ○ FPL tendon is the most common flexor tendon to rupture from attrition by a bony spur in the carpal tunnel

4. Swan neck deformities (SND)

   — Lateral bands are constrained in their dorsal position, upsetting the flexor-extensor balance
   — In this position, the lateral bands increase the pull of the long extensor tendon's central slip, which attaches to the dorsal base of the middle phalanx
   — The increase of flexor profundus tension resulting from hyper-extension of the PIP joint leads to a reciprocal flexion of the DIP joint
   — Progressive disease causes joint destruction and fixed contracture

5. Boutonnière deformities (BND)

   — The boutonniere deformity occurs when the extensor tendon attachment to the middle phalanx is injured (central slip)
   — The central slip may simply be damaged from prolonged inflammation in the proximal interphalangeal (PIP) joint from rheumatoid arthritis, which stretches and eventually ruptures the central slip forcing the PIP joint to bend
   — With time, the lateral bands migrate volarly and eventually causes hyperextension of the distal interphalangeal (DIP) joint

D. Muscles

1. Intrinsic muscle atrophy from disuse
2. Inflammation
3. Cervical myopathy for nerve compression

   — Median and posterior interosseous nerves (PIN)

E. Nerves

1. Inflammatory tenosynovitis involving carpal, cubital and/or radial tunnels

   — Example: PIN compression and/or paralysis from radiohumeral joint synovitis

F. Vessels

1. Vasculitis
2. Raynauds phenomenon

G. Systemic/extraarticular involvement

1. Respiratory
   — Nodules
   — Pleuritis
2. Cardiac
   — Valvular
   — Pericarditis
   — Myocarditis
3. Hematologic
   — Anemia
   — Felty's syndrome
4. Ocular
   — Uveitis
   — Iritis
5. Neurologic
   — Polyneuropathy
6. Multisystem
   — Sjögren's syndrome

II. Laboratory tests

A. Positive rheumatoid factor (RF)

— IgM or IgG rheumatoid factors present in 70–80% of RA patients
— Seropositivity indicates less favorable prognosis

B. Positive anti-nuclear antibody (ANA) in 30%

C. Increased erythrocyte sedimentation rate (ESR) and C-reactive protein (CRP)
D. Decreased hemoglobin

III. Imaging studies

A. Radiographs

— Periarticular osteoporosis and soft tissue swelling
— Joint space narrowing
— Marginal erosions
— Symmetric bilateral involvement of joints
— Carpal ankylosis (bones appear fused)

- Translation deformities
- Ulnar translation of carpus

— Ulnar deviation at metacarpophalangeal joints

IV. Disease staging[20]

A. Lister's three stages of Rheumatoid Arthritis

1. *Proliferative*: Synovial swelling causes pain, limited motion, and potential nerve compression
2. *Destructive*: Synovial erosion results in tendon rupture, bone erosion, and capsular/ligament weakness
3. *Reparative*: Extensive fibrosis causes tendon adherence and joint contractures

Medical Management

Medical management is the primary modality in the treatment of rheumatoid arthritis. Improvements in medical management, including the use of anti-TNFα therapy and combination DMARD therapy, have reduced the need for surgical intervention in recent years. Prompt diagnosis of RA is essential in decreasing progression of disease. Goals in management of RA include prevention or control of joint damage, maintenance of joint function, and pain control. Complete remission is the ultimate goal of treatment, but is rarely achieved. Management of RA requires the involvement of an extensive interdisciplinary team that includes a rheumatologist, other physicians, physical and occupational therapists, social workers and patient educators.

Outline for Medical Management of RA:[21]

I. Baseline evaluation

— Radiography of selected involved joints to establish a baseline from which disease progression and therapeutic response can be monitored
— Laboratory studies

- Rheumatoid factor for diagnostic purposes
- Synovial fluid analysis to rule out other etiologies of joint inflammation
- Complete blood cell count, complete metabolic profile, urinalysis, and stool guaiac prior to beginning medications to assess baseline and possible comorbidities
- Baseline erythrocyte sedimentation rate or C-reactive protein level

— Physical examination

- Joint inflammation and mechanical joint problems
- Manifestations of systemic disease

— Subjective patient assessment of symptoms, including joint pain, morning stiffness, function and fatigue

II. Subsequent evaluation

— Evidence of active disease

- Subjective patient assessment of symptoms
- Physical exam for joint inflammation and mechanical joint problems

— Periodic tests

- Radiographs to assess disease progression
- Erythrocyte sedimentation rate or C-reactive protein level to assess elevation[21]

III. Pharmacologic management

A. Non-steroidal anti-inflammatory agents (NSAIDs)

- Act to reduce joint inflammation and improve function
- Do not alter disease course, thus used in conjunction with other drugs for RA
- Gastrointestinal complications are a major concern with chronic NSAID use. Thus, gastroprotective agents including proton-pump inhibitors and oral prostaglandin analogs are often used in conjunction with therapy[22–24]

B. Disease-modifying anti-rheumatic drugs (DMARDs)

- DMARDs alter the course of RA by preventing joint damage and protecting joints, as evidenced by the ability of most drugs to visibly slow radiographic erosions[25–29]
- Agents can be used alone or in a multitude of combinations that are beyond the scope of this chapter. The use of DMARDs in combination has improved results of medical management of RA
- Multiple factors influence choice of therapy, including efficacy, side effect profile, patient comorbidities, and likelihood of patient compliance

1. Methotrexate (MTX)

   - Often selected as first-line treatment due to its well-established efficacy as well as limited toxicity profile[25–27]
   - Most frequent adverse reaction is elevation of liver enzymes, necessitating routine liver function tests[30]
   - Other frequent side effects include stomatitis, nausea and diarrhea, but have been shown to be reduced with simultaneous folic acid or folinic acid supplementation[31,32]
   - Contraindicated in patients with liver disease renal impairment, lung disease, or alcoholism

2. Leflunomide

   — An alternative monotherapy in patients who cannot tolerate or have an inadequate response to MTX. It can also be used with MTX in patients who do not show a complete clinical response with MTX monotherapy
   — Elevation of liver enzymes occurs in 5% of patients on monoterapy and 60% of patients on combination MTX therapy[28,29]
   — Contraindicated in patients with obstructive biliary disease, liver disease, viral hepatitis, severe immunodeficiency, and on rifampin therapy

3. Hydroxychloroquine (HCQ) and sulfasalazine (SSZ)

   — Alternative choice for first-line therapy in patients with milder disease due to reduced toxicity and side effects[33–36]
   — HCQ and SSZ are relatively well tolerated, causing rash, abdominal discomfort, nausea, and diarrhea
   — SSZ therapy can occasionally cause leucopenia and requires routine blood tests[36]

4. Anti-tumor necrosis factor α therapy (infliximab, etanercept)

   — Relatively new and promising agents in the treatment of RA that are effective in newly diagnosed RA as well as MTX-refractory RA
   — Trials have shown that etenercept monotherapy or ifliximab and MTX combination therapy slows radiographic progression of disease to a greater extent than MTX monotherapy[37,38]
   — Long-term safety data does not exist for these agents, but reported effects include increased incidence of infection, demyelinating disorders, and aplastic amenia

5. Less frequently used agents in the treatment of RA include azathioprine, D-penicillamin, gold salts, minocycline, and cyclosporine

C. Glucocorticoids

— Slow the rate of joint damage and alter disease course[39]

1. Local injections

— Provides dramatic but temporary relief of joint pain
— Used to treat joint flares without altering other therapy Ideal therapy when RA is confined to only a few joints
— Recommended that injections to a single joint be given no more than every three months due to risk of joint infection and microcrystalline arthritis

2. Systemic use

— Low-dose glucocorticoids recommended in severe disease for short periods of time
— Adverse effects of glucocorticoids are numerous and include hypertension, hyperglycemia, weight gain, cataracts, and premature arthrosclerosis, among others
— Of particular concern is the risk for osteoporosis, as RA is an independent risk factor for it development[40]
— Adverse effects of glucocorticoids need to be weighed carefully against the potential benefit of steroid therapy

IV. Non-pharmacologic management

— Patient education and understanding of the nature of RA are essential in coping with RA

— Physical therapy and occupational therapy can provide instruction in joint protection, energy conservation and joint range of motion and strengthening exercises, all of which help to maintain joint function[41–43]

— Dynamic and aerobic exercise regimens have been shown to improve joint function as well as psychological well-being in patients with RA[44]

Rheumatoid Arthritis of Digits

Surgical correction and treatment of rheumatoid wrist, metacarpophalangeal (MCP) joint and thumb deformities take priority of surgical correction, as these procedures significantly improve the quality of life. Although surgical results are unpredictable, correction of more proximal deformities may improve digital function in RA patients. Untreated rheumatoid digital deformities transform from passively correctible flexible deformities to deformities with limited motion and fixed in position.

Flexible Deformities

— Initial inciting factor is synovitis, digital deformity then progresses from a combination of synovitis, adhesions, shortening and/or rupture of the ligaments, intrinsic muscles and extrinsic tendons leading to poor joint position and ankylosis

Fixed Deformities

— Aim to recover flexibility first

Classic Deformities in Rheumatoid Arthritic Digits

Swan Neck Deformity

— Results from synovitis at the wrist, MCP joint, PIP joint or DIP joint
— Difficulty in making a full fist due hyperextended posture of PIPJ

- Causes functional problems

  — Surgical treatment will place the digit in a functional posture

Boutonnière Deformity

- — Always results from PIPJ synovitis
- — Patient has the ability to make a fist, however is unhappy with flexed posture of PIPJ on when the digit is extended
    - More of an aesthetic concern than functional
        - — Surgical treatment risks changing the flexed PIPJ posture into a functionally limiting extended posture[45]

Musculotendinous System of Digitis

Extensor Tendons

- — Flat and band like as it passes over MCPJ
    - Divides into 3 slips at junction of proximal and middle third of proximal phalanx

        A. Central slip

        - — Continues in midline, at level of neck of proximal phalanx, it receives the medial band of intrinsic tendons bilaterally
        - — Continues as central-band which inserts on the base of the dorsal aspect of middle phalanx
        - — Terminal tendon formed when conjoint lateral bands on both sides join eachother on the dorsum of the finger at the level of the middle and distal third of the middle phalanx which then inserts on the dorsal aspect of the base of the distal phalanx
        - — Other extensor tendon insertions on the digit
            - Lateral aspect of volar plate via the sagittal band
            - Inconstant slip from the deep surface of the tendon to the base of the dorsal aspect of the proximal phalanx

        B. 2 lateral slips

Interossei

- Originate from the metacarpal shafts and insert onto the base of the proximal phalanx via the lateral band
- Interosseous ligament passes volar to the MCPJ and remains dorsal to the deep transverse ligament and contributes to the sagital band
- At junction of proximal and middle third of the proximal phalanx, each intrinsic tendon divides into the medial and lateral bands
    - Medial band joins with the central slip for form the central band
    - Lateral band joins with lateral slips of the extensor tendon to form the conjoint lateral band
        - 3 palmar muscles
            - Digital adductors
            - Flexion of Index, ring and small finger at MCPJ
            - No insertion on the long finger
        - 4 dorsal muscles
            - Digital abductors
            - Flexion of index, long and ring fingers at MCPJ
            - No insertion on the small finger[46]

Lumbricals

- Originates from the Flexor Digitorum Profundus (FDP) muscle in the palm. After passing the MCPJ volarly, in joins the interosseous tendon to form the intrinsic tendon
- Only present on the radial aspect of the digit and contributes only to the formation of the radial intrinsic tendon
- Radially, the intrinsic tendon passes dorsally to the deep transverse metacarpal ligament, the lumbrical passes volarly
- Flexes MCPJ and extends interphalangeal (IP) joints
    - Extends IP joints irrespective of MCPJ position due to the mobile origin on the FDP[47]

Ligamentous System of Digitis

Sagittal Band

— Fibrous sheeth that invests the extensor tendon on the dorsum of the MCPJ

- Principal function is to extend the proximal phalanx
- Maintains the extensor tendon in the midline

Triangular Ligament

— Situated dorsally over proximal half of middle phalanx
— Transverse fibers extend between medial sides of conjoint lateral bands

- Maintains dorsal position of the conjoint lateral bands and limits palmar and lateral shift during flexion of the PIPJ

Transverse Retinacular Ligament (TRL)

— Situated on the lateral aspect of the proximal half of the middle phalanx
— Consists of transverse fibers that extend from the lateral side of the conjoint lateral band to the PIPJ volar plate and fibrous flexor sheath. The transverse fibers continue to the dorsum and merge with the fibers of the triangular ligament

- Main function is to prevent dorso-medial shift of the conjoint lateral band when the finger is extended

Oblique Retinacular Ligament (ORL)

— Coordinates movement of the interphalangeal joints and acts as a dynamic tenodesis to aid the conjoint lateral band in extention of the Distál interphalangeal joint
— Extension of the PIPJ places the ORL under tension and prevents easy active or flexion of the DIPJ
— Begins on the lateral aspect of the proximal phalanx and flexor sheath at the neck of the proximal phalanx and courses distally and dorsally

- Passes volar to the axis of the PIPJ, superficial to the collateral ligament, deep to the TRL along the side of the middle phalanx and then inserts into the conjoint lateral band at the level of the neck of the middle phalanx[48,49]

Pathology and Treatment

Swan Neck Deformity (SND)

- Key to treatment and diagnosis of a SND is to determine the joint that is responsible for the SND

Pathogenesis

— Primary PIPJ pathology

- Synovium become inflamed which forms a hyperplastic pannus. Joint streches on the dorsal surface of the volar plate, check rein ligaments and dorsal FDP
- Volar plate stretches and gets destroyed, PIPJ hyperextends, FDP under tension which causes DIPJ flexion (loss of ORL mechanical advantage in extending the DIPJ)[50]

— Primary MCPJ pathology

- Synovitis weakens insertion on dorsal base of proximal phalanx. Extensor forces transmitted to middle phalanx causing hyperextension of PIPJ
- Volar subluxation of MCPJ due to volar plate attenuation. Intrinsics tighten and cause PIPJ flexion and eventually SND

— Primary DIPJ pathology

- Terminal extensor tendon ruptures to do weakening from inflammation and synovitis
- Mallet deformity develops
- Proximal migration of the terminal extensor tendon cause the lateral bands to become lax
- All force is transmitted towards the central slip on middle phalanx

— Primary wrist pathology

- Synovitis leads to carpal collapse, carpal supination, and ulnar translation
- Flexion deformity of wrist and MCPJ results which eventually causes shortening of the intrinsic tendons

Management

Full passive range of PIPJ motion

— Intrinsic tightness assessed using the Finochietto-Bunnell Test[51]

Treatment

— Priority given to patients with abnormal MCPJ (articular damage)
— Intrinsic release for intrinsic contracture and/or MCPJ implant arthroplasty for MCPJ articular damage or volar subluxation
— Ulnar drift, MCPJ with no articular damage: Release radial intrinsic tendon. Crossed intrinsic tendon transfer to correct ulnar drift of the adjacent long, ring and small fingers
— Treatment of DIPJ is joint fusion
— Tenodesis of FDP or conjoint lateral band to prevent PIPJ hyperextension[52]

Limited passive range of PIPJ motion

— Significant disability to patient due to inability to flex PIPJ and grasp objects
— Primary cause is adhesion between the central band and dorsally translated conjoint lateral bands of the PIPJ dorsum

Treatment

— Release with manipulation under anesthesia.
— Essential to correct contributing deformities of MCPJ and DIPJ and ensure there is no advanced intra-articular PIPJ changes
— Examine presence of digitial flexor tenosynovitis. Patients with flexor tenosynovitis will have good passive range of motion, but poor active range of motion. Patient with joint damage will have limitation of both active and passive range of motion[53]

No passive PIPJ motion

- — Usually results from articular cartilage damage or an unstable/dislocated joint
- — Treatment is limited to joint implant arthroplasty or joint fusion. Chung *et al.* recommend joint fusion as it is more reliable in RA patients[45]

Boutonnière deformity

- Flexion deformity of PIPJ with Extension of MCPJ and DIPJ

  Pathogenesis

  - — Synovitis of PIPJ causes synovial proliferation intra-articularly leading to distension of the capsuloligamentous apparatus and stretching of the central band
  - — Conjoint lateral bands are stretched laterally, breaking through between the central band and conjoint lateral bands leading to a volar displacement of the conjoint lateral bands
  - — Conjoint lateral bands assume the role of flexors of the PIPJ rather than extenders (normal role)
  - — Stretched central band is unable to maintain full PIPJ extension. Head of the proximal phalanx prolapses through the attenuated central slip
  - — Central slip rupture causes the loss of lumbrical and interossei function at the base of the middle phalanx. This results in hyperextension of the PIPJ[45]

Management

Full passive range of PIPJ motion

- — Splinting PIPJ in extension. Splint should not extend the DIPJ
- — PIPJ synovitis not responsive to oral medications, an injection of corticosteriods in to the PIPJ maybe beneficial
- — Extensor tenotomy is required for patients who are unable to flex their DIPJ while the PIPJ is maintained in full extension due to a tight Oblique retinacular ligament (ORL)

Limited passive range of PIPJ motion

- Usually chronic inflammation resulting in soft tissue changes
- Trial of splinting in attempts to stretch collateral ligaments, volar plate, joint capsule and volar skin
- Surgical repair is difficult, involves restoring extensor force to PIPJ using local tissue. Challenges involve repairing the central band without limiting flexion[54]

No passive PIPJ motion

- Due to bony ankylosis or severe soft tissue contracture
- Attempts may be made to stretch out soft tissue with plaster splints
- Surgical options in patients with articular damage are limited to joint fusion or implant arthroplasty[54]

Flexor tenosynovitis

- Flexor tendons are involved less frequently than extensor tendons[55]
- Index, long and small fingers are most frequently involved
- Rheumatoid nodules are seen more 3 times more frequently on flexor tendons than extensor tendons and are confined to the profundus tendon[56]
- FDS usually ruputures at the PIPJ secondary to synovitis

Management

- Rheumatoid trigger finger presents as intermittent triggering on flexion and extension
- Flexor tenosynovectomy is an effective method for restoring finger function and preventing flexor tenosynovitis or tendon rupture[57]

Rheumatoid Thumb

- The thumb has been estimated at 50% of the "value" of the hand defined by the American Medical Association standards for disability for the thumb[58]
- Patients with carpal-metacarpal (CMC) joints compensate for loss of CMC motion by hyperextending their thumb MCPJ to preserve the span of the first webspace

— Thumb deformites arise from abnormal stretching of ligamentous and capsular structures, as well as from tendon subluxations

Classification of Rheumatoid Thumb Deformities by Nalebuff[59]

Type I

— Boutonnière deformity resulting from metacarpal phalangeal joint (MCPJ) synovitis which results in capsular weakening
— Extensor Pollicis Brevis (EPB) stretches and allows the Extensor Pollicis longus to sublux in a volar-ulnar direction secondary to extensor hood attenuation
— Extensor power is concentrated distally causing interphalangeal joint (IP) hyperextension
— Thumb collapses due to hyperextension at the IP joint when pinch is attempted along with abnormal MCPJ flexion
— MCPJ and IPJ deformites are passively correctable

Type II

— Boutonnière deformity with a fixed MCPJ and CMC joint involvement

Type III

— Swan-neck deformity starting at the CMC joint
— Dorsal and radial thumb base subluxation resulting in adduction of the distal MCPJ distally
— First webspace is narrowed resulting in inability to grasp large objects
— Thumb hyperextends at the MCPJ to compensate for adduction, in doing so, the volar plate competence is lost
— Flexor tendon balance is lost resulting in IP joint flexion and MCPJ hyperextension
— Belt *et al.* found that thumbs with more than a 4 mm of CMC subluxation had an 81% chance of developing a swan neck deformity[60]

Type IV

— Ulnar collateral ligament attrition

Type V

— Swan neck deformity starting with laxity of the MCPJ volar plate and sparing the CMC joint

Type VI

— Described as an "Opera-glass hand"
— Shortening of the digit due to bone reabsorption and loss of the articular surfaces

Management

Medical

— Maximize medical management
— Bracing and splinting to halt the progression of deformities

- Silver ring splint may be used to limit hyperextension or hyperflexion of the interphalangeal joint or MCPJ[61]

— Corticosteroid injections may provide pain relief by reducing inflammation
— Thumb orthotics may improve thumb function[62]

Surgical

— Terrono *et al.* suggest different treatment modalities of a rheumatoid boutonnière thumb bases on status of all the thumb joints and whether the deformity is passively correctable

- 64% recurrence rate with MCPJ synovectomy combined with an EPL rerouting procedure
- Recommendations

  1) Fusing MCPJ and IP joint in advanced cases
  2) MCPJ arthroplasty for low-demand patients with arthritic changes in the IP and CMC joints
  3) MCPJ fusion with moderate deformity and spared IP joint[63]

— Simmons *et al.* guidelines

1) Destruction of all thumb joints (CMC, MCPJ and IP) is rare, thus simplifying surgical correction
2) Soft tissue procedures should not be performed alone to maintain a long term correction, they should be performed in conjunction with joint procedures
3) Maintain mobility in as many joints as possible

   — CMC: Arthroplasty is the only choice procedure
   — MCPJ: Arthroplasty vs. arthrodesis depending on IP joint
   — IP joint: Arthrodesis is the usual option
   — When IP and MCPJ disease is present, it is preferred not to fuse both joints[58]

Boutonnière thumb

— MCPJ flexion with hyperextension or radial deviation of the IP joint. Radiographs may demonstrate MCPJ destruction and potentially IP joint destruction

- Combination of IP joint fusion and MCPJ silicone arthroplasty
- Minimal destruction of IP joint on radiograph: terminal tendon release may be performed
- Correction of the deformity may initially be achieved, however this may result in MCPJ hyperextension and increased deformity

  — For isolated IP pain or deformity, arthrodesis of the joint is the preferred procedure[58]

Swan-Neck Thumb

— MCPJ deformity is usually severe necessitating arthrodesis[64]
— Deformities of the CMC joint are best treated with a trapeziectomy and a tendon interposition with the goal of suspending the attitude of the thumb MCPJ

Rheumatoid Arthritis of the Metacarpophalangeal Joints

The metacarpophalangeal (MCP) joint plays a critical role in performance of activities of daily living. The chronic synovitis of RA leads to an attenuation of soft tissue restraints on joints. Continuous use of the hand and resultant forces on the joint in the background of weakened soft tissue is a major cause of MCP joint deformities in RA, which include joint subluxation that may progress to total dislocation, ulnar deviation and fixed flexion.

Medical management

- Should be fully optimized, as available surgical treatments have shown progressive decrease in function over time
- Resting and dynamic splints can be attempted to reduce pain and correct deformities

Surgical management

- Indications
    - Severe rheumatoid involvement of the MCP joints, often including joint subluxation or dislocation, affecting activities of daily living
        - Deformity alone is not considered an indication for surgery
        - Pre-operative evaluation
        - Measurement of ulnar drift, active flexion and extension arc of motion
        - Radiographs to evaluate degree of proximal subluxation and migration
- Procedures
    1. MCP joint arthroplasty
        - Surgical treatment of choice for MCP deformities
        - Involves exposure and resection of the metacarpal head and neck followed by insertion of an implant between the metacarpal and proximal phalynx base[65]

- Shown to improve MCP joint motion and ulnar drift immediately after surgery, but these measurements progressively worsen over time[66]
- Swanson silicone implant is most commonly used
- Newer pyrolytic carbon implants have been developed but have not been shown to improve outcomes when compared to Swanson implants. They are still being evaluated for long-term outcomes[67,68]

2. MCP joint synovectomy and joint realignment

   - Historic treatment no longer commonly used due to improvements in medical management of RA
   - Involves incision of the capsule on the radial side and synovectomy with preservation of the joint capsule followed by extensor tendon release and relocation onto the metacarpal head[65]

Rheumatoid Arthritis of the Wrist

Patients diagnosed with rheumatoid arthritis often develop wrist pain within 2 years of diagnosis.[69,70]

Although it is less disabling than rheumatoid arthritis of the hand and fingers, it can be a cause of pain and disability. Rheumatoid arthritis may progress to cause bony destruction and synovitis of the wrist, which may eventually lead to tendon ruptures.[19,71]

Diagnosis and Evaluation

- Functional limitation combined with pain are typical reasons for a patient to present to a physician for an evaluation. Occasionally they may present for evaluation of a deformity, mainly that of the distal radioulnar joint[69]

  - Synovitis of the dorsal wrist my result in cartilage destruction, and attenuation of the stabilizing ligaments leading to dorsal displacement of the ulna and the caput ulna syndrome[72]

  - Wrist may deform due to attrition of supporting soft tissues. The carpus translates ulnarly and supinates, resulting in radial deviation of the wrist. This contributes to the classic zig-zag deformity of the wrist-hand complex[73]

- Workup will include radiographs of the region in question as well as cervical spine imaging and electromyography in patients with radicular symptoms

  - Synovitis of the elbow may result in posterior interosseous nerve dysfunction which may be confused with an extensor tendon rupture
  - Intial presenting symptom may be attritonal flexor tendon rupture secondary to synovitis, bony destruction and osteophytosis of the carpus[19]
  - If a patient has lower extremity disease, it is advisable to address the lower extremity disease before upper extremity surgery/reconstruction because the patient will likely need crutch assistance for their lower extremity[69]

Clinical Evaluation

- Assessment of pain, range of motion, swelling, grip and pinch strength, deformity, stability and crepitus
- Pain with resisted flexion and extension will reflect not only joint disease, but may also suggest tenosynovitis
- Passive versus active motion may help reflect the source of pathology. Inability to actively extend a finger may be a sign of secondary tendon rupture[74]

Radiographs

- Critical to determine what can and cannot be done from a surgical standpoint
- Joint space narrowing is commonly noted as the early finding at the distal radioulnar and radioscaphoid joints[75,76]
  - Midcarpal radiographic disease is typically a later finding[77,78]

Non-Operative Treatment

— Static and dynamic splinting is an established treatment for pain relief, functional improvement and hopefull correction of a deformity[69]
— Intra-articular steroid injection has been shown to improve swelling, pain and patient perceived outcomes[79]
— Intra-articular injections of anti-tumor necrosis factor (TNF) agents are now determined to be generally safe[80]

Operative Treatment

Procedures

— Synovectomy
— Tenosynovectomy
— Tendon repair/reconstruction
— Treatment of an arthritic distal radioulnar joint
— Partial/complete arthrodesis of the radiocarpal joint
— Wrist arthroplasty

Indications

— Persistent symptoms, synovitis or swelling despite a 3 to 6 month course of conservative treatment[81,82]
— Prophylactic surgery to prevent tendon ruptures or irreversible soft-tissue injury
— Progression of the wrist deformity (zig-zag deformity)[83,84]
— Tendon rupture

Relative Contraindications

— History of previous infections (arthroplasty)
— Insufficient bone stalk
— Long standing fixed wrist deformity
— Poor or insufficient proximal arm function that is not correctible

Contraindications

— Comorbidities and poor general health

Synovectomy and Tenosynovectomy

— Indicated for patients with well preserved wrist motion, moderate swelling and relative absence of joint disease

- Dorsal

    - Extensor tendons are exposed after extensor retinaculum is elevated from the fourth or fourth-fifth compartment interval
    - Tenosynovectomy can be performed
    - Posterior interosseous neurectomy may be performed deep into the 4th compartment for pain
    - Radiocarpal joint may be exposed, bone disease and spurs can be removed from the carpus, distal ulna and radius[69]
    - Patients with wrist collapse, lengthening or transfer of the extensor carpi radialis longus (ECRL) tendon to the extensor carpi ulnaris (ECU) tendon can help correct the radial deviation of the wrist and ulnar drift of the digits[85,86]
    - Tendon ruptures are not amenable to primary repair. Tendon grafting are used to restore hand function. EPL at listers tubricle, the extensor digiti minimi at the distal radioulnar joint (DRUJ) and the extensor digitorum communis are the most commonly affected[87]

— Volar

— Flexor pollicis longus followed by flexor digitorum profundus to the index finger are most prone to rupture[19,88]

- Tendon grafting maybe necessary to restore thumb function
- Tendon transfer or grafting maybe needed for a FDP rupture

— Synovectomy and debridement maybe performed via a carpal tunnel release incision

Distal Radioulnar Joint (DRUJ)

— Rheumatoid arthritis may cause instability and dorsal subluxation of the distal ulna. Carpal supination further exaggerates the ulnar prominence

— Distal Ulna Resection (Darrach Procedure)

- Ulnar head is resected via 5th extensor compartment

Indications

— Refractory DRUJ synovitis with concomitant arthritis
— Ulnar extensor tendon ruputure
— Caput ulna syndrome with arthritis
— Patients with ulnocarpal impingment in association with radiocarpal arthrodesis, total wrist arthrodesis or arthroplasty

Contraindications

— Excessive carpal supination
— Risk of ulnar translation of carpus following distal ulna resection[69]

Complications

— Ulnar drift of carpus
— Distal ulna instability[89]

Sauvé-Kapandji Procedure

— Distal radioulnar arthrodesis between the distal radius and ulnar head. A segment of ulna is removed proximal to the arthrodesis site to allow for forearm pronation and supination

Complications

○ Impingement of convergence of the proximal ulnar stump with the radius
○ Non-union of fusion site
○ Dorsal sensory branch of ulnar nerve irritation
○ Regrowth of ulna
○ Tendon rupture[90]

Ulnar Head Arthroplasty

Indications

- Comminuted distal ulnar fracture

- Post traumatic DRUJ arthritis
- Osteoarthritis
- Rheumatoid arthritis
- Failed Sauvé-Kapandji procedures
- Instability of DRUJ in arthritic patients

Contraindications

- Advanced destruction and uncorrectable instability of DRUJ.
- Uncorrected malunion of the distal radius.
- Skeletal immaturity.
- prior infection.
- Known sensitivity or allergy to implant materials.[69]

Partial Wrist Arthrodesis

— Most commonly used partial wrist arthrodesis procedures include radiolunate and radioscapholunate arthrodesis
— Has advantage of some wrist motion preservation

Indications

— Disease of radiocarpal joint with sparing of midcarpal joint
— Progressive ulnar translation of the carpus
— Palmar subluxation of wrist
— Radiocarpal instability

Contraindications

— Midcarpal arthrosis.
— Rapidly progressing inflammation[69,91]

Total Wrist Arthrodesis

Indications

— Diffuse or advanced wrist disease
— Pan-carpal disease
— Pain
— Severe deformity
— Poor soft tissue support

Complications

— Non-union (especially carpo-metacarpal joints)
— Painful hardware
— Hardware failure
— Tendon irritation
— Limited finger range of motion[92]

Total Wrist Arthroplasty

— Has the primary advantage is preservation of wrist motion
— Disadvantage is durability and reliability of the prosthesis
— When successful, patients prefer arthroplasty over arthrodesis primarily because of improved ease of activities of daily living and hygiene[93,94]

References

1. Entezami P, Fox DA, Clapham PJ, Chung KC (2011). Historical Perspective on the etiology of rheumatoid arthritis. *Hand Clin* **27**: 1–10.
2. Landré-Beauvais AJ. (2001) The first description of rheumatoid arthritis. Unabridged text of the doctoral dissertation presented in 1800. *Joint Bone Spine* **68**: 130–142.
3. Rogers J, Dieppe P. (1990) Skeletal palaeopathology and the rheumatic diseases: where are we now? *Ann Rheum Dis* **49**: 885–886.
4. Ortner DJ, Tuross N, Stix AI. (1992) New approaches to the study of disease in archeological New World populations. *Hum Biol* **64**(3): 337–360.
5. Reveille JD. (1998) The genetic contribution to the pathogenesis of rheumatoid arthritis. *Curr Opin Rheumatol* **10**: 187–200.
6. Condemi JJ.(1992) The autoimmune diseases. *JAMA* **268**(20): 2882–2892.
7. Moreland LW. (2001) *Rheumatoid Arthritis: Epidemiology, Pathogenesis and Treatment*. ReMEDICA Publishing, London.
8. Andersson AK, *et al.* (2008) Recent developments in the immunobiology of rheumatoid arthritis. *Arthritis Res Ther* **10**: 204.
9. Barr J. (1913) An address on rheumatoid arthritis. *Br Med J* **1**(2728): 733–735.
10. Bennike P. (1985) *Paleopathology of Danish Skeletons: A Comparative Study of Demography, Disease and Injury*. Akademisk Forlag, Copenhagen (Denmark).

11. Álvarez-Lafuente R, Fernández-Gutiérrez B, Miguel S, *et al.* (2005) Potential relationship between herpes viruses and rheumatoid arthritis: analysis with quantitative real time polymerase chain reaction. *Ann Rheum Dis* **64**: 1357–1359.
12. Balandraud N, Roudier J, Roudier C. (2004) Epstein Barr virus and rheumatoid arthritis. *Autoimmun Rev* 3: 362–367.
13. Klareskog L, Stolt P, Lundberg K, *et al.* (2006) A new model for an etiology for rheumatoid arthritis: smoking may trigger HLA-DR (shared epitope) restricted immune reactions to autoantigens modified by citrullination. *Arthritis Rheum* **54**(1): 38–46.
14. Imboden JB. (2009) The immunopathogenesis of rheumatoid arthritis. *Ann Rev Pathol Mech Dis* **4**: 417–434.
15. Brown FE, Collins ED, Harmataz AS. (2000) Rheumatoid arthritis of the hand and wrist. In: Achauer BM, Elof E, Guyron B (eds.), *Plastic Surgery: Indications, Operations and Outcomes*, Vol. 4. Mosby, St. Louis, pp. 2249–2274.
16. Feldon P, Terrono AL, Nalebuff EA. (1998) Rheumatoid arthritis in the hand and wrist. In: Green DP, Hotchkiss RN, Pederson WC (eds.), *Operative Hand Surgery*, Vol. 2, 4th Edn. Churchill Livingstone, Philadelphia, pp. 1651–1739.
17. Ghavami A. (2007) Rheumatoid arthritis. In: Janis J. (ed.), *Essentials of Plastic Surgery: A UT Southwestern Medical Center Handbook.* QMP Publication, pp. 707–716.
18. Linscheid RL, Lipscomb PR. (1962) Advances in surgical treatment of the rheumatoid hand. *Minn Med* **45**: 273.
19. Mannerfelt L, Norman O. (1969) Attrition ruptures of flexor tendons in rheumatoid arthritis caused by bony spurs in the carpal tunnel. A clinical and radiological study. *J Bone Joint Surg Br* **51**(2): 270–277.
20. Lister G. (2002) Rheumatoid arthritis, its variants, and osteoarthritis. In: Smith P (ed.), *Lister's The Hand*, 4th Edn. Churchill Livingstone, London, pp. 331–397.
21. American College of Rheumatology Subcommittee on Rheumatoid Arthritis Guidelines. (2002) Guidelines for the management of rheumatoid arthritis: 2002 update. *Arthritis Rheum* **46**(2): 328–346.
22. Yeomans ND, Tulassay Z, Juhasz L, Racz I, Howard JM, van Rensburg CJ, *et al.* (1998) for the Acid Suppression Trial: Ranitidine versus Omeprazole for NSAID-Associated Ulcer Treatment (ASTRONAUT) Study Group. A comparison of omeprazolewith ranitidine for ulcers associated with nonsteroidal antiinflammatorydrugs. *N Engl J Med* **338**: 719–726.

23. Hawkey CJ, Karrasch JA, Szczepanski L, Walker DG, Barkun A, Swannell AJ, *et al.* (1998), for the omeprazole versus misoprostol for NSAID-induced ulcer management (OMNIUM) study group. Omeprazole compared with misoprostol for ulcers associated with nonsteroidal antiinflammatory drugs. *N Engl J Med* **338**: 727–734.
24. Silverstein FE, Graham DY, Senior JR, Davies HW, Struthers BJ, Bittman RM, *et al.* (1995) Misoprostol reduces serious gastrointestinal complications in patients with rheumatoid arthritis receiving nonsteroidal anti-inflammatory drugs: a randomized, doubleblind, placebo-controlled trial. *Ann Intern Med* **123**: 241–249.
25. Bologna C, Viu P, Picot MC, Jorgensen C, Sany J. (1997) Long-term follow-up of 453 rheumatoid arthritis patients treated with methotrexate: an open, retrospective, observational study. *Br J Rheumatol* **36**: 535–540.
26. Kremer JM. (1997) Safety, efficacy, and mortality in a long-term cohort of patients with rheumatoid arthritis taking methotrexate: followup after a mean of 13.3 years. *Arthritis Rheum* **40**: 984–985.
27. Drosos AA, Tsifetaki N, Tsiakou EK, Timpanidou M, Tsampoulas C, Tatsis CK, *et al.* (1997) Influence of methotrexate on radiographic progression in rheumatoid arthritis: a sixty-month prospective study. *Clin Exp Rheumatol* **15**: 263–267.
28. Strand V, Cohen S, Schiff M, Weaver A, Fleischmann R, Cannon G, *et al.* (1999) Treatment of active rheumatoid arthritis with leflunomide compared with placebo and methotrexate. *Arch Intern Med* **159**: 2542–2550.
29. Sharp JT, Strand V, Leung H, Hurley F, Loew-Friedrich I. (2000) On behalf of the Leflunomide Rheumatoid Arthritis Investigators Group. Treatment with leflunomide slows radiographic progression of rheumatoid arthritis: results from three randomized controlled trials of leflunomide in patients with active rheumatoid arthritis. *Arthritis Rheum* **43**: 495–505.
30. Kremer JM, Alarćon GS, Lightfoot RW Jr, Willkens RF, Furst DE, Williams HJ, *et al.* (1994) Methotrexate for rheumatoid arthritis: suggested guidelines for monitoring liver toxicity. *Arthritis Rheum* **37**: 316–328.
31. Morgan SL, Baggott JE, Vaughn WH, Young PK, Austin JV, Krumdieck CL, *et al.* (1990) The effect of folic acid supplementation on the toxicity of low-dose methotrexate in patients with rheumatoid arthritis. *Arthritis Rheum* **33**: 9–18.
32. Shiroky JB, Neville C, Esdaile JM, Choquette D, Zummer M, Hazeltine M, *et al.* (1993) Low-dose methotrexate with leucovorin (folinic acid) in the management of rheumatoid arthritis: results of a multicenter randomized, double-blind, placebo-controlled trial. *Arthritis Rheum* **36**: 795–803.

33. Van der Heijde DM, van Riel PL, Nuver-Zwart IH, Gribnau FW, van de Putte LB. (1989) Effects of hydroxychloroquine and sulfasalazine on progression of joint damage in rheumatoid arthritis. *Lancet* **1**: 1036–1038.
34. Van der Heide A, Jacobs JW, Bijlsma JW, Heurkens AH, van Booma-Frankfort C, van der Veen MJ, *et al.* (1996) The effectiveness of early treatment with "second-line" antirheumatic drugs: a randomized, controlled trial. *Ann Intern Med* **124**: 699–707.
35. Esdaile JM, Suissa S, Shiroky JB, Lamping D, Tsakonas E, Anderson D, *et al.* (1995) A randomized trial of hydroxychloroquine in early rheumatoid arthritis: the HERA study. *Am J Med* **98**: 156–168.
36. Hannonen P, Möttönen T, Hakola M, Oka M. (1993) Sulfasalazine in early rheumatoid arthritis: a 48-week double-blind, prospective, placebo-controlled study. *Arthritis Rheum* **36**: 1501–1509.
37. Lipsky PE, van der Heijde DM, St. Clair EW, Furst DE, Breedveld FC, Kalden JR, *et al.* (2000) for the Anti-Tumor Necrosis Factor Trial in Rheumatoid Arthritis with Concomitant Therapy Study Group. Infliximab and methotrexate in the treatment of rheumatoid arthritis. *N Engl J Med* **343**: 1594–1602.
38. Bathon JM, Martin RW, Fleischmann RM, Tesser JR, Schiff MH, Keystone EC, *et al.* (2000) A comparison of etanercept and methotrexate in patients with early rheumatoid arthritis. *N Engl J Med* **343**: 1586–1593.
39. Kirwan JR. (1995) The arthritis and rheumatism council low-dose glucocorticoid study group. The effect of glucocorticoids on joint destruction in rheumatoid arthritis. *N Engl J Med* **333**: 142–146.
40. Buckley LM, Leib ES, Cartularo KS, Vacek PM, Cooper SM. (1995) Effects of low dose corticosteroids on the bone mineral density of patients with rheumatoid arthritis. *J Rheumatol* **22**: 1055–1059.
41. Bell MJ, Lineker SC, Wilkens AL, Goldsmith CH, Badley EM. (1998) A randomized controlled trial to evaluate the efficacy of community based physical therapy in treatment of people with rheumatoid arthritis. *J Rheumatol* **25**: 231–237.
42. Komatireddy GR, Leitch RW, Cella K, Browning C, Minor M. (1997) Efficacy of low resistance muscle training in patients with rheumatoid arthritis functional class II and III. *J Rheumatol* **24**: 1531–1539.
43. Neuberger GB, Press AN, Lindsey HB, Hinton R, Cagle PE, Carlson K, *et al.* (1997) Effects of exercise on fatigue, aerobic fitness, and disease activity measures with rheumatoid arthritis. *Res Nurs Health* **20**: 195–204.
44. Van den Ende CH, Vliet Vlieland TP, Munneke M, Hazes JM. (1998) Dynamic exercise therapy in rheumatoid arthritis: a systematic review. *Br J Rheumatol* **37**: 677–687.

45. Sebastin SJ, Chung KC. (2011) Reconstruction of digital deformites in rheumatoid arthritis. *Hand Clin* **27**: 87–104.
46. Tubiana R, Thomine JM, Mackin E. (1996) Movements of the hand and wrist. In: Tubiana R, Thomine JM, Mackin E (eds.), Examination of the hand and wrist. Mosby, St. Louis (MO), pp. 78–111.
47. Doyle J. (2003) Hand. Surgical anatomy of the hand and upper extremity. In: Doyle J, Botte M (eds.), Lippincott Williams & Wilkins, Philadelphia, pp. 533–667.
48. Haines RW. (1951) The extensor apparatus of the finger. *J Anat* **85**: 251–259.
49. Rockwell WB, Butler PN, Byrne B. (2000) Extensor tendon: anatomy, injury and reconstruction. *Plast Reconstr Surg* **106**: 1592–1603.
50. Harrison SH. (1971) The proximal interphalangeal joint in rheumatoid arthritis. *Hand* **3**(2): 125–130.
51. Bunnell S, Doherty E, Curtis R. (1946) Ischemic contracture, local, in hand. *Plast Reconstr Surg* **3**(4): 424–433.
52. Littler J. (1967) The finger extensor mechanism. *Surg Clin North Am* **47**: 4115–4132.
53. Boyer MI, Gelberman RH. (1999) Operative correction of swan-neck and boutonniere deformities in the rheumatoid hand. *J Am Acad Orthop Surg* **7**(2): 92–100.
54. Nalebuff EA, Millender LH. (1975) Surgical treatment of the boutonniere deformity in rheumatoid arthritis. *Orthop Clin North Am* **6**(3): 753–763.
55. Schindele D, Kloss D, Herren D. (2006) Options in extensor tendon reconstruction in rheumatoid arthritis. In: Trail I, Hayton M (eds.), *Surgery of the Rheumatoid Hand and Wrist*. Elsevier, Amsterdam, pp. 94–106.
56. Saffar P. (2006) Flexor tendon synovectomy in rheumatoid arthritis. In: Trail I, Hayton M (eds.), *Surgery of the Rheumatoid Hand and Wrist*. Elsevier, Amsterdam, pp. 107–117.
57. Millender LH, Nalebuff EA. (1975) Preventive surgery — tenosynovectomy and synovectomy. *Orthop Clin North Am* **6**(3): 765–792.
58. George SMD, Barry PS. (2011) Rheumatoid thumb. *Hand Clin* **27**: 73–77.
59. Nalebuff EA. (1968) Diagnosis, classification and management of rheumatoid thumb deformities. *Bull Hosp Joint Dis* **29**(2): 119–137.
60. Belt E, Kaarela K, Lehtinen J, *et al.* (1998) When does subluxation of the first carpometacarpal joint cause swan-neck deformity of the thumb in rheumatoid arthritis: a 20-year follow-up study. *Clin Rheumatol* **17**(2): 135–138.
61. Zijlstra TR, Heijnsdijk-Rouwenhorst L, Rasker JJ. (2004) Silver ring splints improve dexterity in patients with rheumatoid arthritis. *Arthritis Rheum* **51**(6): 947–951.

62. Silva PG, Lombardi I Jr, Breitschwerdt C, *et al.* (2008) Functional thumb orthosis for type I and II boutonniere deformity on the dominant hand in patients with rheumatoid arthritis: a randomized controlled study. *Clin Rehabil* **22**(8): 684–689.
63. Terrono A, Millender L, Nalebuff E. (1990) Boutonnière rheumatoid thumb deformity. *J Hand Surg Am* **15**(6): 999–1003.
64. Nalebuff EA, Millender LH. (1975). Surgical treatment of the swan-neck deformity in rheumatoid arthritis. *Orthop Clin North Am* **6**(3): 733–752.
65. Burke FD. (2003) The rheumatoid metacarpophalangeal joint. *Hand Clin* **27**: 79–68.
66. Goldfarb CA. (2003) Metacarpophalangeal joint arthroplasty in rheumatoid arthritis. *J Bone Joint Surg Am* **85**: 1869–1878.
67. Parker WL, Rizzo M, Moran SL, *et al.* (2007) Preliminary results of non-constrained pyrolytic carbon arthroplasty for metacarpophalangeal joint arthritis. *J Hand Surg Am* **32**: 1496–1505.
68. Cook SD, Beckenbaugh RD, Redondo J, *et al.* (1999) Long-term follow-up of pyrolytic carbon metacarpophalangeal implants. *J Bone Joint Surg Am* **81**: 635–648.
69. Marco R, Cooney W. (2011) Current concepts and treatment for the rheumatoid wrist. *Hand Clin* **27**: 57–72.
70. Trieb K. (2008) Treatment of the wrist in rheumatoid arthritis. *J Hand Surg Am* **33**: 113–123.
71. Vaughan-Jackson OJ. (1948) Rupture of extensor tendons by attrition at the inferior radio-ulnar joint; report of two cases. *J Bone Joint Surg Br* **30**: 528–530.
72. Backdahl M. (1963) The caput ulnae syndrome in rheumatoid arthritis. A study of the morphology, abnormal anatomy and clinical picture. *Acta Rheumatol Scand Suppl* 5: 1–75.
73. Stack HG, Vaughan-Jackson OJ. (1971) The zig-zag deformity in the rheumatoid hand. *Hand* **3**: 62–67.
74. Wilson RL, DeVito MC. (1996) Extensor tendon problems in rheumatoid arthritis. *Hand Clin* **12**: 551–559.
75. Bywaters EG. (1960) The early radiological signs of rheumatoid arthritis. *Bull Rheum Dis* **11**: 231–234.
76. Martel W, Hayes JT, Duff IF. (1965) The pattern of bone erosion in the hand and wrist in rheumatoid arthritis. *Radiology* **84**: 204–214.
77. Taleisnik J (1987) Combined radiocarpal arthrodesis and midcarpal (lunocapitate) arthroplasty for treatment of rheumatoid arthritis of the wrist. *J Hand Surg Am* **12**: 1–8.

78. Hindley CJ, Stanley JK. (1991) The rheumatoid wrist: patterns of disease progression. A review of 50 wrists. *J Hand Surg Br* **16**: 275–279.
79. Lopes RV, Furtado RN, Pamigiani L, *et al.* (2008) Accuracy of intra-articular injections in peripheral joints performed blindly in patients with rheumatoid arthritis. *Rheumatology* (*Oxford*) **47**: 1548–1553.
80. Bieber EJ, Linscheid RL, Dobyns JH, *et al.* (1988) Failed distal ulna resections. *J Hand Surg Am* **13**: 193–200.
81. Millender LH, Nalebuff EA. (1975) Preventive surgery-tenosynovectomy, and synovectomy. *Orthop Clin North Am* **6**: 765–792.
82. Ryu J, Saito S, Hona T, *et al.* (1998) Risk factors and ruptures in rheumatoid hand. *J Hand Surg Br* **23**: 658–661.
83. Mannerfelt L. (1989) On surgery of the rheumatoid hand: consensus and controversy. *J Hand Surg Br* **14**: 259–260.
84. Shapiro JS. (1996) The wrist in rheumatoid arthritis. *Hand Clin* **12**: 477–498.
85. Clayton ML, Ferlic DC. (1974) Tendon transfer for radial rotation of the wrist in rheumatoid arthritis. *Clin Orthop Relat Res* **100**: 176–185.
86. Ito J, Koshino T, Okamoto R, *et al.* (2003) Radiologic evaluation of the rheumatoid hand after synovectomy and extensor carpi radialis longus transfer to extensor carpi ulnaris. *J Hand Surg Am* **28**: 585–590.
87. Norris SH. (1990) Surgery for the rheumatoid wrist and hand. *Ann Rheum Dis* **49**(Suppl 2): 863–870.
88. Ertel AN, Millender LH, Nalebuff E, *et al.* (1988) Flexor tendon ruptures in patients with rheumatoid arthritis. *J Hand Surg Am* **13**: 860–866.
89. Field J, Majkowski RJ, Leslie IJ. (1993) Poor results of Darrach's procedure after wrist injuries. *J Bone Joint Surg Br* **75**: 53–57.
90. Scheker LR. (2008) Implant arthroplasty for the distal radio-ulnar joint. *J Hand Surg Am* **33**: 1639–1644.
91. Borisch N. Haussmann P. (2002) Radiolunate arthrodesis in the rheumatoid wrist: a retrospective clinical and radiological longterm follow-up. *J Hand Surg Br* **27**: 61–72.
92. Toma CD, Machacek P, Bitzan P, *et al.* (2007) Fusion of the wrist in rheumatoid arthritis: a clinical and functional evaluation of two surgical techniques. *J Bone Joint Surg Br* **89**: 1620–1626.
93. Vicar AJ, Burton RI. (1986) Surgical management of the rheumatoid wrist-fusion or arthroplasty. *J Hand Surg Am* **11**: 790–797.
94. Murphy DM, Khoury JG, Imbriglia JE, *et al.* (2003) Comparison of arthroplasty and arthrodesis for the rheumatoid wrist. *J Hand Surg Am* **28**: 570–576.

CHAPTER 18

CONGENITAL HAND ANOMALIES

Sara Yegiyants and Zubin J. Panthaki

Illustrative Case

1 year old child with post axial polydactyly (Figs. 1–3), type B. Simple excision was performed with good results.

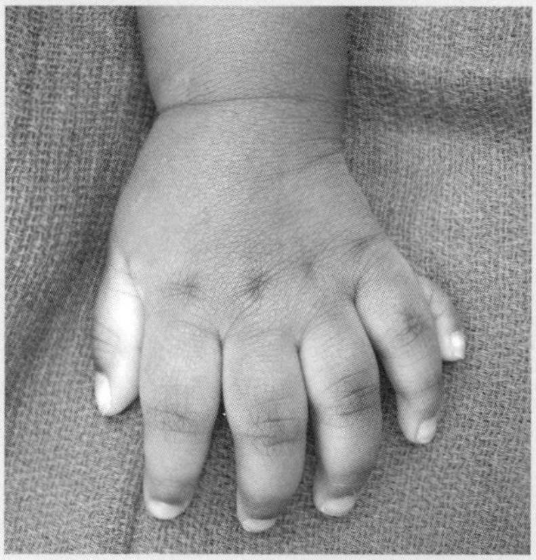

Fig. 1. Polydactily.

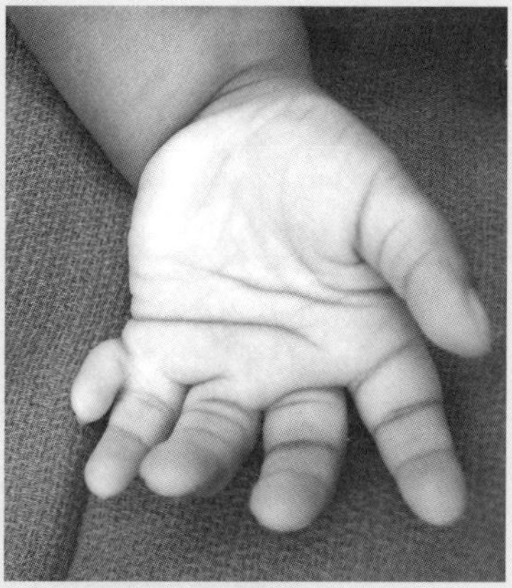

Fig. 2. Polydactily.

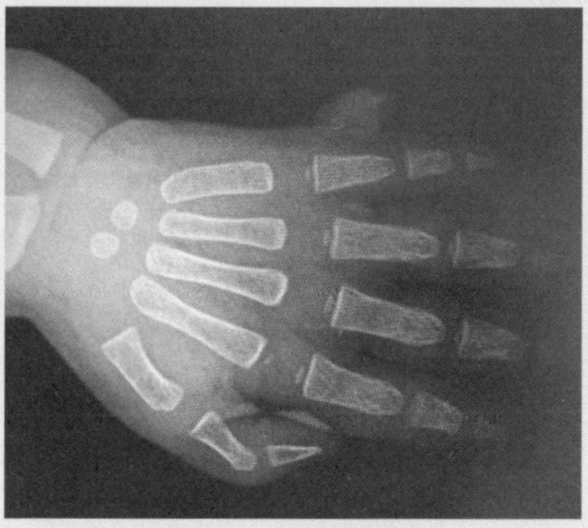

Fig. 3. Polydactily.

Embryology[1,2]

— Limb bud formation begins approximately at 4 weeks and completes by 8 weeks after gestation
— Limb bud is an outgrowth of mesoderm under the overlying ectoderm
— Somatic mesoderm gives rise to muscle, nerve, and vascular elements
— Lateral plate mesoderm gives rise to bone, cartilage, and tendon
— 3 signaling centers, each in a different spatial axis, are responsible for the characteristic limb growth and differentiation
— HOX and T-BOX genes encode transcription factors that are central in limb formation
— Congenital disorders may also be associated with genetic mutations in these families of genes
— During development, disturbance of limb formation may affect other organ formation

Classification of Anomalies[3]

I. Failure of formation

   A. Transverse arrest
   B. Longitudinal arrest

      1. Radial

         a) Thumb hypoplasia (5 types)
         b) Radial deficiency (4 types)

      2. Central

Table 1. Limb Formation Embryogenesis.

Signaling Center	Axis	Substance	Action
Apical ectodermal ridge	Proximodistal	Fibroblast growth factors	Proximal to distal limb development
Zone of polarizing activity	Anteroposterior	Sonic hedgehog protein	Radioulnar limb formation
Wnt pathway	Dorsoventral	Lmx-1	Dorsalization of the limb

3. Ulnar
4. Entire limb (phocomelia)

II. Failure of differentiation

1. Syndactyly
2. Carpal coalition
3. Arthrogryposis
4. Symphalangism
5. Camptodactyly
6. Clinodactyly

III. Duplication

A. Preaxial

1. Thumb

a) Wassel classification
b) 7 types of thumb duplication, Type 4 most common

B. Central

1. Index, long, ring fingers
2. Mirror hand

C. Postaxial

1. Small finger

IV. Overgrowth

1. Gigantism
2. Macrodactyly

V. Undergrowth

1. Brachydactyly

VI. Constriction band syndrome

VII. Generalized skeletal abnormalities

1. Dyschondroplasia
2. Marfan's syndrome

3. Achondroplasia
4. Dystrophic dwarfism

Deformities of the Hand and Fingers[4]

Syndactyly (Figs. 4 to 6)[5]

1. Description
   — Digital separation and web space formation fail to some degree
2. Epidemiology
   — 1 in 2000 incidence
   — 50% bilateral
   — 10–40% inherited via autosomal dominance
3. Pathology
   — Variable fusion of soft tissue and/or skeletal elements of adjacent digits
   — Nails, digital neurovascular bundles, and tendons may be involved

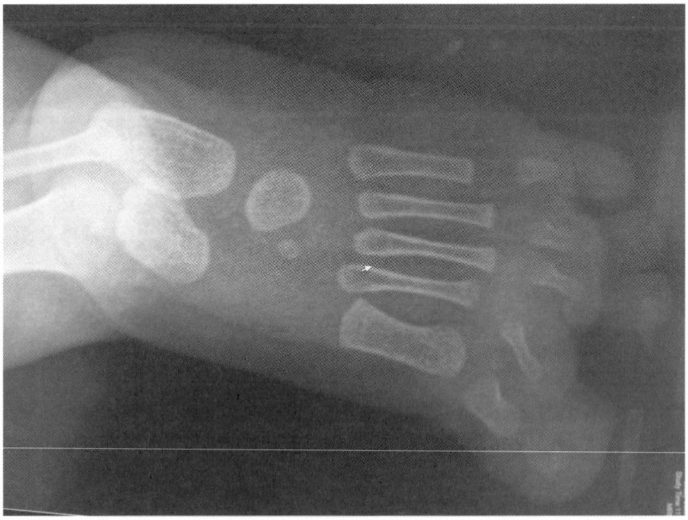

Fig. 4. Syndactily.

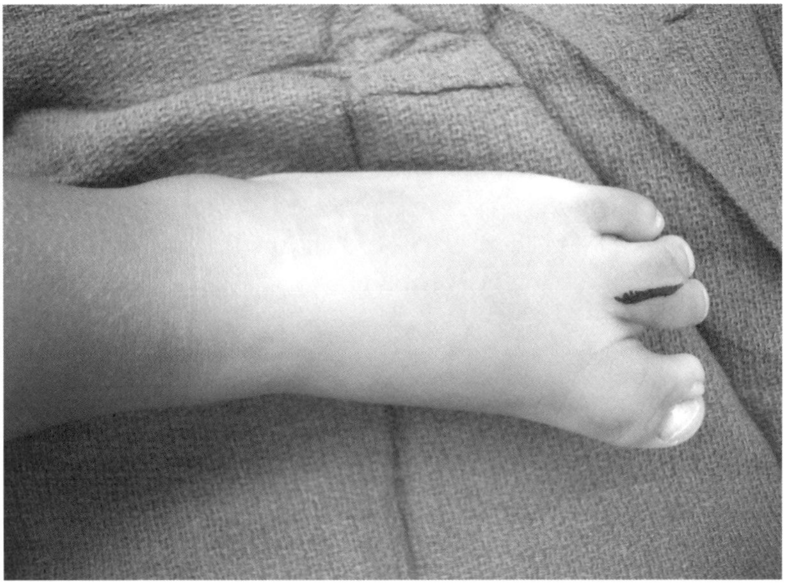

Fig. 5. Syndactily.

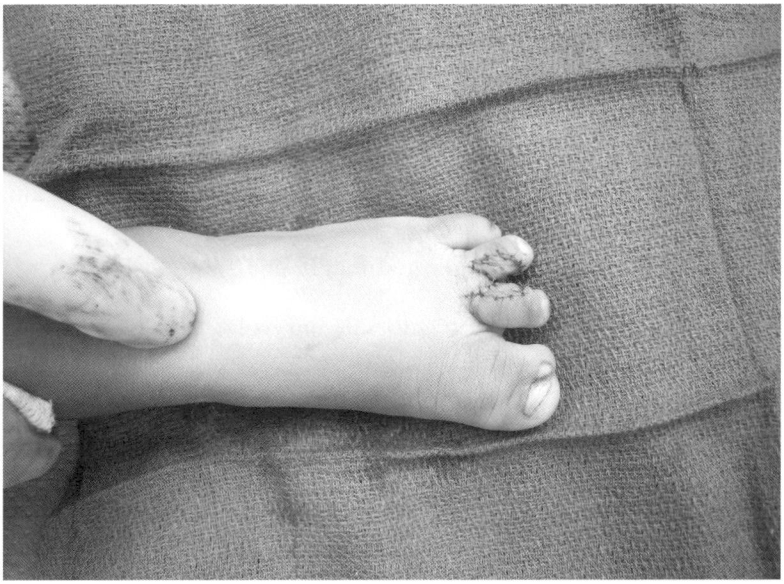

Fig. 6. Syndactily.

— Distal phalangeal fusion results in synonychia with loss of paronychial fold

4. Clinical Features

— Commonly affected web spaces in decreasing order: third, fourth, second, first
— Features to consider: extent of syndactyly, involvement of nail, differential motion between digits

5. Classification

— Complete: web space extends to include fingertip
— Incomplete: web space occurs between normal commisure and fingertip
— Simple: involvement of only skin
— Complex: involvement of skeletal anomalies
— Acrosyndactyly: fusion of distal tips of fingers with fenestration proximally in web space

6. Etiology

— Failure of digital patterning, apoptosis, or AER regression

7. Management

— Surgery is indicated except for mild incomplete syndactyly or complex syndactyly with risk for further impairment due to surgery
— Surgical intervention: approximately at 12 months of age[6]

a. Separation of digits: dorsal and volar zigzag incisions for interdigitating flaps
b. Identify NVB prior to separation
c. Dorsal flaps or triangular flaps form dorsal and volar aspects.
d. Commisure reconstruction: Z-plasty; X-M plasty
e. Skin coverage: Full thickness grafts from either inguinal site, cubital fossa, hypothenar border of hand, skin of an accessory digit
f. Careful defatting is possible to avoid use of skin grafting[7]

g. Paronchial fold: laterally based triangular flaps from the hyponychium of the conjoined digital mass are folded around to form the lateral nail fold
h. Syndactyly involving multiple web spaces requires staging to avoid vascular compromise of the skin flaps or digits

   — Syndactyly of all web spaces is usually treated in two stages. The first procedure separates the thumb/index finger and long/ring finger web spaces
   — Three months later, a second procedure separates the index/long finger and ring/small finger web spaces

i. Immobilization: above elbow cast

Ulnar Polydactyly (Figs. 1 to 3)[4]

1. Description

   — Duplication of the postaxial digit (5th finger)

2. Epidemiology

   — Inherited via autosomal dominance with variable penetrance
   — More common in African Americans

3. Classification

   — Type A: well developed supernumerary digit
   — Type B: rudimentary or pedunculated skin tag

4. Management

   — Type A: digital ablation

   a. Elliptical incision around digit with proximal extensions for exposure
   b. Tendons removed, nerves incised, and arteries coagulated
   c. If abductor digiti quinti or ulnar collateral ligament exists, muscle and tendon should be transferred to adjacent digit

   — Type B: ligated

Central Polydactyly[4]

1. Description

    — Duplication of index, long or ring fingers

2. Epidemiology

    — Inherited via autosomal dominance

3. Management

    — Treatment is to ablate the duplicated digit with augmentation of the retained digit
    — Multiple operations required

Mirror Hand[4]

1. Description

    — Symmetrical duplication of the limb at the midline

2. Classification/Clinical Features

Table 2. Classification and Clinical Features of Mirror Hand.

Type	Name	Clinical Features
1	Ulnar dimelia	Multiple fingers with two ulnae Type A: Ulna well formed Type B: Hypoplastic ulna
2	Intermediate form	Multiple fingers with two ulnae and a radius
3	Intermediate form	Multiple fingers with one ulna and a radius Type A: Radius well formed Type B: Hypoplastic radius
4	Syndromic form	Type A: Sandrow's syndrome — two ulnae Type B: Martin's syndrome — an ulna and radius
5	Multiple hand	Complete duplication of the hand with thumb

3. Etiology

   — Transplantation or replication of ZPA from posterior to anterior margin

4. Management

   — Surgically reduce digit number to four and reconstruct thumb using ablated digit

Brachydactyly (Figs. 7 and 8)[4]

1. Description

   — Shortened finger with preservation but reduced size in digital skeleton

2. Epidemiology

   — Common congenital hand anomaly
   — May be an isolated or syndromic anomaly

3. Classification

Table 3. Classification of Brachydactyly.

Type	Description
A	Middle phalanges of one or more fingers and/or toes are shortened
B	Distal phalanges and nails of fingers and/or toes are shortened
C	Middle phalange of all fingers are affected with fourth finger being longest
D	Distal phalange of thumb and/or great toe is short and broad
E	Metacarpals and/or metatarsals are shortened

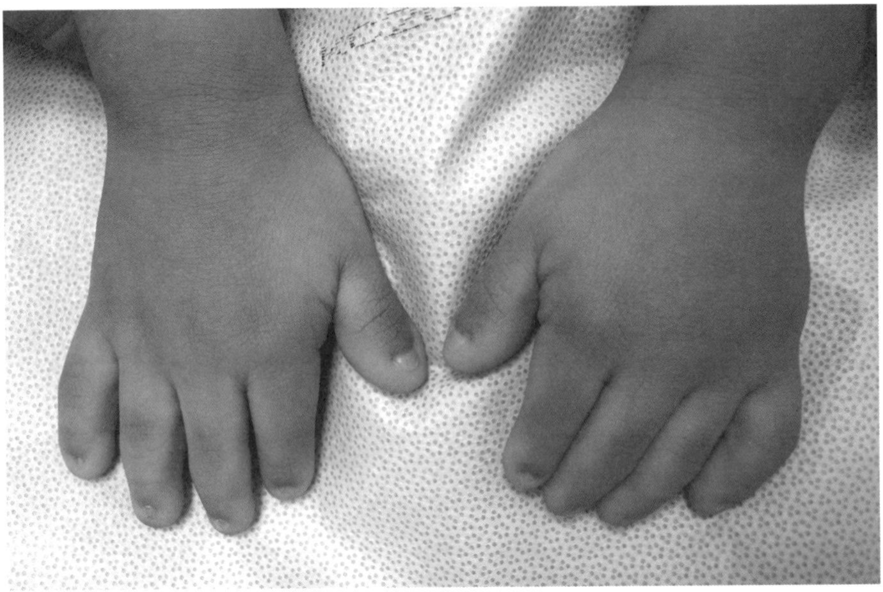

Fig. 7. Brachydactily.

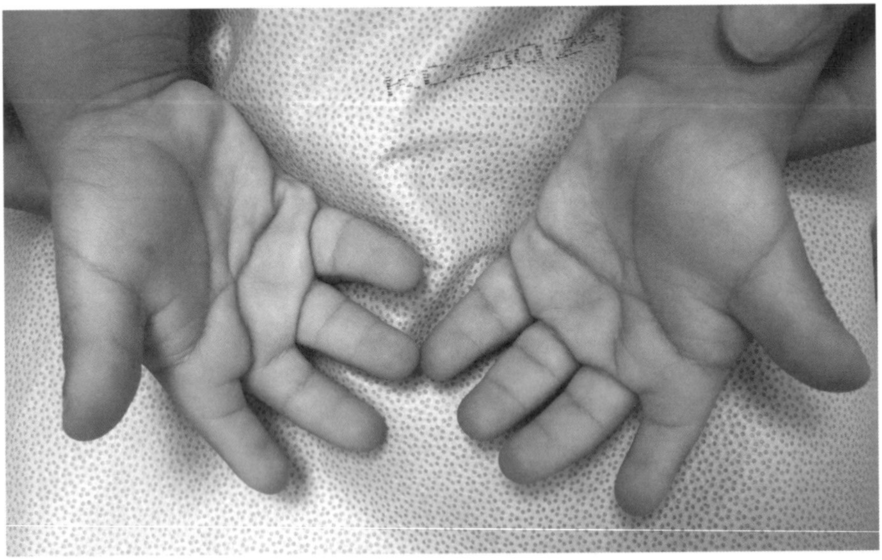

Fig. 8. Brachydactily.

4. Clinical Features

— Small and index fingers are most commonly affected

5. Management

— Lengthening of shortened digit through osteotomy
— Distraction to desired length
— Bone graft or bone regeneration
— Potential complications include joint stiffness, contracture, and loss of hand function

Central Hand Deficiency[4]

1. Description

— Deficiency of central rays creating a cleft hand

2. Epidemiology

— Inherited via autosomal dominance
— Variable expressivity and reduced penetrance
— 1 in 90,000 births

3. Etiology

— Defect of AER of limb bud

4. Clinical Features

— One to four limbs involved
— "V" shaped cleft
— No finger "nubbins"
— Syndactyly (esp. first web)

5. Classification

— Typical cleft hand is V-shaped central defect secondary to hypoplasia
— Atypical cleft hand is associated with symbrachydactyly

Table 4. Manske's Classification of Central Deficiency Based on Thumb Web Space

Type	Description
I	Normal web
IIA	Mildly narrowed web
IIB	Severely narrowed web
III	Syndactylized web
IV	Merged web
V	Absent web

6. Management

— Surgery is indicated for (1) progressive deformity; (2) the first web space; (3) cleft hand; (4) absent thumb; (5) feet

— Most non-urgent indications can be corrected at 1–2 years of age

a. Removal of transverse bones that occupy the cleft
b. Early release of syndactyly to prevent progressive deviation of rays
c. Release of first web space and closure of cleft

i. Cleft is raised as palmar based flap
ii. First web space is released and metacarpal is transposed and fixed
iii. Palmar flap is transferred and new commisure is recreated

— Absent thumb: some cleft hands have two digital rays fused

a. One may be separated and rotated to re-create a thumb
b. Complete absence replaced by free toe transfer; high complications

Amniotic Disruption Sequence: Constriction Ring Syndrome[8]

1. Description

— Partial or complete circumferential constriction around limbs or digits

2. Clinical Features

   — Mechanical strangulations from the ring constrictions
   — Important to examine whether proximal structures of hand are normal
   — Distal edema and reduced viability may be present

3. Classification

   — Simple constriction rings
   — Rings accompanied by distal deformity, with or without lymphedema
   — Rings accompanied by distal fusion; acrosyndactyly
   — Amputation

4. Management

   — Proximal ring may cause distal ischemia or nerve palsy
   — Treatment is aimed at functional and aesthetic improvement
   — Excision of ring and subcutaneous tissue combined with "Z"-plasty or "W" plasty
   — Acrosyndactyly, skin protuberances, and digital absence are commonly seen in amniotic disruption sequence and can be surgically treated

Symbrachydactyly (Figs. 9 to 12)[4]

1. Description

   — Fused and shortened fingers characterized as a pattern of digital loss
   — Presence of finger nubbins and nails distinguishes this from transverse absence

2. Etiology

   — Mesodermal defect thus explaining preservation of ectodermal structures (pulp, nail fold, and nail)

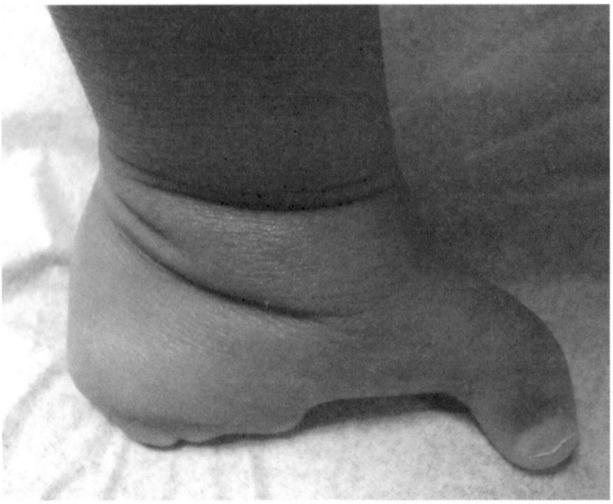

Fig. 9. Transverse arrest.

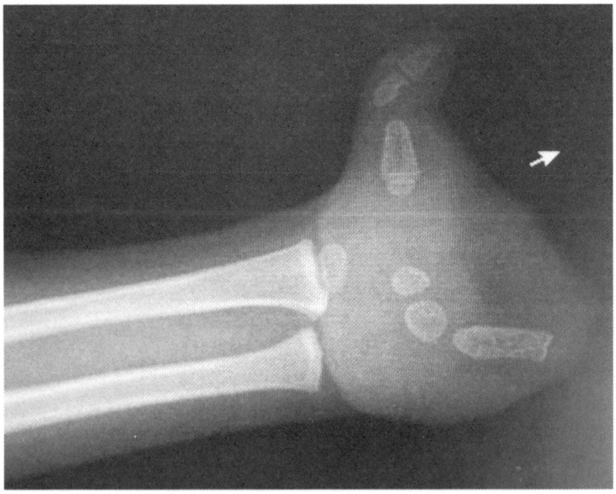

Fig. 10. Transverse arrest.

3. Clinical Features

— Spectrum of deficiency
— Progresses from short middle phalanges, to central rays, to the absence of entire hand

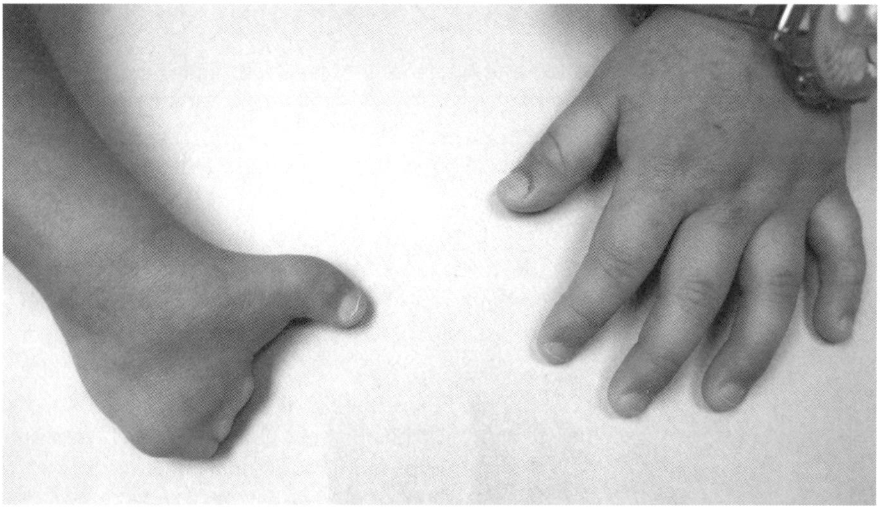

Fig. 11. Transverse arrest.

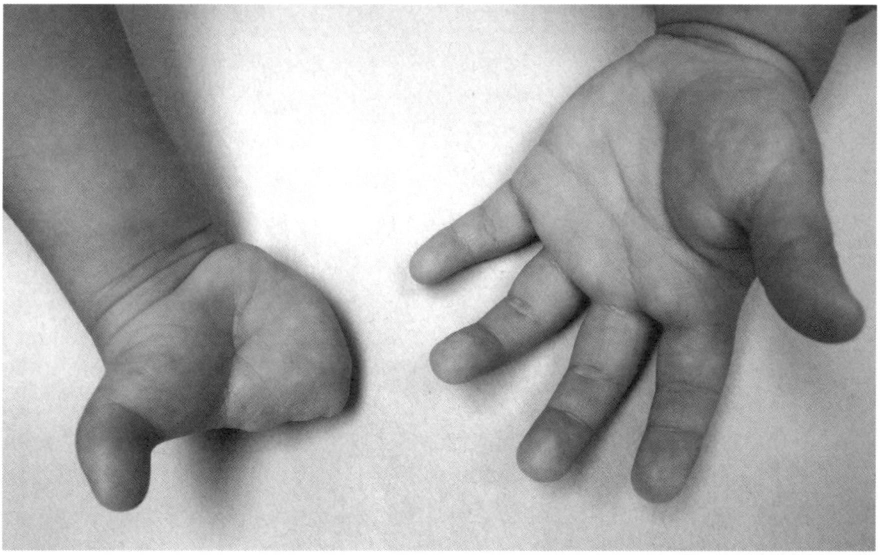

Fig. 12. Transverse arrest.

4. Classification/Management

Table 5. Classification and Management for Symbrachydactyly.

Type	Description
Short finger (Types 1, 2, 3)	Short fingers with small or absent middle phalanges. Function is maintained and surgery is rarely indicated
Oligodactylic (Type 4)	(Few Fingers) A degree of absence of central three rays. Fifth digit lacks middle phalanx but has intact MCP joint. Thumb is also variable in form
Monodactylic (Type 5)	(Single Finger) Lacks all fingers and has only a thumb. Digits present as metacarpal bases and finger nubbins. Wrist is functional
Peromelic (Type 6)	(Short Limb) Hand has only finger nubbins

Clinodactyly

1. Description
   — Curvature of a digit in a radioulnar plane
2. Epidemiology
   — 1–20% incidence
   — Associated with many syndromes and complex hand anomalies
3. Pathology
   — C-shaped epiphyseal plate forms a bracket that restricts longitudinal growth
   — Early ossification prematurely stops growth leading to the "delta phalanx"
   — The epiphyseal bracket can affect other phalanges presenting as angulation of the finger
4. Clinical Features
   — Commonly radial deviation of little finger at DIP

— Radiographic trapezoid shaped middle phalanx seen
— Rarely interferes with function and may only be cosmetic

5. Management

— Surgical correction indicated for severe deformities or with thumb involvement
— Correction requires osteotomy to realign digit or resection of longitudinal epiphyseal bracket to reduce growth potential
— For soft tissue deficit: "Z" plasty, rotational flap, or step advancement flap may be used

Kirner's Deformity

1. Description

— Progressive palmar-radial curvature skeletal deformity of distal phalanx of small finger

2. Epidemiology

— Autosomal dominant with incomplete penetrance–inheritance pattern.
— 2:1 female to male

3. Clinical Features

— Develops in late childhood or adolescence
— Initial swelling along dorsum of distal phalange
— Development of palmar-radial curvature of finger tip
— Joint motion is preserved
— Radiographic appearance varies with stage
— Consider traumatic injury to physis or physeal injury as consequence to frostbite or burns in differential

4. Management

— Deformity has little functional effect; correction not indicated
— Splinting small finger into extension has shown to relieve discomfort and prolonged splinting may correct the deformity
— Distraction lengthening may be used

Symphalangism

1. Description

   — Failure of differentiation of the interphalangeal joint

2. Clinical Features

   — No joint capsule
   — Radiographically seen as clear joint space

3. Management

   — Options: (1) arthrodesis; (2) arthroplasty

Camptodactyly

1. Description

   — Congenital flexion deformity of proximal interphalangeal joint

2. Classifications

   — Type I: Present at infancy
   — Type II: Present at adolescence or acquired
   — Type III: Syndromic

3. Clinical Features

   — Function is rarely impaired
   — Skin shortening, tight retinaculus cutis, short sublimis, abnormal lumbricals, lateral band adhesions, central slip anomalies and bony defects may be present

4. Management

   — Splinting
   — Surgical intervention only indicated in rapidly progressing deformity.
   — Skin shortage treated with Z-plasties

— Abnormal retinaculum and lateral bands are freed from phalanx
— Short sublimis is lengthened
— Abnormal lumbrical insertion is released

Macrodactyly

1. Description

   — Macrodactyly is enlargement of all elements of the digit(s)

2. Epidemiology

   — About 1% incidence

3. Classification

   — Type I: Gigantism and lipofibromatosis
   — Type II: Gigantism and neurofibromatosis
   — Type III: Gigantism and digital hyperostosis
   — Type IV: Gigantism and hemihypertrophy

4. Clinical Features

   — Present at birth or develops within first 3 years
   — Associated with lipofibromatous hamartomas
   — Multiple digits may be involved; commonly index finger
   — Static macrodactyly: enlargement at birth and grows proportionally
   — Progressive macrodactyly: increasingly disproportionate enlargement with age
   — Radiograph reveals enlarged skeleton with advanced bone age
   — Soft tissue swelling may be present on palmar aspect
   — Compression neuropathy with fatty infiltration

5. Management

   — Difficult to treat, often require multiple surgeries to remove extraneous tissues
   — Limiting digital growth: digital nerve stripping or epiphysiodesis
   — Digit reduction: Soft tissue debulking
   — Distal amputation for severe cases

Arthrogryposis

1. Description

   — Syndrome of non-progressive joint contractures present at birth
   — Multiple forms with various presentations

2. Clinical Features

   — Sporadic symmetrical positioning of limbs: shoulder abduction and internal rotation, elbow extension, forearm pronation, wrist flexion, and hand ulnar deviation
   — Digits are flexed and stiff; clasped contracted thumb

3. Management

   — Goals are individualized to each patient
   — Early treatment is passive movements and use of splints
   — Surgical management ranges across the entire upper extremity
   — Surgical treatment regarding thumb and fingers

      a. Osteotomy to realign poorly positioned fingers
      b. Clasped thumb release

Deformities of the Thumb[9,10]

Thumb Hypoplasia

1. Description

   — Represents a spectrum of deficiencies from a slightly smaller thumb to complete absence of thumb
   — Frequently part of radial deficiency
   — Systematic evaluation for syndromes: Holt-Oram, thrombocytopenia absent radius (TAR), VACTERL, Fanconi's anemia

2. Clinical Features

   — Examination varies with age of child
   — Affected neonates typically avoid using thumb when grasping
   — Inspection and palpation of thumb for size, consistency, stability, status of muscles, and stability of MCP and CMC joints
   — Presence or absence of stable CMC joint dictates retention versus ablation

3. Classification/Management

Table 6. Classification and Management of Thumb Hypoplasia.

Type	Findings	Treatment
I	Minor generalized hypoplasia	Augmentation
II	Absence of intrinsic thenar muscles First web space narrowing Ulnar collateral ligament insufficiency	Opponensplasty First web release UCL reconstruction
III	Similar as Type II Extrinsic muscle and tendon abnormalities Skeletal deficiency A: Stable CMC joint B: Unstable CMC joint	A: Reconstruction B: Pollicization
IV	Floating thumb	Pollicization
V	Absence	Pollicization

Thumb Duplication

1. Description

— Pre-axial polydactyly; supernumerary thumb

2. Epidemiology

— High prevalence in white populations

3. Classification

— Classified by degree of skeletal replication
— Defined by whether components are attached proximally (bifid) or are completely separated (duplicated)

4. Clinical Features

— Radiographs define extent of duplication
— Components are palpated for bony elements, joint stability, and motion

5. Management

— No urgency for surgery
— Reconstruction aligns thumb along a longitudinal axis, stabilizes joints, balances motor functions, provides adequate nail plate, and restores sufficient thumb size

Triphalageal Thumb

1. Description

— Thumb with an extra phalanx

2. Epidemiology

— Inherited via autosomal dominance with variable expressivity and penetrance

3. Classification

— First type: extra phalanx with variable size
— Second type: fully developed phalanx in the plane of fingers

4. Clinical Features

— Extra phalanx shape in a triphalangeal thumb: triangular, trapezoidal, or rectangular
— The growth rate of extra phalanx is variable; initial treatment consists of observation to assess growth potential

5. Management

— Small middle phalanx that causes progressive deviation requires excision with ligament reconstruction
— Larger extra phalanx requires fusion of the abnormal phalanx with an adjacent phalanx along with bone removal
— The joint with greatest motion is preserved
— Five fingered hand is treated with pollicization

Congenital Trigger Thumb[11]

1. Description

— Inablity to extend interphalangeal joint of thumb

2. Clinical Features

— Nodule palpable over flexor aspect of metacarpophalangeal joint (Notta node)
— Fixed flexion contracture of the IP joint

3. Management

— Spontaneous resolution by 1 year of age
— Surgical correction before 3 years. Division of A-1 pulley confirming full mobility of interphalangeal joint

Clasped Thumb

1. Description

— Thumb abnormalities ranging from mild deficiency of extensor mechanism to thenar muscles, web space, and soft tissues

2. Classification

Table 7. Classification of Clasped Thumb.

Type	Description
I	Supple with absence or hypoplasia of extensor mechanism
II	Complex with additional joint contracture, collateral ligament abnormality, first web space contracture, and thenar muscle abnormality
III	Associated with arthrogryposis

3. Clinical Features

— Thumb rests in flexion with extension lag
— Lag at MCP joint implies hypoplasia of extensor pollicis brevis muscle tendon unit
— Lag at the IP joint indicates concomitant deficiency of extensor pollicis longus

4. Management

— Initial treatment for children younger than 1 year of age is splinting

— Over the age of 2 or with MCP joint or thumb-index web space contracture, surgical correction is indicated
— Correct soft tissue contracture with four-flap "Z"-plasties along with tendon transfers to enhance extensor mechanism

Deformities of Wrist and Forearm[12]

Radial Deficiency

1. Description

— Wide spectrum of radial involvement presenting as radial club hand
— Shortening of forearm with radial deviation at wrist

2. Epidemiology

— 1 in 55,000 births

3. Clinical Features

— Skeleton, musculotendinous units, joints, neurovascular structures, and soft tissue involvement
— Commonly right-sided
— Radial neurovascular deficiency
— Median nerve displacement toward concavity
— Associated syndromes must be evaluated prior to surgical intervention

4. Pathology

— Radial deviation: inadequate radial support to carpus plus pull from forearm flexors

5. Classification

— Type I: Short Radius
— Type II: Hypoplastic Radius
— Type III: Partial Absence of Radius
— Type IV: Total Absence of Radius

6. Management

— Early stage: emphasize elbow flexion and ulnar deviation of wrist
— Mild Type I: splinting may be sufficient
— Type I and II: distraction lengthening recommended
— Severe Type II to IV: Repair between 6–12 months of age

a. Preoperative splinting
b. Centralization
c. Radialization

Ulnar Deficiency

1. Description

— Similar to radial deficiency, but with ulnar involvement

2. Epidemiology

— 1 in 100,000 incidence
— 4–10 times less common than radial deficiency

3. Clinical Features

— Hypoplasia of entire upper extremity
— Elbow is malformed or fused in majority
— Hands are missing digits, have syndactyly, and thumb abnormalities
— Radiographs are required to determine extent of deficiency
— Rare, unilateral, left-sided ulnar deviation
— Short, bowed radius with hypoplastic or absent ulna

4. Management

— No consensus
— Treat hand deformities for improved function by syndactyly release and reconstruction of thumb and first web space

Intercalary Deficiency — Phocomelia

1. Description

— Intervening segment of limb is absent

2. Probable Cause
   — Thalidomide use in first trimester
3. Management
   — No indication for surgery

Madelung's Deformity

1. Description
   — Excessive radial and palmar angulation of distal radius
2. Clinical Features
   — Distal ulna of affected wrist is dorsally prominent
   — Shorter forearm than normal
   — Confirmed by radiograph
3. Etiology
   — Growth disturbance of palmar and ulnar portion of distal radial physis
4. Management
   — No treatment indicated for painless deformity
   — Pain: physiolysis combined with release of Vickers ligament may improve deformity during growth
   — For skeletally mature patients:
      a. Ligament resection and dome osteotomy
      b. Radial closing wedge osteotomy and ulnar shortening
      c. Radial opening wedge osteotomy
      d. Radial osteotomy and distal ulna resection
      e. Radial osteotomy

Associated Syndromes and Disorders[13]

Apert's Syndrome

1. Description
   — Combination of craniofacial deformity of bicoronal craniosynostosis and midfacial hypoplasia with severe complex syndactyly of hands and feet

2. Apert Hand Abnormalities
   - Type 1: Thumb and little fingers are free; other digits form a central mass
   - Type 2: Only the thumb is free; there is a central digital mass with a common nail and fourth web syndactyly

Table 8. Congenital Hand Disorder Associated Syndromes and Disorders.

Congenital Disorder	Associated Syndromes
Syndactyly	Amniotic Disruption Syndrome Symbrachydactyly, Cleft Hand, Synpolydactyly, Poland Syndrome, Dystrophic Epidermolysis Bullosa, Apert's Syndrome
Central Polydactyly	Grebes' Chondrodysplasia, Synpolydactyly
Brachydactyly	Syndactyly, Clinodactyly, Symphalangism
Central Hand Deficiency	Split Hand/Split Foot, EEC (Ectrodactyly, Ectodermal dysplasia, and Cleft lip/palate), Cornelia de Lange Syndrome, Acrorenal Syndrome, Focal Dermal Hypoplasia
Kirner's Deformity	Cornelia de Lange Syndrome, Silver's Syndrome, Turner's Syndrome, Down's Syndrome
Ulnar Polydactyly	Chondroectodermal Dysplasia, Ellis van Creveld Syndrome
Macrodactyly	Neurofibromatosis (Von Recklinghausen's Disease), Hemihypertrophy
Thumb Hypoplasia	Holt-Oram Syndrome, Thrombocytopenia-Absent Radius (TAR) Syndrome, VACTERL, Fanconi's Anemia
Triphalangeal Thumb	Holt-Oram Syndrome, Fanconi's Anemia, Congenital Heart Disease
Ulnar Deficiency	Musculoskeletal Anomalies, Proximal Femoral Focal Deficiency, Fibular Deficiency, Phocomelia, Scoliosis
Madelung's Deformity	Leri-Weill Dyschondrosteosis, Nail Patella Syndrome
Radial Deficiency	Fanconi's Anemia, Thrombocytopenia Absent Radius (TAR) Syndrome, Holt-Oram Syndrome (Associated with Cardiac Septal Defects), and VATER Syndrome.

   — Type 3: Thumb and the digital mass are fused together and share a common nail

3. Management

   — Type 1 and 2:

      a. Stage 1: Thumb is properly positioned with an osteotomy to create 3 fingered hand
      b. Stage 2: Second stage separation of remaining digits

   — Type 3: Nail separation prior to syndactyly correction

References

1. Zguricas J, Bakker W, Heus H, Lindhout D, *et al.* (1998) Genetics of limb development and congenital hand malformations. *Plast Reconstr Surg* **101**(4): 1126–1135.
2. Kozin SH. (2011) Embryology of the upper extremity. In: Wolfe SW, Hotchkiss RN, Pederson WC, Kozin SH (eds.), *Green's Operative Hand Surgery*, 6th Edn. Elsevier, Philadelphia, pp. 1295–1301.
3. Bates SJ, Hansen SL, Jones NF. (2009) Reconstruction of congenital differences of the hand. *Plast Reconstr Surg* **124**(1): 128e–143e.
4. Kay SP, McCombe DB, Kozin SH. (2011) Deformities of the hand and fingers. In: Wolfe SW, Hotchkiss RN, Pederson WC, Kozin SH (eds.), *Green's Operative Hand Surgery*, 6th Edn. Elsevier, Philadelphia, pp. 1303–1369.
5. Kozin SH. (2001) Syndactyly. *J Am Soc Surg Hand* **1**: 1–13.
6. Sharma RK, Tuli P, Makkar SS, Parashar A. (2009) End-of-skin grafts in syndactyly release: description of a new flap for web space resurfacing and primary closure of finger defects. *Hand (NY)* **4**: 29–34.
7. Greuse M, Coessens BC. (2001) Congenital syndactyly: defatting facilitates closure without skin graft. *J Hand Surg Am* **26**: 589–594.
8. Kawamura K, Chung KC. (2009) Constriction band syndrome. *Hand Clin* **25**: 257–264.
9. Takashi O, Pushman AG, Chung KC. (2010) Treatment of common congenital hand conditions. *Plast Reconstr Surg* **126**(3): 121e–133e.
10. Kozin SH. (2011) Deformities of the thumb. In: Wolfe SW, Hotchkiss RN, Pederson WC, Kozin SH (eds.), *Green's Operative Hand Surgery*, 6th Edn. Elsevier, Philadelphia, pp. 1371–1403.

11. Dunsmuir RA, Sherlock DA. (2000) The outcome of treatment of trigger thumb in children. *J Bone Joint Surg Br* **82**: 736–738.
12. Bednar MS, James MA. (2011) Malformations and deformities of the wrist and forearm. In: Wolfe SW, Hotchkiss RN, Pederson WC, Kozin SH (eds.), *Green's Operative Hand Surgery*, 6th Edn. Elsevier, Philadelphia, pp. 1405–1434.
13. Panthaki ZJ, Armstrong MB. (2003) Hand abnormalities associated with craniofacial syndromes. *J Craniofac Surg* **14**(5): 709–712.

CHAPTER 19

UPPER EXTREMITY TRAUMA

Deniz Dayicioglu and Derek Ulvila

Fingernail Injuries

- Fingernail offers protection for the fingertip, imparts a counterforce against the finger pad which subsequently results in increased tactile sensation, and provides the ability to pick up small objects
- Crush injuries are the most common hand injuries seen in children
- After injury, nail growth can be blunted or absent for up to 21 days
- The entire nail bed is active in the generation and migration of the nail and can take from 70–160 days (approx. 100 days) for longitudinal growth to occur along the length of the entire nail

Physical exam	• Complete sensory, motor, and vascular exams • Check for disruption of the nail or nail border, any laceration to nail bed (linear, stellate, flap), subungual hematoma, active bleeding • Note finger position or deformity which may represent fracture, dislocation, or tendon injury • Foreign bodies (glass, metal, wood, etc.)
Imaging	• AP, lateral, and oblique x-rays of injured fingers ○ Rule out fractures, dislocations, and foreign bodies • Fifty percent of nail bed injuries will have an associate distal phalangeal fracture ○ Most commonly a comminuted tuft fracture

(*Continued*)

(*Continued*)

Injury classification	• Sublingual hematoma • Simple laceration • Stellate laceration • Severe crush • Avulsion
Treatment	• Nail intact without any disruptions of the nail or nail margins; no displaced distal phalanx fracture ○ Nonoperative – no significant difference in outcome compared to nail plate removal and primary laceration repair for patients meeting the above listed criteria ■ Observation — sufficient for most ■ Nail plate trephination to decompress subungual hematoma — utilized if patient complains of pain • Digital block using 1% lidocaine without epinephrine • Use 18 gauge needle or battery-powered microcautery (ophthalmic) unit to bore through nail plate to evacuate subungual hematoma • Irrigate • Nonadherent dressing and gauze • Finger splinted if tuft fracture present • Antibiotic prophylaxis • Disruption of the nail, nail margins, or displaced phalanx fracture ○ Operative — Simple and Stellate Lacerations ■ Informed consent ■ Digital block using 1% lidocaine without epinephrine and if deemed necessary intravenous sedation (IV sedation often useful for children) ■ Remove nail plate with iris scissors or freer elevator ○ Operative — Nail Bed Avulsions and Severe Crush Injuries ■ Digital block and exposure same as previously described

Distal Amputations

No bone exposed =	Bone exposed =
Secondary intention	Completion amputation
Primary closure	Bone shortening
Skin graft (STSG, FTSG)	Fingertip flaps

Fingertip Flaps

Dorsal Oblique Injury	Transverse Injury	Lateral Oblique Injury
Volar V-Y advancement flap (Atasoy)	Volar V-Y advancement flap (Atasoy)	Lateral pulp flap
	Bilateral lateral advancement flaps (Kutler)	Revisions amputation when >50% of phalanx amputated
	Oblique triangular neurovascular island flap	
	Hueston flap	

Volar Oblique Injury

Thumb	Index Finger	Middle Finger	Ring and Small Fingers
Volar neurovascular advancement flap (Moberg)	Volar neurovascular advancement flap (Moberg)	Thenar flap	Cross-finger flap
Pedicled littler neurovascular island flap	Oblique triangular neurovascular island flap		
First dorsal metacarpal artery flap (Kite flap)	Thenar flap		

Major Fingertip Flaps

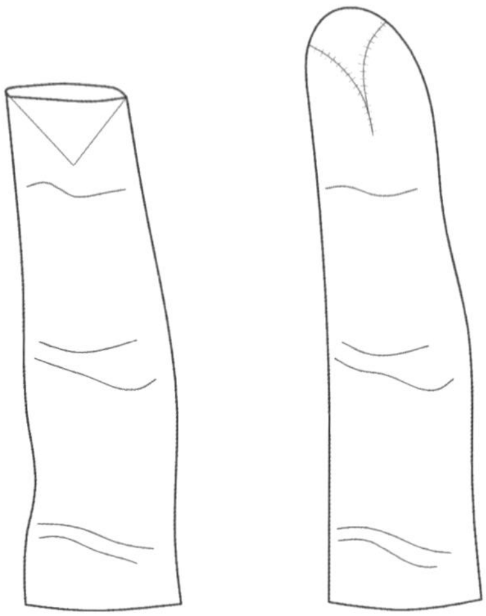

Fig. 1. Atasoy V-Y advancement flap.

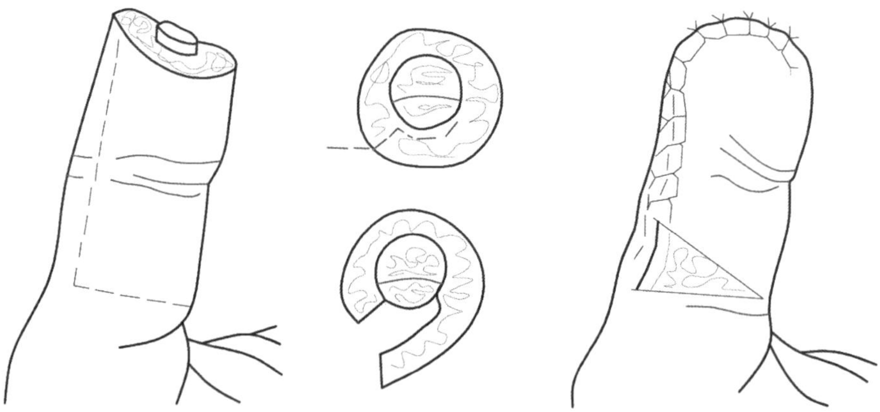

Fig. 2. Hueston flap.

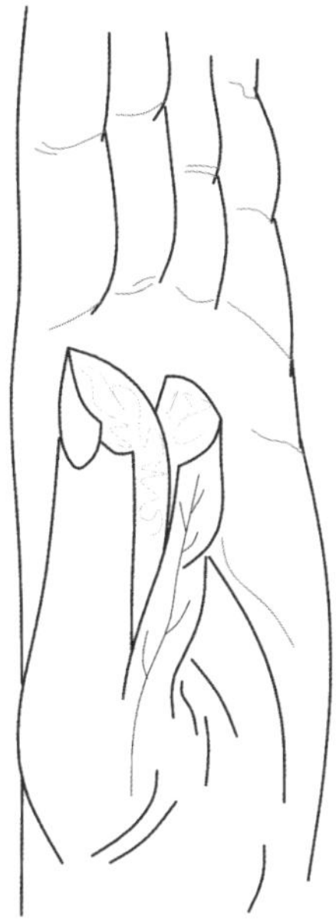

Fig. 3. Moberg flap.

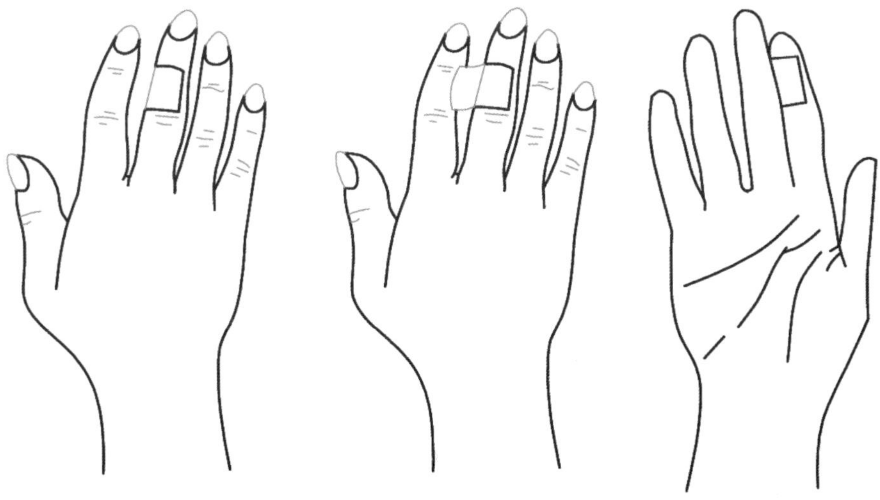

Fig. 4. Cross-finger flap.

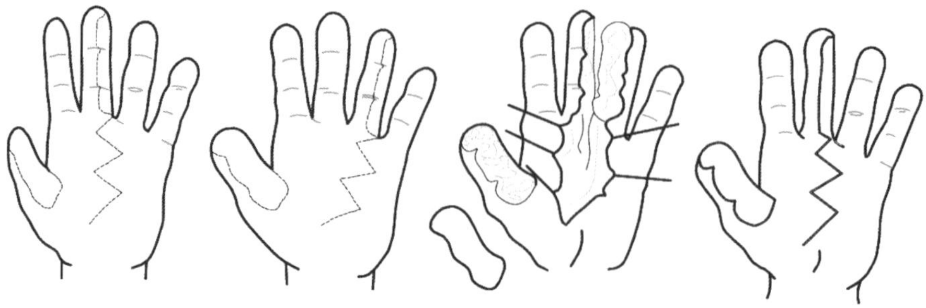

Fig. 5. Neurovascular island flap.

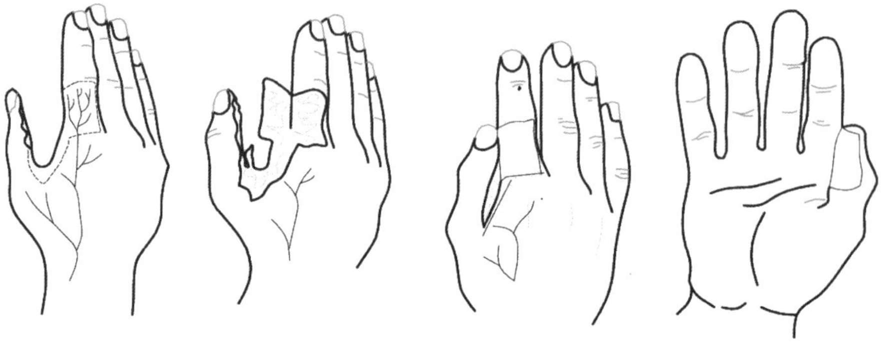

Fig. 6. First dorsal metacarpal artery flap.

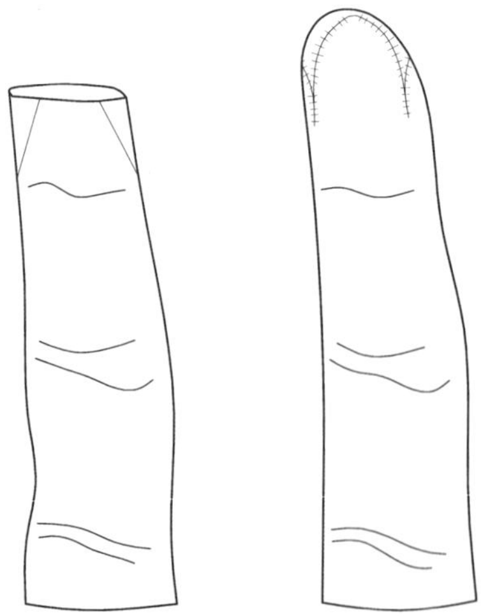

Fig. 7. Kuttler flap

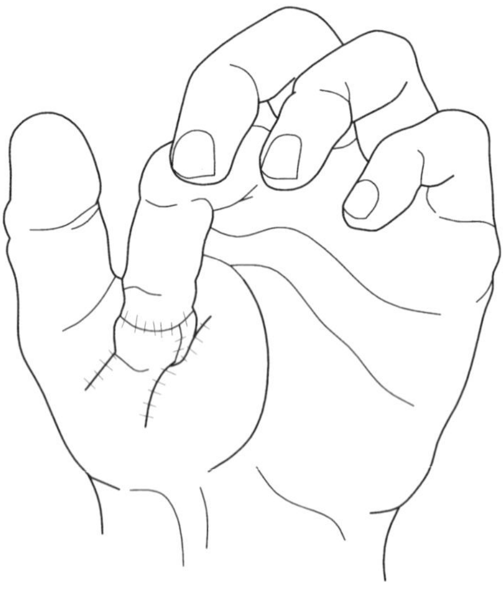

Fig. 8. Thenar flap

Flexor Tendon Injuries

- Flexor tendon injuries should be repaired in the operating room
- Best results associated with early repair
- Avoid FDP advancement (no more than 1 cm) which can lead to quadrigia effect: incomplete FDP flexion of uninjured fingers when the shortened FDP reaches maximal flexion too early
- Proper splint placement and postoperative rehabilitation are as important as operative technique

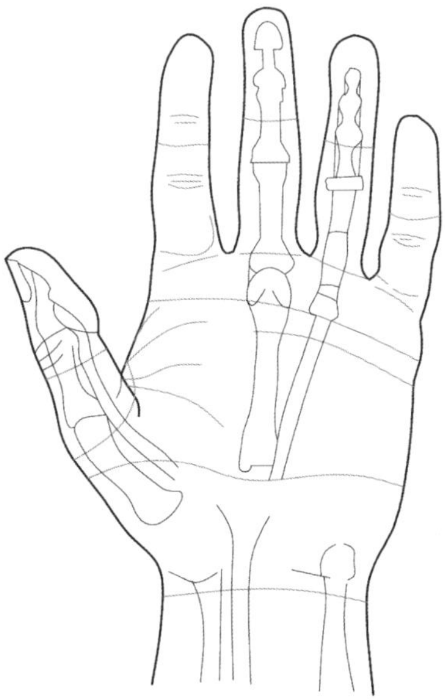

Fig. 9. Flexor tendon zones.

Zone of Injury	Treatment
Zone 1:	**Sharp Injuries:** • Repair DIP volar plate if necessary • Core sutures placed if sufficient FDP length • If distal FDP length not available, reinsert with pull-out suture tied over dorsal button or direct fixation to bone with suture anchors **Avulsion Injuries:** Forced extension during maximal FDP contraction Type 1: FDP retracts into palm; rupture of both vincula • Repair early due to lack of nutrition by vincula or synovial diffusion • Treatment same as sharp injuries Type 2: FDP with small fragment of distal phalanx and retracts to PIP; long vinculum remains intact • Pull-out suture or suture anchor Type 3: FDP with large bony fragment which prevents tendon retraction beyond A4 pulley • Open reduction and wire fixation if fragment permits • Pull-out suture secured over dorsal button Type 4: Avulsion fracture of distal phalanx combined with tendon avulsion from bony fragment with tendon retraction
Zone 2:	"No Man's Land" — due to high risk of adhesions and poor rehabilitation outcomes • Acute repair recommended • Repair of both FDP and FDS recommended • 4-6 core strands of 3–0 or 4–0 nonabsorbable suture Improved strength and gliding are added with epitendinous suture of running 5–0 or 6–0 monofilament polypropylene
Zone 3:	Repair same as zone 2 • Prognosis better for zone 3 • Examine for common digital nerve injury
Zone 4:	Repair same as for zone 2 • Examine for median nerve injury Repair transverse carpal ligament following tendon repair to prevent bowstringing
Zone 5:	Repair same as for zone 2 but epitendinous sutures not necessary

Extensor Tendon Injuries

- Nine extensor tendon zones of injury. Odd zones are over joints and even zones are over bones.

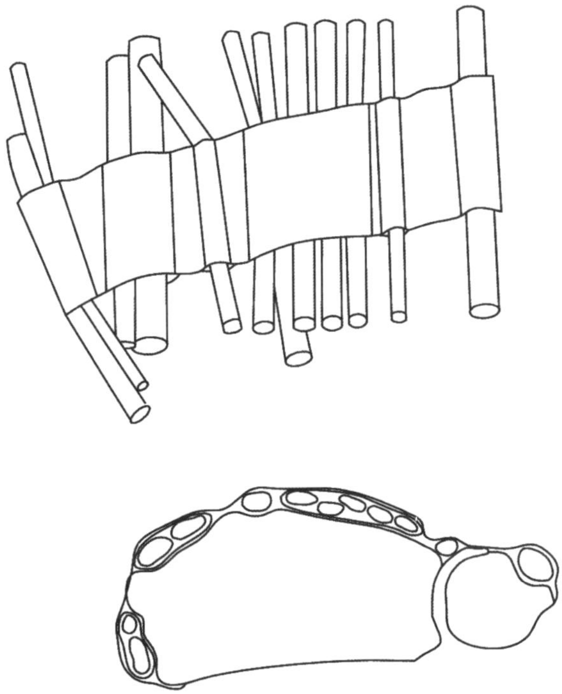

Fig. 10. Extansor Tendon Compartments.

Zone of Injury	Treatment
Zone 1 (Over DIPJ): Mallet finger deformities	Type 1: Closed rupture of tendon at insertion • Immobilization of DIP joint only in full extension for 6 weeks Type 2: Laceration with loss of tendon continuity • Repair with running monofilament suture incorporating skin and tendon, remove suture after 10-14 days, splint as for type 1 Type 3: Abrasion with soft tissue injury and tendon loss • Tendon graft or joint fusion as well as soft tissue coverage (typically requires flap) Type 4: Avulsion fracture • Closed reduction and percutaneous K-wire fixation, if possible • Open reduction with transarticular K-wire and pull-out suture or fracture fragment fixation **Splint as for type 1 followed by removal of K-wires
Zone 2 (Over middle phalanx):	Partial Lacerations: Less than 50% of tendon substance • Conservative treatment — wound care or provide closure, tendon repair not required • DIP splinted in extension until 14 days when sutures are removed at which time active and gentle passive motion begun Lacerations greater than 50% of tendon substance • Repair tendon with running suture, followed by epitendious cross-stitch • Splint DIP joint in full extension for 6 weeks
Zone 3 (Over PIPJ): Untreated Zone 3 injuries can lead to Boutonniere deformity	Closed Injuries: Often represents avulsion of central slip from attachment • Splint PIP joint in extension with DIP joint freely movable for 8 weeks ○ At 3 weeks, switch to spring loaded splint allowing for active flexion and passive extension for remaining 5 weeks

	○ For weeks 8 to 11, switch to night splinting and begin active/passive range-of-motion exercises • In addition, If central slip avulsed with bony fragment from middle phalanx with volar subluxation of joint, treat operatively ○ Dorsal approach with anatomic reduction and fixation. If bony fragment too small, place micro bone anchors into dorsal middle phalanx Lacerations: • Primarily repaired followed by splinting of PIP joint in extension with DIP join freely movable for 8 weeks ○ At 3 weeks, switch to spring loaded splint allowing for active flexion and passive extension for remaining 5 weeks ○ For weeks 8 to 11, switch to night splinting and begin active/passive range-of-motion exercises
Zone 4 (Over proximal phalanx):	Partial Lacerations: Less than 50% of tendon substance • Conservative treatment — wound care or provide closure, tendon repair not required • Range-of-motion exercises begun after wound healed Lacerations greater than 50% of tendon substance • Repair tendon with figure-of-eight sutures • Early, active range-of-motion protocols may be instituted to minimize need for secondary tenolysis
Zone 5 (Over MCP joint): Human bites commonly occur over zone 5 as a result of striking someone in the mouth with a closed fist	Partial Lacerations: Less than 50% of tendon substance • Explore MCP joint because joint involvement is common • Thoroughly irrigate, leave contaminated tendon laceration unrepaired because tendon does not retract at this level • Institute splinting regimen • Provide appropriate antibiotic prophylaxis pending wound culture results

(*Continued*)

Zone of Injury	Treatment
	Lacerations greater than 50% of tendon substance • Should be repaired and inspected for sagittal band involvement ○ Unrepaired sagittal band lacerations will lead to subluxation of the tendon over the MCP joint and loss of effective joint excursion Sagittal Band Injury: Pain & swelling over MCP joint, patient often describes "snapping" and "locking" with active extension, unable to fully extend MCP joint, once passively extended able to hold finger in full extension • Closed Sagittal Band Injury: ○ Acute (less than 2 weeks): ▪ Splint MCP joint in full extension for 3 weeks with PIP joint free ▪ After 3 weeks, remove the splint several times a day for active MCP joint flexion and passive extension ○ Late (greater than 2 weeks) ▪ Primary repair or use of surrounding tendon tissue • Open Sagittal Band Injury: ○ Primary repair, careful to restore correct length to prevent imbalance
Zone 6 (Over metacarpal bones):	Tendons in zone 6 have a more cord-like structure similar to flexor tendons • Repair with core sutures and epitenon sutures ○ Careful attention must be given to tendon length because abnormal tension in one finger may affect the flexion-extension arc of other fingers, via junctureae tendineae ○ However, junctureae tendineae allow for easier tendon retrieval because the tendon ends rarely retract

- Splint with static volar splint with wrist in 30 degrees of extension, MCP joints in 0–15 degrees of flexion, and IP joints in full extension. Wrist extension provides majority of "unloading" of tension off the repair
    - Patient may begin passive hyperextension of MCP joints
    - Between 3–6 weeks, change to dynamic splint during day, static splint at night
    - Between 6–8 weeks, may begin rehab exercises
    - Between 8–12 weeks, wean from splints

Zone 7 (Involve extensor retinaculum): At this level, often many tendons are involved. Carefully identify correct distal and proximal ends

- Repair with core sutures and epitenon sutures
- After repair of tendons, the extensor retinaculum directly overlying the repair should be released to prevent postoperative adhesion formation
    - Portions of the distal and proximal extensor retinaculum should be left intact to prevent bowstringing
- Splint as for zone 6

**Fractures of the distal radius may cause rupture of the extensor tendons in zone 7, these injuries should be ruled out when evaluating these fractures

Zone 8 (Proximal to extensor retinaculum): Carefully identify correct distal and proximal ends

- Repair with core or figure-of-eight sutures
- Splint as for zone 6

Zone 9 (Through extensor muscle substance): Injuries through extensor muscle substance with denervation of muscle distal to the injury. Therefore, return of function after primary repair may be limited.

- Muscle fascia should be directly approximated with figure-of-eight sutures
- Splint as for zone 6

Thumb Extensor Tendon Injuries

Zone of Injury	Treatment
Zone T1 (Over DIPJ): Mallet thumb	Closed injury: • Splint in extension for 6 weeks Open injury: • Primary repair • Splint in extension for 6 weeks
Zone T2 (Over proximal phalanx):	• Primary repair, EPL can usually hold core suture, add epitendinous suture • Splint IP joint for 6 weeks
Zone T3 (Over MCP joint):	Possible injury to either EPL, EPB or both • Primary repair with core sutures • Splint wrist in 30 degrees of extension, IP and MCP joints in extension for 3 weeks
Zone T4 (Over metacarpal):	• Repair same as for zone 3
Zone T5 (Over metacarpal-carpal joint)	Possible injury to either APL, EPB, or both • Repair same as for zone 3 ○ May have concomitant injury to superficial radial nerve or radial artery

Swan Neck Deformity	Flexion of the DIP joint + Hyperextension of the PIP joint Extensor tendon imbalance = Lateral bands contract dorsal to PIP joint Etiology: Untreated mallet finger, congenital or traumatic volar plate laxity
Treatment	Make sure joints are functional — If not arthrodesis If functional joints- • Correct mallet finger • PIP volar plate laxity tenodesis (free tendon graft or FDS rerouting) Splinting and Occupational Therapy after surgery
Boutonierre Deformity	Hyperextension of the DIP joint + Flexion of the PIP joint Etiology: Disruption of the central slip from the base of the middle phalanx Trauma or arthritis
Treatment Conservative	Static extension splinting of PIP with leaving DIP free

(*Continued*)

(*Continued*)

Treatment Operative	When conservative treatment fails Fowler procedure: Release of the extensor mechanism is divided at the junction of proximal and middle thirds on the middle phalanx Littler procedure: Division of the lateral bands dorsally and shifted dorsally, sutured together on the dorsum to the central tendon

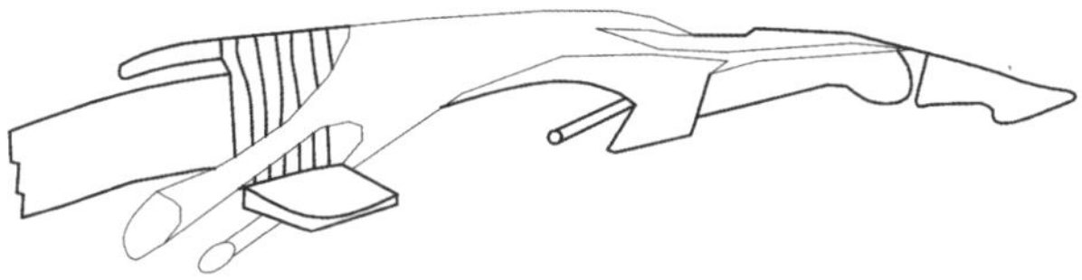

Fig. 11. Extensor apparatus.

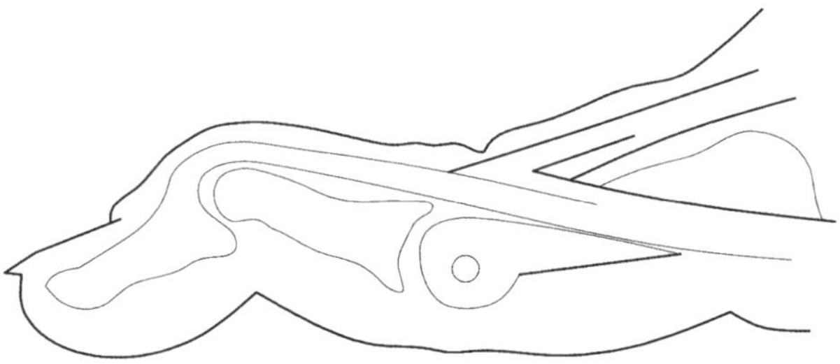

Fig. 12. Swan neck deformity.

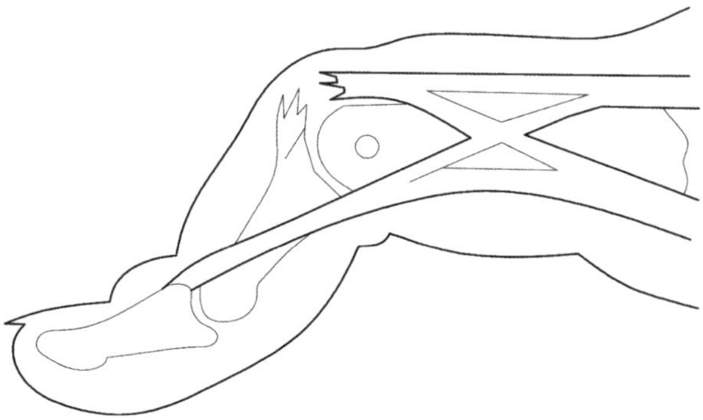

Fig. 13. Boutonierre deformity.

Fractures, Dislocations

Fracture	Treatment

Distal phalanx	Evaluate for associated nailbed injury
	• Tuft
	  ○ Most treated closed with splinting of DIP joint, begin DIP joint motion after 3–4 weeks
	  ○ ORIF
	• Shaft
	  ○ Nondisplaced
	    ▪ Splint DIP joint for 3–4 weeks
	  ○ Displaced
	    ▪ K-wire fixation — single axial K-wire transfixing DIP joint in extension for 4 weeks
	• Base
	  ○ Avulsion of extensor tendon with one-third to one-half of articular surface displaced and/or volar subluxation of the distal phalanx
	    ▪ Treat like Type 4, Zone 1 extensor tendon injury

Middle and proximal phalanx	• Condylar
	  ○ Nondisplaced
	    ▪ Treated closed with extension splinting
	  ○ Displaced — displacement may occur early or late
	    ▪ Unicondylar
	      • If possible, may treat closed with at least two k-wires (due deforming forces from collateral ligaments)
	      • ORIF — midaxial incision, fixation with 1.0–1.2 mm screw, K-wires, or both
	    ▪ Bicondylar
	      • Inherently too unstable for closed reduction
	      • ORIF — dorsal approach between central slip and lateral band to preserve central slip
	        ○ Short oblique intercondylar and shaft fracture pattern — may use lag screws
	        ○ Transverse fracture pattern at condylar shaft interface — may use oblique K-wire or 1.3 mm T plate

(*Continued*)

(*Continued*)

Fracture	**Treatment**
	• Shaft ○ Nonoperative — stable fracture without rotational deformity ■ Buddy taping to adjacent uninjured finger ■ Intrinsic plus position (includes all fingers) — finger MCP joints placed in flexion with IP joints in extension in a well-moled cast ○ Operative — rotational deformity and/or unstable fracture ■ Tranverse or short oblique fracture • Percutaneous crossed K-wire fixation ■ Long oblique fracture • Interfragmentary screw fixation ■ Comminuted fracture or fracture with severe bone loss • Plating — with early protected motion ■ Open fracture • External fixation • Plating — with early protected motion • Base ○ Extra-articular ■ Stable without rotional deformity • Closed reduction with casting of MCP joints in 70 degrees of flexion with PIP joints in neutral ■ Rotational deformity • ORIF using dorsal approach with excision of sagital band — small cortical screws, K-wires, interrosseous wires ○ Intra-articular ■ Nondisplaced • Closed reduction with casting of MCP joints in 70 degrees of flexion with PIP joints in neutral • If oblique fracture pattern, must stabilize with percutaneous fixation even if nondisplaced ■ Displaced • ORIF using dorsal approach with excision of sagital band and capsulotomy — small cortical screws, K-wires, interrosseous wires • External fixation may be required for more complex fracture patterns

(*Continued*)

(*Continued*)

Fracture	Treatment
Metacarpal	• Head — uncommon, can be associated with collateral ligament injury ○ Nonoperative — nondisplaced, less than 20% of articular surface ▪ Immobilization ○ Operative — greater than 1 mm displacement of intra-articular fracture or greater than 20% of articular surface ▪ ORIF • Neck — common, apex dorsal angulation ○ Closed reduction — use hematoma block or local anesthesia ▪ Indications: • Index and middle fingers — angulation greater than 15 – 30 degrees • Ring and small fingers — angulation greater than 40–70 degrees, can tolerate more angulation due to mobility at the corresponding CMC joints • Any rotational deformity ("scissoring") — upon flexion, digits overlap **Increased fracture angulation is associated with protrusion of metacarpal head into the palm ▪ Jahss Maneuver — flexion of MCP and PIP joints to 90 degrees to relax intrinsic muscles and tighten collateral ligaments, apply upward pressure at PIP joint and downward pressure on metacarpal proximal to fracture ▪ Splint with MCP joint in 90 degrees flexion and PIP joint in extension • May use gutter splint for ring or small finger fractures • If unstable, may use crossed K-wires or transverse K-wires into adjacent uninjured metacarpal proximal and distal to fracture site ○ Open reduction — unacceptable closed reduction or open fractures ▪ Dorsal approach with use of K-wires, plates, or intramedullary nails ▪ Splint as for closed reduction

(*Continued*)

(*Continued*)

Fracture	Treatment
	**Boxer's Fracture — small finger metacarpal neck fracture resulting from a blow to the distal-dorsal aspect of a closed fist such as when punching. Loss of the metacarpal head prominence is often seen. ⇒ Be aware of possible MCP joint contamination via a "fight bite" — skin laceration with possible joint involvement from collision of closed fist with teeth • Shaft **Acceptable angulation and shortening post-reduction ⇒ Index and middle fingers = less than 15 degrees ⇒ Ring and small fingers = less than 40 degrees, can tolerate more angulation due to mobility at the corresponding CMC joints ⇒ More than 5 mm shortening may affect extensor mechanism ○ Closed reduction ■ Transverse fracture • Percutaneous medullary nails or K-wires ■ Short oblique fracture • Intramedullary nails or crossed K-wires with longitudinal wire post reduction • Transverse K-wires into adjacent uninjured metacarpal can be use to stabilize fractures of border digits ■ Comminuted • External fixation or transverse K-wires to maintain length ○ Open reduction ■ Multiple transverse fractures ■ Short oblique fracture • Dorsal approach either centered over injured metacarpal or in the intermetacarpal space when adjacent fractures present • 2.0 or 2.4 mm plates

(*Continued*)

(*Continued*)

Fracture	Treatment
	■ Long oblique fracture • Plate fixation as described for short oblique with compression screws • Fixation screws — may be used if length of fracture twice the diameter of metacarpal • Base ○ Extra-articular ■ Closed reduction • If reduction not maintained, K-wire fixation ■ Open reduction • Plate or K-wire fixation ○ Intra-articular ■ Closed reduction — less than 20% articular surface • Splint wrist in extension ■ Open reduction — greater than 20% articular surface • K-wires, T or Y miniplate ****Bennett's Fracture** — Oblique intra-articular fracture from the volar-ulnar metacarpal base of the thumb. The volar oblique ligament holds the fracture fragment in anatomic position. With fracture at this site the distal metacarpal fragment is displaced dorsally and radially by the pull of the abductor pollicis longus. ⇒ Closed reduction — longitudinal traction and pressure on metacarpal base with pronation, stabilize with transarticular K-wire from thumb metacarpal to trapezium or second metacarpal ⇒ If unacceptable reduction (greater than 1 mm articular step-off), ORIF with K-wires, screw, or plate fixation. Radial approach between abductor pollicis and thenar muscles ⇒ Thumb immobilized in thumb spica cast for 4 weeks

(*Continued*)

(*Continued*)

Fracture	Treatment
	****Rolando Fracture** — Comminuted fracture of the thumb metacarpal base with at least 3 fracture fragments. Classic Rolando fracture is T or Y shaped with 3 fragments. Goal of treatment to restore articular surface and metacarpal length. ⇒ ORIF with condylar T or Y plate, K-wires, interosseous wiring ⇒ External fixation for severely comminuted fractures ****Reverse Bennett's Fracture** ("Baby Bennett") — Oblique intra-articular fracture from the volar-ulnar metacarpal base of the thumb. The volar oblique ligament holds the fracture fragment in anatomic position. With fracture at this site the distal metacarpal fragment is displaced dorsally and radially by the pull of the abductor pollicis longus. ⇒ Closed reduction — I

Scaphoid Fracture	
Physical exam	• Anatomical snuffbox tenderness
Imaging	• CT • MRI: To evaluate the vascularity of the proximal pole
Injury classification	• Herbert classification Type A: Incomplete, A1 stable fracture through the waist or A2 through the tubercle Type B: B1 Distal oblique fracture, B2 displaced fracture through the waist, B3 proximal pole fracture, B4 transscaphoid perilunate fracture dislocation Type C: Delayed union Type D: Established nonunion D1: Fibrous union, D2: Pseudoarthrosis

(*Continued*)

Scaphoid Fracture (*Continued*)	
Treatment	• Stable undisplaced fractures = • Short arm cast — longarm cast 3–6 months. • Instead of long term casting operative treatment could be advisable Unstable fractures, stable fractures where longterm casting is not wanted = Dorsal approach Volar approach Novel techniques: Bone grafting, Herbert screw

Gamekeeper's thumb, Skier's thumb	• Torn ulnar collateral ligament of thumb MCP, MCP joint dislocation
Physical exam	• Compare with the uninjured hand
Imaging	• Plain radiographs: May show volar subluxation • MRI: For identifying Stener lesion for complete ligamentous disruption
Injury classification	• Complete or partial tears
Treatment	• Partial tears: Immobilise for 6 weeks in thumb spica cast • Complete tears: Direct repair, anchor suture, pull out suture, bony fixation if avulsion fracture is present

Distal Radius Fractures	
Physical exam	• Soft tissue injuries • Neurovascular exam • EPL • Other bone injuries (carpal, humeral, elbow)
Imaging	• Radial length (11 mm) • Radial inclination (22 degrees) • Palmar tilt (11 degrees) • Intra-articular step off • Ulnar variance • Dorsal comminution • Carpal fractures • Ulnar styloid fracture • Ulnar shaft or head fracture

(*Continued*)

Distal Radius Fractures (*Continued*)

Injury classification	• Multiple classification systems available Extra-intraarticular Stable-unstable Displaced-undisplaced Reducible-irreducible Unstable fracture: La Fontaine criteria (3 or more findings: unstable following closed reduction and plaster) • Associated distal ulnar fracture • Age more than 60 • Dorsal metaphyseal comminution • Intra-articular radiocarpal fracture • Initial dorsal angulation more than 20 • Shortening more than 5 mm • Dsiplacement of more than 2/3 of the width of the shaft
Treatment	Closed reduction and casting Operative treatment
Closed reduction and casting: Nondisplaced fractures Displaced, reducable fractures with acceptable alignment	
Operative treatment: Unstable fractures	Closed reduction and percutaneous pinning (CRPP) Bridging external fixation Nonbridging external fixation Internal distraction bridge plating Arthroscopically assisted reduction and fixation Open reduction and internal fixation (ORIF) ORIF and external fixation
Closed reduction and casting complications: Soft tissue necrosis Stiffness Median nerve injury EPL rupture Malunion	*Operative treatment complications:* Infection Pin tract infection Implant failure

(*Continued*)

Distal Radius Fractures (*Continued*)

Tendon rupture
Extensor tendon irritation
Superficial radial nerve injury

Complications of operative and nonoperative treatment:
Complex regional pain syndrome
Nonunion
Arthritis
Compartment syndrome
DRUJ disorders

Associated injuries:
DRUJ
Ulnar styloid fractures
Scaphoid fractures
Median nerve injury
Ulnar head fracture

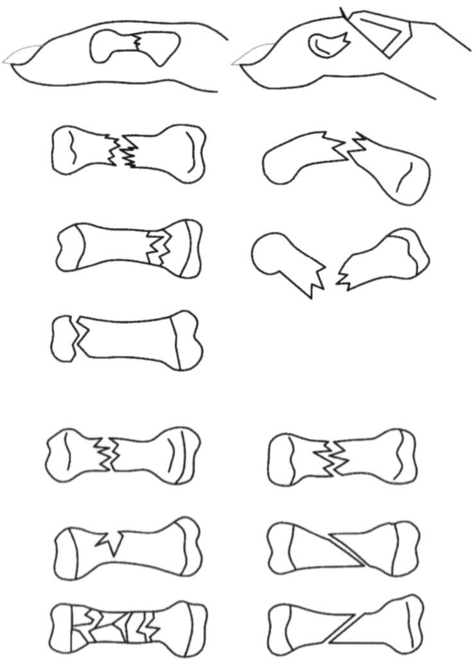

Fig. 14. Different types of phalangeal fractures.

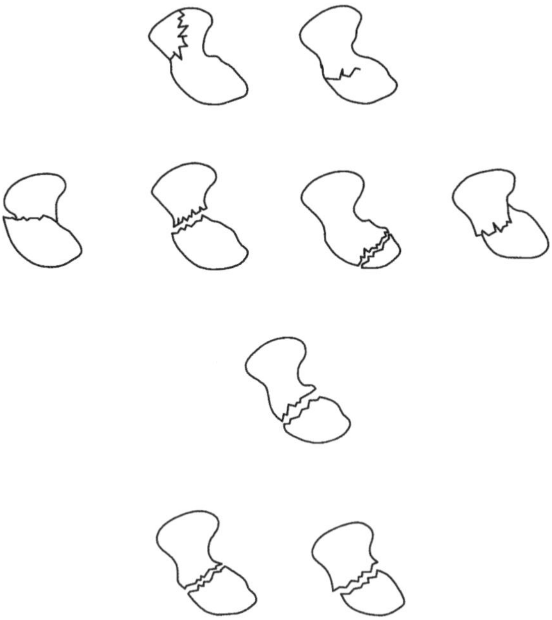

Fig. 15 Herbert classification of scaphoid fractures.

Replantation

- Replantation is the restoration of an amputated part of the upper extremity
- The goal is not the survival of the amputated finger but rather improving long term function and appearance with preservation of quality of life
- Consultation with a hand surgeon is important to determine whether a replantation should be performed
- Replantation determined on individual basis involving patient age, occupation, co-morbidities, mechanism of injury, level of amputation, status of amputated part
    - Ideal patient is young without any co-morbidities having sustained a sharp guillotine-type amputation with minimal tissue destruction and contamination
- Final judgement should not be made until microscopic evaluation of vessels

<table>
<tr><td>Indications:</td><td>• Thumb amputations
• Multiple finger amputations
• Any amputation in a child
• Amputation at the level of the palm, wrist, forearm, upper arm
• Single digit amputations distal to FDS insertion</td></tr>
<tr><td>Contraindications:</td><td>• Significant life-threatening associated injuries
• Co-morbidities precluding prolonged operative time or general anesthesia
• Excessive ischemia time
○ Proximal replantation — muscle ischemia limiting factor
■ Greater than 6 hours warm ischemia time
■ Greater than 12 hours cold ischemia time
○ Digital replantation
■ Greater than 12 hours warm ischemia time
■ Greater than 24 hours cold ischemia time
**Note: Longer times have been reported to be successful
• Crush or avulsion injuries
• Amputated part with multiple levels of injury
• Extensive contamination: often involved in farm or industrial injuries (e.g. oil or grease)
○ Poses risk of infection or sepsis
• Psychologic problems: self-inflicted amputations
• Single-digit amputations in flexor tendon zone 2
○ Digital motion impaired secondary to flexor tendon adhesions associated with zone 2 repairs
○ Replantation of index finger unrewarding, brain excludes index finger and uses middle finger to pinch with thumb
○ Replantation of single middle, ring, or small fingers may interfere with other 2 fingers because of common FDP tendons</td></tr>
<tr><td>Young patients</td><td>• Better overall functional outcome
• Plasticity and regeneration potential are greater
• The digit will continue to grow
• Children technically more demanding due to small caliber of vessels and increased vasospasm</td></tr>
</table>

(*Continued*)

(*Continued*)

Older patients:	• The recovery of tendon and nerve function usually poorer • Added risk of producing stiffness in the uninjured fingers • Atherosclerosis may complicate outcome of vascular anastomoses
Management:	• Use pressure dressing to stop bleeding and tourniquet for upper arm injuries, do not use vessel clamps which can cause vessel injury and decrease final usable vessel length • Amputated part should be wrapped in moist gauze, placed in plastic container, then container placed on ice ○ Avoid direct contact of amputated part with ice which may lead to frostbite compromising a successful replantation • Radiographs of both proximal and amputated parts • Debridement and irrigation of both proximal and amputated parts ○ All foreign material must be removed prior to replantation • Reperfusion is the utmost priority for upper arm and forearm amputation to prevent muscle ischemia ○ Temporary vascular shunts may be useful
Order of repair and operative technique	• Tourniquet should be applied to upper arm at beginning of procedure • Identification of involved structures ○ Meticulous exploration, debridement, irrigation, identification and tagging of all vital structures ○ Assess vessel damage ○ Normal vessel — pearly gray with no petechiae ○ Ribbon sign ("corkscrew") — tortuous appearing vessel caused by stretch and torsion of the vessel ▪ Red-line sign — red streak (multiple hemorrhages) along vessel, implying distal vessel damage **Red-line sign and ribbon sign are poor prognostic indicators

(*Continued*)

(*Continued*)

- Spurt test — must have strong head pressure
- Patency test — milk vessel to check back-bleeding and inflow patency

  - Preserve all amputated but nonreplantable tissue as it may be considered for use in the reconstruction as sources of free nerve, vessel, tendon, bone, or skin grafts
- Bony fixation
  - Anatomic bone stabilization is key
  - Methods of fixation:
    - K-wires
    - 90-90 interosseous wiring
    - Dorsal or lateral miniplates
    - Lag screws
    - Intramedullary implants
- Extensor and flexor tendon repair
  - Usually repaired next because range-of-motion to allow tendon apposition may disrupt microvascular repair
  - Flexor tendons may have retracted and require retrieval
- Nerve repairs
  - Primary nerve repair
  - Primary nerve grafting
    - Nerve graft donor sites
      - Terminal branch of posterior interosseous
      - Antebrachial cutaneous nerves
      - Sural nerve
  - Tag nerve ends for secondary repair
- Arterial anastomoses
  - If signs of vessel damage, cut back vessel to healthy intimal level
  - Avoid tension on anastomoses
  - If tension-free vascular repair cannot be accomplished use:
    - Bone shortening
    - Vein grafts
      - Donor sites: forearm, dorsum of foot, leg
  - For digits, both arteries should be repaired, however, most will survive with one good artery

(*Continued*)

(*Continued*)

- The thumb ulnar artery is usually the largest and most commonly repaired
  - Use xylocaine or papaverine solution for vasospasm
- Venous anastomoses
  - Repair similar to arteries
  - Use vein grafts when needed
  - Use at least 2 veins to avoid venous congestion
    - Dorsal veins are larger and don't impede repair of volar structures
  - Use arteriovenous fistula when venous outflow in distal amputations is not possible
  - In case of venous insufficiency, may use heparinize gauze or leeches to improve venous outflow

**Note: Nerve, arterial, and venous repairs often are done in different orders depending on the level of amputation and physician preference.

- ➢ For proximal replantations where muscle ischemia is critical, vascular repair should be performed after bony fixation to prevent muscle necrosis
- ➢ Some may perform the arterial anastomoses, then repair nerves to allow toxic metabolites to be flushed out before repairing venous anastomoses
  - ➢ If venous repair after arterial repair, reperfusing arterial anastomoses will fill digital veins allowing for easier identification

- Closure
  - Hemostasis is essential to avoid a hematoma that could press on the vascular anastomoses and compromise blood supply to replanted tissue
  - If proximal amputation, decompressive fasciotomies are indicated to prevent compartment syndrome due to muscle swelling after reperfusion
    - Fasciotomies are not required for digital replants
  - Skin closures should be loose, use skin grafting or local flaps if needed

(*Continued*)

(*Continued*)

	• Dressing ○ Antibiotic ointment ○ Petroleum-impregnated gauze placed over incisions with fluffy/bulky dressing ■ Avoid circumferential placement ○ Protective splinting ○ Maintain access to fingertips for postoperative monitoring
Postoperative Care	• Monitoring ○ Clinical ■ Color ■ Capillary refill ■ Temperature ■ Bleeding ■ Turgor ○ Doppler ■ Surface ■ Implantable ○ Pulse oximeter ○ Temperature probes • Pharmacologic ○ Antibiotics ○ Heparin, LMWH ○ Dextran ○ Aspirin ○ Leeches (Hirudin) ■ Infection with *Aeromonas hydrophila* secondary to leech usage may occur, provide prophylaxis with 3rd generation cephalosporin, quinolones (not recommended for children), or bactrim • Warm ambient temperature and extremity temperature • Adequate IV hydration • Smoking cessation • Outpatient rehabilitation

Acknowledgments

Authors would like to thank Ceren Dayicioglu Isil for medical illustrations.

Further Reading

1. Morrison WA. (2007) Digital replantation. *Hand Clin* **23**(1): 1–12.
2. Hanel DP, Chin SH. (2007) Wrist level and proimal upper extremity replantation. *Hand Clin* **23**: 13–21.
3. Mullett H, Hausman M. (2006) Fractures and ligamentous injuries of the wrist In: Thorne CH, *et al.* (eds.), *Grabb and Smith's Plastic Surgery*. Lippincott William and Wilkins, New York, pp. 782–789.
4. Friedman DW, Kells AMY, Aviles A. (2006) Fractures, dislocations and ligamentous injuries of the hand. In: Thorne CH, *et al.* (eds.), *Grabb and Smith's Plastic Surgery*. Lippincott William and Wilkins, New York, pp. 790–809.
5. CME/Moc (2008): *Plastic and Reconstructive Surgery* (Hand) **121**(4): 1–12.
6. Extensor tendon CME (2009): /Moc: *Plastic and Reconstructive Surgery* (Hand) **123**(2): 52–57.
7. Extensor tendon CME (2008): /Moc: *Plastic and Reconstructive Surgery* (Hand) **121**(3): 109–120.
8. Metacarpal fractures CME (2008): /Moc: *Plastic and Reconstructive Surgery* (Hand) **121**(15): 1–13.
9. Wrist injuries CME (2007): /Moc: *Plastic and Reconstructive Surgery* (Hand) **120**(5): 73–89.

CHAPTER 20

DUPUYTREN'S DISEASE

Sara Yegiyants and Zubin J. Panthaki

Illustrative Case

52 year old right hand dominant man with several years history of right small and ring finger flexion contractures, palmar nodules and cords, and worsening function with time. On examination has positive table top test.

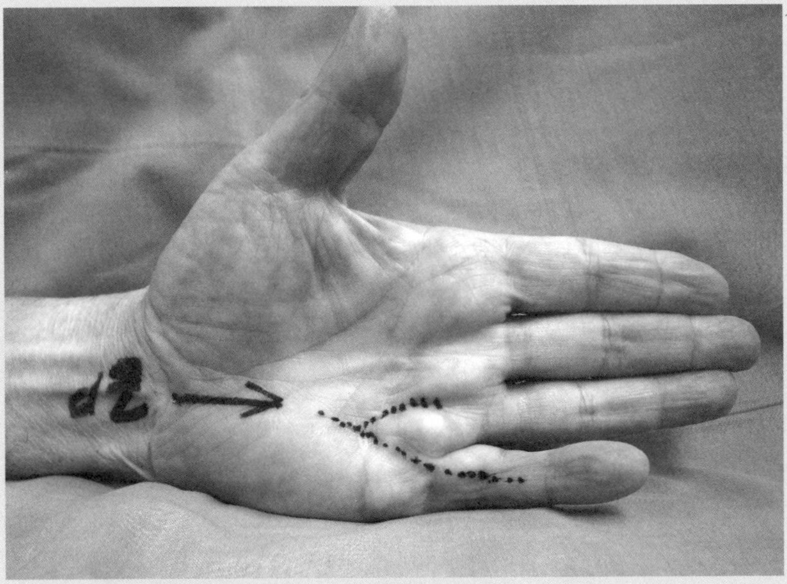

Operative technique: Palmar fasciectomy

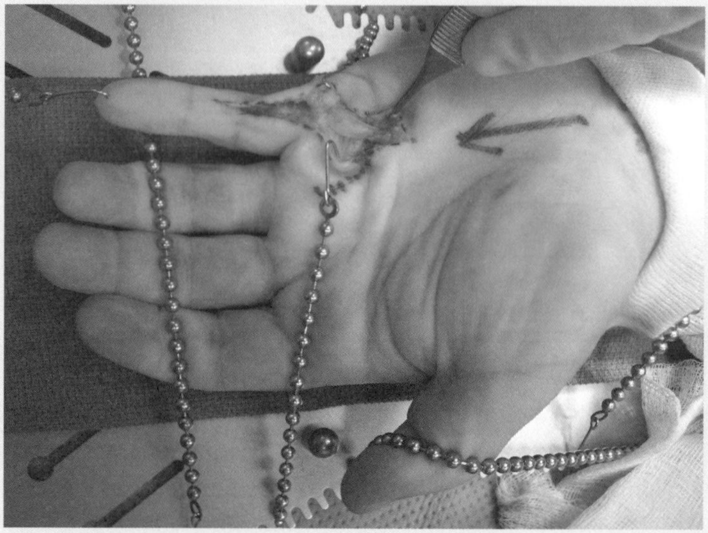

Variety of incisions can be employed
Dissection is began proximal in normal tissue
Neurovascular structures are identified and protected

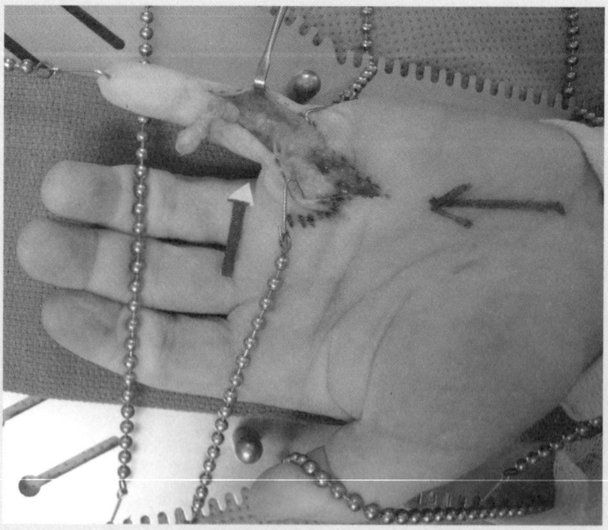

Diseased cords are divided proximally and dissected distally

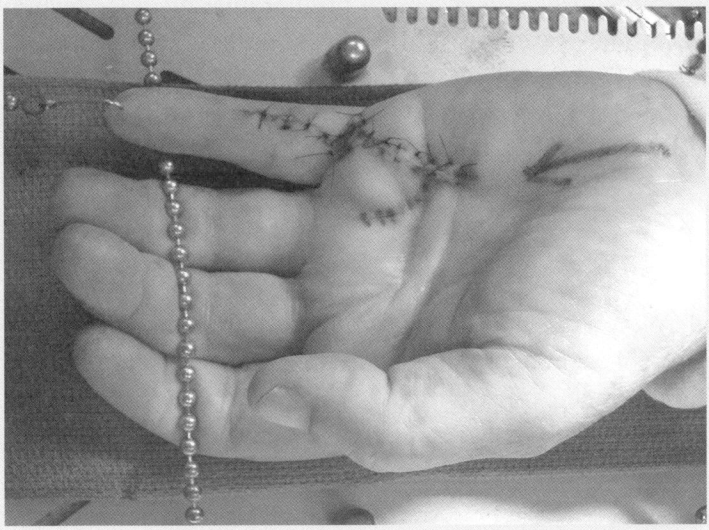

Closure with Z-plasty at MP flexion crease

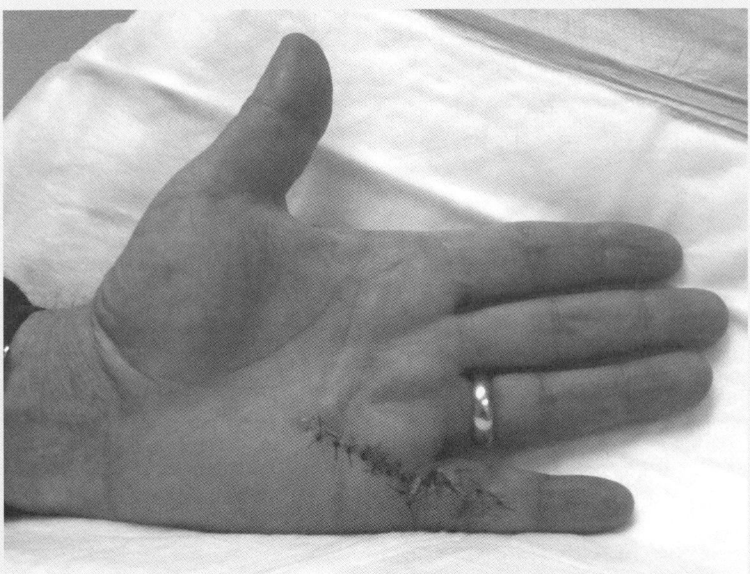

Sutures removed in 10 to 14 days

Dupuytren's disease is a benign proliferative disorder involving palmar and digital fascia resulting in nodules, cords, and disabling contractures.[1]

The eponym was coined after Dupuytren performed a fasciotomy using an open transverse incision in 1831.

I. Epidemiology

- Primarily affects older men of northern European descent
- Autosomal dominant Mendelian inheritance pattern with variable penetrance and expressivity
- Associated with diabetes mellitus, seizure disorders, alcohol use, tobacco use, heavy manual labor

II. Pathophysiology

- Proliferation of fibroblasts
- Dedifferentiation into myofibroblasts
- Increased type III collagen
- Increased expression of growth factors
  - FGF, TGF, PDGF, IL-1

III. Presentation

- Usually bilateral
- Ring finger most commonly involved
- Nodules occur first followed by formation of cords
- Progresses from palm to digits, from ulnar to radial
- Skin changes may be present (pitting, dimpling)
- Ectopic deposits
  - Knuckle pads (Garrod's nodes)
  - Plantar fibromatosis (Lederhosen's disease)
  - Penile fibromatosis (Peyronie's disease)

IV. Normal Anatomy of Palmar Fascia[2]

- Three-dimensional matrix of transverse, longitudinal, and vertical skin ligaments
- Allows the hand to withstand shear forces and movement of tendons

A. Most palmar cords cause MCP joint flexion deformity

1. Pretendinous cord most common

B. Digital cords cause PIP joint contracture

1. Central cord most common
    - Originates from pretendinous band
    - Spiral cords displace the neurovascular bundle to the midline

V. Treatment[3]

A. Surgical — 50% of patients will develop recurrence within 5 years

Indications

1. 30 degree MP contracture
2. PIP contracture of 20 degrees
3. Positive Table Top test
4. Nodule over trigger finger requiring surgery

Surgical options

1. Fasciotomy
    - Divides diseases cords
    - High recurrence rate
2. Percutaneous fasciotomy[4]
    - Recurrence rate of 58% at 3 years
3. Limited fasciectomy
    - Removes portion of diseased tissue
    - High recurrence rate

4. Regional fasciectomy
    - Excision of diseased palmar fascia and longitudinal cord
5. Dermatofasciectomy
    - Wide excision of palmar and digital skin and fascia
    - May necessitate skin grafting
    - May leave open to heal by secondary intention (McCash technique)

Anesthesia

1. Local, axillary block, general

Postoperative care

1. Early OT with range of motion exercises
2. Splinting to maintain correction

Complications

1. 17% of cases
2. Hematoma, skin loss, tendon damage, nerve injury, vascular damage and digital ischemia, chronic regional pain syndrome "Dupuytren's flare"

B. Nonsurgical

- Collagenase[5]
    1. Xiaflex©
        - Clostridium histolyticum collagenase
        - FDA approved February 2010
        - Indicated when MP joint contracture is greater than 30 degrees, PIP joint contracture is greater than 20 degrees and progressing
        - Injections into the cord at the level of the affected joint
        - 0.58 mg in 0.25 ml used for MP cords, 0.58 mg in 0.20 ml used for PIP cords

    - Patient returns next day for manipulation of fingers
    - Recurrence rate of 10% for MP, 20% for PIP at 5 years
    - Tendon rupture rate of 0.2%

- Steroids
- Calcium channel blocker
- Ultrasound
- Radiotherapy

References

1. Shaw RB, Chong KS, Zhang A, Hentz VR, Chang J. (2007) Dupuytren's Disease: history, diagnosis, and treatment. *Plast Reconst Surg* **120**(3): 44–54.
2. Hurst L. (2011) Dupuytren's contracture. In: Wolfe SW, Hotchkiss RN, Pederson WC, Kozin SH (eds.), *Green's Operative Hand Surgery*, 6th Edn., Elsevier, Philadelphia.
3. Swartz WM, Lalonde DH. (2008) Dupuytren's disease. *Plast Reconstr Surg* **121**(4): 1–10.
4. Foucher G, Medina J, Navarro R. (2003) Percutaneous needle aponeurotomy: complications and results. *J Hand Surg* **28**: 427–431.
5. Gilpin D, Coleman S, Hall S, Houston A, *et al.* (2010) Injectable collagenase Clostridium histolyticum: a new nonsurgical treatment for Dupuytren's disease. *J Hand Surg Am* **35**(12): 2027–2038.

CHAPTER 21

MICROSURGERY: GENERAL PRINCIPLES

Harvey W.-M. Chim and Christopher J. Salgado

Illustrative Case

- A middle-aged man presents with an ulcer involving the left tongue. This is diagnosed as a squamous cell carcinoma
- Following resection by the oncologic surgeon, a defect is left in the left tongue and floor of mouth. What is the next step in management?
- This patient was treated with a free radial forearm flap transferred using microsurgical technique to reconstruct the left tongue and floor of mouth

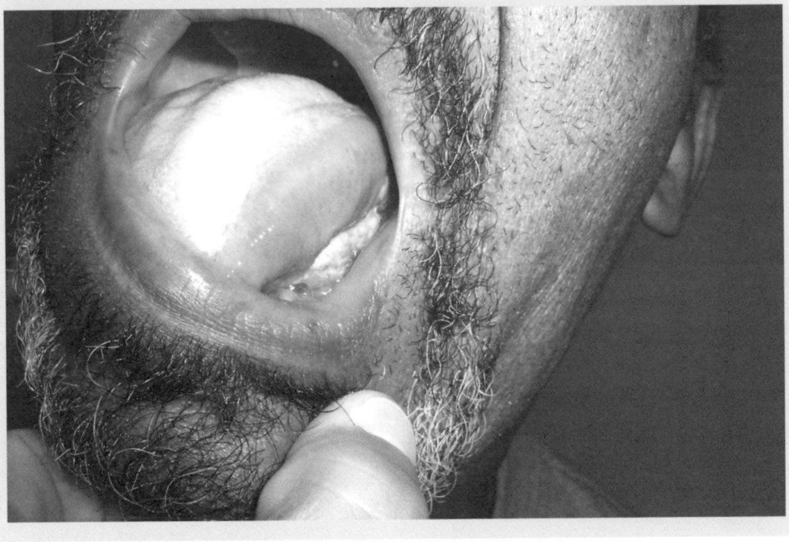

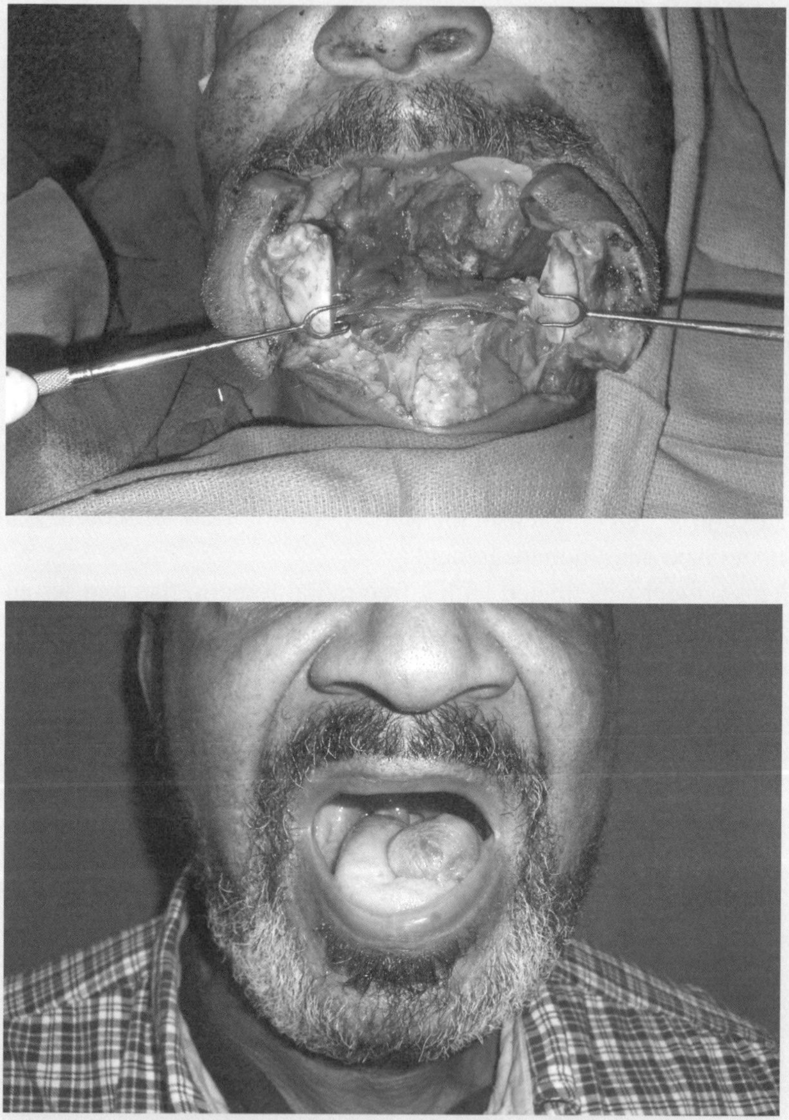

Definition

- Microsurgery allows transfer of free tissue from one part of the body to another
- Survival of the tissue relies on a single pedicle artery and draining vein
- The donor and recipient vessels are connected through microsurgical technique to re-establish flow to the expendable tissue

Overview

- Indications for microsurgery
  - Free tissue transfer
  - Replantation
  - Transplantation (hand, face)
- Indications for free tissue transfer
  - Reconstruction of complex wounds and tissue loss
  - Reconstruction after tumor resection
  - Trauma
  - Congenital defects
- Indications for replantation
  - Thumb amputations
  - Multiple finger amputations
  - Proximal (palm, wrist) amputations
  - Pediatric finger amputations
- Indications for hand and face transplantation
  - Complex tissue defects not reconstructable by conventional free tissue transfer or other techniques
- Success rate >95% for free tissue transfer and >90% for replantation in most centers
- Commonly used fasciocutaneous flaps

- Radial forearm flap: workhorse flap for head and neck, upper extremity reconstruction. Supplied by radial artery
- Scapular and parascapular flap: large volume of tissue available. Supplied by circumflex scapular vessels
- Deep inferior epigastric perforator (DIEP) flap: commonly used for breast reconstruction. Supplied by deep inferior epigastric vessels
- Groin flap: older flap based on superficial circumflex iliac artery
- Dorsalis pedis flap: soft pliable tissue available for reconstruction. Supplied by first dorsal metatarsal artery and dorsalis pedis

- Commonly used myocutaneous flaps
  - Transverse rectus abdominis myocutaneous flap (TRAM): commonly used for breast reconstruction. Supplied by deep inferior epigastric vessels
  - Rectus abdominis flap: applications in upper and lower extremity, trunk reconstruction. Based on deep inferior epigastric vessels
  - Latissimus dorsi flap: large volume of muscle available. Supplied by thoracodorsal vessels
  - Gracilis flap: used to extremity reconstruction, facial reanimation and functional free muscle transfers. Based on medial circumflex femoral vessels

- Commonly used osteocutaneous flaps
  - Fibular flap: used for head and neck reconstruction. Supplied by peroneal vessels
  - Deep circumflex iliac artery (DCIA) flap: allows harvest of large segment of iliac crest, backup option for head and neck reconstruction
  - Radial forearm flap: segment of bone can be harvested for use in phalloplasty
  - Great toe flap: used for thumb reconstruction. Supplied by first dorsal metatarsal artery in 70% of cases

Classification

- Mathes and Nahai classification of muscle flaps according to vascular supply:
    - Type I: single pedicle
    - Type II: dominant pedicle(s), with minor pedicle(s)
    - Type III: two co-dominant pedicles
    - Type IV: segmental pedicles
    - Type V: dominant pedicle, with secondary segmental pedicles

- Examples of muscle flaps per Mathes and Nahai classification:

    - Type I: tensor fascia lata, gastrocnemius
    - Type II: gracilis
    - Type III: gluteus maximus, serratus anterior
    - Type IV: sartorius

- Type V: latissimus dorsi

Technical Considerations

- Microsurgery is performed using an operating microscope or occasionally high powered loupe magnification
- 9-0 or 10-0 nylon interrupted sutures are used to reapproximate donor and recipient artery and vein
- Coupled anastomosis involves the use of a microvascular coupler, which does not require sewing. Patency rates appear similar to hand-sewn anastomoses, with the advantage of savings in time
- Coupled anastomoses are more easily performed on veins as thin pliable walls allow eversion around the prongs of the coupler
- Absence of tension and pressure on the anastomosis is required to prevent flap failure
- Muscle does not tolerate warm ischemia more than 2 hours
- Skin and fasciocutaneous flaps can tolerate up to 4–6 hours of ischemia
- Cooling of the flap on the operative field can increase tolerance of tissue to ischemia

- Methods to relieve spasm of vessels
    - Topical lidocaine
    - Topical papaverine
    - Irrigation with heparinized saline
    - Mechanical dilation
- Technical errors which may lead to flap failure:
    - Loose suture placement, resulting in media exposure and clotting
    - Tight suture placement, resulting in intimal distortion and clotting
    - Anastomosis in the zone of injury
    - Excessive tension
    - Compression on pedicle
    - Hematoma formation and compression of the pedicle
    - Twisting of pedicle from poor placement

Breast Reconstruction

- Common flaps used are deep inferior epigastric perforator (DIEP) and transverse rectus abdominis (TRAM) flaps
- Other flaps used include superior gluteal artery perforator (SGAP), inferior gluteal artery perforator (IGAP), transverse gracilis and anterolateral thigh flaps
- Recipient vessels most commonly used are internal mammary vessels or thoracodorsal vessels

Head and Neck Reconstruction

- Defects may involve tongue, floor of mouth, lip, mandible or maxilla
- Flaps most often used are fasciocutaneous or osseocutaneous where bone is required for reconstruction of the facial skeleton
- Fasciocutaneous flaps most commonly used for soft tissue reconstruction include radial forearm flap, scapular flap and anterolateral thigh flap
- Osseocutaneous flaps used include fibular flap and parascapular flap

- Recipient vessels which may be used include facial, transverse cervical, lingual or superior thyroid. Anastomoses to the superficial temporal vessels may be performed for scalp reconstruction

Upper Extremity Reconstruction

- This may involve reconstruction of digits to recreate a functional hand or coverage of defects
- Reconstruction of the hand may involve toe to thumb or toe to finger transfers
- Microsurgical options for soft tissue coverage include fasciocutaneous flaps such as anterolateral thigh, dorsalis pedis and lateral arm flaps

Lower Extremity Reconstruction

- Free tissue transfer is most often required for reconstruction of defects involving the distal one-third of the leg, with exposed bone. Alternatively, very large defects often resulting from trauma or oncologic resection may also require free tissue transfer for limb salvage
- Options include muscle flaps such as latissimus dorsi and rectus flaps, with overlying skin graft. These have the advantage of large bulk to cover the defect and obliterate dead space
- Fasciocutaneous flaps such as anterolateral thigh flaps may also be used for coverage of defects
- In the leg, it is essential to check the patency of vessels (anterior tibial, posterior tibial and peroneal) prior to microsurgery. Options include duplex ultrasound or CT angiogram. This will determine the feasibility of free tissue transfer and perhaps requirement for vascular surgery intervention prior to definitive coverage

Postoperative Care and Monitoring

- Vigilant postoperative monitoring is essential to detect early thrombosisand impending flap failure

- The flap is perfused only through the microvascular anastomosis immediately post-operatively
- Endothelialization occurs across the anastomosis and is complete by around 2 weeks
- Reperfusion of the flap also occurs from the periphery and wound bed through vasculogenesis and angiogenesis
- Risk of flap failure is greatest in the first 3 to 5 days postoperatively
- Hourly flap checks are required for at least the first 24 to 48 hours. This should be performed in an ICU setting or a specialized microsurgery floor
- Postoperative monitoring techniques for flap checks:
    - Clinical assessment
    - Doppler: external and internal
    - Continuous monitoring of tissue oxygen partial pressure (PaO_2)
    - Laser Doppler flowmetry with spectrophotometry
    - Positron emission tomography (PET)
    - Microdialysis
- Clinical assessment and doppler are most commonly used for monitoring
- Clinical monitoring involves assessment of color, temperature, swelling and capillary refill. A healthy flap is pink and warm, minimally swollen in the immediate postoperative period and well-perfused
- A congested flap indicative of venous compromise will be blue, swollen and warm, with a shortened capillary refill time
- An ischemic flap indicative of arterial compromise will be pale in color, cold, not swollen and with a delayed capillary refill time
- The "pinprick" test can be used to monitor flaps with a skin paddle. The flap is pricked with a small 25 to 30 gauge needle. Immediate flow of bright red blood indicates a healthy and well perfused flap. A congested flap will result in rapid flow of dark venous blood. An ischemic flap will not have significant blood return
- Keeping patients "nothing by mouth" and on bedrest for the first 24 hours is routine to prevent complications, and also in the event that OR re-exploration is required
- Venous congestion can be treated with medicinal leech therapy or systemic heparin

- Leeches work by secreting hirudin, a selective thrombin inhibitor
- Leeches commonly transmit *Aeromonas hydrophilia*. Hence prophylaxis with ciprofloxacin or bactrim should be used with leech therapy.
- Salvage rate of flaps that require re-exploration for flap ischemia: around 50%
- In the event of microvascular thrombosis causing flap failure, thrombolytic agents such as tissue plasminogen activator (tPA), streptokinase or urokinase can be used to restore flap perfusion

Anticoagulation

- Anticoagulation is commonly used after free tissue transfer. However, the exact regimes differ between surgeons
- Some agents include aspirin, heparin and dextran
- The exact regime used for anticoagulation has not been shown to affect overall flap survival. However, dextran is associated with increased systemic concentrations
- Aspirin has been shown to decrease incidence of macrovascular graft occlusion, as well as result in increased vessel patency and decreased platelet aggregation[1]
- Subcutaneous or low molecular weight heparin was shown to have a statistically significant effect on prevent of postoperative flap thrombosis in a large prospective study[2]
- No difference in flap survival and complications was found between use of aspirin and low molecular weight heparin[3]
- Intraoperative heparin has not been shown to be useful, with no difference in incidence of microvascular thrombi and complications between treated and control patients[4]
- Aspirin: blocks endothelial cyclooxygenase pathway and subsequently thromboxane A2 preventing vasoconstriction and thrombus formation
- Heparin: increases activation of antithrombin-3, inactivating thrombin. Prevents conversion of fibrinogen to fibrin and decreases platelet adhesion
- Dextran: volume expander that prevents platelet adhesion. Inactivates von Willebrand factor

References

1. Salemark L, Wieslander JB, Dougan P, Arnlijots B. (1991) Effects of low and ultra low oral doses of acetylsalicylic acid in microvascular surgery: an experimental study in rabbits. *Scand J Plast Reconstr Surg Hand Surg* **25**: 203–211.
2. Khouri RK, Cooley BC, Kunselman AR, *et al.* (1998) A prospective study of microvascular free flap surgery and outcome. *Plast Reconstr Surg* **102**: 711–721.
3. Ashjian P, Chen CM, Pusic A, Disa JJ, Cordeiro PG, Mehrara BJ. (2007) The effect of postoperative anticoagulation on microvascular thrombosis. *Ann Plast Surg* **59**: 36–39.
4. Chen CM, Ashjian P, Disa JJ, Cordeiro PG, Pusic AL, Mehrara BJ. (2008) Is the use of intraoperative heparin safe? *Plast Reconstr Surg* **121**: 49e–53e.

PLASTIC SURGERY OF THE LOWER EXTREMITY

CHAPTER 22

LOWER EXTREMITY RECONSTRUCTION

John R. Barbour and Milton B. Armstrong

Illustrative Case

A 25 year-old female school teacher was involved in a single vehicle collision. She sustained an open tibia fracture [Gustilo IIIb] but maintained intact distal sensation and pulses (Fig. 1A). She was treated initially at an outside facility and transferred to a tertiary care center with plastic surgery and reconstructive expertise following medical stabilization, serial operative débridements, and external fixation of the bony fragments (Fig. 1B). Four days following transfer, seven days

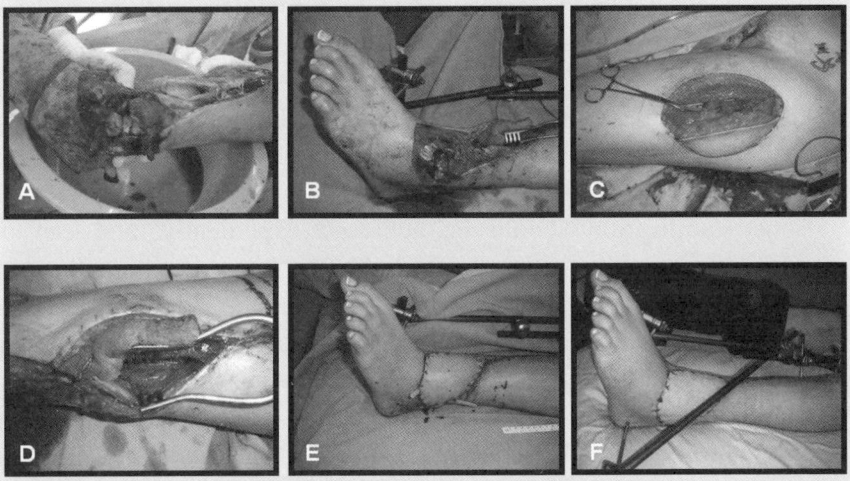

Fig. 1. Operative sequence from initial presentation through final operative debulking.

following the injury, an anterior-lateral thigh fasciocutaneous flap was performed (Fig. 1C), plugged into the anterior tibial artery and vein proximally (Fig. 1D). The bulky excessive tissue was later debulked in the operating room (Figs. 1E and 1F). The patient has now achieved full weight-bearing status on this extremity and is fully ambulatory, having returned to work and full activity.

Principles of Lower Extremity Reconstruction

- The modern dilemma that reconstructive surgeons face is no longer how to salvage an extremity but knowing whether or not attempting salvage is the best treatment for the patient.
- The goal in the reconstruction of lower extremity trauma is to restore the anatomy of the altered segment and to achieve functional recovery.
- Primary factors influencing outcomes of lower extremity injuries include degree of soft tissue damage, absence of plantar sensation, and severity of vascular injury.
- Indications for primary amputation include complete anatomic division of the posterior tibial nerve in adult patients, crush injuries with > 8 hours of warm ischemia, and an unstable patient.
- Preservation of mobility of the knee and ankle joints and restoration of the sensation and proprioception of the plantar surface of the foot allow for a functional extremity.
- Bone stabilization should be achieved expediently, and can be achieved internally with screws, rods, or plates or externally with percutaneous pins.
- Early flap coverage of wounds has demonstrated improved results if accomplished within the first 72 hours following injury.
- Limb reconstruction should be reserved for patients with reasonable expectation of ambulation within one year of the injury.
- Amputation may result in a more functional limb, as it can result in a quicker return to ambulation, activity, and work.

Evaluation

- Evaluation of a patient with a significant extremity injury should focus on the patient as a whole, with assessment and treatment following standard guidelines of the Advanced Trauma Life Support system.
- Severe open fractures treated at dedicated trauma units with both orthopedic and plastic surgery services have lower complication rates and lower need for revision surgery compared with those treated initially at local hospitals without such services.[1]

History

- The exact mechanisms of injury including any foreign material which could be present within the wound or crush-type patterns are significant.
- Details which would suggest potential for bacterial contamination should be gathered.
- Previous surgical procedures on that limb or the vascular system as well as a smoking history would be important in determining the likelihood of success of any soft tissue coverage procedure.
- Diabetes, vascular disease, obesity, and nicotine use are known to diminish the likelihood of success.

Physical Exam/Triage

- A detailed peripheral vascular exam including both lower extremities is needed on initial presentation, as obvious as well as occult vascular injuries may occur in association with lower extremity trauma.
- Angiographic techniques (CT vs MRA) may be necessary to evaluate for arterial injury.
- A neurovascular exam must be conducted noting any insensibility or diminished pulses.
- Ipsilateral examination of stability and range-of-motion of all joints should be documented, examining at least one joint on either side of the injury.

- Exposure of vital structures (nerves, vessels, joints) must be addressed by soft-tissue reconstruction.
- Patients with a fracture and a deep laceration should be treated as if there is an open fracture.
- Tetanus prophylaxis should be administered to patients with open fractures.
- Antimicrobial therapy based on cultures should be initiated.
- Reduction and temporary stabilization of fractures precedes or accompanies wound closure, as internal fixation devices must be covered at the time of wound closure.

Wound assessment

Fully probe the extent of the wound	• Exposed nerves, vessels, bone • Open or exposed joints • Prosthetic material or orthopaedic hardware
Determine the bacterial contamination	• Degree • Chronicity • Cultures from previous debridements
Examine for autologous usage	• Possibility of "spare parts"
Determine the patient's expectations	• Long-term outcome • Possible prolonged rehabilitation

Osteomyelitis

- *Staphylococcus aureus* is the most common organism seen in osteomyelitis seeded from areas of contiguous infection, but anaerobes and Gram-negative organisms, including *Pseudomonas*, *E. coli*, and *Serratia marcescens* are also common.
- Mixed infections are the rule rather than the exception.
- The diagnosis of osteomyelitis is often based on radiologic studies (lytic center).
- Cultures from a bone biopsy are needed.
- Antibiotic therapies involve nafcillin and ciprofloxacin or a cephalosporin with anti-pseudomonal activity.

- Diagnostic tests include:
    - Erythrocyte sedimentation rate (ESR), which effectively rules out osteomyelitis if normal
    - Bone cultures
    - Bone biopsy
    - MRI (T1-weighted images show decreased signal)
- MRI not an option in patients with metallic implantable devices (complicates multi-trauma patient).
- Treatment involves IV antibiotics (six weeks) with high penetration into the bloodstream, and debridement of all non-viable tissue including bone.

Compartment Syndrome

- Compartment syndrome can occur in any crush injury or closed fracture.
- Incidence is approximately 5–10% of all tibial fractures.
- Increased pressure within a closed osteo-fascial compartment rises above capillary pressure (usually 30 mm Hg) leading to muscle and nerve necrosis.
- Ischemic muscle releases myoglobin which is renally toxic (precipitates within the tubules).
- Renal toxicity can be minimized by alkalinizing the urine (pH >8.0) and aggressive intravenous fluid hydration to increase urine output.
- Lack of distal pulses is frequently the last sign to present and muscle and nerve death can occur in the presence of pulses, so vascular exam should not be the decision-making factor to perform a fasciotomy.
- Indications for four-compartment fasciotomy:
    - Compartment pressure greater than 30 mm Hg
    - Prolonged time to revascularization
    - Simultaneous arterial and venous injuries
    - High clinical suspicion

Wound Debridement

- Management of the open fractures should consist of early debridement and skeletal stabilization.

- Studies comparing external fixation with intra-medullary nails have shown no difference with respect to union, delayed union, deep infection, and chronic osteomyelitis.[2,3]
- The most critical step in the treatment of a severely injured upper limb is immediate debridement of all doubtfully viable tissue and extension to live bleeding tissue.
- Wound closure is advised only when all criteria are met:
    - Treatment of limb-threatening vascular injury
    - Removal of all devitalized tissue
    - Control of infection
    - Stabilization of fractures

Limb Salvage versus Amputation

- For smaller wounds with no exposure of vital structures, healing by secondary intention may be preferable.
- Any wound unlikely to heal by secondary intention in 3 weeks should be skin grafted.
- Larger wounds with exposed vital structures should be closed using a local flap or free tissue transfer.
- The decision whether or not to amputate must be individualized, taking into consideration not only the wound but also associated injuries, age, and socioeconomic status.
- Multiple injury severity scores have been designed to assist the surgeon in making the decision whether to amputate a severely injured lower extremity.
    - Mangled Extremity Severity Score (MESS)
    - Predictive Salvage Index (PSI)
    - Limb Salvage Index (LSI)
    - Nerve Injury, Ischemia, Soft Tissue Injury, Skeletal Injury, Shock, and Age of Patient Score (NISSSA)
    - Hanover Fracture Scale-97 (HFS-97)[4–6]
- The Lower Extremity Assessment Project (LEAP) was undertaken by surgeons who prospectively studied five different scoring systems in an attempt to assess outcomes after lower extremity trauma.

- Systems for scoring the severity of lower extremity injury have limited usefulness and cannot be used as the sole criterion by which amputation decisions are made.

Predictors of Poor Outcome

Medically Related	• Presence of severe soft tissue injury[7] • Absence of plantar sensation on presentation[7] • Involvement of three or more compartments within the leg • Injury to two or more of the tibial vessels • Cadaveric foot on presentation[7]
Non-Medically Related	• Major complication[7] • Low education level[7] • Non-white race[7] • Low socio-economic level of the patient • Lack of health insurance • Poor social support network[7] • Low self-sufficiency prior to the traumatic event[7]

- One component which does not correlate with an increased risk of amputation is bony skeletal deficit, as bone grafting and vascularized free bone transfer has improved the outcomes in many patients.[7]
- Patients with limb reconstruction have equal functional outcomes as those who undergo amputation.
- Reconstruction should be offered provided there is hope for the patient to ambulate within the first year.

Contraindications to Reconstruction

- Absolute contraindications to any attempts at limb salvage include medical instability of the patient without the ability to tolerate the procedure and any limb which would not reasonably be salvaged despite the best possibly surgical outcome.
- Crush injuries with massive tissue damage and prolonged warm ischemia (over six hours) of the distal portion do not allow for reconstructive efforts.

- An insensate foot alone is not an absolute contraindication to limb salvage.

Indications for Primary Amputation

Absolute indications for primary amputation	• Inability to medically tolerate salvage procedures • Complete disruption of the posterior tibial nerve in adults • Crush injuries with warm ischemia time greater than six hours
Relative indications for primary amputation	• Serious associated poly-trauma • Severe ipsilateral foot trauma • Massive burns with an open fracture in the wound • Devascularized limb with an open fracture • Protracted course to obtain coverage/reconstruction (>6 hours)

- The consequences of failed limb reconstruction are often overwhelming, leading to greater tissue loss, functional deficits, or eventual amputation. It is best to choose the initial procedure with the least morbidity and the greatest chance of overall success.

Anatomy

- The tibia and fibula are connected along their length by the interosseous membrane and divide the leg into two anatomic compartments, the anterior and posterior.
- The anterior compartment contains four muscles (all inervated by the deep peroneal nerve):
  - Extensor digitorum longus
  - Extensor hallucis longus
  - Peroneus
  - Tibialis anterior
- The antero-lateral compartment contains two muscles (innervated by the superficial peroneal nerve):
  - Long peroneus
  - Short (brevis) peroneus

- The posterior compartment is subdivided into superficial and deep portions by a thin inter-muscular fascia.
- Three muscles are located within the superficial compartment (innervated by the tibial nerve):
    - Gastrocnemius
    - Soleus
    - Plantaris
- The deep compartment contains four muscles (innervated by the tibial nerve):
    - Popliteus (flexion of the knee and medially rotating the leg)
    - Flexor digitorum longus
    - Flexor hallucis longus
    - Tibialis posterior (extend and medially rotate the foot and flex the toes)
- The tibial nerve courses deep in the proximal portion of the leg and then moves medially and superficially. The blood supply of the area is provided by the posterior tibial and the peroneal arteries.
- Small bone defects of the tibia are best treated with external fixation and cancellous bone grafting. The management of extensive and complex defects is more challenging.
- Segmental, comminuted tibial fractures or extensive bone defects require vascularized bone grafts to overcome infection and restore bone continuity and blood supply.

Injury Classification

- The classification of lower extremity fractures considers the mechanism of the trauma, the location, the extent and type of fracture, involvement of soft tissues, and neurovascular impairment.
- Crush injuries, avulsions, or high-speed bursting injuries typically lead to more complex defects.
- Clinical classification methods also consider the involvement of soft tissues injuries associated with open fractures. The most frequently utilized is the Association of Osteosynthesis (OA) classification proposed by Gustilo[8] (Table 1).

Table 1. Gustilo Classification System.

Grade I	Skin lesions smaller than 1 cm; clean; bone fracture with minimal comminution
Grade II	Skin lesions larger than 1 cm in size; no extensive soft tissue damage; minimal crushing; moderate comminution and contamination
Grade III	Extensive skin damage/loss with muscle and neurovascular involvement; high speed injuries; comminution of the fracture; instability
Grade IIIA	Extensive laceration of soft tissues with bone fragments covered; severe comminution or segmental fractures
Grade IIIB	Extensive deficit of soft tissues with periosteal stripping, contamination, and severe comminution; exposed bone must be replaced with a local or free flap as coverage
Grade IIIC	Exposed fracture with arterial injury necessitating repair

Table 2. Byrd Classification Scale.

Type I	Low energy fractures; oblique or spiral fracture with laceration smaller than 1 cm
Type II	Medium-energy trauma; displaced or comminuted fracture with laceration larger than 2 cm and myocutaneous contusion
Type III	High-energy trauma; severely displaced or comminuted fracture; segmental fracture or bone defect with laceration larger than 2 cm and loss of skin and muscle substance
Type IV	High-energy trauma; crush/avulsion with arterial damage requiring microvascular repair

- A separate classification of fractures has suggested by Byrd and is based on the mechanism of trauma and the bone and soft tissue lesion[9] (Table 2).

Primary Reconstruction

Timing

- Traditionally, soft-tissue cover has been delayed to allow for edema to settle, as well as to facilitate a second-look operation to assess tissue viability.

- Studies evaluating free tissue transfers in the treatment of trauma have clearly revealed advantages of radical debridement and early wound closure with vascularized tissue.[10]
- Studies have demonstrated an increased chance of infection and a high rate of thrombosis in patients undergoing delayed flap closure.[11]
- All wounds must be clean and adequately débrided of all infectious and non-viable tissue prior to any attempt at closure.
- Certain wounds, such as severely contaminated wounds and electrical burns benefit more from serial debridements and delayed reconstruction than early flap coverage.

Debridement

- Serial operative debridement of the wound and surrounding soft tissues allow for time for marginally viable tissue to become evident, and an interval of two days between debridements is ideal.
- Bedside dressing changes allow for removal of bacteria and debris and prevent desiccation.
- In the case of exposed bone or extremely contaminated wounds, consider tobramycin beads.
- Quantitative cultures should be taken intra-operatively to gauge contamination level.
- Less than 10×10^5 colony-forming units/gm of tissue should be obtained prior to wound closure.
- Following avulsion or/and de-gloving injury, the damage may be under-estimated at the first examination. Consider using the avulsed skin as a full-thickness graft following debridement.

Bony Stabilization

- Stabilization of the bony structures of the lower limb is needed for adequate healing.
- External fixation can be limb saving in the setting of high-energy trauma with soft tissue damage in the medically unstable patient and/or when definitive fracture treatment must be delayed.
- Bones as well as joints can be stabilized in the acute setting of trauma or limb reconstruction.

- Proper bone healing requires an adequate blood supply from nutrient arteries and the periosteum. Prevent excessive periosteal stripping, maximizing perfusion to the healing bone.
- In many centers, inter-medullar rod fixation has become first-line therapy in the immediate setting, replacing external fixation.
- A key component for successful bone healing is early weight bearing and functional activity.
- Weight bearing provides axial loading to the fracture, nonunion, or osteotomy site that stimulates osteogenesis. A lack of axial loading in the presence of normal blood supply and adequate bony stability will cause resorption at the bone gap site.[12]
- Bony contact at the gap site dramatically augments frame stability and the ability to bear weight.
- When compared with internal plates and intra-medullary (IM) nails, external fixators cause less disruption of the soft tissues, blood supply, and periosteum, and allow post-operative adjustability.
- Pin site infections respond well to aggressive local pin care and empiric oral antibiotics.
- Internally placed hardware can become colonized by bacteria, and may prove difficult to salvage with antibiotic therapy alone.
- The mobility afforded to patients by early ORIF or external fixation helps with early rehabilitation and prevention of venous stasis, decreasing the incidence of deep vein thrombosis.

Revascularization

- Distal perfusion may be improved following reduction of fractures through resolution of any actively spasmodic or kinked vessel.
- Revascularization of any damaged vessels should be undertaken as soon as bony stabilization is achieved to optimize odds of limb survival.
- Revascularization can be accomplished temporarily through the use of a prosthetic shunt if fixation of the limb will be prolonged and if there is concern for limb ischemia.
- Definitive vascular repair should be delayed until after bony stabilization has been achieved, so as not to risk damage during reduction. If primary anastomosis of the injured vessel is not possible, interposition

grafting should be considered, most commonly using the contralateral saphenous vein. The re-establishment of blood supply to an ischemic limb brings risk for reperfusion injury, thus one should maintain a low threshold for fasciotomy in this setting.

Soft tissue coverage

- In many cases, due to complexity and extent of injury, the "reconstructive ladder" is not feasible in the management of lower extremity trauma and rather a "reconstructive elevator" is needed.
- Wound coverage options are determined by the characteristics of that specific wound, including the size and state of the wound, the type of tissue (ski, muscle, bone) which is deficient, the location of injury, and the length of vascular pedicle needed.
- Critical structures are frequently exposed in larger wounds and complicate treatment with observation and dressing changes.
- Primary closure is rarely achievable due to a lack of sufficient healthy tissue required to achieve tension-free closure.
- Tissue expanders in the lower extremity have yielded poor results, with high complication rates.[13]
- Negative pressure dressings have been shown to reduce bacterial counts and encourage granulation tissue, thus providing a clean, vascularized tissue bed.[14]
- Local muscle flaps, such as the gastrocnemius or soleus, are useful; however they will not cover defects larger than 25 square cm or those on the distal third of the leg, ankle, or foot.
- Free tissue transfer allows for coverage of a greater area, as the flap generally provides more bulk, and is less likely to be dependent on blood vessels within the "zone of injury."
- Fasciocutaneous flaps are supplied by means of numerous branches of the trunk arteries that pierce and then coalesce with each other above the deep fascia, and are particularly suited for small to moderate-sized defects in the distal third of the leg.
- Local factors can also prevent the prudent use of a free flap, such as single arterial vessel run-off or instances in which long vein grafts are needed for an anastomosis outside the zone of injury.

- A fasciocutaneous flap can additionally be used in combination with a muscle flap such as a proximal third tibial defect in which the gastrocnemius is used to fill the bony concavity while lateral fasciocutaneous flap provides additional coverage. The success rates of fasciocutaneous flaps are high (over 90 percent). difference can be explained in that a more severe fracture is likely associated with a greater degree of soft-tissue damage, and a free tissue transfer may be able to reconstruct the larger defect with greater success, given its bulk and better blood supply.
- Choices for soft tissue coverage in the lower extremity include usage of local flaps, regional flaps, and free tissue transfer.
- Local flaps are pedicled tissue immediately adjacent to the wound; and may include skin, fascia, muscle, or bone in nearly any combination. Regional flaps involve pedicled tissue separated from the immediate surrounding area of the wound.
- Cross-leg flaps can be preformed and may be an excellent resource in otherwise difficult patient management scenarios.
- Free flaps can be extremely helpful in wounds complicated by osteomyelitis, radiation, and bony non-union. Contour abnormalities after surgery frequently improve with time as the bulky muscle atrophies due to disuse and denervation.
- When reconstructing a soft tissue defect following trauma, locate the anastamosis outside the zone of injury, and an end-to-side anastomosis is historically preferred.

Regional coverage

- Reconstruction should not be attempted until local vascularity is ensured and the wound has been appropriately débrided, and is free of gross contamination, necrotic debris, and infection.
- Split or full-thickness skin grafts frequently are all that is needed for coverage within the thigh if an adequate wound bed is present.
- Local muscle flaps may be needed for coverage of exposed bone or neurovascular structures without sufficient blood supply to support skin grafting.
- For skin and subcutaneous tissue deficits in the region of the knee, skin grafting alone is also acceptable if joint is not violated. In the

absence of an available gastrocnemius muscle, strong consideration for a free-flap is encouraged.

Local Flaps for Leg Defects

Proximal Third

- The more frequently used local flaps for proximal-third injuries are the gastrocnemius and tibialis anterior muscles.
- Blood supply to the medial gastrocnemius is through the medial sural artery, whereas the lateral sural artery supplies the lateral gastrocnemius.
- Either head, or both, can be transposed without loss of foot dorsiflexion, provided the soleus muscle is functional.
- Lateral defects are more easily covered using the lateral gastrocnemius, whereas larger wounds of the proximal tibia and knee are more amenable to coverage with the medial gastrocnemius.
- The medial head of the gastrocnemius is longer and thus often preferred for knee wounds.
- Both heads of the gastrocnemius muscle may be used to cover large soft tissue deficits.
- Although either muscle head must be elevated carefully to avoid adjacent structure injury, the peroneal nerve is at greater risk of injury when elevating the lateral head.

Middle Third

- Lying deep to the gastrocnemius muscle, the soleus can be elevated and transposed into wounds of the proximal and middle thirds of the leg.
- The dominant vascular pedicles of the soleus are branches of the popliteal artery (proximal, near origin), branches of the posterior tibial artery (medial belly), and branches of the peroneal artery (lateral belly).
- If the wound to be closed is small, the muscle can be split longitudinally and used as a hemi-soleus flap.
- If the soleus is transposed, foot plantar flexion is usually preserved as long as the gastrocnemius muscle is functional.

Distal Third

- Recently, while free flaps are occasionally required, the development of local fasciocutaneous flaps has allowed for less morbidity in treating these difficult wounds.
- The vascular plexus accompanying cutaneous nerves can supply areas of overlying skin and soft tissue.
- A variable supply of small-vessel arteries (one to three) runs alongside the sural nerve subcutaneously in the calf.
- When dissecting the reverse sural fasciocutaneous flap, a line is drawn from halfway between the Achilles tendon and the lateral malleolus at the ankle and extended to a midline point between the heads of the gastrocnemius.
- Including a cuff of muscle during elevation may prevent damage to the vessels accompanying the nerve.
- The most distal point of safe flap elevation is precisely five-centimeters proximal to the tip of the lateral malleolus.
- A fasciocutaneous flap from the posterior calf up to 14 centimeters in diameter can be elevated as part of a distally based flap, and may be transposed to cover distal leg and foot wounds.

Foot Defects

- For foot defects, the choice in wound coverage should be based on whether the wound is on a weight-bearing or non-weight-bearing surface.
- The instep of the foot is non-weight-bearing and may be covered with a thick split-thickness skin graft.
- In the case of isolated heel wounds, local fasciocutaneous flaps can be used.
- When dealing with larger defects, a medial or lateral plantar flap may be used.
- The reverse sural nerve flap can be used for coverage of the non-weight-bearing heel.

- When a wound is present on the plantar surface of the forefoot, a toe fillet flap may be used.
- Small soft tissue deficits of the lateral malleolus can be addressed with a pedicled extensor digitorum brevis flap and coverage with a skin graft.
- Wounds of the medial or lateral malleolus can be treated by rotation of a dorsalis pedis flap.
- Larger foot wounds, particularly those involving the plantar surface of the heel, can frequently be closed utilizing a muscle flap and in conjugation with a split-thickness skin graft.

Free Tissue Transfer

- Local flap options may be precluded by trauma in the immediate vicinity.
- Laceration or crush superior to the lateral malleolus may damage the blood supply to the sural nerve flap.
- If the wound is too large to be covered by a single local flap, a free flap should be considered.
- If a large amount of tissue is required for coverage of a large defect, the latissimus dorsi muscle is a suitable option.
- The rectus abdominis flap has a long vascular pedicle and provides a large amount of tissue, similar to the latissimus, although its width is narrow.
- Morbidity from the rectus abdominis donor site, abdominal wall weakness, may be significant.
- A gracilis flap is an excellent option for smaller defects and conveys less donor-site morbidity.
- General reconstructive principles involve attempting to anastomose the vessels outside the zone of injury and to reconstruct the soft tissues prior to skeletal structure.
- Single-tissue and composite flaps may include an osseous component for large bony defects.
- Free fibula flaps with an associated skin paddle are an option in wounds with concurrent bony and soft-tissue deficits.[15]

Vascular Anastomoses

- The vascular anastomosis should be performed outside the zone of injury, most commonly proximal in the leg to the anterior tibial or posterior tibial vessels.
- The arterial anastomosis should be performed in an end-to-side manner, whereas the venous anastomosis is usually performed as end-to-end.
- Superficial veins are more susceptible to vasospasm and should be avoided if possible.

Secondary Reconstruction

- Delayed treatment of nerve and bone deficits can be addressed.
- The sural nerve is a common source for nerve grafting as it leaves minimal donor morbidity (numbness on lateral ankle and foot).
- The sural nerve is positioned within the groove between the lateral malleolus and the Achilles tendon, as it travels bordering to lesser saphenous vein.
- Nerve repair is more likely to result in a favorable outcome in children than in adults.
- Bone grafting is delayed past the first 6–12 weeks following soft tissue coverage.
- Options for bone reconstruction include cancellous bone grafts (<3 cm deficit), Ilizarov bone lengthening (3–6 cm), and vascularized bone grafts (>6 cm deficit).
- The fibula mid-shaft can be used as a pedicled local flap or a vascularized free flap and can include the adjacent lateral skin paddle for skin coverage.
- The proximal and distal 6 cm should be preserved for knee and ankle motion.
- The arterial supply is via the peroneal artery and up to 25 cm of bone can be harvested in the average adult.
- Conventional treatments (i.e., bone grafting, Ilizarov technique) are best indicated for limited (<6 cm) defects because of the prolonged time needed for newly formed bone to consolidate.

- Microsurgical bone transfers are indicated when conventional treatments are unlikely to be sufficient (bone defect >6 cm, poorly vascularized or infected wounds) or have previously failed.
- The primary indication for free bone transfer to tibial defects remains severely comminuted fractures or extensive bone loss greater than 6 cm (Gustillo grade III).
- Additional reasons for free bone transfer include:
  — Bone resection to address pseudoarthrosis or chronic osteomyelitis
  — Limb length discrepancy (>6 cm difference) following fractures or replantation
  — Severe amputation stump lengthening
  — Extensive soft tissue and bone defects (<6 cm) of the lower third of the leg (osteocutaneous-myo-osteocutaneous flap)

Vacuum-Assisted Closure of Lower Extremity Wounds

- Clinical studies have shown vacuum-assisted closure (VAC) increases blood flow, rates of granulation tissue formation, and random-pattern flap survival and decreases bacterial counts.[16]
- VAC therapy is not indicated in heavily contaminated wounds with devitalized tissue.
- If a wound is clean, bony stability is present, and no vital structures are exposed, VAC therapy can facilitate dressing of the wound and often promotes healing without surgical intervention.
- Importantly, VAC should be used as a temporizing measure before definitive closure.
- Reports of arterial erosion and hemorrhage during the use have occurred, and it should not replace adequate surgical debridement.

Complications

- Surgical treatment of chronic osteomyelitis requires radical debridement followed by wound coverage and obliteration of dead space with vascularized tissue.

- Studies have shown that well-vascularized skin flaps, including pedicled muscle flaps and free tissue transfer, are equally effective in the treatment of chronic osteomyelitis.[17,18]
- Success is dependent on debridement and using well-vascularized tissue to obliterate the dead space.
- The most common early complications at the donor site are infection, decreased flexion of the great toe, paresthesias of the dorsum of the foot, and loss of foot dorsiflexion.
- Among late complications, the most common are edema, pain with ambulation, ankle stiffness, scarring, and instability and tibial curvature in children.
- Fibular harvesting does not usually cause any significant functional deficit to adults.
- Early complications at the recipient site include anastomotic thrombosis, venous congestion, infection, wound breakdown, limb shortening/lengthening, and posterior tibial artery thrombosis.
- Late recipient site complications include fractures, bony instability, delayed union, non-union, mal-alignment, and pain and/or edema after walking.
- Microvascular complications usually manifest within hours of the operation.
- The bone flap may tolerate venous thrombosis because of bleeding from the medullary canal, but impaired venous drainage of the skin paddle must be addressed with leech therapy.
- Placement of wound drains may be helpful in reducing the risk of hematomas.
- Any concern for flap vascular compromise demands urgent examination.
- In the event of a cellulitic infection, a course of antibiotics may be warranted.
- Should an abscess develop, drainage accompanied by culture-specific antibiotics may resolve the infection.
- In the patient who has a retained orthopedic fixation device, the likelihood of bacterial eradication is reduced. Removing devitalized bone or involved prosthetic plates, closure with vitalized tissue, and long-term antibiotic therapy may control the infection.

Amputation Principles

- Preservation of as much length as possible of the extremity is important in rehabilitation.
- A patient with a below-knee amputation (BKA) is far more functional and uses less work-of-energy when compared to an above-knee amputation (AKA).
- Quality of life is improved in BKA versus AKA patients, due to psychological factors and increased mobility.
- Conserve otherwise viable tissue distal to the injury and consider full or split-thickness grafts from the amputated portion, minimizing additional donor-site morbidity for the patient.

Conclusions

- Free tissue transfer using microsurgical techniques has moved limb salvage into a new era.
- Ideally, the patient with a complicated lower extremity wound will experience stable healing with restoration of adequate function and satisfactory cosmetic appearance.
- Amputation is the last resort, although informing the patient of the likely outcome, particularly if the result promises poor function, makes the decision for amputation easier.
- The ultimate aim is to restore limb function and return patients to normal life.

References

1. Naique SB, Pearse M, Nanchahal J. (2006) Management of severe open tibial fractures: the need for combined orthopaedic and plastic surgical treatment in specialist centres. *J Bone Joint Surg Br* **83**(3): 351–357.
2. Bhandari M, Guyatt GH, Swiontkowski MF, Schemitsch EH. (2001) Treatment of open fractures of the shaft of the tibia. *J Bone Joint Surg Br* **83**(1): 62–68.
3. Yokoyama K, Itoman M, Uchino M, Fukushima K, Nitta H, Kojima Y. (2008) Immediate versus delayed intramedullary nailing for open fractures of the tibial shaft: a multivariate analysis of factors affecting deep infection and fracture healing. *Indian J Orthop* **42**(4): 410–419.

4. Shawen SB, Keeling JJ, Branstetter J, Kirk KL, Ficke JR. (2010) The mangled foot and leg: salvage versus amputation. *Foot Ankle Clin* **15**(1): 63–75.
5. Bosse MJ, MacKenzie EJ, Kellam JF, *et al.* (2001) A prospective evaluation of the clinical utility of the lower-extremity injury-severity scores. *J Bone Joint Surg Am* **83**-A(1): 3–14.
6. Ly TV, Travison TG, Castillo RC, Bosse MJ, MacKenzie EJ. (2008) Ability of lower-extremity injury severity scores to predict functional outcome after limb salvage. *J Bone Joint Surg Am* **90**(8): 1738–1743.
7. MacKenzie EJ, Bosse MJ, Kellam JF, *et al.* (2002) Factors influencing the decision to amputate or reconstruct after high-energy lower extremity trauma. *J Trauma* **52**(4): 641–649.
8. Gustilo RB, Mendoza RM, Williams DN. (1984) Problems in the management of type III (severe) open fractures: a new classification of type III open fractures. *J Trauma* **24**(8): 742–746.
9. Byrd HS, Spicer TE, Cierney G, III. (1985) Management of open tibial fractures. *Plast Reconstr Surg* **76**(5): 719–730.
10. Moda SK, Kalra GS, Gupta RS, Maggu NK, Gupta RK, Kalra MK. (1994) The role of early flap coverage in the management of open fractures of both bones of the leg. *Injury* **25**(2): 83–85.
11. Arnez ZM. (1991) Immediate reconstruction of the lower extremity — an update. *Clin Plast Surg* **18**(3): 449–457.
12. Ilizarov GA. (1971) Basic principles of transosseous compression and distraction osteosynthesis *Ortop. Travmatol Protez* **32**(11): 7–15.
13. Borges Filho PT, Neves RI, Gemperli R, *et al.* (1991) Soft-tissue expansion in lower extremity reconstruction. *Clin Plast Surg* **18**(3): 593–599.
14. Herscovici D Jr, Sanders RW, Scaduto JM, Infante A, DiPasquale T. (2003) Vacuum-assisted wound closure (VAC therapy) for the management of patients with high-energy soft tissue injuries. *J Orthop Trauma* **17**(10): 683–688.
15. Lee KS, Han SB, Baek JR. (2004) Free vascularized osteocutaneous fibular graft to the tibia in 51 consecutive cases. *J Reconstr Microsurg* **20**(4): 277–284.
16. Thompson JT, Marks MW. Negative pressure wound therapy. *Clin Plast Surg* **34**(4): 673–684.
17. Kawakatsu M, Ishikawa K, Sumiya A. (2010) Free latissimus dorsi musclocutaneous flap transfer for chronic osteomyelitis of the tibia: 16-year follow-up. *J Plast Reconstr Aesthet Surg* **63**(9): e691–e694.
18. Park G, Kim H. (2010) Treatment of chronic osteomyelitis using the medial sural perforator flap. *J Plast Reconstr Aesthet Surg* **63**(1): 153–159.

CHAPTER 23

REDUCTION MAMMAPLASTY, AUGMENTATION MAMMAPLASTY, AND MASTOPEXY

John C. Oeltjen

Illustrative Case

A 30-year-old female presented to clinic with long standing history of back pain, neck pain, bra tension on the shoulders, social anxiety, and inability to exercise due to her large breasts. The patient stated that she was approximately a "DD" cup in bra size and would like to be a "C" cup. Her discomfort was only temporarily relieved with over-the-counter pain medications and attempts at weight loss had not helped with her symptoms. She has no family history of breast cancer and had not noted any masses, nipple discharge, or other changes in her breasts. She desired a breast reduction.

On examination the patient had bilateral Grade III ptosis with the right breast being larger than her left breast. Her inframammary fold to nipple distance was 14.5 cm on the right and 13 cm on the left. Palpation demonstrated extensive glandular tissue but no specific palpable masses, palpable lymphadenopathy, or nipple discharge. Her BMI was 29.87 kg/m^2. After extensive consultation, the patient was offered a reduction mammaplasty via an inferior pedicle Wise pattern technique.

The surgical procedure went without incident. A total of 740 g of tissue was removed from the right breast and 520 g of tissue was removed from the left breast. At 6 month follow up the patient continued to be happy with the results and noted a drastic improvement in her symptoms and quality of life (see Fig. 1).

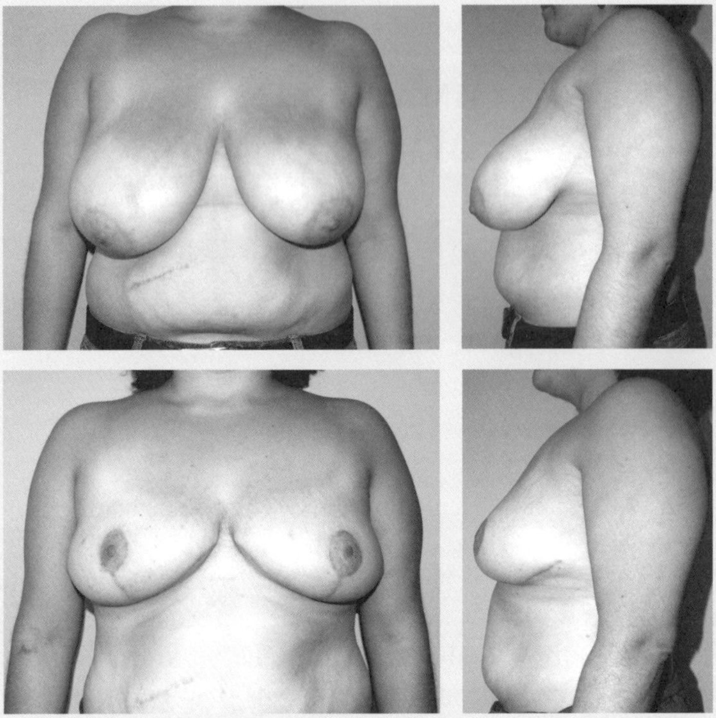

Fig. 1. Preoperative and 6 months postoperative photos of a patient who underwent bilateral breast reduction mammaplasty via a Wise pattern with an inferior pedicle reduction pattern.

Breast Anatomy

- Gentle superior convexity and inferior concavity in shape
- Anterior most projection is marked by the nipple areolar complex
  - Marks the transition between the superior convexity and inferior concavity
- Inframammary fold marks the inferior border between the breast and the chest wall
  - Generally situated at the mid-humeral level, the Pitanguay point, rarely higher, sometimes as low as the level of the junction between the proximal 2/3 of the humerus and distal 1/3 of the humerus

- At the level of confluence of the anterior and posterior capsule of the breast (see below)
- Does not have distinct fascial attachments from the skin or dermis to the chest wall
- Gentle curvature from the central chest proceeding lateral to merge with the lateral superior border of the pectoralis muscle

- Breast bud develops into glandular tissue
  - Develops within the superficial fascial system — Scarpa's fascia
  - Splits the fascia into an anterior and posterior fascial layers
    - Encompasses the breast tissue within fascia — breast capsule
  - Inferior confluence of anterior and posterior fascial layers is at the inframammary fold
- Breast is a combination of glandular tissue and fatty deposition
  - Internal support structure is provided by Cooper's ligaments
  - Cooper's ligaments weaken and lengthen with age
  - Amount of glandular tissue increases with pregnancy and decreases with age
- Breast ptosis is measured in grades (see Fig. 2)
  - Grade I — nipple is at or within 1 cm below the inframammary fold and above the lower convexity of the breast mound
  - Grade II — nipple is within 1 to 3 cm below the inframammary fold and above the lower convexity of the breast mound
  - Grade III — nipple is positioned greater than 3 cm below the inframammary fold and/or at the dependent position on the convexity of the lower pole of the breast mound

General Considerations with Breast Surgery

- Human culture places a strong emphasis and importance on the breast
  - Considered central to the female form
  - Associated with fertility

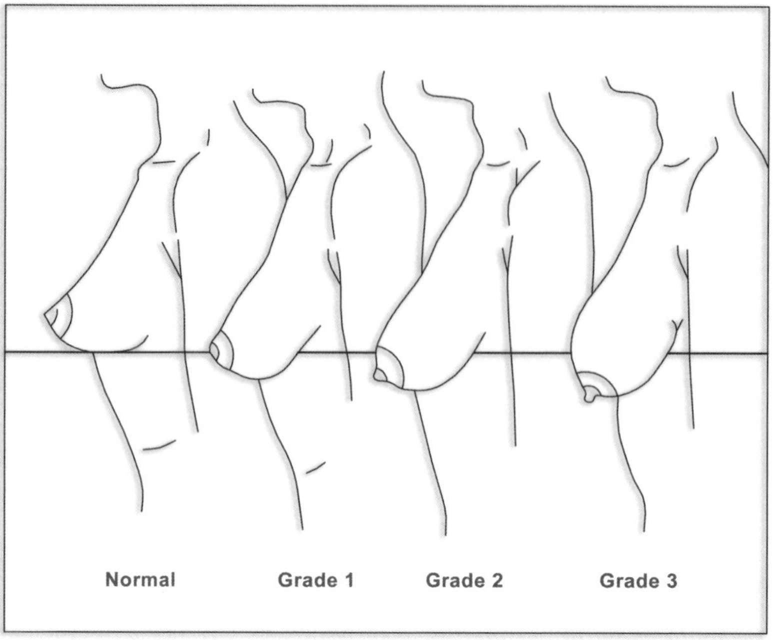

Fig. 2. Breast ptosis — an illustration demonstrating the progressive grades of breast ptosis in relation to the inframammary fold.

  - Scars, asymmetry, poor aesthetic results, and post-operative complications can be very emotionally charged
    - Good physician/patient relationships are important
    - Thorough and adequate consents are imperative
- In general is elective surgery
  - No nutritional deficiencies
  - Consider no surgery unless tobacco use stopped
  - Medically stable and optimized
- Breast cancer is prevalent
  - 1 in 8 women develop breast cancer[1]
  - Proper preoperative evaluation for evidence of cancer
    - Yearly mammograms after the age of 45 in individuals with no family history of breast cancer
    - Yearly follow-up with primary care physician

- With a strong family history of breast cancer, may consider consultation with a breast oncologist prior to elective surgery
- Scars from breast surgery result in calcifications that may distort future mammograms
- Implant placement results in a 17 to 50% reduction in the amount of breast parenchyma visualized in mammography
  - Dependent upon subglandular versus subpectoral placement
  - Dependent upon severity of capsular contracture
  - Has not resulted in an increased rate of cancer in augmented individuals[2]

- Breast surgery is considered clean non-contaminated surgery
  - Intraoperative first generation cephalosporin or equivalent antibiotics should be sufficient
    - No prospective double blind studies are available investigating appropriate perioperative antibiotic prophylaxis, especially with the placement of implants
    - *Staphylococcus epidermidis* is naturally found in the breast glandular tissue and can result in infections
    - Many surgeons have a preferred approach to antibiotic prophylaxis in breast surgery
      - Triple antibiotic irrigation solution utilized in implant placement
        - 1 gm Ancef
        - 5,000 units Bacitracin
        - 80 mg Gentamicin in 500 mL of normal saline[3]
      - Others utilize povidone-iodine within the implant pocket however this may void the implant warranty
    - Similarly no consensus for postoperative prophylactic antibiotic therapy exists
- Blood loss can be significant
  - Breast is highly vascular

- Perforators from the pectoralis muscle
- Perforators through the muscle from the internal mammary artery

- Hematomas can be large due to absence of restrictive fascial compartments
- Meticulous hemostasis can keep the need for transfusion minimal
- Postoperative care
  - Involves drains, support garments, implant care, wound healing
  - Accomplished primarily in an outpatient setting or as an overnight admission
  - Pain generally well tolerated
    - Pain medications by mouth
    - Some physicians advocate local anesthetic delivery devices (pain pumps) — supported by anecdotal evidence only

Physical Exam Specifics for Breast Surgery

- Height, weight, BMI
  - Important in the documentation for breast reduction insurance reimbursement
- Visual characteristics to note
  - Ptosis grade
  - Striae
  - Asymmetries
  - Height of nipple areolar complex in relation to humerus
  - Chest wall abnormalities or asymmetries
  - Fullness of superior, medial, and lateral aspects of breast mound
  - Axillary fullness including folds of skin and subcutaneous tissue excess
- Breast measurements including
  - Sternal notch to nipple distance

- Inframammary fold to nipple distance
- Nipple to midline distance and nipple to nipple distance
- Nipple areola complex diameter
- Base width — width of the footprint of the breast on the chest wall
- Superior pole pinch thickness
- Medial breast pinch thickness
- Confirm with the patient any preoperative asymmetries

- Skin exam
  - Scars
  - Skin changes indicative of underlying processes including malignancy
  - Striae indicative of loss of skin elasticity
  - Vein prominence indicative of thin skin and overall loss of elasticity

- Palpation
  - Systematic evaluation of the breast mound palpating for masses or abnormalities
  - Evaluation of the nipple areolar complex and any expressible nipple discharge
  - Evaluation of the axilla for an palpable lymphadenopathy

Reduction Mammaplasty: Patient Selection and Preoperative Considerations

- Surgical goals of breast reduction surgery
  - Reduce the size of the breast
  - Elevate the remaining breast tissue on the chest wall resulting in an appropriate breast form
  - Place the nipple areolar complex at the anterior most projection of the breast mound

- Patient goals for breast reduction surgery
  - Relief of pain
    - Neck, back, and shoulder

- Compression from bra straps
- Improved physical activity
  - Large breasts make running and other high impact sports difficult
  - Large breast can interfere with efforts to exercise and loose weight
- Improved appearance
  - Increased selection of clothing
  - Breast lift
  - Weight loss
  - Psychosocial relief

- Patient/doctor relationship
  - Must establish congruence and discrepancies between perceived goals and achievable surgical results
    - Patients must understand scars that will be present
    - Patients must understand that generally "lifts" achieved with breast reduction will have a finite existence
      - With time the breasts will descend due to the weight of the remaining breast tissue on the skin and fascia
      - Stretch marks on the skin preoperatively are a strong indicator that the lift will not be retained postoperatively
    - Patients must understand that "cup" size (A, B, C, D, etc.) is not an industry standard
      - Different vendors have different measurements of cup size
      - Cup size discussed preoperatively is only a guideline, not a specific measurable result
      - Numerical measurement is chest wall circumference and will rarely change with breast reduction surgery
    - Patients also must understand
      - Possible need for a free nipple graft in instances of nipple areolar complex vascular compromise

        - Especially in ptotic breasts where the distance planned to transpose the nipple areolar complex is greater than 22 cm[4]
        - Free nipple graft
            - Has an increased risk of nipple areolar loss
            - Results in loss of sensation and erectile properties of the nipple areolar complex
            - May result in nipple pigmentation changes especially in darker pigmented individuals
    - Possible detrimental effect of reduction on breast feeding
    - Postoperative pregnancy
        - May result in recurrent breast hypertrophy
        - Post-pregnancy involution will result in recurrent breast ptosis

- Many reduction mammaplasty patients are obese
    - Weight loss may decrease the size of the breasts but exercise can be difficult with macromastia
    - Morbidly obese individuals
        - Often have underlying nutritional deficiencies resulting in poor wound healing
        - Have associated medical conditions that require adequate preoperative optimization
            - Cardiovascular disease
            - Respiratory disease
                - Asthma
                - Sleep apnea
            - Diabetes

- Reimbursement
    - Insurance carriers are steadily reducing coverage of breast reduction procedures
        - The physician must document that the procedure is medically indicated
            - Relief of pain in the neck, back and shoulder

        - Relief of intertriginous infections
        - The above symptoms have failed medical therapy
    - The physician must remove "enough" breast tissue to reduce the breast size and weight
        - Trying to avoid reimbursement for a veiled mastopexy procedure
        - Minimal resection volumes in the past have been 500 gm per breast
        - More recently, minimal resection vary between insurance carriers and are often connected with body mass index (BMI) and can be more than 500 gm per breast
    - Many carriers have policy riders specifically excluding coverage of breast reductions
  - If insurance coverage is refused after the procedure is performed, the patient will be responsible for a large bill including
    - Hospital operative time and supplies
    - Anesthetic provider
    - Surgeon
  - If realistic concerns exist over coverage, the patient can be offered a cosmetic package price for the procedure as an alternative

Reduction mammaplasty — operative considerations

- Many different patterns exist for breast reduction
  - All are aimed at achieving the above states goals
  - Results vary between surgeons for the different methods
    - All tout their way of accomplishing the end result
    - All are dependent upon an interaction of many different variables, many of which the surgeon does not control
      - Weight of the breasts
      - Elasticity of the skin
      - Scarring
      - Inherent support structure of the breasts

- Each surgeon should keep a couple of the methods in his/her armamentarium for use in appropriate situations
- More popular approaches include
    - Wise pattern reduction mammaplasty
    - Vertical reduction mammaplasty
    - Superior pedicle mammaplasty
- Wise pattern reduction mammaplasty (see Fig. 3)
    - Based on the pattern used to cut cloth for a brassiere
    - New position of the nipple areolar complex is placed on the anterior projection of the inframammary fold
        - Around 21 cm from the sternal notch
        - Length varies dependent upon individuals trunk/chest size
        - A difficult problem to fix is surgical superior misplacement of the nipple areolar complex

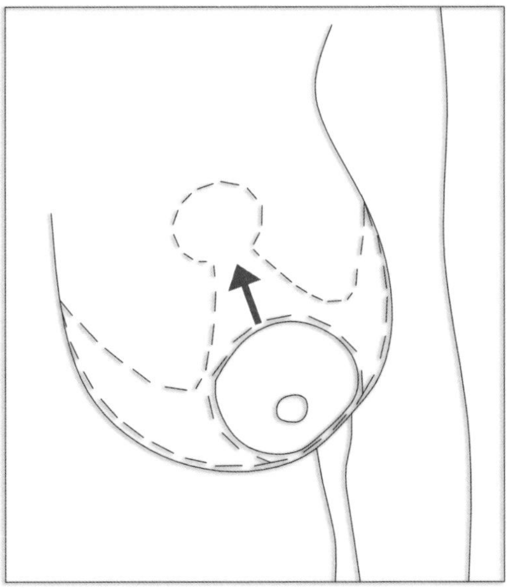

Fig. 3. Wise pattern reduction — preoperative skin incision marking.

  - A "keyhole" incision is either drawn from a template or free-handed on the breast mound while in the standing position
  - The new size of the nipple areolar complex is a diameter of 38 to 45 mm dependent upon patient request, surgeon preference, and resultant size of the breast mound
  - The standard length of the keyhole limb is 5 cm making the resultant distance from the nipple to the inframammary fold 5 cm
  - The divergence of the keyhole limbs determines the amount of resection, tightening of the skin envelope, and conical shape of the resultant mound
    - Narrow divergence results in less excision and less projection
    - Wider divergence results in more excision and more projection
    - Amount of divergence possible in the procedure is limited by tension on the skin closure
  - Advantages
    - Standardized approach to reduction mammaplasty — relative ease of use
    - Can be used on a variety of different breast sizes including macromastia
    - Fairly uniform and predictable preservation of the neurovascular supply to the nipple areolar complex
    - "On table" results are predictive of final results
  - Disadvantages
    - Large scar
    - Trifurcation incision point at the site of maximum wound tension often results in minor wound healing issues
    - Inframammary incision can result in discomfort when irritated by a brassiere
    - A "boxy" resulting appearance of the breast mound and bottoming out with loss of superior pole fullness over time.
- Vertical reduction mammaplasty (see Fig. 4)
  - Lassus procedure as modified by Lejour and Hall-Findlay[5–9]

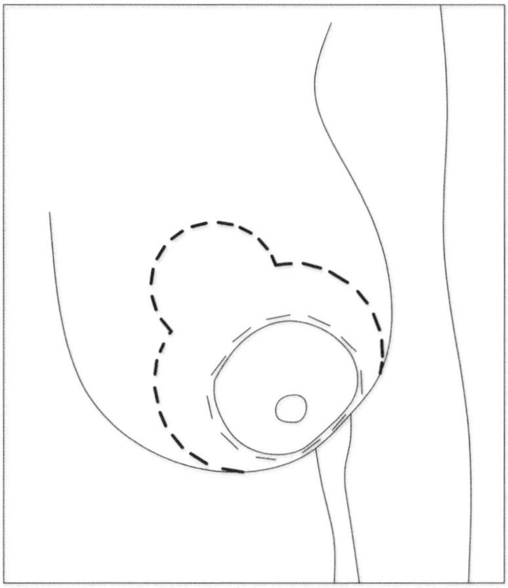

Fig. 4. Vertical pattern reduction — preoperative skin incision marking.

- Based on removal of parenchyma from the inferior aspect of the breast
  - Amount of resection directly influences the size of the reduction and the amount of "coning" of the resultant mound
  - Remaining tissue inferiorly is arranged to create "pillars" of support for the breast hopefully avoiding bottoming out
  - May require small horizontal extensions but generally is performed without a horizontal incision
  - Nipple areolar complex neurovascular supply is based on a superior or medial pedicle
  - Closure of the vertical incision
    - Often results in a nipple to inframammary fold distance greater than 5 cm
    - Requires "cinching" to shorten the length and remove vertical "dog ear" deformities
- The new position of the nipple is at the anterior projection of the inframammary fold

  - The new size of the nipple areolar complex is a diameter of 38 to 45 mm
  - Advantages
    - Avoids the uncomfortable horizontal inframammary incision of the Wise pattern
    - Less of a bottoming out and "boxy" appearance of the resultant breast mound
    - Good aesthetic results for moderate breast reductions up to 1000 gm
  - Disadvantages
    - On table results are not as predictive as Wise pattern of final results
      - Longer learning curve for the physician
      - Requires "hand-holding" with the patient until tissues settle and final results are apparent, up to 6 months after the surgery
    - In obese individuals does not allow for addressing of axillary fullness
    - Is generally considered less applicable to macromastia patients requiring reductions greater than 1500 gm

- Superior pedicle with inferior breast resection mammaplasty, Pitanguay reduction
  - Based on removal of parenchyma from the inferior aspect of the breast
    - Results in a periareolar, vertical and inframammary horizontal incision, Wise pattern
    - Nipple areolar complex neurovascular supply is based on a superior pedicle
  - The new position of the nipple is at the anterior projection of the inframammary fold
  - The new size of the nipple areolar complex is a diameter of 38 to 45 mm

- Advantages
  - Generally a faster operation than the inferior pedicle due to less time required to de-epithelialize the inferior pedicle
  - The superior base of the breast parenchyma has less difficulty with bottoming out and "boxy" appearance of the resultant breast mound than the Wise pattern reduction
  - Nice aesthetic results for moderate breast reductions
- Disadvantages
  - On table results are not as predictive as Wise pattern of final results
  - Difficult lengthy transposition of the nipple areolar complex in larger breasts
    - Not as easily applied to macromastia
    - Superior pedicle difficult to fold on itself in patients with glandular breast parenchyma[4]

Reduction mammaplasty — postoperative care and complications

- Can be performed as an outpatient procedure, reasons for admission can include
  - Large amount of intraoperative blood loss — observe for stability
  - Pain management — admission for intravenous (IV) medications
  - Concern of vascular supply to nipple areolar complex — observation
  - Drain management
- Drain placement and subsequent removal are dependent upon surgeon preference
- Possible complications
  - Vascular compromise of the nipple areolar complex
    - Congestion
      - If noticed intraoperatively consider free nipple graft
      - Postoperatively
        - Observation
        - Release of sutures

        - Leech therapy
        - Return to operating room for conversion to free nipple graft

    - Ischemia
        - If noticed intraoperatively consider free nipple graft
        - Postoperatively
            - Observation
            - Release of sutures
            - Nitro paste
            - Return to operating room for conversion to free nipple graft
    - Can result in partial loss of the nipple areolar complex
        - Dressing changes and secondary healing
            - Multiple follow up appointments
            - Physician patient relationship maintenance important
        - Eventual revision including reconstruction and tattooing
- Changes in nipple sensation
    - Paresthesia
        - May return with time
        - Is a known risk factor in reduction surgery, up to 9%, dependent upon
            - Reduction pattern utilized
            - Amount of tissue excised[10]
    - Hyperesthesia
        - Thought to result from decreased tension and traction on the sensory nerves
        - Generally improves with time
- Asymmetry
    - Important to try to achieve symmetry intraoperatively
    - Some asymmetry may result from variance in post operative edema
        - Wait at least 6 months prior to considering a revision

    - Important to stress preoperatively that some asymmetry is natural
    - If changing in the immediate postoperative period consider hematoma or seroma formation

- Wound healing issues

    - Often at areas of tension or multiple incisions meeting at a single point — i.e. trifurcation points
    - Generally heal secondarily with wound management
    - Scars can be revised later

- Hypertrophic scarring, especially at the medial and lateral horizontal inframammary incisions
- Axillary fullness

    - Especially in the obese patient, important to emphasize preoperatively that the breast does not include excess tissue in the axilla and the reduction focuses anteriorly
    - Excision in the original operation or in a revision surgery may be considered cosmetic and potentially not reimbursed by insurance carriers

- Poor positioning of the nipple areolar complex

    - Important to note intraoperatively and fix
    - Too low can be raised with crescentic excision
    - Too high is much more difficult to repair

        - Nipple areolar complex is not covered by bathing suits/bras
        - May require insertion of tissue expanders
        - Best is to avoid

- Poor shape or aesthetic result
- Insufficient or too large of a reduction

    - Preoperative assessment of patient expectations important

- Postoperative recurrent ptosis

    - Natural process

        - Preoperative assessment of patient expectations and procedure limitations important

        — Highly glandular/heavier breasts will descend more readily
      - Preoperative assessment of skin quality can be predictive

Augmentation Mammaplasty: Patient Selection and Preoperative Considerations

- Surgical goals of augmentation surgery
  - Increase the size of the breast mound
  - Correct any gross asymmetry
  - Mastopexy — limited to Grade I ptosis
- Patient goals for breast augmentation mammoplasty surgery — improved appearance
  - Psychosocial
  - Increased selection of clothing
  - Breast lift
- Patient/doctor relationship
  - Must establish congruence and discrepancies between perceived goals and achievable surgical results
    - Patients must understand scars that will be present
    - Realities of implants must be stressed to the patient
      - Implants have a finite lifetime and will most likely have to eventually be replaced due to failure
      - Implants have an inherent risk of infection
        - Greatest risk is in the perioperative period
        - May also "spontaneously" become seeded from transient bacteremia at any point in time resulting in an infection
      - As a foreign object placed within the body, the implant causes a natural reaction of the body that is to "wall off" the implant with a layer of scar tissue, a capsule
        - A soft capsule is the desired result
        - Pathologic proliferation of the capsule results in a capsular contracture

- Grading of capsular contracture
  - Grade I — no palpable capsule, breast is soft and natural appearing
  - Grade II — minimal firmness of the implant palpated, implant not visible
  - Grade III — moderate firmness, harder, implant profile is visible
  - Grade IV — severe firmness, breast is hard, tender, painful, cold, and distorted[11]
- Causes of capsular contracture are still being elucidated
  - May be related to formation of a biofilm on the implant[12]
  - Higher risk of formation associated with
    - Perioperative hematoma
    - Implant infection[13]
- Tightening of the capsular contracture results from myofibroblasts present in the capsule[14]

— The implant causes physical changes

- Gradual and progressive thinning of the overlying breast parenchyma
- Flattening of the underlying ribs
- Thinning and stretching of the skin resulting in visible striae

— With time the implants will descend due to their weight, they are not anchored to or attached to the chest wall

— Stretch marks on the skin preoperatively are a strong indicator that the lift achieved with implant will not be retained postoperatively

- Patients must understand that "cup" size is not an industry standard

  — Implants do not come in "cup" sizes, rather in cubic centimeters, a rough estimate in a "normal" sized individual is that 125 cc equals an increase in 1 level of cup size

        - Different bra vendors have different measurements of cup size
        - Cup size discussed preoperatively is only a guideline, not a specific measurable result
      - Postoperative pregnancy will affect the aesthetic result obtained in the surgery
    - Understanding the desired postoperative size
      - Tools to elucidate
        - Photos supplied by the patient of other individuals with desired breast appearance
        - Desired cup size with an understanding "cup" size limitations described above
        - Diagrams of breast profile with increasing superior pole fullness
          - Natural concave superior pole — minimal implant projection
          - Unnatural but possibly more desired convex superior pole — maximum implant projection
        - Photos supplied by surgeon of different patient results
        - During the consultation, use of implants in a bra to estimate desired size
      - Important to reinforce the limitations or sequelae in patient's requesting "unnatural" or "large" augmentations
        - Increasing trend of placement of greater than 300 cc, high profile, or extra high profile implants
        - Can exceed the limits of the natural tissue envelope
          - Excessive tissue atrophy and ptosis
          - Chest wall deformities
          - Permanent and irreparable damage[15]
- Reimbursement
  - Purely a cosmetic procedure
  - Patient may be responsible for postoperative complications necessitating medical intervention

        - Many insurance carriers have policy riders specifically excluding coverage of complications resulting from cosmetic procedures
            - Hospital admission, operative time and supplies
            - Anesthetic provider
            - Surgeon — fee possibly waived
        - Commercial insurance specific for cosmetic surgery is available

Augmentation mammaplasty — operative considerations

- Anesthetic
    - Monitored anesthesia with intercostal block
        - Risk of pneumothorax
        - Pectoralis muscle not paralyzed
    - General anesthetic
        - Increased cost
        - Anesthetic sequelae including nausea
        - Longer postoperative care and observation
- Implant choice — highly dependent on surgeon preference
    - Saline versus silicone
        - Saline
            - Silicone rubber shell filled with injectable normal saline
            - More popular in the United States for aesthetic procedures due to previous silicone moratorium
            - Advantages
                - Cheaper
                - Smaller incision required for insertion
                - If implant ruptures, body absorbs the saline and patient's breast becomes smaller
                - Allow for small adjustments in fill to achieve symmetry

        - Increased superior pole projection for a less natural but often desired "augmented" appearance
    - Disadvantages
        - More rippling — implant folds visible in the augmented breast skin surface, usually superior medial breast
        - Harder, less natural "feel"

- Silicone
    - Silicone rubber shell filled with viscous silicon polymer
    - Increasing popularity in the United States after moratorium lifted in 2006
    - Advantages
        - Softer, more natural "feel"
        - Newer cohesive implants retain shape even with failure of the silicone rubber shell
        - Decreased superior pole fullness for a more natural appearance
        - Less rippling
    - Disadvantages
        - More expensive
        - Previous litigation history
        - Requires a larger incision for insertion
        - Prefilled standardized sizes preventing fine adjustments for small asymmetries
    - Federal Food and Drug Administration (FDA) Requirements[16]
        - Physician must undergo training in order to place silicone implants
            - Provided by manufacturing companies
            - Discusses results of studies evaluating implant safety
        - Prior to placement, physician required to supply the patient with booklet published by manufacturer informing the patient on the risks of surgery
        - Manufacturer required to keep registry of implants

- As stated by FDA, suggested periodic evaluation of implant integrity by MRI
  - 3 years after placement
  - Every 2 years afterwards
  - May not be covered by insurance

- Textured versus smooth implant outer silicone shell
  - Textured implants
    - Advantages
      - Less movement
        - Shell integrates into capsule
        - Important for anatomic shaped
      - Decreased incidence of capsular contracture
        - With implant placed in subglandular plane
        - No significant difference in subpectoral position[17]
    - Disadvantages
      - More palpable due to increased thickness of shell[18]
      - Higher incidence of spontaneous rupture thought to be due to increased incidence of "fold flaw" (see below for explanation of fold flaw)[19]
  - Smooth implants
    - Advantages
      - Less palpable
      - Less incidence of spontaneous rupture
      - Decreased rippling in comparison to textured
    - Disadvantages
      - Movement
      - Increased capsular contracture in subglandular position[17]

- Round versus anatomic shape
  - Round implants
    - More common for cosmetic augmentation
    - Advantages
      - Ease of insertion — no polarity
      - Increased superior pole projection for a less natural but often desired "augmented" appearance

        - Disadvantages
            - Unnatural appearance due to superior pole projection
    - Anatomic implants
        - Silicone anatomic implant use in the United States currently restricted to study protocols
        - More commonly used in breast reconstruction
        - Pocket design and dissection more precise to prevent malposition and rotation
        - Advantage — more natural shape due to decreased superior pole fullness
        - Disadvantages
            - More difficult to place
                - Precise pocket
                - Additional variables including height, width, and multiple levels of projection
            - Malrotation resulting in an abnormal appearing breast shape
- Size and profile
    - Size measured in cubic centimeters (cc)
    - Profile is manufacturer dependent but spans from low to high
    - Size selection dependent upon
        - Patient desires
        - Physician preference
        - Patient physical characteristics
            - Base width — foot print of the breast on the chest wall
                - Implant width cannot exceed the width of the chest
                - Maximum implant width is the difference between the measured base width of the breast and twice the medial pinch thickness of the breast
            - Tissue elasticity

            - More elastic tissue allows for placement of larger implant
            - Overly lax tissue may not be able to support larger implant
            - Less elastic tissue will provide better support for a larger implant but will restrict shape and size
        - Location of the nipple areolar complex
        - Location of inframammary fold

    - Profile selection dependent upon
        - Patient desired projection
        - Physician preference
        - Projection dependent on volume, implant profile, tissue envelope, amount of breast parenchyma
        - Increased amount of parenchyma overlying implant will increase projection
        - Goal of increasing profile is to increase breast projection however a tight overlying skin envelope can negate this

- Submuscular versus subglandular placement
    - Submuscular
        - Superiorly the implant is beneath the pectoralis major muscle
            - Most approaches include the release of the inferior and the inferior medial attachments of the pectoralis major muscle
            - Implant pocket is then dissected in the loose areolar plane posterior to the muscle
        - Inferiorly the implant is beneath the glandular tissue
        - Advantages
            - Provides increased healthy soft tissue coverage of the implant
            - Used to camouflage the superior pole of the round implant providing the more natural concave shape
            - Less palpability of harder saline implant
            - Results in a decreased capsular contracture rate[20]

    - Disadvantages
      - Over aggressive release of the medial attachments of the pectoralis muscle results in a synmastia deformity
      - Insufficient release of the muscle results in "window shading" — a visible deformity of the implant with flexion of the pectoralis muscle
      - Increased risk of bleeding with incision of muscle
      - Increase postoperative pain with muscle incision
  - Subglandular
    - Implant is placed above the pectoralis major muscle
    - More common with silicone implants
    - More common in patients desiring prominent superior pole fullness
    - Requires sufficient soft tissue coverage of the implant — at least 2 cm in pinch test of superior pole
    - Advantages
      - Less postoperative discomfort
      - No deformity with pectoralis muscle flexion
    - Disadvantages
      - Increased risk of capsular contracture[17]
      - Increase implant infection risk
      - Increase visibility and palpability of implant
- Access incision
  - Axillary
    - Incision is hidden within the axilla posterior to the pectoralis muscle
    - Implant can be placed either in submuscular or subglandular plane
    - Can be assisted endoscopically
    - Advantages — nearly imperceptible scar
    - Disadvantages
      - Difficult placement of silicone implant through the axilla due to larger incision needed

        - Difficult controlled dissection of the implant pocket due to visualization
        - Any postoperative adjustments or implant exchanges have to be done through a periareolar or inframammary incision

- Periareolar
    - Incision is made along the inferior border of the nipple areolar complex
    - Implant can be placed either in submuscular or subglandular plane
    - Advantages
        - Direct visualization of dissection of implant pocket
        - Incision can be incorporated into a periareolar mastopexy
    - Disadvantages
        - Possibly visible scar on the anterior most aspect of the breast
        - Difficult placement of silicone implant in women with small areola
        - Potentially increased risk of changes in nipple sensation
        - Possible vascular compromise of the nipple areolar complex
        - Incision through glandular tissue
            - Higher risk of infection
            - May affect ability to lactate

- Inframammary
    - Incision made in or slightly above the inframammary fold over the breast meridian, often laterally displaced
    - Implant can be placed either in submuscular or subglandular plane
    - Advantages
        - Best direct visualization of dissection of implant pocket
        - Incision can be incorporated into an inverted "T" mastopexy
        - No incision through breast glandular tissue

        - Disadvantages
            - Visible scar on the breast
            - Incision at a site of tension — possibility of poorer healing
    - Umbilical
        - Incision is made in the umbilicus and tract bluntly dissected to the breast
        - Implant pocket is dissected via blunt dissection with a balloon
        - Implant is then placed via the umbilicus into the pocket
        - Advantages
            - Nearly imperceptible scar in the umbilicus
        - Disadvantages
            - Complete dissection performed blindly and bluntly
                - Minimal control of pocket
                - Difficult to achieve hemostasis
            - Revisions and implant replacements require an incision on the breast
            - Increased possibility of violation of abdominal or thoracic cavity during blunt dissection from the umbilicus
            - Cannot be used for placement of silicone implants

- Pocket dissection pearls
    - Lateral and superior dissection
        - Perform primarily with blunt dissection in order to avoid injury to the innervation of the nipple areolar complex
        - Keep to a minimum to avoid superior and lateral displacement of the implant
    - Inframammary fold adjustment
        - Inframammary fold can be lowered for symmetry or proper placement of the breast mound on the chest wall
        - Violation of the inframammary fold can result in postoperative descent of the implant to undesirable location

Augmentation mammaplasty — postoperative care and complications

- Considered an outpatient procedure
- Drain placement and subsequent removal are dependent upon surgeon preference but are rarely used
- Possible complications
    - Vascular compromise of the nipple areolar complex
        - Congestion or ischemia
            - Rare
            - Most commonly a result of previous incisions or placement of too large of an implant
            - Treatment
                - Release sutures
                - Downsize implant
    - Changes in nipple sensation
        - Paresthesia
            - Injury to the 3rd–5th lateral intercostal nerve during dissection of the implant pocket
            - May return with time
            - Is a known risk factor in augmentation surgery, 3–5% for all approaches[21]
        - Hyperesthesia
            - Thought to result from tension and traction on the sensory nerves
            - Generally improves with time
    - Asymmetry
        - Important to try to achieve symmetry intraoperatively
        - Some asymmetry may result from variance in post operative edema
            - Wait at least 6 months prior to considering a revision
        - Important to stress preoperatively that some asymmetry is natural

    - If changing in the immediate postoperative period consider hematoma or seroma formation or implant deflation
  - Wound healing issues
    - Rare unless comorbidities present or too much tension on the wound
    - Generally heal secondarily with wound management
  - Poor positioning of the nipple areolar complex
    - Important to note intraoperatively and fix
    - Too low can be raised with crescentic excision or lowering of the inframammary fold
    - Too high
      - Consider raising the inframammary fold to its original position if it had been lowered or decreasing the size of the implant
      - Direct surgical lowering or the nipple areolar complex difficult and results in a superior breast pole scar
  - Too small — a common reason for reoperation, communication is important
  - Poor shape
    - May require reoperation
    - Gross deformity raises concerns over hematoma or seroma
  - Postoperative ptosis
    - Important to predict preoperatively through assessment of tissue envelope quality
    - Natural process — preoperative assessment of patient expectations and procedure limitations important
    - Larger implants will place more tension on the natural tissues

Mastopexy

Patient selection and preoperative considerations

- Surgical goals of mastopexy surgery
  - Elevate the breast tissue on the chest wall resulting in an appropriate breast form restoring superior pole fullness

- Place the nipple areolar complex at the anterior most projection of the breast mound

- Patient goals for mastopexy surgery
  - Improved appearance
    - Increased selection of clothing
    - Increased cleavage
    - Youthful look
  - Relief of pain
    - Decreases strain on bra to provide lift
    - Decreases moment arm of weight of breast on neck, back, and shoulder

- Patient/doctor relationship
  - Must establish congruence and discrepancies between perceived goals and achievable surgical results
    - Patients must understand scars that will be present
    - Patients must understand that generally "lifts" have a finite existence
      - With time the breasts will descend due to the weight of the breast tissue on the skin and fascia
      - Stretch marks on the skin preoperatively are a strong indicator that the lift will not be retained postoperatively
      - The heavier the breast, the shorter the longevity
    - Patients must understand the size of the breast can decrease up to a "cup" size with the mastopexy surgery
      - Removal of skin decreases size of breast
      - Compression and tightening of remaining breast tissue and skin decreases apparent volume
      - Additionally, patient must understand that "cup" size is not an industry standard (see details above)

        - Patients also must understand risks
            - Possible neurovascular compromise of the nipple areolar complex
                - Rare
                - May result in partial nipple areolar loss requiring wound care and eventual revision
            - Possible detrimental effect of mastopexy on breast feeding — less probable than in reduction mammaplasty since mammary ducts are not interrupted
            - Postoperative pregnancy will result in recurrent breast ptosis
            - Weight loss after the mastopexy will result in decreased breast volume and recurrent ptosis

- Reimbursement — mastopexy is purely a cosmetic procedure and will not be reimbursed by insurance carriers

Mastopexy — operative considerations

- Many different patterns exist for the mastopexy procedure
- All are aimed at achieving the above states goals
- Results vary between surgeons for the different methods
    - All tout their way of accomplishing the end result
    - All are dependent upon an interaction of many different variables, many of which the surgeon does not control
        - Weight of the breasts
        - Elasticity of the skin
        - Scarring
        - Inherent support structure of the breasts
- Each surgeon should keep a couple of the methods in his/her armamentarium for use in appropriate situations
- May be combined with an augmentation
    - Difficult surgery

        - Increasing weight and size of breast while trying to tighten and decrease the size of the overlying skin
            - Increased tension leads to increased healing difficulty
            - Multiple incisions for mastopexy with dissection for implant placement can compromise neurovascular supply to nipple areolar complex
        - Higher complication rate than the individual procedures
        - High surgeon learning curve
    - Can be performed in two stages, especially in difficult patients
- More popular approaches include
    - Wise pattern mastopexy
    - Vertical mastopexy
    - Periareolar mastopexy
    - Crescentic mastopexy
- Wise pattern mastopexy
    - Based on the pattern used to cut cloth for a brassiere
    - New position of the nipple areolar complex is placed on the anterior projection of the inframammary fold
        - At least 21 cm from the sternal notch
        - Length varies dependent upon individuals trunk/chest size
        - A difficult problem to fix is superior misplacement of the nipple areolar complex
    - A "keyhole" incision is either drawn from a template or free-handed on the breast mound while in the standing position
    - The new size of the nipple areolar complex is a diameter of 38 to 45 mm dependent upon patient request, surgeon preference, and resultant size of the breast mound
    - The standard length of the keyhole limb is 5 cm making the resultant distance from the nipple to the inframammary fold 5 cm
    - The divergence of the keyhole limbs determines the amount of resection, tightening of the skin envelope, and conical shape of the resultant mound
        - Narrow divergence results in less excision and less projection

        - Wider divergence results in more excision and more projection
        - Width is limited by tension on the skin closure

    - Advantages

        - Standardized approach to mastopexy — relative ease of use
        - Can be used on a variety of different breast shapes and sizes
        - "On table" results are predictive of final results

    - Disadvantages

        - Trifurcation incision point at the site of maximum wound tension often results in minor wound healing issues
        - Inframammary incision can result in discomfort when irritated by a brassiere
        - Support dependent on skin alone, increasing likelihood of recurrent ptosis
        - Multiple scars for a cosmetic procedure

- Vertical mastopexy

    - Based on removal of skin excess from the inferior aspect of the breast with release of the inferior breast parenchyma, suture reshaping of the parenchyma, and suture anchoring the parenchyma superiorly to the pectoralis fascia

        - Amount of skin and parenchyma resection directly influences the amount of "coning" of the resultant mound
        - May require small horizontal inframammary extensions but generally is performed without a horizontal incision
        - Nipple areolar complex neurovascular supply is based on superior or medial pedicle
        - Closure of the vertical incision

            - Often results in a nipple to inframammary fold distance greater than 5 cm
            - Requires "cinching" to shorten the length and remove vertical "dog ear" deformities

    - The new position of the nipple is at the anterior projection of the inframammary fold

- The new size of the nipple areolar complex is a diameter of 38 to 45 mm
- Advantages
    - Avoids the uncomfortable horizontal inframammary incision of the Wise pattern
    - Less of a bottoming out and "boxy" appearance of the resultant breast mound due to internal reshaping
    - Good aesthetic results for moderate mastopexies
- Disadvantages
    - On table results are not as predictive as Wise pattern of final results
        - — Longer learning curve for the physician
        - — Requires "hand-holding" with the patient until tissues settle and final results are apparent in up to 6 months
    - Is generally considered less applicable severely ptotic breasts

• Periareolar mastopexy or doughnut mastopexy
- Based on removal of skin circumferentially around the nipple areolar complex with a purse string suture to tighten the remaining breast envelope
    - Limited superior transposition of nipple areolar complex compared to more invasive techniques
    - Purse string suture
        - — Permanent suture provides lasting strength and tension
            - Commonly use Gore Tex or Mersilene suture
            - Can become exposed with wound breakdown or slow erosion to the surface
                - Once exposed, will become colonized with bacteria and has to be removed
                - Removal will relax the associated breast causing asymmetry and loss of the lift
        - — Absorbable suture

        - Safer in that it has lower risk of exposure necessitating removal
        - Once is absorbs, the tension of the lift is transferred to the scar resulting in widening and relaxation of the lift

    - Results in a scar around the nipple areolar complex
    - New size of the nipple areolar complex is a diameter of 38 to 45 mm
    - Advantages
        - Faster operation than the above mastopexies
        - Easily and safely combine with an augmentation
    - Disadvantages
        - More limited longevity
        - Limited to small lift procedures
        - Will flatten the anterior breast shape
    - Benelli mastopexy modification and extension of the doughnut mastopexy
        - Treats skin and parenchyma separately
        - Skin envelope is dissected off of the parenchyma
        - Parenchyma is reshaped with a combination of incisions and sutures including anchoring parenchyma superiorly to the pectoralis fascia[22,23]

- Crescentic mastopexy
    - Limited excision of a crescent shaped piece of skin superior to the nipple areolar complex with primary closure
    - Applicable to fine adjustments to the height of the nipple areolar complex
        - Limited superior transposition of nipple areolar complex
        - No adjustment of the circumference of the nipple areolar complex

- Advantages
  - Fast
- Disadvantages
  - Does not tighten the envelope
  - More appropriately termed as a transposition of the nipple areolar complex
  - Limited longevity

Mastopexy — postoperative care and complications

- Usually performed as an outpatient procedure — admission primarily for complications noted during the procedure
- Rare drain placement
- Possible complications
  - Vascular compromise of the nipple areolar complex
    - Congestion
      - Release sutures and adjust tension and pressure
      - Observation
    - Ischemia — rare
    - Can result in partial loss of the nipple areolar complex
      - Dressing changes and secondary healing
        - Multiple follow up appointments
        - Physician patient relationship maintenance important
      - Eventual revision including reconstruction and tattooing
  - Changes in nipple sensation
    - Paresthesia — may return with time
    - Hyperesthesia — generally improves with time
  - Asymmetry
    - Important to try to achieve symmetry intraoperatively
    - Some asymmetry may result from variance in post operative edema
      - Wait at least 6 months prior to considering a revision

        - Important to stress preoperatively that some asymmetry is natural
        - If changing in the immediate postoperative period consider hematoma or seroma formation

    - Wound healing issues

        - Often at areas of tension or multiple incisions meeting at a single point — i.e. trifurcation points
        - Generally heal secondarily with wound management
        - Scars can be revised later

    - Poor positioning of the nipple areolar complex

        - Important to note intraoperatively and fix
        - Too low can be raised with crescentic excision
        - Too high is much more difficult to repair

            - Nipple areolar complex is not covered by bathing suits/bras
            - May require insertion of tissue expanders
            - Best is to avoid

    - Poor shape or aesthetic result
    - Insufficient lift — preoperative assessment of patient expectations important
    - Postoperative recurrent ptosis

        - Natural process

            - Preoperative assessment of patient expectations and procedure limitations important
            - Highly glandular/heavier breasts will be more difficult

        - Preoperative assessment of skin quality can be predictive

Acknowledgements

Author would like to thank Ceren Dayicioglu for illustrations.

References

1. National Cancer Institute — Surveillance Epidemiology and End Results website, http://seer.cancer.gov/statfacts/html/breast.html.

2. Handel N, Silverstein MJ, Gamagami P, *et al.* (1993) Factors affecting mammographic visualization of the breast after augmentation mammaplasty. *JAMA* **14**: 1913–1917.
3. Adams WP Jr, Rios JL, Smith SJ. (2006) Enhancing patient outcomes in aesthetic and reconstructive breast surgery using triple antibiotic breast irrigation: six-year prospective clinical study. *Plast Reconst Surg* **117**: 30–36.
4. Jones G. (2006) Breast reduction. In: Mathes S (ed.), *Plastic Surgery,* 2nd Edn. Elsevier, Philadelphia, PA, pp. 539–584.
5. Lassus C. (1970) A technique for breast reduction. *Int Surg* **53**: 69–72.
6. Lassus C. (1987) Breast reduction: evolution of a technique — a single vertical scar. *Aesthetic Plast Surg* **11**: 107–112.
7. Lejour M, Abboud M. (1990) Vertical mammaplasty without inframammary scar and with breast liposuction. *Perspect Plast Surg* **4**: 67.
8. Lejour M. (1994) Vertical mammaplasty and liposuction of the breast. *Plast Reconstr Surg* **94**: 100–114.
9. Hall-Findlay EJ. (1999) A simplified vertical reduction mammaplasty: shortening the learning curve. *Plast Reconstr Surg* **104**: 748–759.
10. Gonzalez F, Brown FE, Gold ME, *et al.* (1993) Perioperative and postoperative nipple sensibility in patient undergoing reduction mammaplasty. *Plast Reconstr Surg* **92**: 809–814.
11. Baker JL Jr. (1975) Classification of spherical contractures. Presented at the Aesthetic Breast Symposium, Scottsdale, Arizona.
12. Pajkos A, Deva AK, Vickery K, *et al.* (2003) Detection of subclinical infection in significant breast implant capsules. *Plast Reconstr Surg* **111**: 1605–1611.
13. Williams C, Aston S, Rees TD. (1975) The effect of hematoma on the thickness of pseudosheaths around silicone implants. *Plast Reconstr Surg* **56**: 194–198.
14. Baker JL Jr, Chandler ML, LeVier RR. (1981) Occurrence and activity of myofibroblasts in human capsular tissue surrounding mammary implants. *Plast Reconstr Surg* **68**: 905–912.
15. Tebbetts JB, Teitelbaum S. (2010) High- and extreme-high-projection breast implants: potential consequences for patients. *Plast Reconstr Surg* **126**: 2150–2159.
16. U.S. Food and Drug Administration website, http://www.fda.gov/MedicalDevices/ProductsandMedicalProcedures/ImplantsandProsthetics/BreastImplants/ucm063871.htm.
17. Barnsley GP, Sigurdson LF, Barnsley SE. (2006) Textured surface breast implant in the prevention of capsular contracture among breast augmentation patients. A meta-analysis of randomized controlled trials. *Plast Reconstr Surg* **117**: 2182–2190.

18. Burkhardt BR, Dema CP. (1994) The effect of Siltex texturing and povidone-iodine irrigation on capsular contracture around saline inflatable breast implants. *Plast Reconstr Surg* **93**: 123–128.
19. Handel N, Cordray T, Gutierrez J, Jensen JA. (2006) A long-term study of outcomes, complications, and patient satisfaction with breast implants. *Plast Reconstr Surg* **117**: 757–767.
20. Asplud O, Gylbert L, Jurell G, Ward C. (1996) Textured or smooth implants for submuscular breast augmentation. *Plast Reconstr Surg* **97**: 1200–1206.
21. Maxwell GP, Hartley RW. (2006) Breast augmentation. In: Mathes S (ed.), *Plastic Surgery,* 2nd Edn. Elsevier, Philadelphia, PA, pp. 1–31.
22. Benelli L. (1990) A new periareolar mammaplasty: the "round block" technique. *Aesthetic Plast Surg* **107**: 93–100.
23. Benelli LC. (1998) Periareolar Benelli mastopexy and reduction. In: Spear SL (ed.), *Surgery of the Breast: Principles and Art.* Lippincott-Raven, Philadelphia, PA, pp. 685–696.

CHAPTER 24

BREAST RECONSTRUCTION

John C. Oeltjen

Illustrative Case

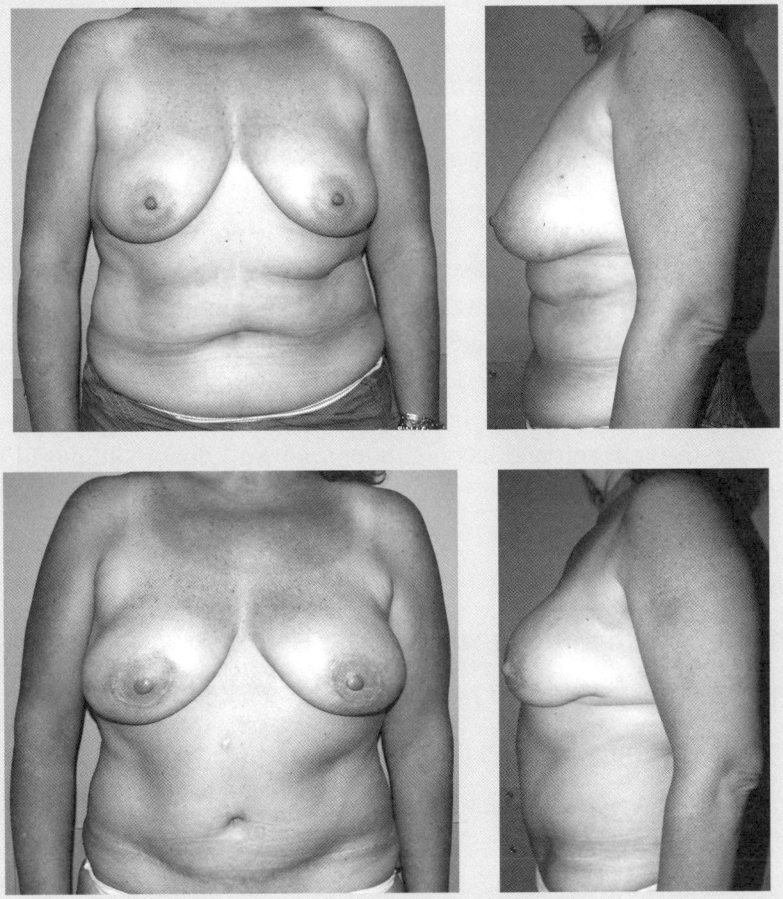

Fig. 1. Preoperative and 2 year postoperative photos of a patient who underwent a bilateral DIEP free flap breast immediate reconstruction.

48 year old G0P0 female presented to clinic with a clinical diagnosed T1N0Mx left breast cancer with a strong family history of breast cancer, BRCA1 and 2 negative, desiring breast reconstruction after a pending left modified radical mastectomy and right prophylactic mastectomy. The stated that she was a "B" cup in breast size and wanted to remain that size. The patient had no history of hypertension, diabetes, or any abdominal surgeries. On exam, the patient had bilateral Grade I ptotic breasts with no palpable masses or expressible nipple discharge. Her abdomen had skin and soft tissue excess without an overt pannus, scars, or hernias. Her BMI was 27.59 kg/m^2.

After a complete review of her history and physical exam, the patient was counseled extensively on the reconstructive options from implant to autologous tissue based reconstruction. The patient elected to undergo an immediate reconstruction with autologous tissue from the abdomen.

The patient underwent a bilateral mastectomy with immediate bilateral deep inferior epigastric artery perforator flap reconstruction. Her postoperative course was uneventful. 6 months following, she returned for an abdominal incision revision and bilateral nipple areolar reconstruction. Later she underwent bilateral nipple areolar tattooing. 2 years in follow up from her original surgery she continues to be happy with the result and has no abdominal wall donor site morbidity (see Fig. 1).

General Considerations with Breast Reconstruction Surgery

- Surgeon goals for breast reconstruction
    - Do not interfere with the patient's cancer treatment
        - May have to delay reconstruction until treatments are completed
        - If reconstructing the breast in the immediate setting, may have to change plan dependent upon pathology results

- Reconstruct a breast mound so that the patient appears normal within clothes
- Reconstruct a breast mound so that the patient or an observer cannot tell that the patient has had a mastectomy
    - Ideal
    - In reality, all surgery results in scars, with skin sparing mastectomy the scar is on the anterior aspect of the breast
    - Mastectomy is associated with removal of sensation and this is not routinely restored in the reconstructive process

- Human culture places a strong emphasis and importance on the breast
    - Considered central to the female form
    - Associated with fertility
    - Scars, asymmetry, poor aesthetic results, and postoperative complications in the context of cancer can be very emotionally charged
        - Good physician/patient relationships are important
        - Thorough and adequate consents are imperative
- As opposed to cosmetic breast surgery, is not entirely elective especially with immediate reconstruction
    - In patient's with multiple co-morbidities, may want to delay or not perform the reconstruction
    - Ideally patient will cease tobacco use
- Breast cancer is prevalent
    - 1 in 8 women develop breast cancer[1]
    - With a strong family history of breast cancer, may consider consultation with a geneticist prior to surgery
        - May elect to undergo a contralateral prophylactic mastectomy
        - May elect to undergo a hysterectomy and salpingo-oopherectomy
- Breast surgery is considered clean non-contaminated surgery
    - Intraoperative first generation cephalosporin or equivalent antibiotics should be sufficient

- No prospective double blind studies are available investigating appropriate perioperative antibiotic prophylaxis, especially with the placement of implants or tissue expanders
- *Staphylococcus epidermidis* is naturally found in the breast glandular tissue and can result in infections
- Many surgeons have a preferred approach to antibiotic prophylaxis in breast surgery
    - Triple antibiotic irrigation solution utilized in implant placement
        - 1 gm cefazolin
        - 5,000 units bacitracin
        - 80 mg gentamicin
        - In 500 mL of normal saline[2]
    - Others utilize povidone-iodine within the implant pocket however this may void the implant warranty
- Similarly no consensus for postoperative prophylactic antibiotic therapy exists[3]
- Lymphadenectomy may increase risk for infection due to increased rates of seroma formation and decreased lymphatic system associated immunity

- Blood loss can be significant
    - Breast is highly vascular
        - Perforators from the pectoralis muscle
        - Perforators through the muscle from the internal mammary artery
    - Hematomas can be large due to absence of restrictive fascial compartments
    - In immediate reconstruction, blood loss with the reconstructive portion of the procedure may be low but the patient may have already had significant blood loss from the preceding mastectomy
    - Axillary dissection with exposed axillary vessels and large branches can result in rapid large volume blood loss

  - Patient's having completed neo-adjuvant chemotherapy may be anemic preoperatively
- Postoperative care
  - Involves drains, support garments, implant care, wound healing
  - Pain generally well tolerated
    - Pain medications by mouth
    - Some physicians advocate local anesthetic delivery devices (pain pumps) — supported by anecdotal evidence only

History and Physical Exam Specifics for Breast Reconstructive Surgery

- History — specifics in breast reconstruction
  - Tumor staging — both clinical and pathologic
  - Planned course of cancer therapy
    - Mastectomy versus lumpectomy with radiation
    - Prophylactic mastectomy
    - Chemotherapy
    - Radiation therapy
  - Surgical history specific for breast and potential donor sites
    - Reduction mammaplasty, mastopexy, augmentation, lumpectomy, biopsies
    - Abdominal surgeries including laparotomy, hysterectomy, open cholecystectomy, cesarean section
    - Back or shoulder surgery
    - Previous thoracotomy
  - Physical exam
    - Breast — see similar section in reduction mammaplasty, augmentation mammaplasty, mastopexy chapter
    - Abdomen
      - Surgical scars
      - Skin and subcutaneous tissue excess and laxity

- Hernias, importantly midline and umbilical
- Diastasis

- Buttock and thighs
  - Surgical scars
  - Skin and subcutaneous tissue excess and laxity
- Back and axilla
  - Surgical scars
  - Scoliosis
  - Skin and subcutaneous tissue excess and laxity
  - Functional latissimus dorsi muscle and atrophy or paralysis from denervation during previous axillary lymph node dissection

Patient Selection and Preoperative Considerations

- The initial consultation for breast reconstruction can be very emotional
  - Patient has just learned of a life threatening diagnosis
  - The proposed treatment for that life threatening illness is also very disfiguring
  - The patient has multiple different issues, not just the reconstruction, to concentrate on
- Patient goals for reconstruction need to be elucidated during the consultation process but may include
  - Restoration of normalcy and feeling of "wholeness"
  - Breast size change, either larger or smaller
  - Improvement in breast appearance such as a lift
- Patient/doctor relationship
  - Must establish congruence and discrepancies between perceived goals and achievable surgical results
    - Patients must understand scars that will be present

        - Patients must understand that generally "lifts" achieved with breast reconstruction may have a finite existence
            - The support structure of the breast, Cooper's ligaments, have been removed
            - With time the breasts will descend due to the weight of the implants or transferred tissue on the skin and fascia
            - Stretch marks on the skin preoperatively are a strong indicator that the lift will not be retained postoperatively
        - Patients must understand that "cup" size is not an industry standard
            - Different vendors have different measurements of cup size
            - Cup size discussed preoperatively is only a guideline, not a specific measurable result
            - Numerical measurement is chest wall circumference and will rarely change with breast surgery
        - Patients also must understand
            - Reconstruction by any method is usually a series of staged procedures taking up to 1 year
            - The sensation of the breast will not be restored
            - Even after mastectomy, there remains the possibility of cancer recurrence
            - Symmetry is difficult to achieve in unilateral mastectomies and reconstruction

- Reimbursement
    - By federal law, insurance carriers are responsible for covering reconstruction and symmetry procedures
        - The extent of coverage, for example, how many procedures and revisions, is not dictated by law
        - Some insurance companies are refusing reconstruction after lumpectomies
            - States are passing legislation addressing the "loop hole"
            - Important to pre-certify partial breast reconstruction

- With continuing budget shortages, government subsidized health care may place limitations on reconstruction for patients without insurance

Approaches to Reconstruction

- Consists of three main approaches to reconstruction
  - Implant based reconstruction including the use of tissue expanders and permanent implants
  - Implant based reconstruction along with autologous flap transposition generally including latissimus dorsi myocutaneous flap with an implant
  - Autologous reconstruction without the use of implants including donor sites from the abdomen, buttocks, or thighs
- Can be combined with symmetry procedures on the contralateral breast the specifics of which can be found in the previous chapter
  - Reduction mammaplasty
  - Augmentation mammaplasty
  - Mastopexy
- Nipple reconstruction is usually left until after an optimal breast mound has been formed
  - Is optional, many patient elect not to undergo nipple reconstruction
  - Includes a surgical procedure to create a nipple mound
    - Local tissue rearrangement of flaps to project a nipple
      - Multiple different patterns exist
      - In general difficult to achieve long lasting projection
    - Grafting of tissue from either the groin or labia
    - May include the placement of autologous cartilage or various collagen products in order to increase longevity of projection
    - Can often be performed under local anesthetic
  - May be preceded or followed by tattooing pigment to the areola
    - Camouflages scars
    - Achieves a more realistic appearance of the areola

- Reconstruction in a patient who will be receiving or has received radiation
    - Radiation results in
        - Increased wound healing difficulty
        - Increased infections
        - Increased capsular contracture rates in implant reconstruction
        - Increased fibrosis of the veins and fragility of the arteries
    - Traditionally breast reconstruction has been delayed in patients who will be likely receiving radiation
        - The paradigm is shifting as improved surgical techniques and more focused radiation becomes available
        - Still associated with higher complication rates in comparison to non-irradiated patients
    - Delayed reconstruction of irradiated patients
        - Irradiated tissue does not expand easily or well
        - Usually requires transfer of some form of autologous tissue to the region to achieve a stable breast mound

Implant Based Breast Reconstruction

- Replaces the volume of breast parenchyma with implant volume
- Either one or two stages
    - One stage
        - Placement of a non-adjustable silicone or saline implant
        - Placement of an adjustable saline implant with removable port
        - More technically challenging operation
        - Limited size of implant placement — cannot put tension on the fresh mastectomy flaps
    - Two stages
        - Placement of a tissue expander followed by expansion to an appropriate size

        - Second operation where the tissue expander is exchanged for a non-adjustable implant
        - Allows for adjustment of size with expansion
        - Allows for adjustment of pocket position placement at the second operation

- Either in the immediate or delayed setting

    - Immediate

        - Combined with a skin sparing or nipple sparing operation
        - Can be one or two stages

    - Delayed

        - Routinely reconstruction after a mastectomy without skin or nipple preservation
        - Requires the use of a tissue expander followed by a second surgery

- Patient selection

    - Not indicated in patients who are adverse to having implants placed
    - Relatively contraindicated in patient who have had radiation or will be undergoing radiation (see radiation section)
    - Relatively contraindicated in women with large and or ptotic breasts

        - Current maximum available implants are 800 mL in silicone and 1100 mL in saline
        - These maximum implant sizes may only produce a small breast mound in obese large breasted women
        - Implants will not provide a unilateral breast reconstruction symmetric with a contralateral ptotic breast

            — May require a combination of contralateral mastopexy with implant placement for symmetry in unilateral procedure

            — In bilateral procedure, concomitant mastopexy or mastectomy skin envelope reduction procedure is required to remove excess skin and create an appropriate skin envelope over the implant

- Operative specifics
  - Implant placement (see Fig. 2)
    - Submuscular — implant placed underneath pectoralis major muscle superiorly and serratus anterior muscle inferolaterally
      - Limited muscle coverage inferiorly due to limited muscle availability
      - Difficult inferior pole expansion due to resistance of fascia
    - Partial submuscular — implant placed under the pectoralis major muscle superiorly and dermis of inferior mastectomy flap inferiorly
      - Allows for better inferior pole expansion than total submuscular
      - Depends upon the inferior mastectomy flap for support of the implant while placing tension on that flap
    - Partial submuscular with an acellular dermal matrix inframammary sling
      - Allows for better inferior pole expansion than total submuscular
      - Utilizes acellular dermal matrix to support the implant and shape the implant pocket
      - Associated with higher infection and seroma rate when compared to implant reconstruction without its use[4–6]
  - Requires drain placement
    - Large operative void is created and filled with a foreign object
    - Accumulation of seromas
      - Places increased tension on surgical incisions
      - Distorts the shape
      - Increases the risk of infection
  - Implant choice
    - Tissue expander
      - All are saline filled

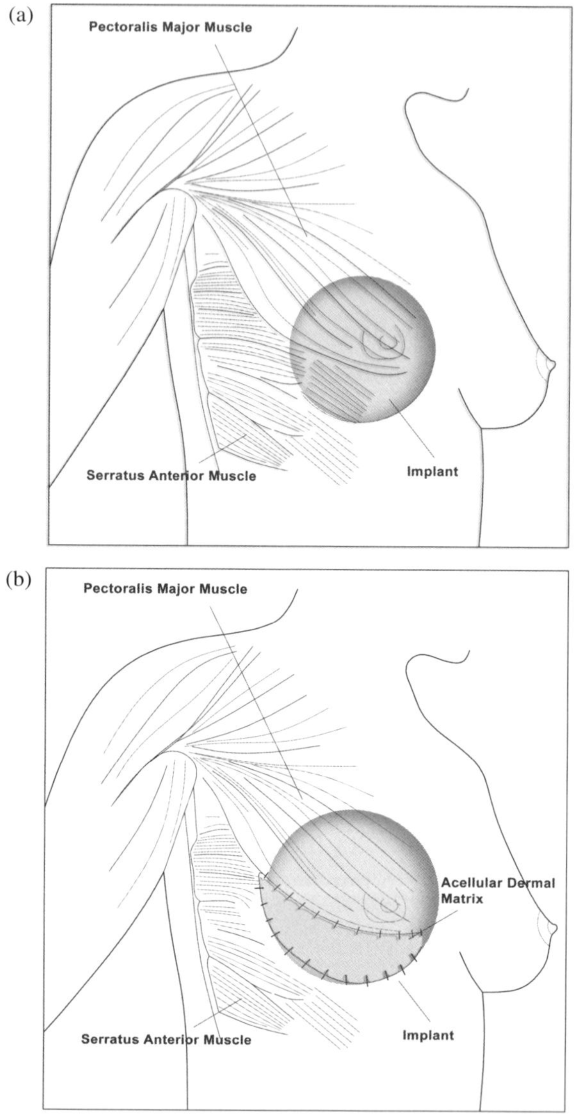

Fig. 2. Submuscular versus partial submuscular with acellular dermal matrix inframammary sling tissue expander placement. (a) The tissue expander is placed beneath the pectoralis major muscle, serratus anterior muscle, and fascia of the anterior chest wall. (b) The tissue expander is placed beneath the pectoralis major muscle superiorly and inferiorly underneath a "sling" fashioned out of acellular dermal matrix.

- Surgeon preference between remote and integrated port however integrated port more popular
- Size used is based primarily on base width of the breast footprint on the chest wall or width of the mastectomy pocket
- Profiles used, low, moderate, and high, are surgeon preference

- Saline implants
  - Silicone rubber shell filled with injectable normal saline
  - More popular in the United States for aesthetic procedures due to previous silicone moratorium, less popular in reconstructive patients
  - Advantages
    - Cheaper however cost is usually not an issue as most reconstruction is considered a "medically necessary" procedure and is reimbursed by insurance carriers
    - Smaller incision required for insertion however mastectomy incisions are not usually size limiting
    - If implant ruptures, body absorbs the saline and patient's breast becomes smaller
    - Allow for small adjustments in fill to achieve symmetry
    - Increased superior pole projection for a less natural but often desired "augmented" appearance
  - Disadvantages
    - In comparison to silicone implants, increased difficulty with visible rippling, (implant folds visible in the augmented breast skin surface, usually superior medial breast) due to lack of overlying breast parenchyma
    - Harder, less natural "feel"
  - Appropriate for patients in which follow up may be difficult to perform or in patients who do not want silicone implants

- Silicone implants
  - Silicone rubber shell filled with viscous silicon polymer

- Advantages
  - Softer, more natural "feel"
  - Newer cohesive implants retain shape even with failure of the silicone rubber shell
  - Decreased superior pole fullness for a more natural appearance
  - Less rippling in comparison to saline implants
- Disadvantages
  - More expensive however cost usually not an issue due to insurance carrier reimbursement of a "medically necessary" procedure
  - Previous litigation history
  - Requires a larger incision for insertion however mastectomy incisions are not usually size limiting
  - Prefilled standardized sizes preventing fine adjustments for small asymmetries
- Federal Food and Drug Administration (FDA) Requirements[7]
  - Physician must undergo training in order to place silicone implants
    - Provided by manufacturing companies
    - Discusses results of studies evaluating implant safety
  - Prior to placement, physician required to supply the patient with booklet published by manufacturer informing the patient on the risks of surgery
  - Manufacturer required to keep registry of implants
- As stated by FDA, suggested periodic evaluation of implant integrity by MRI
  - 3 years after placement
  - Every 2 years afterwards
  - Covered by insurance if the implant is placed as a reconstruction

- Textured versus smooth implant outer silicone shell
  - Textured implants

    - Limited to use in reconstruction primarily with anatomic implants
    - Advantages
      - Less movement
        - Shell integrates into capsule
        - Important for anatomic shaped implant placement stability
      - Decreased incidence of capsular contracture (see below section for description of capsular contracture)
    - Disadvantages
      - More palpable due to increased thickness of shell[8]
      - Increased rippling[9]
  - Smooth implants
    - Advantages
      - Less palpable
      - Less incidence of spontaneous rupture[10]
      - Less rippling[9]
    - Disadvantages
      - Movement
      - Increased capsular contracture rates

- Round versus anatomic shape
  - Round implants
    - Advantages include ease of insertion since there is no polarity
    - Disadvantages include unnatural appearance due to superior pole projection
  - Anatomic implants
    - Use of silicone anatomic implants in the United States currently restricted to study protocols
    - More commonly used in breast reconstruction
    - Ideally, pocket design and dissection is more precise to prevent malposition and rotation however pocket is large in a mastectomy

        - Advantage includes more natural shape due to decreased superior pole fullness
        - Disadvantages
            - More difficult to place because of additional variables including height, width, and multiple levels of projection
            - Malrotation resulting in an abnormal appearing breast shape

    - Size and profile
        - Size selection dependent upon
            - Patient desires
            - Physician preference
            - Patient physical characteristics
                - Base width is the foot print of the breast on the chest wall, implant width cannot exceed the width of the chest
                - Tissue elasticity, more elastic tissue allows for placement of larger implant
                - Size of expanded pocket
        - Profile is manufacturer dependent but spans from low to high
        - Profile selection dependent upon
            - Patient desired projection
            - Physician preference
            - Profile of implants placed is not dependent upon profile of tissue expander placed
            - Generally high profile implants are placed in reconstruction to try to make up for lack of projection resulting from the mastectomy

- Timing
    - Tissue expansion can begin 2 weeks after tissue expander is placed if wounds show good healing
    - Expansions can be performed weekly
    - Amount of expansion at the visit is limited by
        - Patient's pain experience

        — Assessment of the viability of the mastectomy flaps during the expansion

    - After expansion is completed, a period of consolidation/healing of several weeks is allowed prior to undergoing removal of the tissue expander and exchange with a non-adjustable implant

- Advantages of implant based reconstruction
    - Limited surgical site
        - Operation limited to breast and chest region
        - Other donor sites not created
        - Results in an overall quicker recovery and less discomfort for the patient
    - Limited operative time in comparison to other reconstructive approaches
    - Great variety in implant shape and size
        - Allows for tailoring of the breast reconstruction to the desires and wishes of the patient
        - Not limited by size of the donor site as in autologous reconstruction
- Disadvantages of implant based reconstruction
    - In a unilateral procedure, difficult to create a natural appearing breast with ptosis similar to the contralateral native breast
    - Implants have a finite lifetime and will most likely have to eventually be replaced due to failure
        - Longevity of implants is variable
        - About a 10% failure at 10 years
    - Implants have an inherent risk of infection
        - Higher risk of infection than in augmentations due to vascular compromise of overlying mastectomy with removal of breast parenchyma
        - Greatest risk is in the perioperative period

        - May also "spontaneously" become seeded from transient bacteremia at any point in time resulting in an infection

    - As a foreign object placed within the body, the implant causes a natural reaction of the body that is to "wall off" the implant with a layer of scar tissue, a capsule

        - A soft capsule is the desired result
        - Pathologic proliferation of the capsule results in a capsular contracture

            — Causes of capsular contracture are still being elucidated
                - May be related to formation of a biofilm on the implant[11]
                - Higher risk of formation associated with
                    - Perioperative hematoma
                    - Implant infection[12]
                - Tightening of the capsular contracture results from myofibroblasts present in the capsule[13]

            — Higher risk of capsular contracture in reconstruction as compared to augmentation
            — Anecdotal evidence points to a decreased capsular contracture rate with the use of acellular dermal matrix[14]

- Postoperative care and complications

    - Generally an overnight admission for immediate reconstruction, possibly outpatient procedure for delayed reconstruction
    - Drain placement and subsequent removal are dependent upon surgeon preference
    - Possible complications

        - Infection
        - Mastectomy flap loss or poor wound healing

            — Dependent upon
                - Thinness of the mastectomy flaps
                - Tension of the underlying implant on the skin
                - Patient factors such as history of radiation or smoking

            — Can be difficult to predict intraoperatively

    - Wound breakdown with implant exposure often results in an infection requiring removal of the implant

- Asymmetry
    - Difficult to achieve symmetry in unilateral procedures
    - Natural "ptosis" of native contralateral breast is difficult if not impossible to achieve
        - Contralateral mastopexy may help
        - Contralateral augmentation achieves better symmetry
        - Symmetry procedures should be delayed until second stage for optimum result
    - Important to stress preoperatively that some asymmetry is natural and expected
    - If changing in the immediate postoperative period consider hematoma or seroma formation or implant deflation

- Poor shape
    - May require reoperation and adjustment of implant pocket
    - Gross deformity raises concerns over hematoma or seroma

- Postoperative ptosis
    - Important to predict preoperatively through assessment of tissue envelope quality; thin skin in elderly patients will provide little lasting support of an implant reconstruction
    - Larger implants will place more tension on the natural tissues

Latissimus Dorsi Myocutaneous Flap with Implant Based Breast Reconstruction

- Replaces the volume of breast parenchyma with both autologous tissue transposed from the back along with an implant
- Provides healthy well vascularized tissue over an implant
- Latissimus dorsi muscle is transposed from the back based upon an intact thoracodorsal artery and vena comitantes (see Fig. 3)
    - Pedicle may be damaged during a sentinel lymph node dissection, axillary node dissection, or thoracotomy

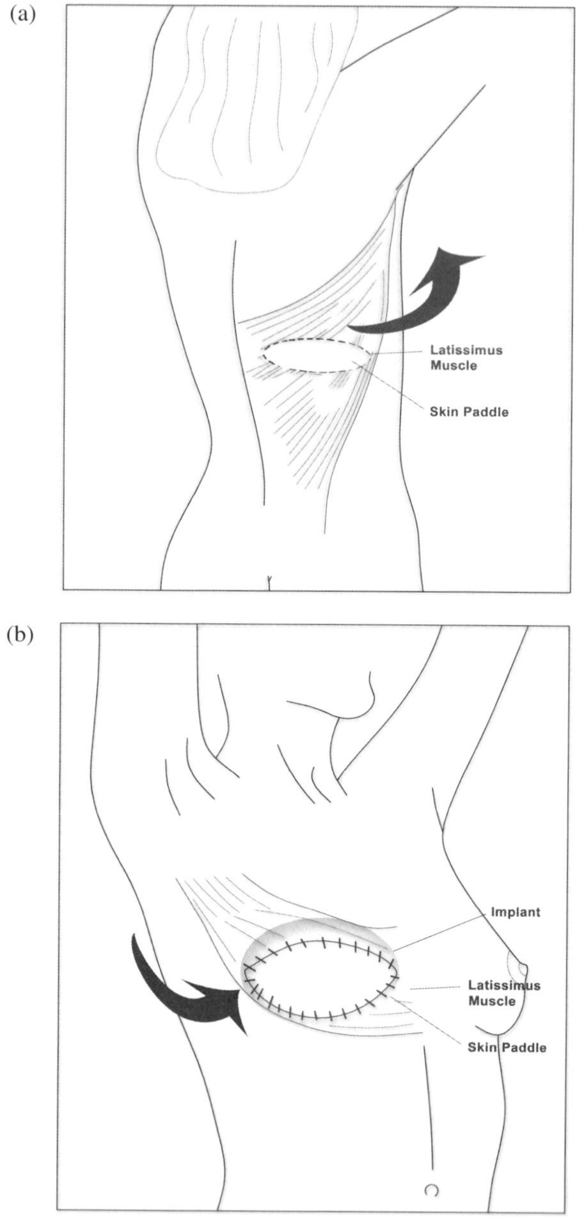

Fig. 3. Latissimus dorsi breast reconstruction. The ipsilateral latissimus dorsi muscle is harvested with a skin paddle and then transposed to the anterior chest utilizing the skin paddle to increase skin coverage of the breast mound.

- For delayed reconstruction, atrophy of the ipsilateral latissimus dorsi muscle or "winging" of the scapula are an indication that the pedicle may be damaged
- If the thoracodorsal artery is ligated proximally, the latissimus dorsi muscle may survive via backflow from an intact serratus anterior branch

- Patient selection
  - Not indicated in patients who are adverse to having implants placed
  - Relatively contraindicated in athletic individuals that depend upon upper extremity strength
    - Rowers
    - Rocks climbers
  - Relatively contraindicated in individuals with pre-existing ipsilateral or contralateral shoulder limitations
  - Relatively contraindicated in patient who will be undergoing radiation (see radiation section)
  - As opposed to implant alone reconstruction, latissimus dorsi with implant based reconstruction can match larger breasts in obese women
- As with implant alone based reconstruction, the implant placed can be performed in either one or two stages
  - One stage
    - Usually performed in the immediate reconstruction setting
    - Placement of a non-adjustable silicone or saline implant
    - Placement of an adjustable saline implant with removable port
    - Limited size of implant placement — cannot put tension on the fresh mastectomy flaps
  - Two stages
    - Placement of a tissue expander followed by expansion to an appropriate size

        - Second operation where the tissue expander is exchanged for a non-adjustable implant
        - Allows for adjustment of size with expansion
        - Allows for adjustment of pocket position placement at the second operation

- Either in the immediate or delayed setting
    - Immediate
        - Combined with a skin sparing or nipple sparing operation
        - In skin sparing, the cutaneous paddle from the back replaces the removed nipple areolar complex
        - Can be one or two stages
    - Delayed
        - Routinely reconstruction after a mastectomy without skin or nipple preservation
        - Cutaneous paddle from the back use to replace or augment the breast mound skin envelope
        - Unless a small breast mound is the desired result, often requires the use of a tissue expander followed by a second stage
- Operative specifics
    - Patient positioning — each operation requires at least one change in patient position
        - Supine positioning — for the mastectomy and for the inset of the flap and placement of the implant
        - Lateral decubitus — for harvesting of a unilateral latissimus dorsi myocutaneous flap
        - Prone — for harvesting of a bilateral latissimus dorsi myocutaneous flap
    - Implant placement
        - Superiorly implant is placed beneath the pectoralis major muscle
        - Inferiorly the implant is placed beneath the transposed latissimus dorsi muscle

- Requires drain placement
  - Large operative void is created and filled with a foreign object
  - Accumulation of seromas
    - — Places increased tension on surgical incisions
    - — Distort the shape
    - — Increase the risk of infection
- Implant choice is as detailed in above section
  - Tissue expander, saline implant, or silicone implant
  - Textured versus smooth
  - Anatomic versus round
  - Size and profile
- Timing is as detailed above

- Advantages of latissimus dorsi with implant based reconstruction
  - Increase of healthy robust vascularized tissue overlying the implant
    - Soft tissue of the breast mound is augmented by the flap while projection is provided by the breast implant
    - Provides a more natural appearing breast reconstruction; it is easier to achieve symmetry to the contralateral breast in a unilateral reconstruction
    - In an irradiated individual, provides needed vascularized tissue for creation of the breast mound
    - Overall low donor site morbidity — function of the latissimus dorsi muscles can be substituted by other muscles in the region including the rhomboids
    - Relatively low risk of flap ischemia
  - With the use of an implant, the great variety of implant shapes and sizes are included in the surgeon's armamentarium
    - Allows for tailoring of the breast reconstruction to the desires and wishes of the patient
    - Not limited by size of the donor site

- Disadvantages of latissimus dorsi with implant based reconstruction
  - Requires intraoperative position change increasing overall operative time
  - Results in a back scar
    - Accompanied by hollowing with removal of the muscle
    - Back asymmetry in a unilateral procedure
  - Implant complications, as detailed above, remain
    - Finite lifetime of the implants
    - Infections
    - Capsular contracture
- Postoperative care and complications
  - Generally the patient is admitted for 2–3 days for pain control and mobilization
  - Drain placement and subsequent removal
    - Dependent upon surgeon preference
    - High risk of donor site seroma formation; should leave in place until patient is fully mobilized
- Possible complications
  - Infection — specifically implant related, may consider more than a single dose perioperative antibiotic prophylaxis
  - Seroma — back donor site seroma is one of the most common complications in latissimus dorsi breast reconstruction procedure
  - Mastectomy flap loss or poor wound healing
    - Dependent upon
      - Thinness of the mastectomy flaps
      - Tension of the underlying implant on the skin
      - Patient factors such as history of radiation or smoking
    - With additional latissimus dorsi muscle covering the implant, wound breakdown is less likely than implant alone reconstruction to result in implant exposure
    - Can be difficult to predict intraoperatively

- Asymmetry
  - Natural "ptosis" of native contralateral breast is difficult if to achieve due to presence of implant
    - Contralateral mastopexy may help
    - Contralateral augmentation achieves better symmetry
    - Symmetry procedures should be delayed until second stage for optimum result
  - Important to stress preoperatively that some asymmetry is natural and expected
  - If changing in the immediate postoperative period consider hematoma or seroma formation or implant deflation
- Poor shape
  - May require reoperation and adjustment of implant pocket
  - Gross deformity raises concerns over hematoma or seroma
- Shoulder morbidity[15]
  - Patient will be reluctant to mobilize shoulder postoperatively due to pain especially with a concomitant axillary node dissection
  - Important to utilize physical therapy early in the postoperative period to help move the patient
  - Latissimus dorsi myocutaneous flap breast reconstruction is relatively contraindicated in patient's with previous history of shoulder difficulties

Autologous Tissue Flap Based Breast Reconstruction

- Replaces the volume of breast parenchyma with autologous tissue whether transposed as a pedicled flap or transplanted as a free flap from a donor site
  - Abdominal donor site — transverse rectus abdominis myocutaneous flap (TRAM) (see Fig. 4)
    - Pedicled depends upon superior epigastric artery

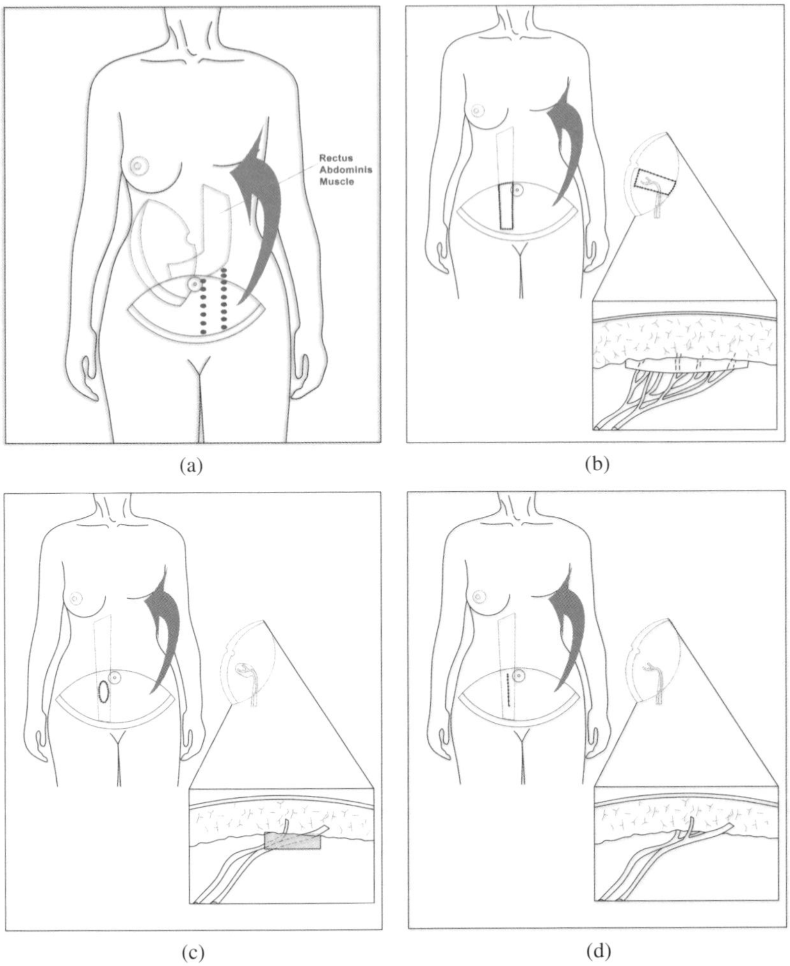

Fig. 4. Pedicled versus perforator based harvest of abdominal skin and subcutaneous tissue for breast reconstruction. (a) Pedicled TRAM — the rectus abdominis muscle is utilized as the conduit to transpose the abdominal skin and subcutaneous tissue based on the superior epigastric artery. (b) Free TRAM — the inferior rectus abdominis muscle is harvested along with the deep inferior epigastric artery to transfer the abdominal skin and subcutaneous tissue. (c) Muscle and fascial sparing free TRAM — only muscle surrounding a select number of perforators is harvested along with the deep inferior epigastric artery to transfer the abdominal skin and subcutaneous tissue. (d) DIEP — the perforators are dissected free of the surrounding muscle and harvested with the deep inferior epigastric artery to transfer the abdominal skin and subcutaneous tissue.

    - Free flap depends upon deep inferior epigastric artery
        - Standard TRAM
        - Muscle and fascial sparing TRAM
        - Deep inferior epigastric artery perforator flap (DIEP)
        - Superficial inferior epigastric artery flap (SIEA)
  - Gluteal donor site free flap depends upon gluteal artery
    - Superior gluteal artery perforator flap (SGAP)
    - Inferior gluteal artery perforator flap (IGAP)
  - Thigh donor site free flap
    - Transverse gracilis myocutaneous flap (TUG) depends upon medial circumflex femoral artery
    - Anterior lateral thigh fasciocutaneous flap (ALT) depends upon descending branch of the lateral circumflex femoral artery
- Goal is to replace entire volume of tissue removed by the mastectomy with autologous tissue
- In autologous free flap reconstruction, the recipient vessels include
  - Thoracodorsal artery and vena comitantes
    - Traditional approach
    - With less prevalence of axillary node dissection, there has been a decrease in the use of the thoracodorsal vessels[16]
    - Artery and vena comitantes may be damaged during the axillary node dissection or thoracotomy
  - Internal mammary artery and vena comitantes[16]
    - Increasing popularity
    - Avoids axillary dissection
    - Often larger artery in comparison to thoracodorsal
    - Position allows for more freedom of positioning of free flap during inset
    - Standard approach includes removal of a portion of the cartilaginous third or fourth rib
        - Possible pneumothorax
        - Increased postoperative discomfort
    - If used, is no longer available for coronary bypass grafting

- Patient selection
  - Not indicated in patients who are not medically stable enough to undergo a lengthy anesthetic time
  - Abdominal flaps may be contraindicated in individuals with previous abdominal surgery
    - Previous abdominoplasty is a definite contraindication
    - Open cholecystectomies, chevron incisions, aggressive Pfannensteil incisions may interrupt required blood supply
    - Ostomies through the rectus muscle obviate the harvest of ipsilateral tissue
  - Muscle harvesting procedures are relatively contraindicated in athletic individuals dependent upon abdominal wall, gluteal or thigh strength.
  - Relatively contraindicated in patient who will be undergoing radiation (see radiation section)
  - May have wound healing issues associated with obesity but obesity alone is not a contraindication
- Usually performed as a single stage reconstruction
  - Often requires a shorter revision surgery
  - Bilateral breast gluteal and thigh flap reconstruction can be performed in two stages, reconstructing one breast at a time
  - Bilateral abdominal based reconstruction is performed as a single operation.
- Either in the immediate or delayed setting
  - Immediate
    - Combined with a skin sparing or nipple sparing operation
    - In skin sparing, the cutaneous paddle from the donor site replaces the removed nipple areolar complex
  - Delayed
    - Routinely reconstruction after a mastectomy without skin or nipple preservation
    - Cutaneous paddle from the donor site used to replace inferior skin on the breast mound

- Operative specifics
  - Patient positioning
    - For abdominal and thigh donor sites the entire operation performed in supine position
    - Gluteal donor sites
      - Supine positioning for the mastectomy and for the microsurgical anastamosis and inset of the flap
      - Lateral decubitus or prone for harvesting of a the flap, prone is needed if performing bilateral
  - Flap inset
    - Superiorly flap is inset anterior to the pectoralis major muscle but posterior to the superior mastectomy flap
    - Inferiorly
      - In immediate reconstruction, the flap is inset posterior to the inferior mastectomy flap
      - In delayed reconstruction, the cutaneous portion of the flap replaces the inferior mastectomy flap
  - Requires drain placement both at the donor and recipient sites
  - Microsurgery requires a stable and controlled environment
    - Larger operating room for manipulation and positioning of microscope
    - Staff knowledgeable in microsurgical instruments
    - Stable patient
      - Warm
      - Normotensive, specifically no vasoconstrictors needed to maintain blood pressure
      - Isovolemic with good urine output
- Pedicled versus free TRAM based breast reconstruction
  - Advantages of pedicled flap reconstruction
    - Overall faster operation
    - No microsurgery involved
      - Shorter operative time
      - Postoperative close monitoring of the flap not required

- Advantages of free TRAM reconstruction
  - Deep inferior epigastric artery is larger than the superior epigastric artery
    - Improved blood supply to transferred tissue with successful microsurgical anastamosis
    - Less flap fat necrosis
    - Can reliably transfer more tissue
  - Decreased abdominal wall morbidity
    - From standard to fascial/muscle sparing techniques less muscle is removed in a free flap than with a pedicled TRAM[17]
      - Less postoperative abdominal pain
      - Less postoperative abdominal wall morbidity including abdominal hernia, bulging, or weakness
    - Especially in a bilateral procedure with fascial/muscle sparing approach, the abdominal wall strength is preserved in comparison to a bilateral pedicled approach
  - Improved shaping of the breast mound
    - Inframammary fold is not violated in order to allow passage of the pedicled flap
    - Pedicle of the free flap allows for more freedom of rotation and placement of the flap for the breast mound

- Advantages of autologous tissue based breast reconstruction
  - Provides the most natural reconstruction of the breast mound
    - "Like is replaced with like"
    - Provides natural ptosis and feel
  - In an irradiated individual, provides needed vascularized tissue for creation of the breast mound
  - Donor sites are chosen to have low donor site morbidity
    - Rectus muscle function replaced by psoas, external and internal oblique muscles
    - Gluteal muscle is spared in gluteal flaps

        - Gracilis muscle function replaced by other thigh adductors
        - Lateral thigh flap does not include sacrifice of the vastus lateralis muscle

    - No implant related complications
    - Primarily a one stage operation to create a breast mound

- Disadvantages of autologous tissue based breast reconstruction

    - More technically demanding, especially with microsurgical reconstruction
    - Longer operative and recovery time
    - Some of the procedures require intraoperative position change increasing overall operative time
    - Results in additional scars

        - Abdominal donor site results in

            - A periumbilical incision
            - A transverse hip bone to hip bone incision

        - Gluteal donor site results in a transverse incision at the superior or inferior aspect of the buttock with associated indentation and contour deformity
        - Transverse gluteal flap result in a medial superior thigh horizontal incision
        - Anterior lateral thigh flap results in a vertical incision along the anterolateral thigh with central flattening of the normal convex contour of the thigh

- Postoperative care and complications

    - Generally the patient admitted for 4–7 days for flap observation and vascular checks, pain control and mobilization
    - Drain placement and subsequent removal are dependent upon surgeon preference

- Possible complications

    - Infection — without implants there is reduced perioperative antibiotic requirements in relation to implant based breast reconstructions.

- Seroma — donor site seroma is a common
- Mastectomy flap loss or poor wound healing
  - Dependent upon
    - Thinness of the mastectomy flaps
    - Tension of the underlying implant on the skin
    - Patient factors such as history of radiation or smoking
  - Can be difficult to predict intraoperatively
- Free or pedicled flap loss due to
  - Technical error
  - Tension or pressure on the anastamosis, pedicle, or transferred tissue
  - Patient instability
- Asymmetry
  - Size of reconstruction is limited by tissue available for transfer
  - Easier than implant based reconstructions to achieve ptosis due to natural descent of autologous tissue
  - May require a contralateral mastopexy or reduction mammaplasty to achieve symmetry
  - Symmetry procedures should be delayed until second stage for optimum result to ensure flap survival and allow to postoperative "settling"
  - Important to stress preoperatively that some asymmetry is natural and expected
  - If changing in the immediate postoperative period consider hematoma or seroma formation
- Poor shape
  - May require reoperation with flap revisions
  - Gross deformity raises concerns over hematoma or seroma

References

1. National Cancer Institute — Surveillance Epidemiology and End Results website, http://seer.cancer.gov/statfacts/html/breast.html.
2. Adams WP Jr., Rios JL, Smith SJ. (2006) Enhancing patient outcomes in aesthetic and reconstructive breast surgery using triple antibiotic breast irrigation: six-year prospective clinical study. *Plast Reconstr Surg* **117**: 30–36.
3. Phillips BT, Wang ED, Mirrer J, Lanier ST, *et al.* (2011) Current practice among plastic surgeons of antibiotic prophylaxis and closed-suction drains in breast reconstruction: experience, evidence, and implications for postoperative care. *Ann Plast Surg* **66**: 460–465.
4. Lanier ST, Wang ED, Chen JJ, *et al.* (2010) The effect of acellular dermal matrix use on complication rates in tissue expander/implant breast reconstruction. *Ann Plast Surg* **64**: 674–678.
5. Anthony AK, McCarthy CM, Codeiro PG, Mehrar BJ, *et al.* (2010) Acellular human dermis implantation in 153 immediate two-stage tissue expander breast reconstruction: determining the incidence and significant predictors of complications. *Plast Reconstr Surg* **125**: 1606–1614.
6. Chun YS, Verma K, Rosen H, Lipsitz S, *et al.* (2010) Implant-based reconstruction using acellular dermal matrix and the risk of postoperative complications. *Plast Reconstr Surg* **125**: 429–436.
7. U.S. Food and Drug Administration website, http://www.fda.gov/MedicalDevices/ProductsandMedicalProcedures/ImplantsandProsthetics/BreastImplants/ucm063871.htm.
8. Burkhardt BR, Dema CP. (1994) The effect of Siltex texturing and povidone-iodine irrigation on capsular contracture around saline inflatable breast implants. *Plast Reconstr Surg* **93**: 123–128.
9. Barnsley GP, Sigurdson LF, Barnsley SE. (2006) Textured surface breast implant in the prevention of capsular contracture among breast augmentation patients. A meta-analysis of randomized controlled trials. *Plast Reconstr Surg* **117**: 2182–2190.
10. Handel N, Cordray T, Gutierrez J, Jensen JA. (2006) A long-term study of outcomes, complications, and patient satisfaction with breast implants. *Plast Reconstr Surg* **117**: 757–767.
11. Pajkos A, Deva AK, Vickery K, *et al.* (2003) Detection of subclinical infection in significant breast implant capsules. *Plast Reconstr Surg* **111**: 1605–1611.

12. Williams C, Aston S, Rees TD. (1975) The effect of hematoma on the thickness of pseudosheaths around silicone implants. *Plast Reconstr Surg* **56**: 194–198.
13. Baker JL Jr., Chandler ML, LeVier RR. (1981) Occurrence and activity of myofibroblasts in human capsular tissue surrounding mammary implants. *Plast Reconstr Surg* **68**: 905–912.
14. Salzberg CA, Ashikari AY, Koch RM, Chabner-Thompson E. (2011) An 8-year experience of direct-to-implant immediate breast reconstruction using human acellular dermal matrix (AlloDerm). *Plast Reconstr Surg* **127**: 514–524.
15. Button J, Scott J, Taghizadeh R, Weiler-Mithoff E, Hart AM. Shoulder function following autologous latissimus dorsi breast reconstruction. A prospective three year observational study comparing quilting and non-quilting donor site techniques. *J Plast Reconstr Aesthet Surg* **63**: 1505–1512.
16. Saint-Cyr M, Youssef A, Bae HW, Robb GL, Chang DW. (2007) Changing trends in recipient vessel selection for microvascular autologous breast reconstruction: an analysis of 1483 consecutive cases. *Plast Reconstr Surg* **119**: 1993–2000.
17. Vyas RM, Dickinson BP, Fastekjian JH, Watson JP, *et al.* (2008) Risk factors for abdominal donor-site morbidity in free flap breast reconstruction. *Plast Reconstr Surg* **121**: 1519–1526.

CHAPTER 25

AESTHETIC BODY CONTOURING: ABDOMINOPLASTY

Steven Rueda and Seth R. Thaller

Illustrative Case

A 38 year old Hispanic female presents to your office requesting a "tummy tuck". She says she expected her body to return to her usual habitus after the birth of her last child three years ago but is unhappy with her current physical appearence. She denies any medical conditions or taking any medications. Her past surgical history is significant for an emergency exploratory laparotomy for appendicitis 6 years prior to presentation. She developed no postoperative complications. She delivered her two children via spontaneous vaginal delivery. Her physical exam is remarkable for a BMI of 31kg/m^2. Abdominal inspection reveals a 10-cm vertical scar extending from 2-cm below the

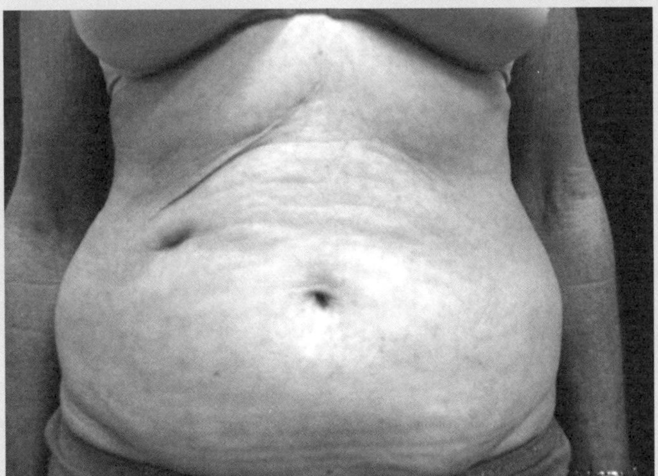

umbilicus towards the pubic region. On palpation of the abdominal wall there is mild skin laxity and lower abdominal flaccidity. The procedure most adequate for this patient's abdominoplasty is?

This patient has the indications for a modified Type II abdominoplasty. The previous scar from her exploratory laparotomy can be used as the means to access her abdominal musculature and remove excess tissue. This patient also has mild skin laxity and lower abdominal wall flaccidity which make the Type IIa an adequate procedure.

Indications

- Loose upper abdominal skin
- Excess abdominal fatty tissue
- Abdominal bulging due to fascia flaccidity
- Damaged lower abdominal skin
- Striae
- Diastasis of rectus muscles

Contraindications

- The contraindications to undergo abdominoplasty include those that limit patients from undergoing any other major surgical procedure
- However, other contraindications that affect outcome or technique are also included. See Table 1

Preoperative Care

Preoperative Interview

- Have a member of the staff or yourself hand the patient documentation describing the procedure of interest in detail including preoperative care, surgical approach, and postoperative care

History and Physical Exam

History

1. Obtain the main problem the patient wants to address
2. Assess the patient's behavior and if expectations are realistic

Table 1. Common Contraindications to Abdominoplasty.

Contraindication	Discussion
Emotional instability and unrealistic expectations	Beware of patients that have an unusual history of previous surgeries, previous litigations for aesthetic surgery, unusual demands and behavior. Screen and refer for psychiatric evaluation when adequate
Selected abdominal scars	Can be relative or absolute contraindications as these can cause avascular necrosis when abdominal wall is elevated during surgery. In general, if the scar can be resected with the pannus it does not pose a risk for necrosis. On the contrary, midline scars that are transected below the umbilicus can be relative or absolute contraindications as the resulting scar can affect blood flow across the midline of the abdomen. Vascular compromise is also seen in classic subcostal incisions like that of open cholecystectomy
Future pregnancy	Can lead to abdominal wall laxity and is thus a relative contraindication to the procedure
Morbid obesity (BMI > 40)	Can lead to difficulty tightening the abdominal wall by abdominoplasty alone
History of thromboembolic disease	A relative contraindication as the procedure puts patients at increased risk for these conditions
Failure to meet preoperative evaluation	Due to severe comorbid condition (heart disease, pulmonary disease, poorly controlled diabetes, etc.) or any other factors
Smoking	It is not advisable to operate on patients who smoke due resulting poor healing and potential ischemia to tissues

3. Past surgical history with emphasis on abdominal interventions and any complications
4. Past medical history to screen for bleeding disorders or comorbid conditions that would put the patient at increased morbidity if they were to undergo the procedure
5. Medication and allergy history with emphasis on intake of NSAIDs, steroids, anticoagulants, herbals, or hormones

6. Always perform a review of systems to ensure no relevant symptoms are being missed

Physical (ideally performed in a three-way mirror)

1. Obtain patients BMI and inspect the body to assess likelihood of operative intervention
2. Examine area of patient's complaint
3. Explain the anatomy in layman's terms and the outcome that is realistically expected
4. Use drawings or software to explain the anatomical cause of the patients deformity and preferred technique to correct it
5. Determine if abdominoplasty alone would result in desired outcomes or if a less invasive procedure like liposuction would be more adequate
6. Examine the abdomen for any hernias (umbilical, inguinal)
7. Perform a basic heart and lung examination
8. Informed consent is important. Never forget to answer any questions the patient has about the procedure, the risks, and the alternative treatments if available
9. Obtain photographs in front, back, right lateral, left lateral, front oblique, back oblique, bending over, and extra skin pictures. These help guide the procedure and are usually repeated after the procedure to analyze the results

Preoperative Tests

- The American Society of Anesthesiologists task force claims most preoperative tests to be ordered should be determined on a case by case basis
- Preoperative evaluation by anesthesiologist and medical specialist is suggested for patients with severe comorbid conditions (ASA III risk)
- Studies 1–2 are suggested for healthy patients; studies 3–6 may also be appropriate, especially for patients older than 40, with comorbid conditions, or suspected of smoking:

    1. CBC
    2. βhCG for female patients

3. PT/PTT/INR
4. Chest X-ray
5. ECG
6. Urine cotinine levels

Nutritional Evaluation

- Many patients seeking body contouring surgery are obese or present following bariatric surgery
- Both types of patients often have preexisting micronutrient/macronutrient deficiencies that lead to increased postoperative complications
- Among the nutritional deficiencies reported are proteins, vitamins, and minerals
- An extensive history is necessary to identify patients at risk of nutritional deficiency. Important parameters to inquire are initial weight, weight loss, rate of weight loss, procedure performed, time since bariatric procedure, and dietary habits.
- Large amount of weight loss rate, total weight loss, malabsorptive procedures, and poor diet should alert the plastic surgeon's attention to a possible nutritional deficiency
- Countouring procedures are recommended once the patient achieves a steady weight which occurs between 18–24 months postop.
- Guidelines for nutrition screening and support after bariatric surgery are shown in Tables 2a and 2b
- Micronutrient deficiencies are less common in band gastroplasty than in Roux-en-Y gastric bypass and biliopancreatic diversion presumably because the small intestine remains intact
- Table 2c describes the nutritional deficiencies, presentation, recommendations, and additional comments to take into account when evaluating the body contouring patient. Additional deficiencies not included in the recommended biochemical surveillance are presented.

Table 2a. Recommended Biochemical Surveillance of Nutritional Status After Malabsorptive Bariatric Surgical Procedures.

Surveillance Factor	Roux-en-Y Gastric Bypass	Biliopancreatic Diversion (± Duodenal Switch)
Time Interval		
1st year	Every 3–6 mo	Every 3 mo
Thereafter	Annually	Every 3-6 mo depending on symptoms
Laboratory tests	CBC, platelets	CBC, platelets
	Electrolytes	Electrolytes
	Glucose	Glucose
	Iron studies, ferritin	Iron studies, ferritin
	Vitamin B12 (MMA, HCy optional)	Vitamin B12 (MMA, HCy optional)
	Liver function (GGT optional)	Liver function (GGT optional)
	Lipid profile	Lipid profile
	25-Hydroxyvitamin D	Albumin and prealbumin
	Optional: Intact PTH Thiamine RBC folate	RBC folate Fat-soluble vitamins (6–12 mo) Vitamin A 25-Hydroxyvitamin D Vitamin E Vitamin K and INR Metabolic bone evaluation Intact PTH (6–12 mo) 24-h urine calcium (6–12 mo) Urine N-telopeptide (annually) Osteocalcin (as hended) Metabolic stone evaluation 24-h urine calcium, citrate, uric acid, and oxalate Trace elements Zinc Selenium Miscellaneous (as needed) Carnitine Essential fatty acid chromatography

Source: Table adapted from Ref. 13.

CBC, complete blood cell count; GGT, γ-glutamyltransferase; HC, homocysteine; INR, international normalized ratio; MMA, methylmalonic acid; mo, months; PTH, parathyroid hormone; RBC, red blood cell.

Table 2b. Routine Nutrient Supplementation After Bariatric Surgery

Supplement	Dosage†
Multivitamin	1–2 daily
Calcium citrate with Vitamin D	l,200–2,000 mg/day + 400–800 U/day
Folic acid	400 μg/day in multivitamin
Elemental iron with Vitamin D*	40–65 mg/day
Vitamin B12	≥350 μg/day orally
	Or 1,000 μg/mo intramuscularly
	Or 3,000 μg every 6 mo intramuscularly
	Or 500 μg/week intramuscularly

Source: Adapted from Ref. 13.
mo, month.
*For menstruating women.
†Patients with preoperative or postoperative biochemical deficiency states are treated beyond these recommendations.

Operative Technique List

- Table 3. Shows seven techniques that are used during abdominoplasty
- The properties of skin, musculofascial system, and quantity of fat are important factors that determine the type of technique to be used

Operative Technique Description

Type I. Suction-Assisted Lipectomy (SAL)

Indications

- Minimal skin laxity and minimal flaccidity of musculofascial system
- Adequate skin tone allows proper retraction and desired results
- Usually 0.5 to 1.0 L of volume removed

Contraindications

- Poor skin tone , significant skin laxity, or moderate to significant musculofascial flaccidity

Table 2c. Nutritional Deficiency Presentation, Recommendation, and Additional Comments.

Nutrient	Clinical Presentation	Recommendations	Comments
Vitamin B12	Mainly subclinical. Neurologic impairment, anemia, megaloblastosis	≥ 350 μg/day orally	Patients after Roux-en-Y gastric bypass cannot maintain B12 levels with diet alone
Folate	Mainly subclinical. Megaloblastic anemia, megaloblastosis	400 μg/day	Common in obese patient without any bypass procedure
Vitamin C	Usually asymptomatic. If severe, patients present with gingivitis, dryhair, nose bleeds, easy bruising	1–2 g/day	Vitamin C important in wound healing collagen synthesis and angiogenesis. Increased susceptibility to infection
Thiamine	Peripheral neuropathy, weakness, Wernicke encephalopatny	50–200 mg/day IV until symptom resolution, 10–100 mg oral daily	Common in vertical banded gastroplasty
Vitamin A	Night blindness, dry skin	25,000–50,000 IU orally or 10,000 IU IV before elective procedures	Common in biliopancreatic diversion. Important for wound healing and immune system

(*Continued*)

Table 2c. (*Continued*)

Nutrient	Clinical Presentation	Recommendations	Comments
Calcium and Vitamin D	Osteoporosis, osteomalacia, secondary hyper-parathyroidism	I,200–2,000 mg/day + 400–800 U/day	Most common in Roux-en-Y gastric bypass
Vitamin K	Bleeding		No manifestations of bleeding in literature. Data lacking about the effects of this vitamin
Vitamin E	Anemia, neurological deficit, cataracts		Not a common deficiency when patients supple-mented with multivitamin
Iron	Fatigue, dizziness, pale skin	40–65 mg/day	Addition of Vitamin C for increased absorp-tion is adequate
Zinc	Subclinical. Hair thinning, hair loss	11 mg/day for men and 8 mg/day for women	Important for wound strength and healing

Source: Table compiled from Refs. 10, 11 and 13 recommendations.

Step-by-Step Procedure (Fig. 1)

1. Excess fat is palpated and marked with surgical marker while patient standing
2. After induction of anesthesia, the super-wet or tumescent method may be used. Super-wet fluid is injected in the subcutaneous tissue until skin blanching is achieved. The amount of fluid injected should be the same or 50% larger than that of expected aspirate. Advantages of super-wet technique are decreased bruising, blood loss, and pain due to the effects of epinephrine and lidocaine. To

Table 3. Abdominolipoplasty Classification System.

Category	Skin	Fat	Musculofascial System	Treatment
Type I	Minimal laxity	Variable	Minimal flaccidity	Suction-assisted lipectomy
Type Ia	*Minimal laxity*	↑↑	*Minimal flaccidity*	*Extended suction-assisted lipectomy*
Type II	Mild laxity	Variable	Mild lower abdominal flaccidity	Miniabdominoplasty
Type IIa	*Mild laxity with vertical scar*	*Variable*	*Mild lower abdominal flaccidity*	*Open miniabdominoplasty*
Type III	Moderate laxity	Variable	Moderate lower and/or upper abdominal flaccidity	Modified abdominoplasty
Type IIIa	*Minimal, mild, or moderate laxity*	*Variable*	*Moderate lower and/or upper abdominal flaccidity*	*Endoscopic modified abdominoplasty*
Type IV	Severe laxity	Variable	Significant lower and/or upper abdominal flaccidity	Standard abdominoplasty with succion-assisted lipectomy

Rows in italic font describe minimal-access variation techniques. Underlined font indicates differences between minimal-access variation techniques and their counterparts.
Source: Table compiled from Refs. 6 and 7.

avoid lidocaine toxicity the amount injected should not be greater than 35 mg/kg.

3. Marked areas undergo liposuction and are contoured as desired. The cannulas of choice for the initial part of the procedure are large bore. It is important to maintain symmetry by removing identical amounts of aspirate volume bilaterally

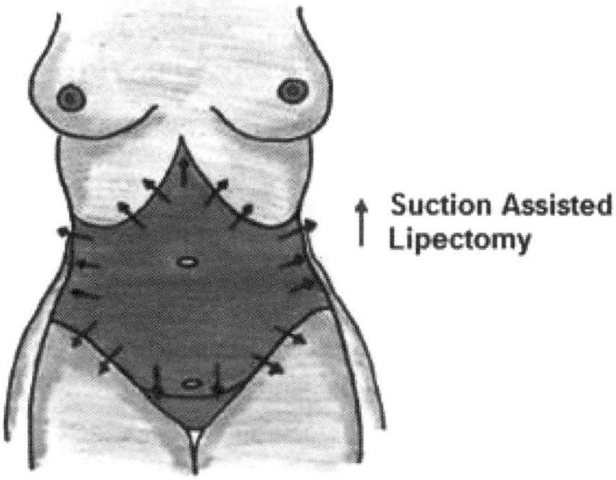

Fig. 1. Type 1.

4. Repeat step 3, however, as suctioning progresses superficially smaller bore cannulas should be used
5. Postoperative care will be discussed in the corresponding section

Type Ia. Extended Suction-Assisted Lipectomy

Indications

- Indications are similar to those of Type I except larger volumes (V > 1.0 L) are to be removed
- Adequate skin tone, minimal laxity, and minimal musculofascial flaccidity

Contraindications

- Poor skin tone, greater than minimal skin laxity or musculofascial flaccidity. Skin retraction would be poor with undesirable results

Step-by-Step Procedure (Fig. 2)

1. Patient should be in prone position
2. Two bilateral incisions lateral to sacral unit and corresponding counterincisions are made below underwear line

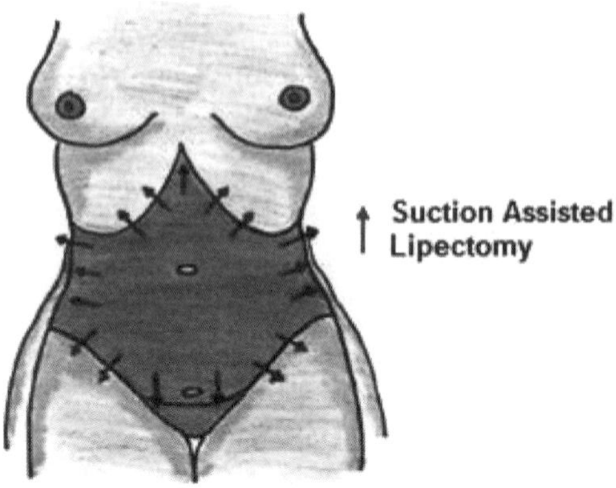

Fig. 2. Type 1a.

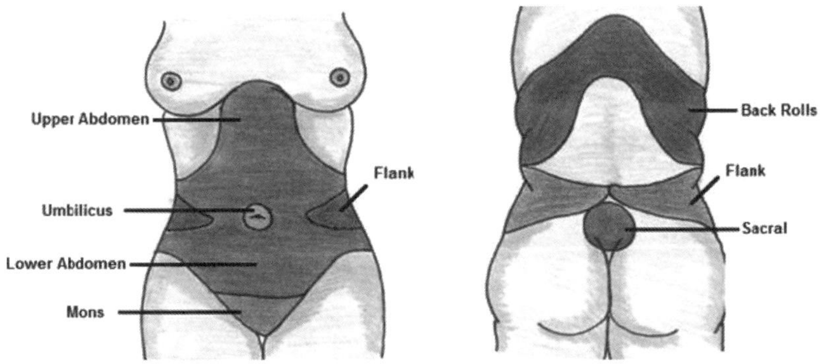

Fig. 3. Aesthetic units.

3. Liposuction is then performed in the waist and flanks in beltlike fashion
4. Repeat suction with smaller cannulas
5. Patient now placed in supine position
6. Two incisions in umbilicus and pubis with corresponding counterincisions are made to suction remaining aesthetic units (see Fig. 3)
7. Repeat suction using smaller cannulas

8. Resulting asymmetries can be treated with symmetric suctioning, autologous fat transplantation, or molding fat into resulting defect among others
9. Postoperative care will be discussed in the corresponding section

Type II. Miniabdominoplasty

Indications

- Patients with mild skin laxity and mild lower abdominal flaccidity for whom SAL is not sufficient
- Primarily for anatomical defects of the lower abdominal region

Contraindications

- Patients with upper or full abdominal skin laxity
- Musculofascial flaccidity in upper abdomen

Step-by-Step Procedure (Fig. 4)

1. As in SAL (Steps 1–4), the patient undergoes liposuction of areas demarcated
2. Upper transverse skin incision is made 5–7 cm superior to anterior vulvar commissure to gain access to the musculofascial system and to create the flap

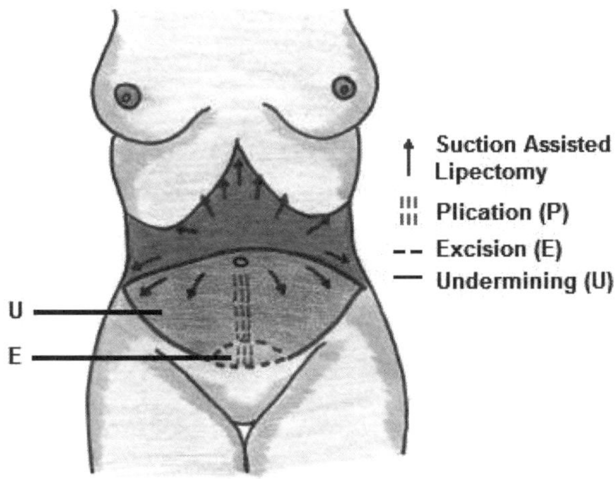

Fig. 4. Type II.

3. The flap is undermined to the level of the umbilicus with the help of a retractor
4. The laxity of the musculofascial system is then evaluated and subsequently vertically plicated to tighten musculature
5. The operating table is then flexed to evaluate and mark excess skin
6. Excess skin is resected to allow skin tightening
7. One Jackson–Pratt drain is inserted
8. Multilayer wound closure laterally to medially
9. Postoperative care will be discussed in the corresponding section

Type IIa. Open Miniabdominoplasty

Indications

- Patients with mild skin laxity and mild lower abdominal flaccidity who underwent a previous surgery that resulted in a vertical scar that cannot be resected by abdominoplasty

Contraindications

- Patients with skin laxity of upper or through entire abdomen
- Musculofascial flaccidity in upper abdomen

Step-by-Step Procedure (Fig. 5)

1. As in SAL (Steps 1–4), the patient undergoes liposuction of demarcated areas

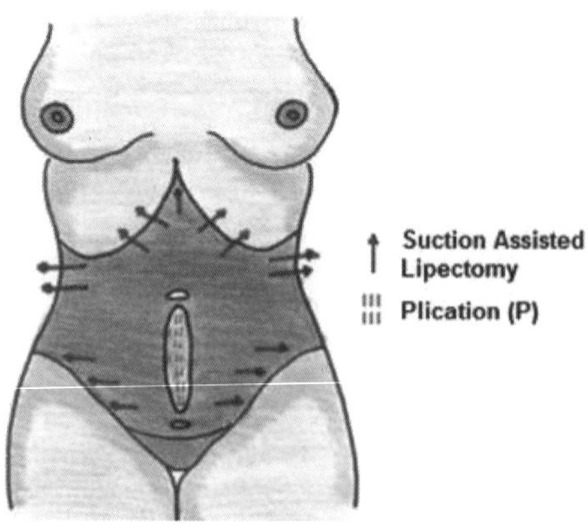

Fig. 5. Type IIa.

2. Excess skin surrounding scar is estimated using ellipse grasping technique and the area demarcated with surgical marker
3. Skin is incised down to muscular fascia and inferiorly extended towards pubis if necessary
4. Skin is resected en bloc from inferior to superior edge
5. Rectus musculofascial system is then plicated vertically
6. One Jackson-Pratt drain is inserted
7. Multilayer wound closure
8. Postoperative care will be discussed in the corresponding section

Type III. Modified Abdominoplasty

Indications

- Ideal for patients with moderate skin laxity and moderate lower and/or upper musculofascial flaccidity
- Consider in patients who cannot undergo a Type IV abdominoplasty because of scars that limit the extent of upper flap undermining

Step-by-Step Procedure (Fig. 6)

1. As in SAL it is important to demarcate areas to undergo liposuction with patient standing
2. With the patient slightly flexed at the waist the incision line is marked in the lower abdominal fold within anterior superior iliac spine (ASIS) boundaries
3. As in SAL Steps (1–4), the patient undergoes liposuction of demarcated areas
4. Incision is made at the previously marked incision line and the flap is undermined superior to the umbilicus
5. The rectus can then be plicated around and superior to umbilicus in an elliptical fashion (if the umbilical stalk is not transected)
6. It may be desirable to transect the umbilicus in patients with excess tissue in upper abdominal and periumbilical regions as this enables rectus plication more superiorly. It is important to make sure no umbilical hernias are present if this procedure is preferred. After

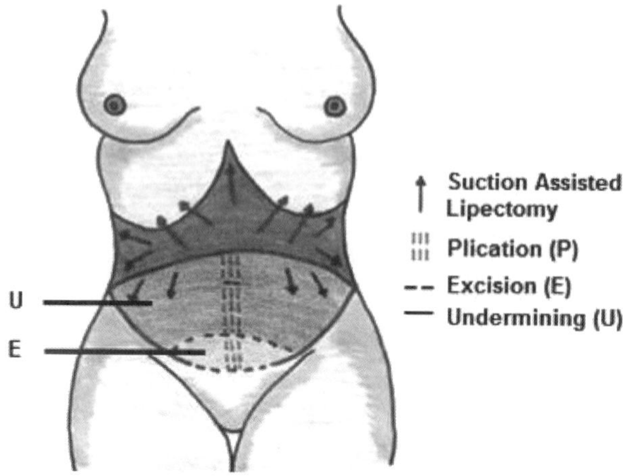

Fig. 6. Type III.

umbilicus is transected and rectus is plicated, the resulting defect from transection is closed with figure of eight sutures and the umbilicus can be reattached in a more aesthetically pleasing location if desired

7. The operating table is the flexed at a 30 degree angle and the flap advanced inferiorly
8. The excess skin is then excised
9. A Jackson–Pratt drain is then inserted
10. Multilayer closure of the wound follows
11. Postoperative care will be discussed in the corresponding section

Type IIIa. Endoscopically Assisted Abdominoplasty

Indications

- Ideal for patients with minimal or mild skin laxity with muscular flaccidity that can be repaired via endoscopic instruments
- The technique is able to address upper abdominal muscles that don't have large width defects. This technique is less desirable for wide defects since it is necessary to perform wider incision and skin undermining become necessary

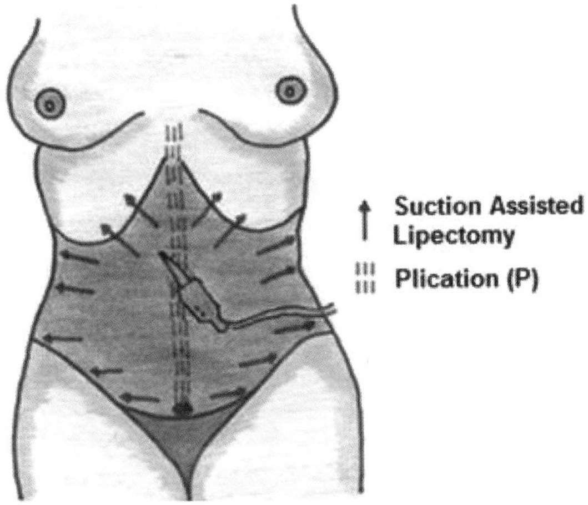

Fig. 7. Type IIIa.

Step-by-Step Procedure (Fig. 7)

1. With the patient on supine position a periumbilical, transumbilical, or pubic incision is made
2. Abdominal skin is retracted at various regions and a cavity is created that allows access of the fiber optic endoscope
3. For umbilical incisions the endoscope is inserted and the musculature plicated percutaneously from superior to inferior aspect using external landmarks as a guide
4. For pubic incision it is necessary to transect the umbilicus and the defect repaired after plication
5. Surface irregularities may arise after endoscopic plication. Undermining of skin adjacent to defect is an excellent means to achieve smooth contour and symmetry
6. Close drains are used to evacuate fluid
7. Postoperative care will be discussed in the corresponding section

Type IV. Full Abdominoplasty

Indications

- Ideal for patients with severe skin laxity and significant upper and/or lower abdominal muscle flaccidity

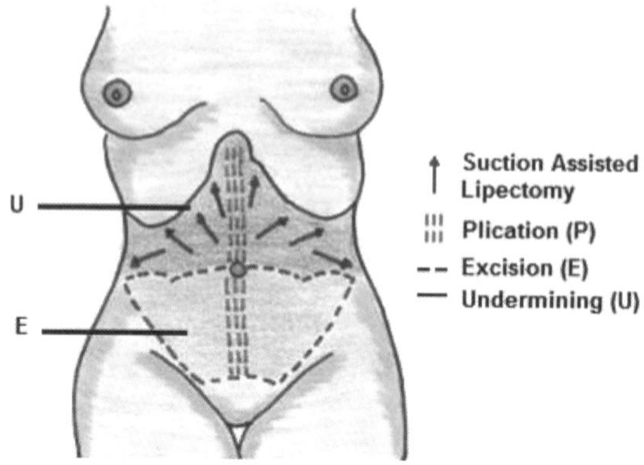

Fig. 8. Type IV.

- If 5–8 cm of skin needs to be excised in vertical dimension it is likely that a full abdominoplasty is the proper procedure

Step-by-Step Procedure (Fig. 8)

1. Preoperative marking should be done with the patient on standing position and wearing their underwear in manner of choice
2. Two transverse lines of identical length should be marked: one perpendicular to rectus muscles just above the umbilicus extending from the lateral side of each rectus muscle; holding the abdominal skin stretched upwards the second line is drawn at a level close to 5 cm above anterior vulvar commissure without laterally extending to the inguinal creases
3. The lateral edges of the inferior line are extended in a curvilinear fashion towards the anterior superior iliac spines (ASIS). Abdominal contour and position of underwear help define the extent of the lines and if their position relative to ASIS. Always remember not to extend the line beyond the inguinal crease
4. The lateral edges of the superior line are then taken to the lateral edges of the newly extended inferior line with mild arching to avoid upper/lower wound discrepancy upon closure
5. Shallow angled lateral edges would be desirable when significant waist narrowing is desired
6. The patient can now be placed supine in the operating table. It is advisable for the patient to elevate legs with pillows at the knee level

to avoid sciatic nerve tension when operating table is in the beach chair position. The surgeon must ensure the operating table can flex to this position

7. The abdomen is injected with necessary amounts of epinephrine and lidocaine
8. Liposuction of required areas
9. A circumferential incision around the umbilicus is done to release it from adjacent abdominal skin
10. For classic full abdominoplasty an incision is made in the previously described inferior line. The panniculus is elevated by use of scalpel, electrocautery, and retractors followed by V-shaped pattern undermining up to the xiphoid process superiorly and costal margins laterally
11. The amount of muscle to be plicated is estimated using hands or forceps. A surgical marker can be used to draw the limits of the area to be vertically plicated (2–0 nylon sutures in a buried or figure of eight pattern are commonly used)
12. Once plication has been done, the operating table is flexed again and excess skin from umbilicus to pubis can be estimated and removed
13. The operating table is flexed again, the flap advanced and sutured with 4–0 polyglactin 910 sutures at the lower margin
14. The umbilicus under the flap is now palpated at the new umbilical position. A vertical incision is made to exteriorize the umbilicus using bovie cautery. The adjacent subcutaneous fatty tissue surrounding the umbilicus is also removed using electrocautery
15. The umbilicus is positioned into place using mattress sutures through skin, fascia, and tied on umbilicus
16. With patient on flexed position, the edges are approximated after further advancing the flap inferiorly. Multilayer closure is done beginning with superficial fascia using 2–0 polyglactin 910
17. Two drains are placed and sutured into place
18. Postoperative care will be discussed in the corresponding section

Postoperative care

- Care mainly concentrates on avoiding ischemia and tension
- Bed flexion is desired for Types II to IV abdominoplasty. Ambulation is suggested with spine in flexion and avoiding full extension

- Regular surgical care is advised with:
  1. Incentive spyrometry encouraged to avoid pulmonary telecasts
  2. Compressive stokings and ambulation due to risk of thromboemoblic disease
  3. NPO except oral meds with gradual diet advancement as bowel recovers
  4. IV Normal saline, 2 ml administered for each 1 ml aspirated in a 24-hr period plus MIVF
  5. Foley catheter until patient is able to void without significant intra-abdominal effort
     - Abdominal binders should be worn for 2 weeks. However, the binder needs to be released occasionally to avoid ischemia or venous insufficiency
     - Drains should removed if patient has been ambulating and amount of fluid drained is less than 30 mL in 24 hrs
     - Patient should be monitored for skin recovery, development fluid collection, etc. once weekly during the first 30 days and once every six months until the patients is one year postoperative
     - Full range activity should be possible one month after procedure

Complications

- Complications range is varied in abdominoplasty: from postoperative pain to death
- There are both local and systemic complications

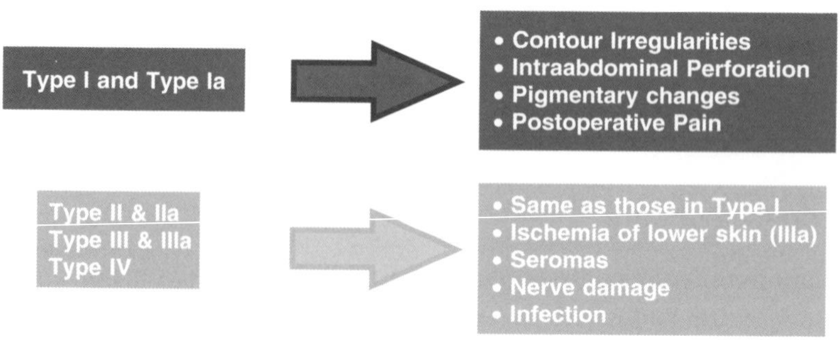

Further Reading

1. Castro CC, Costa JH, Salema R. (1993) How to deal with abdominoplasty in an abdomen with a sear. *Aesthetic Plast Surg* **17**(1): 67–71.
2. Menz P. (1996) Pregnancy after abdominoplasty. *Plast Reconstr Surg* **98**(2): 377–378.
3. Neaman K, Hansen JE. (2007) Analysis of complications from abdominoplasty: a review of 206 cases at a university hospital. *Ann Plast Surg* **58**(3): 292–298.
4. Gravante G, Araco A, Sorge R, Araco F, Delogu F, Cervelli D. (2007) Wound infections in post-bariatric patients undergoing body contouring abdominoplasty: the role of smoking. *Obes Surg* **17**(10): 1325–1331.
5. American Society of Anesthesiologists, Inc. Practice Advisory for Preanesthesia Evaluation. (2002) *Anesthesiology* **96**: 485–496.
6. Matarasso A. (1989) Abdominolipoplasty. *Clin Plast Surg* **16**: 289–303.
7. Matarasso A. (1995) Minimal-access variations in abdominoplasty. *Ann Plast Surg* **34**: 255–263.
8. Trussler AP, Kurkjian TJ, Hatef D, Farkas J, Rohrich RJ. (2010) Refinements of abdominoplasty: a critical outcomes analysis over a 20-year period. *Plast Reconstr Surg* **126**(3): 1063–1074.
9. Matarasso A. (2000) Abdominoplasty. In: Achauer B, *et al.* (eds.), *Plastic Surgery Indications, Operations, and Outcomes.* Mosby, Philadelphia, pp. 2783–2821.
10. Agha-Mohammadi S, BChir MB, Hurwitz DJ. (2008) Nutritional deficiency of post-bariatric surgery body contouring patients: what every plastic surgeon should know. *Plast Reconstr Surg* **122**: 604–613.
11. Agha-Mohammadi S, Hurwitz DJ. (2010) Enhanced recovery after body-contouring surgery: reducing surgical complication rates by optimizing nutrition. *Aesth Plast Surg* **34**: 617–625.
12. Agha-Mohammadi S, BChir MB, Hurwitz DJ. (2008) Potential impacts of nutritional deficiency of postbariatric patients on body contouring surgery. *Plast Reconstr Surg* **122**: 1901–1914.
13. Mechanick JI, Kushner RF, Sugerman HJ, Gonzalez-Campoy JM, Collazo-Clavell ML, Spitz AF, Apovian CM, Livingston EH, Brolin R, Sarwer DB, Anderson WA, Dixon J, Guven S; American Association of Clinical Endocrinologists; Obesity Society; American Society for Metabolic and Bariatric Surgery. (2009) American Association of Clinical Endocrinologists, The Obesity Society, and American Society for Metabolic and Bariatric

Surgery medical guidelines for clinical practice for the perioperative nutritional, metabolic, and nonsurgical support of the bariatric surgery patient. *Obesity (Silver Spring)* **17** Suppl 1: S1–70.

14. Shiffman M, Mirrafati S. (2005) *Aesthetic Surgery of the Abdominal Wall.* Springer-Verlag, New York.

CHAPTER 26

AESTHETIC BODY CONTOURING: ABDOMINOPLASTY BODY CONTOURING AFTER BARIATRIC SURGERY

Benjamin Lemelman, Paul G. Cofnas and Seth R. Thaller

Illustrative Case

A 35 year old black female status post roux-en-y gastric bypass surgery 2 years ago presents to your office with a chief complaint of "sagging skin" secondary to massive weight loss. She has lost a total of 50% of her excess body weight. She has excess skin on her trunk, upper arms and thighs that causes her discomfort when walking and exercising. She is pleased with her weight loss, but embarrassed by the appearance of her skin. She says her low self-esteem and poor body image has discouraged her from dating and going out in public with her girlfriends. Her weight has been stable at 192 lbs. for the past three months.

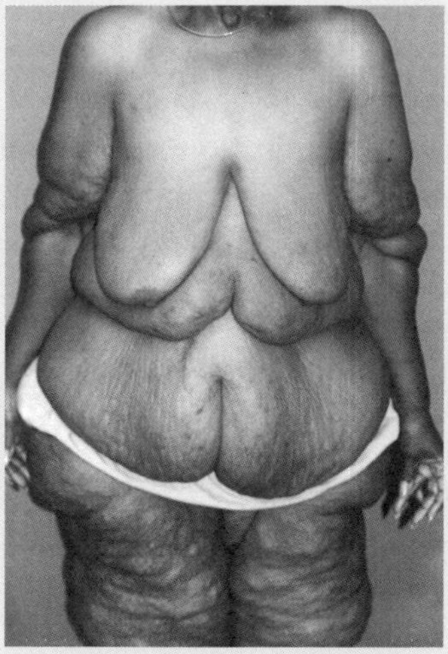

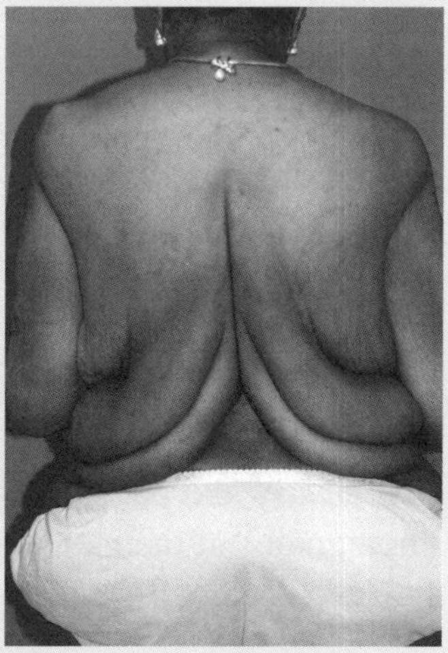

I. Background[1,2]

A. Etiology: In 2008, nearly 220,000 bariatric surgeries were performed in the United States and Canada alone, with the numbers rising for each subsequent year.
B. Indications for bariatric surgery.
   1. Obesity increases morbidity and mortality.
   2. Patient failed multiple weight loss attempts through diet, lifestyle modifications and medications.
   3. BMI ≥ 40.
   4. BMI ≥ 35 with a secondary disease.
C. Reasons to perform body contouring surgery.
   1. Following bariatric surgery, patients are left with unwanted, redundant skin.
   2. This extra tissue can cause physical and emotional discomfort.
   3. Excess skin can also decrease mobility, and cause irritation during walking and exercise.
D. Common procedures performed by the plastic surgeon.
   1. Belt Lipectomy (also known as the Total Body Lift).
   2. Brachioplasty.
   3. Thighplasty.

II. Preoperative Evaluation[3–8]

A. Multidisciplinary approach involving nutritionist, psychologist or psychiatrist, bariatric surgeon and primary care physician.
B. Patients' weight:
   1. Usually plateaus at 16–18 months following bariatric surgery.
   2. Must be stable for at least 3 months prior to body contouring surgery.
C. Full history and physical exam is mandatory.
D. Photographs of the patient from all angles allow for inspection of symmetry and deformities.

E. Risks

1. Malnutrition, vitamin and protein deficiencies.
2. Hypertension and diabetes; stabilize chronic conditions prior to procedure.
3. Ischemia and arrhythmia needs to be evaluated by EKG.

F. Preoperative counseling

1. Patient must understand the risks of surgery, as well as the trade off: unwanted tissue and skin will be replaced with scars.
2. Patient must have realistic expectations.
3. Psychiatric assessment is advised.
4. Stop smoking to prevent wound dehiscence.

G. Prophylaxis

1. Deep venous thrombosis (DVT) prophylaxis must be initiated in the preoperative period and continued postoperatively. This involves the use of both enoxaparin and sequential compression devices placed on the lower extremities.
2. Perioperative antibiotics to minimize infection.

III. Operative Techniques

A. Belt lipectomy[7,8]

1. Prior to surgery place epidural catheter for pain management and foley catheter.
2. Begin by drawing markings in the standing position.
   a. Note the vertical midline both on the anterior and posterior aspects.
   b. Mark the inferior and superior incisions on the anterior surface.
   c. Pinch the excess lateral skin and fat between your thumb and index finger to approximate and mark the lateral closure line; known as "grasp test."

   d. Continue the inferior and superior markings to the posterior side, making sure to adjust the inferior line for a buttocks lift. Also, mark the expected suture line location.
   e. Mark four vertical lines above both the anterior and superior iliac spines. These marks denote the fixation points inferiorly and laterally and are used to ensure symmetry.
   f. Circle the areas to be treated with liposuction, and mark an X in the areas with the highest fat density.

3. Belt lipectomy is a dynamic surgery, and the patient's position must change throughout the procedure.

   a. Best performed with a team of surgeons to minimize the amount of time of patient sedation.
   b. Techniques vary from one surgeon to the other; some begin the operation with the patient in the prone position, others begin with the patient supine.
   c. This chapter will discuss one technique which begins with the patient in:

      i. Supine position.
      ii. Followed by one lateral decubitus position and finally the remaining lateral decubitus position.
      iii. This allows for proper resection of both lateral and posterior portions of the body life and gives the surgeon adequate time to focus on the anterior portion.
      iv. Rolling of the patient must be a team effort involving 5 to 6 people.

4. First, secure the umbilicus with two sutures superiorly and inferiorly.
5. Then dissect downward to the level of rectus fascia.
6. Incise the anterior inferior abdominal marking also to the level of the fascia.
7. At this point the patient's abdominal wall is exposed and must be inspected and treated for possible hernias.

8. Once the flap is ready to be excised, the table must be flexed for removal. The patient is then rolled onto the lateral decubitus position to perform the dissection of the posterior and lateral flaps.
9. Finally, this process is repeated by rolling the patient onto his other side.
10. Closure of the fascia and skin is performed based on the preoperative markings.
11. Jackson Pratt drains on closed suction are placed in the posterior and are important for the healing process.

B. Brachioplasty[8,9]

1. Markings may be drawn while the patient is sitting or standing, with the elbow bent 90 degrees and the shoulder abducted to 90 degrees.

    a. First, mark the bicipital groove.
    b. Then, pull downward on the flap to create tension and mark the superior suture line which will be later approximated to the line of bicipital groove. The distal portion of this line will usually reach the elbow.
    c. The proximal portion of the suture line lies high in the axilla. From this proximal point on the superior suture line, draw another mark 90 degrees into the chest wall.
    d. Next, perform a pinch test to mark the proximal mark for the inferior suture line within the axilla.
    e. Finally, approximate the inferior suture line by performing another pinch test.

2. Begin the procedure by incising the superior marking line as well as the line extending to the chest wall.
3. Elevate this flap of skin and subcutaneous tissue from the fascia.
4. Dissection is continued with caution to preserve nervous and vascular structures including the medial antebrachial cutaneous nerve and the basilic vein.
5. Next, elevate the forearm to avoid tethering of the posterior tissue.

6. Then estimate the final closure line by elevating the newly created flap with heavy forceps and pinching the superior margin of the incision below the elevated flap.

   a. This should be performed at multiple points, usually three, followed by division and excision of the flap.
   b. This technique ensures proper closure.

7. In order to close the incised axilla, secure the proximal inferior point to the superior marking on the clavipectoral fascia using permanent 0-braided nylon suture.
8. The tissue and skin is then closed above a Jackson Pratt drain to avoid seroma formation.

C. Thighplasty[10–12]

1. Often performed by extracting two crescent flaps:

   a. One extends from the buttocks to the medial thigh.
   b. The other extends from the medial thigh to the medial knee.
   c. Both together from an L shaped closure line.

2. The markings may be difficult with the patient in the upright position due to large volumes of hanging skin from the pannus and thighs.

   a. With the patient supine and knees bent with hips slightly open, mark the upper incision between the thigh and labia majora.
   b. Next, with the patient's thigh held in flexed position, displace the loose tissue to mark the inferior line on the midmedial thigh.
   c. The posterior line is marked at the level of the junction between the thigh and buttocks, while the anterior line extends from the level of the mons pubis to the point of maximal resection in the medial thigh. The joining of the two lines creates the first crescent.

d. The second crescent is drawn for the vertical band. This begins with a midmedial thigh marking extending down to the knee.
e. Then perform a pinch test to mark the posterior line of resection.
f. Finally, join the anterior line of the vertical band to that of the initial crescent by moving the former more posterior. This technique allows for the scar to be placed in a more posterior location.
g. It is important to have the patient stand to finalize the markings before surgery.

3. Procedure

a. There are multiple approaches to thighplasty in the massive weight loss patient; this chapter will focus on the vertical thighplasty.
b. May require liposuction prior to the procedure: in the months prior to operation or on the day of the operation, depending upon the laxity of the skin.
c. Perform anterior incision first to the level of the deep facia.
d. Take care to preserve the greater saphenous vein including the fat surrounding the vessel to prevent lymphedema.
e. Posterior branch of the saphenous vein is often ligated.
f. Continue dissection to the level of the posterior markings.
g. Ensure hemostasis using an automatic surgical clip applier.
h. Begin removal of tissue in a distal to proximal fashion by mobilizing the anterior line posteriorly to determine the amount of resected tissue.
i. Join the flaps together with staples prior to closure of each layer.
j. Place a Jackson Pratt drain to prevent seroma.
k. Close superficial fascia using running number 0 suture.
l. Close deep dermis with interrupted suture.
m. Finally, close epidermis using running suture.

IV. Postoperative Care and Complication Prevention

A. Belt lipectomy[7,8]

1. All patients must be admitted to the hospital for acute care.
2. Position patient with flexion at the waist in typical "beach chair" fashion.
3. Average hospital stay is 3–4 days.
4. Remain in flexed position for about 1 week, followed by therapy to improve straightening. Physical therapy is important for patients to return to normal activity.
5. Pain management: epidural shall remain for about 36 hours after surgery, and ultimately controlled with oral pain medication.
6. Discontinue foley catheter about 5 hours after epidural is stopped.
7. With assistance, patient should ambulate on day of surgery.
8. Deep Venous Thrombosis (DVT) prophylaxis must be initiated in the preoperative period and continued postoperatively. This involves the use of both enoxaparin and sequential compression devices placed on the lower extremities.
9. Seroma formation is a common complication.

    a. Remove Jackson-Pratt drains when they decrease output to 30–40 mL per day.
    b. Anterior drains will usually reach this criteria by the first week to 10 days.
    c. Posterior drains will reach criteria more slowly, usually by the end of the second week.
    d. All drains must be removed by two weeks unless output is extremely high (greater than 150 mL per day).
    e. If seroma remains following drain removal, aspiration is required.

10. Use a super wetting solution prior to lipoplasty in order to minimize blood loss.
11. Wound dehiscence is a common complication due to tension of wound closure.

B. Brachioplasty[8,9]

1. The patient must avoid elevation of the arm and abduction of the shoulder beyond 90 degrees.
2. Cover incisions with gauze, wrap with ace bandages and elevate arms on pillows.
3. Drains will remain with their outputs recorded, until they drain less than 30 cc per day.
4. After three days, supply the patient with compressive elastic sleeves. These sleeves may remain for excess of six weeks to ensure healing.
5. Two weeks postoperatively the patient must perform physical therapy exercises in order to reintroduce abduction of the shoulder.
6. Most patients undergoing brachioplasty also endure other procedures at the same time. They must be managed accordingly with DVT and antibiotic prophylaxis.
7. The most common complications of brachioplasty include seromas, hypertrophic scars, controversial scar location, and nerve injury.

C. Thighplasty[10–12]

1. Alternating pressure lower leg stockings are used throughout the procedure and during the patient's hospitalization, usually lasting two to four days.
2. The lower torso drains may be removed when output is less than 50 mL per leg per 24 hours (about 10 days).
3. The patient may gain about 10 pounds due to fluid administration and post-surgical fluid retention.
4. If natural diuresis does not occur by postoperative day 3, begin oral diuretics.
5. Suture lines are covered with steri-strips and checked daily for skin separation.
6. Small gaps are common at the inner thigh-labial junction. Wound care includes cleaning with soap and water as well as dry dressings to reduce irritation and foul odor.

7. Again, seromas are a common complication. These tense or fluctuant asymmetrical swellings are caused by premature removal of drains. Large bore needle aspiration is diagnostic and therapeutic. If serum accumulates, a percutaneous drainage catheter may be placed to a suction bulb for 10 days.
8. Lymphocele is another complication due to disruption of the lymphatics. These may resolve with the use of prolonged closed suction drainage.
9. Descent of labial thigh scars and distortion of labii are avoided by the Colles fascia stitch. However, this suture cannot overcome an over-resection of medial thigh skin. Labial deformities may be resolved by skin graft or vertical band excision if there is a laxity of residual transverse thigh skin.

References

1. Van der Beek ESJ, Te Riele W, Specken TF, Boerma D, van Ramshorst B. (2010) The impact of reconstructive procedures following bariatric surgery on patient well-being and quality of life. *Obes Surg* **20**: 36–41.
2. Bruschi S, Datta G, Bocchiotti MA, Boriani F, Obbialero FD, Fraccalvieri M. (2009) Limb contouring after massive weight loss: functional rather than aesthetic improvement. *Obes Surg* **19**: 407–411.
3. Datta G, Cravero L, Margara A, Boriani F, Bocchiotti MA, Kefalas N. (2006) The plastic surgeon in the treatment of obesity. *Obes Surg* **16**: 5–11.
4. Tang L, Song AY, Choi S, Fernstrom M, Rubin JP. (2007) Completing the metamorphosis: building a center of excellence in postbariatric plastic surgery. *Ann Plast Surg* **58**: 54–56.
5. Gusenoff JA, Rubin JP. Plastic surgery after weight loss: current concepts in massive weight loss surgery. *Aesthet Surg J* **28**: 452–455.
6. Rohrich RJ, Gosman AA, Conrad MH, Coleman J. Simplifying circumferential body contouring: the central body lift evolution. *Plast Reconstr Surg* **18**: 525–535.
7. Neves CGL, Cram AE, Aly AS. (2009) Belt lipectomy: lower body lift. In: Aston SJ, Steibrech DS, Walden JL. (eds.), *Aesthetic Plast Surg*. Elsevier Science Limited, pp. 813–822.

8. Rubin JP, Gusenoff J. (2009) Bodylifts and post-massive weight loss body contouring. In: Guyuron B, Eriksson E, Persing JA, Chung KC, Disa J, Gosain A, Kinney BM, Rubin JP. (eds.), *Plastic Surgery Indications and Practice*. Elsevier Science Limited, pp. 1627–1664.
9. Hurwitz D, Neavin T. (2009) Brachioplasty. In: Aston SJ, Steibrech DS, Walden JL (eds.), *Aesthetic Plast Surg*, Elsevier Science Limited, pp. 805–812.
10. Mathes DW, Kenkel JM. (2008) Current concepts in medial thighplasty. *Clin Plast Surg* **35**: 151–163.
11. Cram A, Aly A. (2008) Thigh reduction in the massive weight loss patient. *Clin Plast Surg* **35**: 165–172.
12. Hurwitz DJ. (2006) Thighplasty in the weight loss patient. *Semin Plast Surg* **20**: 38–48.

CHAPTER 27

BODY CONTOURING VIA SUCTION LIPECTOMY

Michelle De Souza and Garry Martin II

Illustrative Case

39 year old woman desires improvement in her body contour. She sites excess adiposity of her abdomen, flanks, and arms. She does not want any long scars and requests minimal time away from work. She has no significant medical or surgical history, and does not use tobacco products (Figs. 1 to 5).

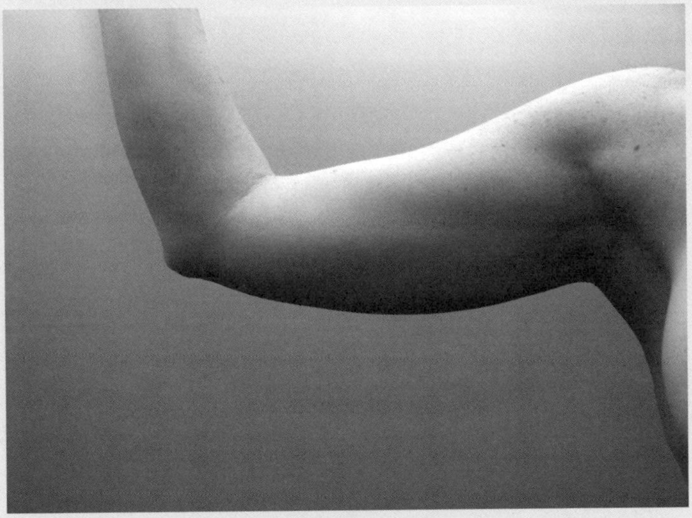

Fig. 1.

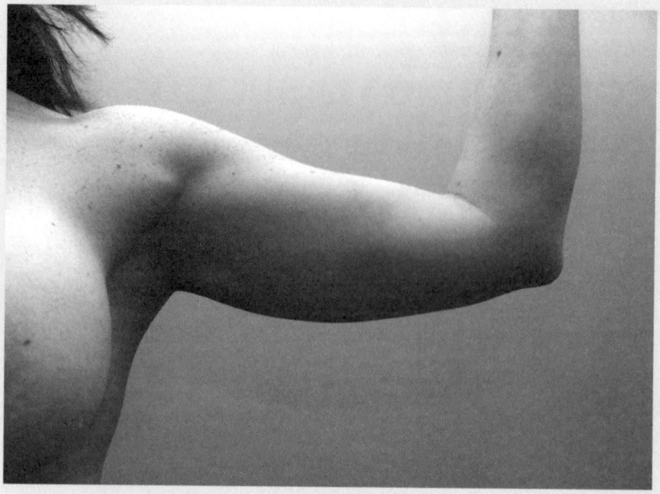

Fig. 2.

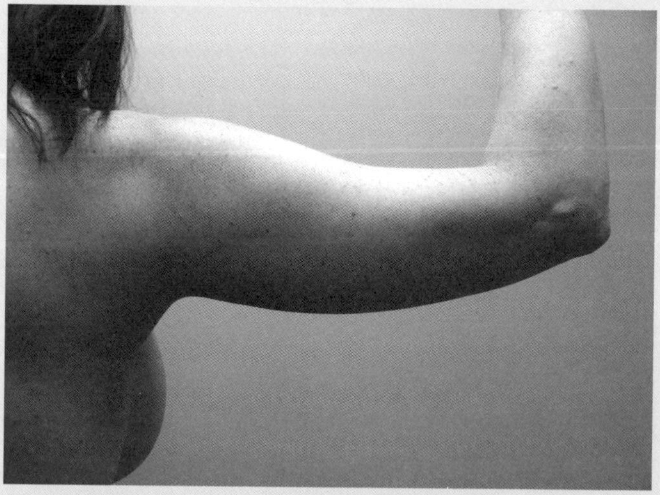

Fig. 3.

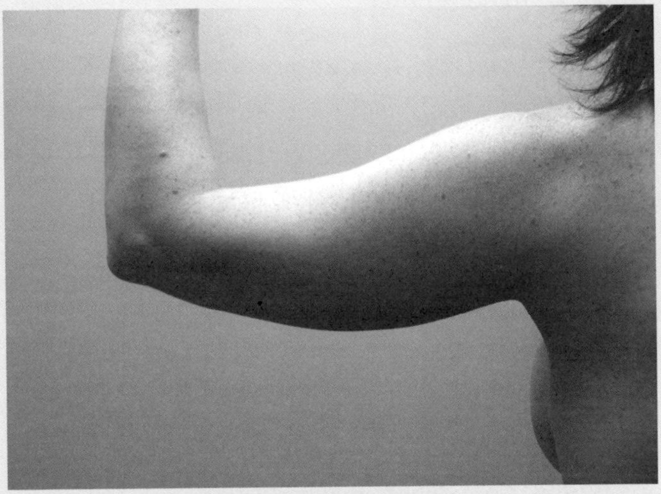

Fig. 4.

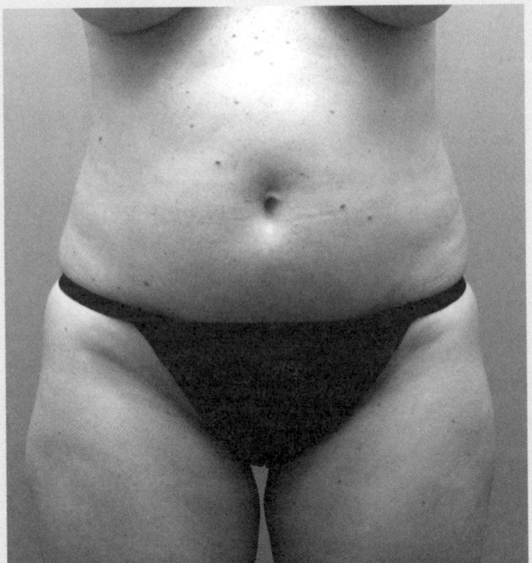

Fig. 5.

I. Preoperative Considerations

A. Patient Selection

1. Assess patient's goals and expectations, making note of the feasibility of reaching such goals; remain cautious of patients with:
    a) Eating disorders
    b) Body dysmorphic disorder
    c) Unhealthy lifestyle choices in regards to weight control
    d) Unrealistic expectations
    e) Significant skin excess or poor skin elasticity
2. Assure stable weight with appropriate diet/exercise program in place for ~1 year
    a) Within 20% ideal bodyweight

B. Physical Exam

1. Contour irregularities
2. Areas of localized adiposity
3. Asymmetry
4. Pinch test to assess thickness of layers of skin and soft tissue
5. Existing scars/surgeries
6. Deformities that are not obvious (i.e. hernias or fascial compromise)
7. Skin quality (tone, elasticity, laxity, dermal thickness)
8. Special attention to inhibitors of proper healing:
    a) Local scars
    b) Radiation
    c) Infections/cellulitis
    d) Significant skin laxity
    e) Neurovascular state of local tissue
    f) Certain medications (i.e. steroids)

II. Anatomy

A. Adipose Anatomy

1. Differences in superficial and deep layers of fat in various regions of the body
    a) Abdomen

(1) Superficial layer — small fat lobules packed tightly between fibrous septa that are perpendicular to the skin, consistent thickness
(2) Deep layer — large lobules packed loosely in widely spaced fibrous septa, thickness tapers medially and laterally

b) Paralumbar

(1) Superficial layer — compact with uniform depth over the area
(2) Deep layer — more irregular, large fatty pockets with varying septa, varying thickness

c) Gluteal-thigh

(1) Superficial — small fat lobules in tight rigid fibrous septa; highly structured
(2) Deep — dense and compact, regularly spaced lobules and sturdy/more rigid, fibrous septa

d) Leg/arm

(1) No discrete or distinct subcutaneous fascia dividing the adipose into two layers; single layer
(2) Similar to the superficial fatty layer of the trunk

2. Where two layers exist, both layers are targeted
3. Contour irregularities will be more apparent in the superficial layer
4. For single layer regions, smaller cannulas will yield a more favorable result

B. Zones of Adherence

1. Regions where facial planes are closely connected to superficial structures, near which contour irregularities are more likely

III. Operative Preparation

A. Patient Marking and Access Sites

1. Create topographic map in standing position
2. Consider marking pre-existing concavities
3. May use different colors for concavities and convexities

B. Positioning and Prepping

1. Prone, supine, or lateral decubitus positioning
2. Standing prep for circumferential liposuction or repeat prep after turning patient
3. Betadine scrub and paint or chlorhexadine
4. External warmer
5. Foley catheter when appropriate (length of procedure and when > 5L aspirate is planned for fluid balance)

C. Wetting Solution

1. 1 liter Lactated Ringer's solution, 1mL epinephrine 1:1,000, 50 mL 1% lidocaine
2. Maximum lidocaine dosage when delivered subcutaneously: 35 mg/kg.
   a) Higher levels may be tolerated, but not suggested
3. Lidocaine peak plasma levels approach 2–3 mcg/mL, 8–16 hrs after infiltrate
   a) Subjective toxicity symptoms begin at 3–5 mcg/mL
4. Local tissue levels of lidocaine are subclinical for analgesia within 4–8 hours of initial infiltration
5. Infiltrate deep and superficial layers in a plied fashion
6. May be beneficial to warm infiltrate solution to avoid hypothermia
7. Allow time (7–10 min) for effective vasoconstriction
8. Consider infiltration with local anesthetic under sterile conditions prior to scrubbing and prepping the patient

D. Fluid Management

1. Large volume liposuction
   a) > 5000 mL of total aspirate during a single procedure
   b) Should observe overnight in a hospital setting
2. Approximately 70% of tumescent volume infiltrated is NOT aspirated when a procedure is completed

3. Use a data sheet to communicate fluid balances in patients with large volume liposuction
    a) In: IVF, tumescent fluid
    b) Out: urine output, lipoaspirate, insensible losses, blood loss
4. Resuscitation guidelines
    a) < 5000 mL – maintenance fluid plus subcutaneous infiltrate
    b) > 5000 mL – maintenance fluid plus subcutaneous infiltrate plus 0.25 mL IVF/mL of aspirate > 5000 mL[11]

IV. Operative Techniques (Techniques and Illustrations)

A. Dry Technique
1. First developed by Yves–Gerard Illouz, MD in 1977
2. No infiltration of subcutaneous solutions prior to insertion of liposuction cannula
3. Aspirate contains 20–45% blood

B. Wet Technique
1. 300 mL of infiltrate per site
2. Blood loss 4–30% of aspirate

C. Super Wet Technique
1. 1:1 infiltrate: aspirate ratio
2. Blood loss 1–2% of aspirate volume

D. Tumescent Technique
1. 2–3: 1 infiltrate: aspirate ratio
2. Blood loss ~1% of aspirate volume

E. Suction Assisted Lipectomy
1. Removes adipose utilizing a hollow blunt-tipped cannula of various sizes attached to a high-powered suction ~1atm
2. Adipocyte architecture is largely preserved

F. Ultrasound Assisted Lipectomy

1. Cannula delivers ultrasound waves subcutaneously which cavitate and lyse adipocytes
2. Good for fibrous areas such as back and flanks, and repeat procedures
3. Keep probe moving when in use to avoid heat conduction burn

G. Laser-Assisted Lipectomy

1. Neodymium:yttrium-alumium-garnet (Nd:YAG) laser targets adipocyte membranes

H. Hand-Aspiration

1. Done via syringe-generated suction
2. Helpful for small areas but can be fatiguing for larger areas

V. Operative Considerations in Various Body Regions

A. Neck/Face

1. An adjunct to rhytidectomy, can assist with flap elevation, or to target localized fat compartments such as jowls
2. Use small diameter cannulas
3. Avoid suctioning cephalad to zygoma
4. Potential access sites: nasolabial crease, postauricular, submental crease, nasal vestibule, intraoral
5. Avoid over-suctioning the neck to avoid the anterior platysmal banding deformity, also known as a cobra deformity

B. Abdomen

1. Superficial and deep fat layers are targeted
2. Keep cannula parallel to abdomen, avoid intra-abdominal injury
3. Caution if hernias are suspected, particularly with pre-existing abdominal surgeries and scars
4. Potential access sites are hidden within pubic area, umbilicus, or inframammary folds

C. Back

1. Superficial and deep fat layers are targeted
2. Deeper fatty layer creates the "love handle" deformity
3. Back skin is thicker than other skin, which tends to show less contour deformity
4. Potential access sites are below underwear line and beneath bra line

D. Chest/Breast

1. More fibrous tissue in gynecomastia is an indication for ultrasound assisted liposuction
2. Thorough liposuction does not remove glandular component, which should be removed surgically

E. Thigh

1. Can address targeted areas such as upper lateral thigh or medial thigh
2. Circumferential thigh liposuction can deliver greater skin contraction
3. Anterior thigh liposuction is technically challenging and prone to show contour irregularities
4. Potential access sites are inguinal crease and infragluteal crease

F. Gluteal/Buttock

1. Follows same principles as back liposuction
2. Potential access sites are gluteal cleft or infragluteal fold

G. Arm

1. Follows same principles as thigh liposuction
2. Circumferential arm liposuction will deliver greater skin contraction
3. Can extend liposuction to forearm
4. Potential access sites are axilla and elbow

H. Lower Legs

1. Follows same principles as thigh liposuction
2. Special locations for liposuction include the knees or ankles

VI. Operative Techniques Description

A. The pre-operative analysis of the patient includes good photographs, according to the photographic standards. A risk assessment with regards to surgery, based on the history and physical. The ASA classification can help with risk stratification as well as the selection of preoperative serum laboratory evaluations
B. Prior to surgery, topographic markings are drawn on the area to be liposuctioned. The patient is then taken to the operating room. The patient is positioned either prone, supine, or in a lateral decubitus position in order to facilitate liposuction. Full excursion of the liposuction cannula and the surgeon's arms should be easy
C. After the patient is in position, the wetting solution is infiltrated. Planned incisions can be used to introduce the wetting solution. Allow time for the hemostatic effect of the wetting solution to take place
D. Incision locations for liposuction should allow for cross hatching of the cannula from multiple angles. A fan-shaped technique is used with the cannula held parallel to the patient's skin
E. Cannulas are selected by location and quantity of fenestrations as well as diameter. Examples include: Las Vegas, Mercedes, etching
F. End point of liposuction is assessed by inspection, palpation, two point pinch test, a gloved wet hand check for smoothness of contour, quality of aspirate (bloody aspirate signals the end of liposuction)

VII. Post Operative Care

A. Closure with non-absorbable suture for larger access sites, fine chromic or fast gut suture for smaller access sites, steri-strips
B. Compression garment to areas that have been suctioned

    1. The use of compression foam or Jones roll under the garment may be beneficial to evenly distribute compression
    2. Garments are worn for up to 4–6 weeks

C. Serosanguinous drainage is expected from incision sites for the first 24–48 hrs

D. Oral narcotics are adequate for outpatient procedures. IV narcotics may be given for inpatients
E. May shower in 1–2 days
F. Drains may be used

1. Indications include:
   a. Gynecomastia
   b. > 2L lipoaspirate from abdomen alone
   c. Large volume liposuction (> 5 L total aspirate)
2. Removed when < 30 mL/24 hrs

G. Follow up protocol:
   1. 5–7 days — suture removal
   2. 2 weeks — increase activity level
   3. 2–4 weeks — wean off compression
   4. 6 weeks — assess edema and results
   5. 3 months — early results
   6. 6 months to 1 year — final results, swelling should be resolved

VIII. Complications

A. Contour Irregularities
   1. Overcorrection
      a) May be treated with fat injection either at the time of surgery if recognized or at a later stage
   2. Undercorrection
      a) May repeat procedure after patient is healed
   3. Abnormal skin retraction
      a) Loose skin may be excised
   4. Embolic phenomenon
      a) Thromboembolism

   b) Fat embolism
   c) Prevented by shorter procedures and early ambulation

5. Fluid collections

   a) Seromas
   b) Hematomas

6. Skin discoloration

   a) Hyperpigmentation, more common
   b) Hypopigmentation possible

7. Burns

   a) Can occur from laser assisted or ultrasound assisted lipectomy

8. End hits

   a) Ecchymoses from the liposuction cannula tip striking the skin on end

9. Infection is uncommon

10. Paresthesias are usually temporary

11. Lidocaine toxicity

   a) 3–5 mcg/mL: Subjective — metallic taste in mouth, paresthesias of lips/tongue, tinnitus, restlessness, lightheadedness
   b) 6–9 mcg/mL: Objective — tremors, twitching
   c) 8–15 mcg/mL: Central Nervous System — seizures, decreased level of consciousness, coma, death
   d) > 20 mcg/mL: Respiratory arrest
   e) > 26 mcg/mL: Cardiac arrest

Acknowledgments

The authors would like to thank Joseph P. Hunstad, MD for the courtesy of his pictures for this chapter.

Further Reading

1. Gingrass MK, *Grabb and Smith*, 6th Edn. 2007, Lippincott Williams and Wilkins.
2. Hughes CE. (1999) Patient selection, planning and marking in ultrasound-assisted lipoplasty. *Clin Plast Surg* **26**: 279–282.
3. Rohrich RJ, *et al.*, An update on the role of subcutaneous infiltration in suction-assisted lipoplasty; *Plast Reconstr Surg* **111**(2): 926–927.
4. Markman B, Barton FE Jr. (1987) Anatomy of the subcutaneous tissue of the trunk and lower extremity. *Plast Reconstr Surg* **80**: 248–254.
5. Rohrich RJ, Smith PD, Marcantonio DR, Kenkel JM. (2001) The zones of adherence: role in minimizing and preventing contour deformities in liposuction. *Plast Reconstr Surg* **107**: 1562–1569.
6. Hunstad JP. (2009) *Atlas of Abdominoplasty*. Saunders, Elsevier, pp. 15–24.
7. Hanke W, Sattler G, Borris S (eds.) (2007) *Textbook of Liposuction*. Series in Cosmetic and Laser Therapy, Informa Healthcare.
8. Francesce G, *et al.* Effects of traditional and ultrasonic liposuction on adipose tissue: a biochemical approach. *Plast Reconstr Surg* **106**(1): 197–199.
9. Illouz Y, Body contouring by lipolysis: a 5-year experience with over 3000 cases. *Plast Reconstr Surg* **72**(5): 591–597.
10. Haeck PC, *et al.* Evidence-based patient safety advisory: liposuction. *Plast Reconstr Surg* **124**(4S): 28S–44S.
11. Rohrich RJ, *et al.* Fluid resuscitation in liposuction: a retrospective review of 89 consecutive patients. *Plast Reconstr Surg* **117**(2): 431–435.
12. Kenkel JM, *et al.* Hemodynamic physiology and thermoregulation in liposuction. *Plast Reconstr Surg* **114**(2): 503–513.
13. Kenkel JM, *et al.* Pharmacokinetics and safety of lidocaine and monoethylglycinexylidide in liposuction: a microdialysis study. *Plast Reconstr Surg* **114**(2): 516–524.

CHAPTER 28

ABDOMINAL AND THORACIC RECONSTRUCTION

Umbareen Mahmood and Deniz Dayicioglu

Illustrative Case

Abdominal Wall Reconstruction

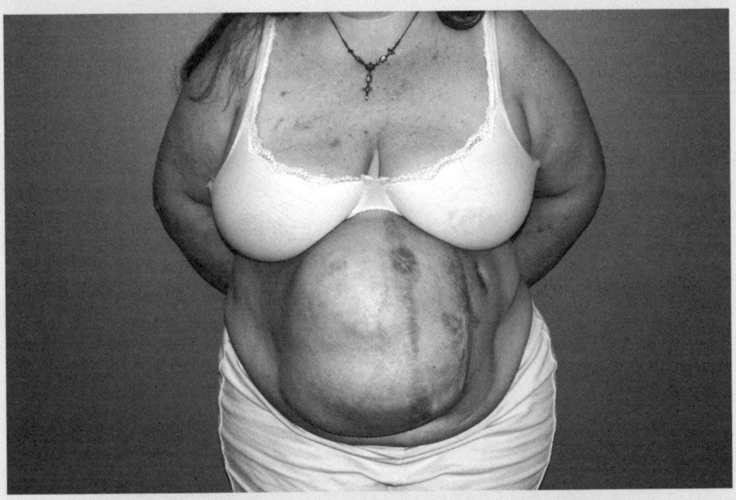

Fig. 1. Preoperative appearance of the patient.

A 46 year-old female patient with a history of low grade liposarcoma that was excised 10 years ago is referred to plastic surgery. Assistance for repair of the ventral hernia is needed after removal of

(*Continued*)

(*Continued*)

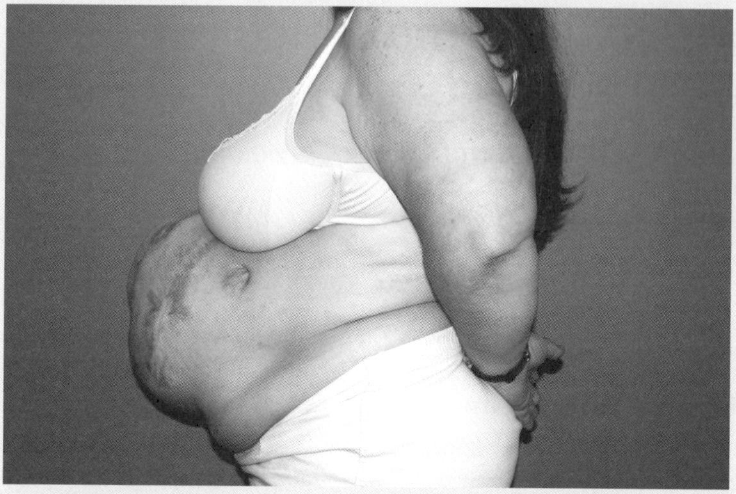

Fig. 2. Preoperative appearance of the patient.

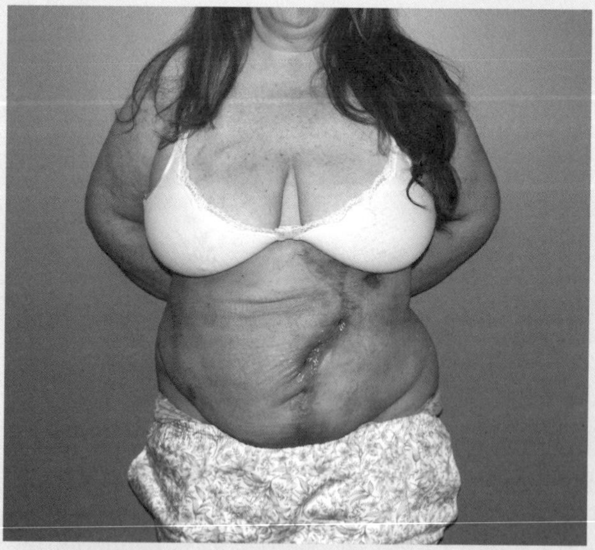

Fig. 3. Postoperative appearance of the patient.

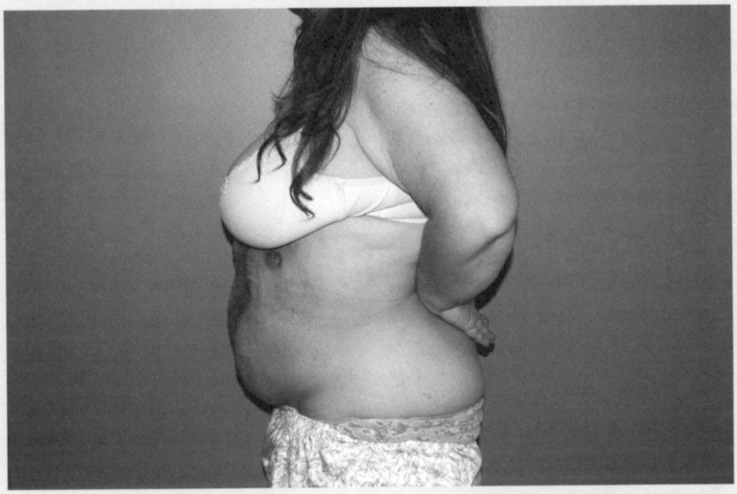

Fig. 4. Postoperative appearance of the patient.

a recurrent tumor by surgical oncology. Past medical history is significant for diabetes. Past surgical history is significant for multiple abdominal surgeries. Her chief complaint is recurrence of the tumor that was diagnosed in routine scans and discomfort, and aesthetic concerns. CT scan demonstrates a 20 cm ventral hernia. Patient states she had been using abdominal binders for support. She was never offered a hernia repair before due to the potential recurrence of the tumor that would mandate further surgical treatments. Upon review of systems, the patient denies any respiratory problems (Figs. 1 and 2).

After the colonic tumor is resected, the hernia is repaired using component separation and porcine mesh. This is covered by marlex mesh. The hernia sac along with the redundant skin is excised. The patient recovered well overall but experienced partial skin necrosis along the incision that eventually healed secondarily (Figs. 3 and 4).

Anatomy

I. Introduction/Anatomy

Goal: structure and functional restoration

1. Functions of abdominal wall
    a. Protect visceral structures
    b. Stabilize trunk
    c. Aid in movement and posture
2. Goals of reconstruction
    a. Restore function and integrity
    b. Prevent evisceration/hernia
    c. Provide dynamic support
    d. Aesthetics
3. Muscles (5 pairs)
    a. 3 flat muscles
        i. External oblique
        ii. Internal oblique
        iii. Transversus abdominis
    b. 2 vertical muscles
        i. Rectus abdominis
        ii. Pyrimadalis
4. Vasculature (Fig. 6)
    a. Zone I (mid-abdomen)
        i. Deep epigastric arcade
        ii. Superior epigastric artery (from internal thoracic artery)
            1. Travels down with the posterior rectus sheath
        iii. Deep inferior epigastric artery (from external iliac artery)
            1. Travels up with posterior rectus sheath
            2. Joins superior epigastric artery above umbilicus
            3. Supply both muscle and skin

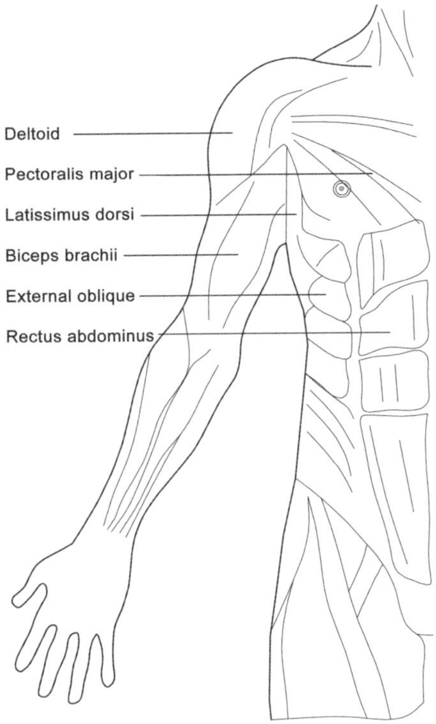

Fig. 5. Abdominal and thoracic musculature.

b. Zone II (lower abdomen)

   i. Epigastric arcade and external iliac artery
   ii. Superficial epigastric artery and superficial external pudendal artery (from femoral artery) superficial to fascia supplies overlying skin
   iii. Inferior epigastric artery (from external iliac artery) supplies underlying muscle
   iv. Deep circumflex iliac artery (from external iliac artery) supplies muscles around ASIS

c. Zone III (flanks and lateral abdomen)

   i. Intercostal, subcostal, and lumbar arteries (from aorta)

      1. Travel between the transversus abdominis and oblique muscles to supply overlying skin

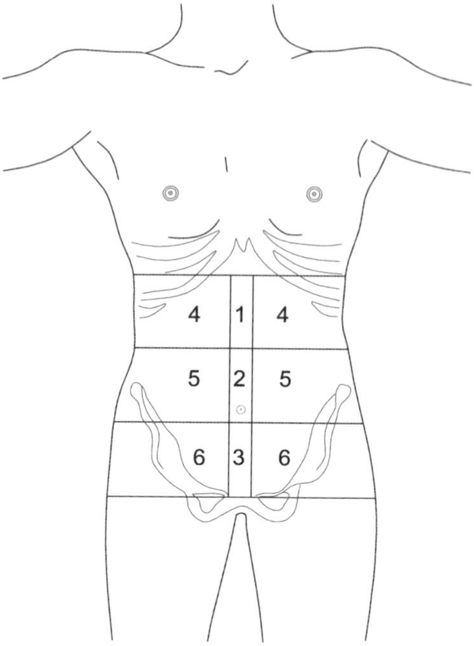

Fig. 6. Zones of the abdomen for vasculature.

5. Important anatomy:

   a. Borders

      i. Superior: xiphoid process, costal cartilage of 7th and 12th ribs
      ii. Inferior: inguinal ligament (lateral), pubic tubercle (medial)
      iii. Lateral: midaxillary line through superior part of iliac crest

   b. Abdominal layers: skin, subcutaneous tissue, superficial fascia (2 layers: camper fascia and scarpa fascia), deep fascia (below level of umbilicus), external oblique muscle, internal oblique muscle, transversus abdominis muscle, extraperitoneal fascia, peritoneum

   c. Other landmarks

      i. Arcuate line (Fig. 7)

         1. Above arcuate line: anterior rectus sheath composed of external oblique aponeurosis and anterior layer of internal oblique aponeurosis; posterior rectus sheath composed of

(a)

(b)

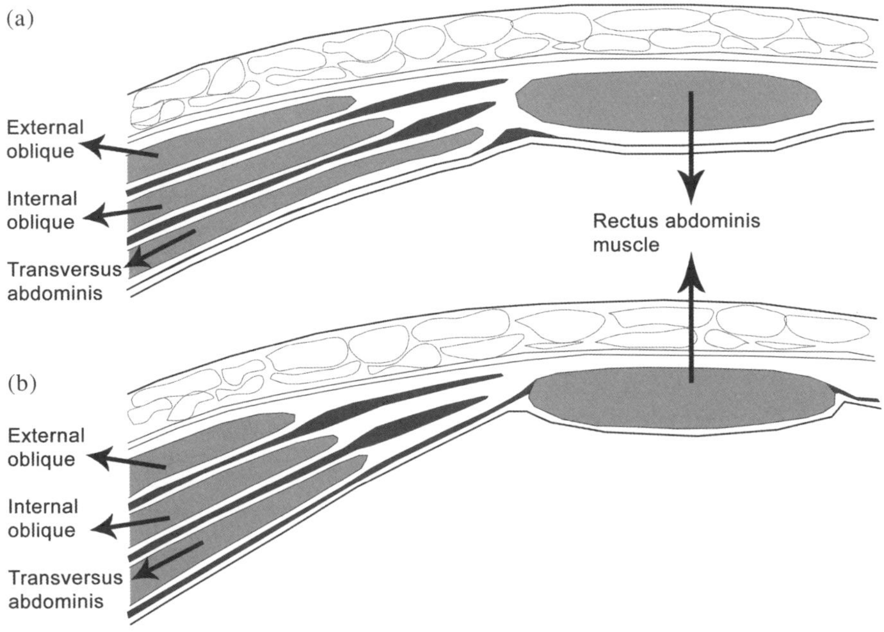

Fig. 7. (**a**) Above arcuate line. (**b**) Below arcuate line.

posterior layer of internal oblique aponeurosis, transversus abdominis aponeurosis, transversalis fascia posterior to rectus muscle

2. Below arcuate line: all 3 aponeuroses form anterior rectus sheath; posterior sheath composed of transversalis fascia only

ii. Linea alba: fusion of anterior and posterior rectus fascia at abdominal midline

iii. Linea semilunaris: aponeuroses of external oblique, internal oblique, transversus abdominis muscles at lateral edge of rectus abdominis muscle

d. Innervation: motor and sensory (T7 to L4)

i. Rectus abdominis: 5 lower intercostal and subcostal nerves

ii. External oblique: intercostal, subcostal, and ilioypogastric nerves

iii. Internal oblique and transversus abdominis: intercostal, subcostal, iliohypogastric, and ilioinguinal nerves
iv. Pubis: iliohypogasric and femoral cutaneous nerves

II. Preoperative Evaluation

1. History
    a. Establish diagnosis, extent and chronicity of problem, etiology, previous treatments, history of abdominal surgery
    b. Address preoperative comorbidities
        i. DM, HTN, COPD, coronary artery disease, peripheral vascular disease, obesity, malnutrition
            1. Cardiac clearance, optimization of nutrition, blood glucose control, PFTs
    c. Social history especially tobacco and alcohol use (impair wound healing and immune function)
    d. Medications
2. Physical examination
    a. Extent of defect: size/location/condition (see chart below)
    b. Patient stability, other abdominal wounds/interventions/scars
    c. Wound preparation/debridement and control of infection
3. Imaging
    a. CXR, CT or MRI, fistulogram if applicable

III. Classifications of Abdominal Wall Defects

Partial

- Loss of skin and subcutaneous or myofascial system
- Skin/subcutaneous defect: correct primarily with regard to size
- Myofascial defect: correct primarily based on position

Partial

  - Partial relative defect: repair with prosthetics or autologous tissue
  - Large absolute defect: repair with flap or free tissue transfer

Position of Defect

- Midline vs. Lateral
  - Midline defect: difficult to reconstruct with local flap, reconstruct with staged mesh or components separation
  - Lateral defect — reconstruct with local and distant flaps, may require mesh
- Upper vs. middle vs. lower third

Size of Defect

- Partial skin and subcutaneous defect
  - <5 cm partial deficit can be closed primarily
  - 5–15 cm partial deficit closed with local flap or STSG
  - >15 cm partial deficit closed with axial skin flap, local flap, fasciocutaneous flap, tissue expansion (after temporizing with STSG)
  - Defect can also be decreased in size with VAC therapy
- Partial myofascial defect
  - <3 cm closed primarily
  - >3 cm with sufficient skin and subcutaneous tissue can be closed with prosthetics
  - >3 cm can also be closed with components release based on position
  - >3–10 cm closed with tissue expansion, local flaps, distant flaps, free flaps

Complete

- Full-thickness loss of both the superficial and musculofascial layers
  - Advance skin if loss <15 cm
  - Immediate vs. delayed reconstruction

Clean vs. Contaminated

- Clean
  - Amenable to immediate reconstruction with skin grafts, flaps, and non-absorbable mesh
- Contaminated
  - Rely on temporary reconstruction with absorbable mesh and delayed skin grafting

IV. Reconstructive Options

A. Immediate closure
B. Delayed closure
    a. Negative pressure wound therapy (VAC: vacuum-assisted closure)
C. Prosthetics
D. Skin grafts
E. Tissue expanders
F. Local/regional flaps
G. Free tissue transfer

V. Immediate Closure vs. Delayed Closure

Immediate closure	Delayed closure
○ First line ○ More cost effective and less time consuming ○ Requires medically stable patient and clean wound	○ Preferred if patient unstable, wound contaminated, or further procedures planned ○ Often used for bowel edema/ trauma
○ Tension-free closure is critical	○ Loss of domain may be initially managed with mesh, skin graft, abdominal binders, etc. ○ Can be facilitated by wet-to-dry dressing changes or VAC therapy

- Negative pressure wound therapy: VAC therapy
    - Facilitates formation of granulation tissue
    - Removes exudate and excess fluid from extravascular space
    - Promotes neovascularization of wound
    - Enhances wound healing in preparation for graft or flap

VI. Prosthetic Mesh

- Partial myofascial defects
- Require sufficient skin and subcutaneous tissue and stable wound bed

- Advantages:
  - No donor site morbidity

  Availability
  - Size
  - Strength
- Absorbable
  - Polyglactin (Vicryl)
    - Advantages:
      - Safe in contaminated fields
      - No removal necessary
      - High tensile strength
      - STSG compatible
      - Can be incised
      - Can be used as temporizing management
    - Disadvantages:
      - Degradation
      - Decreased strength over time
      - Increased risk of hernia formation, ulceration, fistulas
- Disadvantages
  - Cost
  - Infection
  - Seroma
  - Erosion/fistula/extrusion
- Composites (Prolene/ePTFE)
  - Sepramesh, Proceed, Composix, Vypro, Ultrapro
    - Advantages:
      - Inner layer prevents bowel adhesion
    - Disadvantages:
      - Limited long term outcome data
- Nonabsorbable
  - Polytetrafluorethylene (Teflon, Gore-Tex), Polypropylene (Marlex, Prolene)
  - Advantages:
    - Availability
    - Increased fibrovascular ingrowth (polypropylene)
    - Can be placed over viscera
    - Separates from tissue easily
    - Pliable
    - Resistant to bacterial infection (polypropylene)
  - Disadvantages:
    - Decreased fibrovascular ingrowth (Gore-Tex)
    - Increased rate of infection
    - Increased rate of seroma formation (Gore-Tex)
    - Risk of extrusion
    - Risk of fistula formation
    - STSG not supported
- Bioprosthetics
  - Xenograft, Surgisis, Alloderm
  - Advantages:
    - Resistant to infection/contamination
    - Decreased erosion
    - Decreased rate of adhesions
    - Can be incised
    - Easy handling/pliable
    - Increased revascularization
    - Can be used as temporizing management
  - Disadvantages:
    - Cost
    - Size limitation
    - Limited long-term outcome data

VII. Skin Grafts

- Partial skin and subcutaneous defects
  - >5 cm defect that cannot be closed primarily
  - Can be removed later after tissue expansion
- Full-thickness defects
  - Delayed coverage following mesh placement, granulation
    - Prevents evisceration and further retraction of fascial edges
    - Immediate coverage placed directly on bowel
      - Stops insensible losses
      - Necessitates use of abdominal binder
      - No reconstruction if skin graft adherent to bowel or mesh (remove epithelial layer, leave dermal layer)

VIII. Tissue Expanders

- Advantages:
  - Aesthetic — good color and contour match
  - Limits donor site morbidity
  - Enables reconstruction with well-vascularized autologous tissue
- Disadvantages:
  - Requires staged approach
  - Cannot be used in infected wound — risk of extrusion
  - 20% rate of premature exposure and infection cited
- Partial skin and subcutaneous defects
  - Placed in the periphery of the wound in the subcutaneous tissue over ribs, ilium, or lumbar fascia
  - 20% rate of exposure and infection
- Full-thickness defects
  - Placed between the internal oblique and transversus abdominis or between the external oblique and internal oblique
  - Provides approximately 50% innervated, well-vascularized contractile, autologous tissue without need for mesh placement

IX. Local/Regional Flaps

- Cutaneous flaps (fasciocutaneous and musculocutaneous)
  - Primarily for partial skin and subcutaneous defects
- Thoracoepigasric
- Iliolumbar bipedicled flap
- Groin flap
- Superficial inferior epigastric artery (SIEA) flap
- Extended deep inferior epigastric flap (DIEP)

- Thoracoepigastric flap
  - Upper 1/3 of abdomen
  - 25 × 7 cm
  - Most common perforator vessel from superficial epigastric artery
  - Limited arc of rotation

- Iliolumbar bipedicle flap
  - Middle 1/3, lateral abdomen (when combined with tensor fascia lata graft)
  - Superficial circumflex iliac artery and lumbar artery

- Groin flap
  - Lower 1/3 of abdomen, ipsilateral
  - 25 × 10 cm
  - Superficial circumflex iliac artery
  - Large arc of rotation

- Superficial inferior epigastric (SIEA)
  - Lower 1/3 of abdomen
  - 15 x 30 cm
  - Superficial inferior epigastric artery
  - Unreliable location of donor pedicle

- Extended deep inferior epigastric (DIEP)
  - Lower 1/3 of abdomen, groin
  - Musculocutaneous flap
  - Deep inferior epigastric artery

- Muscle flaps
  - Primarily for partial musculofascial defects of lateral abdominal wall > 3 cm

    a. Rectus abdominis
    b. External oblique
    c. Internal oblique

a. Rectus abdominis muscle flap
  - Superiorly based for upper 2/3, inferiorly based for lower 1/3
  - 25 × 6 cm
  - Deep superior and inferior epigastric artery
  - May be myocutaneous

b. External oblique
  - Preferred for upper 2/3 defects
  - 20 × 40 cm
  - Lateral cutaneous branches of inferior 8 posterior intercostal arteries
  - Limited arc of rotation, unreliable pedicle
  - May be myocutaneous

c. Internal oblique
  - Lower 1/3 defects, groin
  - 10 × 20 cm
  - Ascending branch of deep circumflex iliac artery
  - Difficult dissection
  - Unreliable donor vessel

(*Continued*)

(*Continued*)

- Distant muscle flaps
  - Primarily for larger partial or full-thickness defects of the midline and lateral abdominal wall

    a. Latissimus dorsi
    b. Tensor fascia lata
    c. Rectus femoris
    d. Vastus lateralis
    e. Extended rectus
    f. Gracilis

a. Latissimus dorsi
- Upper lateral 1/3 deficits
- 25 × 35 cm
- Thoracodorsal artery
- Harvest pregluteal fascia to increase area of coverage and arc of rotation
- Donor site morbidity
- Used more often for free flap reconstruction

b. Tensor fascia lata
- Lower 2/3 deficit
- 5 × 15 cm
- Ascending branch of lateral circumflex femoral artery
- Can be pedicled or free flap
- Good substitute for fascial defect
- High donor site complication rate; >8 cm harvested needs skin graft closure

c. Rectus femoris
- Lower 2/3 deficit
- 20 × 8 cm
- Descending branch of lateral circumflex femoral artery
- Strong, good for chronic wounds
- Weakens quadriceps function ~20–25%; minimize functional limitation by suturing distal end to vastus medialis and lateralis
- Skin may be unreliable

d. Vastus lateralis
- Lower 2/3 deficit
- 10 × 26 cm
- Descending branch of lateral circumflex femoral artery
- Limited donor morbidity
- Lacks substantial fascial component

e. Extended rectus femoris (mutton chop)
- Epigastric, large defect
- Harvest rectus femoris with posterior fascia and iliotibial tract
- 10 × 30 cm
- Descending branch of lateral circumflex femoral artery
- Weakens quadriceps function

f. Gracilis
- Lower 1/3 deficit
- 6 × 24 cm
- Ascending branch of medial circumflex femoral artery
- Size limitation
- Distal skin island unreliable

(*Continued*)

(*Continued*)

- Free flaps
  - Appropriate conditions:
    - Local tissues inadequate
    - Pedicled flaps cannot reach or are too small
    - Total, full-thickness abdominal defects
    - Previous failed attempt with alloplastic reconstruction
    - Contaminated/infected wounds
  - Tensor fascia lata
  - Latissimus dorsi
  - Anterolateral thigh

X. Operative Techniques

A. Component separation (Ramirez) (Fig. 8)

Release external oblique fascia over internal oblique fascia (4 cm at costal margin, 8 cm at waist, 3 cm at supra pubic area is obtained)

Musculofascial components in continuity with nerve and blood supply

Repair in the midline

Cover the relaxing incisions with mesh

- If necessary release posterior rectus sheath (with this addition 5 cm in costal margin, 10 cm at the waist, 3 cm suprapubic area per side)
- Elevate skin over underlying abdominal musculature laterally
- Make a vertical incision from costal margin to inguinal ligament 2–3 cm lateral to semilunaris
- Dissect between external oblique and internal oblique to anterior or posterior axillary line
- Dissect between rectus abdominis muscle and posterior rectus
- Rectus muscle with the overlying rectus sheath and attached internal oblique-transversus abdominus advanced medially
- Monitor peak airway pressures and for signs of abdominal compartment syndrome

1. Components separation — modifications

- Tissue expanders placed between oblique muscles through lateral wall incision
- Lateral incision directly over linea semilunaris

(*Continued*)

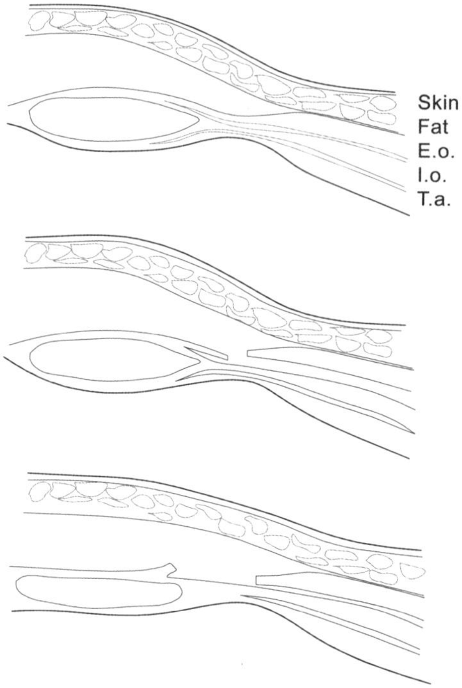

Fig. 8. Component separation.

(*Continued*)

- Endoscopically assisted release of external oblique
- Periumbilical perforator preservation
- Unilateral rectus complex mobility

  4 cm costal margin

  8 cm waist

  3 cm supra pubic area

B. Latissimus dorsi flap

  A lazy S incision is planned along the lateral border of latissimus dorsi muscle. The skin incision is planned according to size of defect

  Anterior edge of the latissmus dorsi muscle is identified

  The skin and subcutaneous tissues are dissected away from the muscle

  The distal insertions of the muscle and paraspinal attachments are released

(*Continued*)

(*Continued*)

The flap is then raised from anterior to posterior and distal to proximal towards the thoracodorsal artery and vein pedicle

The nerve is dissected and divided

Humeral attachment of the muscle is divided to gain more length if necessary depending on the location of the defect

C. Serratus anterior flap

The same steps as for latissimus dorsi are performed

The serratus muscle is identified and only a portion of the muscle is dissected in order to prevent winged scapula

The serratus branch of the thoracodorsal artery and vein are dissected

The muscle can be quite large to cover defects in the posterior trunk

D. Omental flap
E. Pectoralis major flap
F. Scapular and parascapular flaps
G. Transverse rectus abdominis muscle flaps
H. External oblique flap

I. Anterolateral thigh flap :

I. Markings are done according to the perforators with Doppler. A line is drawn between anterior superior iliac spine and superolateral aspect of patella. Midway of this drawing is investigated for the major perforator for the ALT flap. Then 1/3 superior and 2/3 inferior aspect is selected within the flap while keeping other perforators within the flap
II. Anterior incision is made down to the fascia
III. Rectus muscle is retracted medially, septum between rectus and vastus lateralis is identified
IV. The septocutaneous and musculocutaneous perforators are identified and followed. If needed a lateral incision is made
V. The lateral circumflex artery and vein are dissected distal to proximal. The motor nerve is protected in the neurovascular bundle. Artery and vein are dissected and separated from each other. Size match is checked before flap transfer to the recipient area

J. Free flaps

Recipient artery
Extraperitoneal: common femoral; deep circumflex lliac; superior epigastric; inferior epigastric; internal thoracic; saphenous V. loop grafts

Intraperitoneal: gastroepiploic; jejunal; iliac (pedicle length prohibitive)

XI. Postoperative Care

1. Pain control
2. Drains (often more than 1)
3. Abdominal binder
4. Physical/occupational therapy
5. Limitations in physical activity and avoidance of heavy lifting for ≥6 weeks

Further Reading

1. Netter FH. (1989) *Atlas of Human Anatomy*. Ciba-Geigy, New Jersey.
2. Knoetgen J, Johnson CH, Arnold PG. (2006) Reconstruction of the chest. In: Mathes SJ (ed.), *Plastic Surgery: Volume VI — Trunk and Lower Extremity*. Elsevier, Pennsylvania, pp. 411–440.
3. Janis JE. (2007) Abdominal wall reconstruction. In: Janis JE (ed.), *Essentials of Plastic Surgery*. Quality Medical Publishing, Missouri, pp. 434–440.
4. Rohrich RJ, Lowe JB, Hackney FL, *et al*. (2000) An algorithm for abdominal wall reconstruction. *Plast Reconstr Surg* **105**: 202–216.
5. Nozaki M, Sasaki K, Huang TT. (2006) Reconstruction of the abdominal Wall. In: Mathes SJ (ed.), *Plastic Surgery: Volume VI — Trunk and Lower Extremity*. Elsevier, Pennsylvania, pp. 1175–1196.
6. Lowe JB. (2006) Updated algorithm for abdominal wall reconstruction. *Clin Plast Surg* **33**: 225–240.
7. Dumanian GA. (2007) Abdominal wall reconstruction. In: Thorne CH, Beasley RW, Aston SJ, Bartlett SP, Gurtner GC, Spear SL (eds.), *Grabb and Smith's Plastic Surgery,* 6th Edn. Lippincott, Pennsylvania, pp. 670–675.
8. Frye DE, Osler T. (1991) Abdominal wall considerations and complications in reoperative surgery. *Surg Clin North Am* **71**(1): 1–11.
9. Mathes SJ, Steinwald PM, Foster RD, *et al*. (2000) Complex abdominal wall reconstruction: a comparison of flap and mesh closure. *Ann Surg* **232**(4): 586–596.

ABDOMINAL AND THORACIC WALL RECONSTRUCTION

Thoracic Reconstruction

Anatomy of the Thorax

I. Anatomy

1. Sternum, bilateral clavicles, 12 thoracic vertebrae, bilateral scapulae, 10 ribs with associated cartilage, 2 ribs without cartilage
   a. Ribs 1–7 articulate with the sternum = true ribs
   b. Ribs 8–12 no articulation with sternum = false ribs
   c. Ribs 11–12 don't articulate with sternum or superior ribs = floating ribs
   Skeletal chest wall function: protective barrier, dynamic stability, respiratory function
2. Muscles: cover thoracic viscera, anterior chest muscles largely responsible for movement of the upper extremities
   a. Diaphragm — innervated by C3–C5
   b. 3 layers of intercostal muscles: external, internal, innermost
      i. Neurovascular bundle runs inferior to the rib, running between latter two layers of intercostal muscles
   c. Accessory muscles of respiration
   d. Sternocleidomastoid (SCM)
   e. Scalene muscles

II. Mechanics of Ventilation

1. Inspiration: expansion of the thorax → negative intra thoracic pressure → negative intrapulmonary pressure → inflow of atmospheric air into the lungs
   a. Muscles involved in maximal inspiration: SCM, scalenes, external intercostals

2. Expiration: (passive) recoil of the chest wall → contraction of the thorax → positive intrapulmonary pressure which equilizes with atmospheric pressure
    a. Muscles involved in maximal expiration: internal intercostals, external oblique, rectus abdominis, internal oblique, transversalis muscle

III. Defects of Thorax

1. Reconstruction of the chest may involve both skeletal and soft tissue components
2. Etiology: trauma, infection, tumor, congenital, iatrogenic (i.e. radiation)
    A. Chest wall tumors
        1. Primary — rare; most commonly originate from soft tissue
            a. Benign
                i. Most common benign tumor: osteochondroma
                    1. Difficult to differentiate from chondrosarcomas so treatment is aggressive
                ii. Fibrous dysplasia and histiocytosis
                iii. Rarely involve scapula or clavicle
            b. Malignant — more than 96% of primary bone tumors that originate in the sternum are malignant
                i. Most common malignant: myeloma, chondrosarcoma, Ewing sarcoma, osteogenic sarcoma
        2. Metastatic
            a. Primary distant sites: kidney, thyroid
            b. Primary local sites: lung, pleura, mediastimun, breast
            c. Resection includes the tumor, ribs involved with the tumor, ribs superior and inferior to the affected area
            d. Advanced tumors may be complicated by radiation, infections
        3. Soft tissue tumors
            a. Benign: fibromas, lipomas, giant cell tumors, vascular tumors (i.e. hemangiomas)

b. Desmoid tumors — originate in muscle and fascia, tend to aggressively invade adjacent structures, high recurrence rate. 40% tend to occur in the shoulder and chest
c. Malignant: most common — malignant fibrous histiocytoma and rhabdomyosarcoma; also liposarcoma and leiomyosarcoma

4. Most common cause of chest wall defects: breast carcinoma, sarcoma, squamous cell carcinoma, desmoid tumors

B. Sternal wound infections

1. Basic principles: debridement, obliteration of the mediastinal dead space
2. Pairolero classified sternal wounds into 3 types:

a. Type 1: wound separation +/– sternal instability, serosanguinous drainage — within 3 days after sternotomy
b. Type II: mediastinitis, cellulitis, and purulent drainage-within 3 weeks
c. Type III: chronic sinus tracts — within months-years

C. Intrathoracic soft tissue defect.

1. Bronchopleural fistula, empyema, recurrent airleak, leakage from cardiac vessels, erosion, esophageal perforation, intrathoracic irradiation
2. Goal: treat infection and re-establish airtight pleural space
3. Treatmeant: muscle flaps — serratus anterior, latissimus dorsi, pectoralis major, omentum, rectus abdominis

a. Latissimus dorsi generally divided during thoracotomy incision; other muscles are good alternatives and latissimus dorsi can be added for additional bulk

IV. Preoperative Tests for Thoracic Reconstruction

1. Pulmonary function tests (PFTs)

a. In a patient with impaired baseline PFTs a defect <5 cm may cause functional problems

2. Tidal volume
3. Chest X-ray
4. Arterial blood gas
5. MRI; arteriogram

V. Physical Exam

1. Look for previous incisions — possible damage to internal mammary artery or superior epigastric blood supply, previous axillary surgery may have caused damage to thoracodorsal vessels

Congenital syndromes:

   a. Poland syndrome resulting in abnormal latissimus dorsi and serratus muscles
   b. Pectus excavatum (sternal depression), pectus carinatum (sternal protrusion), or previous repair may have jeopardized the blood supply of local flaps

2. Presence of atherosclerotic disease

VI. Skeletal Reconstruction

1. Chest wall defect
   a. Adequate debridement is crucial before reconstruction attempts
   b. <5 cm diameter defect: skeletal reconstruction not required
   c. >5 cm defect or more than 4–5 ribs involved → paradoxical respiratory motion and abnormal respiration: requires rigid reconstruction
      1. Irradiated chest wall becomes stiff and usually doesn't require reconstruction for support even for defects >5 cm
   d. Reconstruction begins with the deepest tissues and proceeds to the most superficial
   e. Generally accepted that an air-tight pleural cavity is essential
2. Autogenous bone
   a. Graft donor sites: ribs, fibula, iliac crest
      1. overlap graft with recipient site trabecular bone to prevent resorption and fibrous encapsulation

b. Bone flaps: fascia lata, intercostal rib, scapular osteocutaneous

3. Prosthetic materials

a. High-density polyethylene (Marlex), PTFE (Teflon), e-PTFE (Gore-tex), polypropylene (Prolene), polyglactin (Vicryl), methylmethacrylate

VII. Soft Tissue Reconstruction

Trapezius flap	▪ Mathes and Nahai type II ▪ Dominant pedicle: transverse cervical artery ▪ Minor pedicle: posterior intercostal arteries, occipital arteries ▪ Innervation: spinal accessory nerve ▪ Defect coverage: posterior midline, posterior neck, proximal paraspinal defects
Parascapular flap	▪ Fasciocutaneous flap ▪ Dominant pedicle: circumflex scapular artery ▪ Innervation: none ▪ Coverage: shoulder, axilla, lateral chest wall
Latissimus dorsi flap	▪ Mathes and Nahai type V ▪ Dominant pedicle: thoracodorsal artery Segmental vessels: posterior intercostal and lumbar arteries ▪ Innervation: thoracodorsal nerve ▪ Coverage: contralateral posterior chest wall, anterior and lateral chest wall defect
Pectoralis major flap	▪ Mathes and Nahai type V ▪ Dominant pedicle: thoracoacromial artery ▪ Segmental: intercostal arteries, perforators from internal mammary artery ▪ Innervation: medial and lateral pectoral nerves ▪ Coverage: midline sternal defect, intrathoracic
Serratus anterior flap	▪ Mathes and Nahai type III ▪ Dominant pedicles: thoracodorsal and lateral thoracic artery ▪ Innervation: long thoracic nerve ▪ Coverage: anterior and posterior chest wall defect, intrathoracic

(*Continued*)

(*Continued*)

External oblique flap	▪ Mathes and Nahai type IV ▪ Segmental: lateral cutaneous branches of inferior posterior intercostal arteries ▪ Innervation: thoracoabdominal nerves ▪ Coverage: anterior chest wall
Rectus abdominis flap	▪ Mathes and Nahai type III ▪ Dominant pedicles: superior and inferior epigastric arteries ▪ Innervation: thoracoabdominal nerves ▪ Coverage: midline, anterolateral chest wall defect
Omental flap	▪ Mathes and Nahai type III ▪ Dominant pedicles: right and left gastroepiploic arteries ▪ Requires laparotomy and tunneling through diaphragm or over costal margin ▪ Coverage: anterior midline, lateral chest wall, mediastinal cavity defects
Osteocutaneous free flaps	
Fibular	▪ Blood supply: peroneal artery ▪ Can harvest flexor hallucis longus to augment ▪ Available length: 25–30 cm of bone ▪ Must evaluate preoperatively for peripheral vascular disease
Scapular	▪ Blood supply: branch of circumflex scapular artery ▪ Can be combined with latissimus dorsi flap, provides large amount of soft tissue ▪ Available length: approx 14 cm of bone (lateral scapula) ▪ Postoperative morbidity includes decreased shoulder range of motion
Iliac crest	▪ Segmental blood supply: deep circumflex iliac artery ▪ Associated skin island often with unpredictable circulation; soft-tissue cumbersome and adherent to bone ▪ Painful donor site
Radial forearm	▪ Blood supply: radial artery ○ Pedicle between brachioradialis and flexor carpi radialis muscles ▪ Good quality skin island (pliable, thin), long vascular pedicle ▪ Poor bone source (need to preserve enough radius to prevent donor site postoperative morbidity) ▪ Available length: approx. 10 cm ▪ Evaluate preoperative with Allen test

VIII. Alloplastic Materials

e-PTFE (Gore-Tex)
Polyproplene (Marlex)
Methyl methacrylate and plastic sandwiches
Vicryl
Marlex mesh
Nylon
Methyl methacrylate
Teflon
Prolene
Silastic

IX. Complications of Alloplastic Materials

1. Infection
2. Flaccidity
3. Extrusion
4. Strong exothermic reaction during application
5. Fibrous capsule formation

X. Congenital Defects

1. Poland Syndrome
   a. Pathology: absent sternal head of pectoralis major muscle, hypoplastic/aplastic breast and subcutaneous tissue, syndactyly/hypoplasia of ipsilateral upper extremity
      i. May have absent/hypoplastic pectoralis minor muscle, abnormality of latissimus dorsi and serratus muscles, and absent anterolateral ribs +/– lung herniation
   b. Reconstruction: ipsilateral latissimus dorsi muscle, breast implant, alloplastic mesh
2. Pectus Excavatum
   a. Pathology: male/female ratio of 4:1, posterior sternal depression
   b. Reconstruction: osteotomies, sternal turnover, sternal strut, Ravitch technique (osteotomy and wedge strut), cartilaginous wedge resections, metal vs. absorbable implants
3. Pectus Carinatum
   a. Pathology: male/female ratio of 4:1, anterior sternal protrusion, less common than excavatum
   b. Reconstruction: resection of costal cartilages, sternal osteotomies, struts

Further Reading

1. Brown DL, Borschel G. (2004) Thoracic Reconstruction. *Michigan Manual* of *Plastic Surgery*. Lippincott Williams and Wilkins, Philadelphia, pp. 344–348.
2. Janis JE. (2007) Chest wall reconstruction. In: Janis JE (ed), *Essentials of Plastic Surgery.* Quality Medical Publishing, Missouri, pp. 423–433.
3. Cohen M, Ramasastry SS. (1996) Reconstruction of complex chest wall defects. *Am J Surg* **172**: 35–40.
4. Chang RR. (2007). Thoracic reconstruction. In: Thorne CH, Beasley RW, Aston SJ, Bartlett SP, Gurtner GC, Spear SL (eds.), *Grabb and Smith's Plastic Surgery,* 6th Edn. Lippincott, Pennsylvania, pp. 665–669.
5. King TC, Smith CR. (1989) Chest wall, pleura, lung, and mediastinum. In: Schwartz SI, Shires GT, Spencer FC (eds.), *Principles of Surgery,* 5th Edn. McGraw-Hill, Inc., New York, pp. 627–770.
6. Netter FH. (1989). *Atlas of Human Anatomy*. Ciba-Geigy, New Jersey.
7. Knoetgen J, Johnson CH, Arnold PG. (2006) Reconstruction of the chest. In: Mathes SJ (ed.), *Plastic Surgery: Volume VI — Trunk and Lower Extremity*. Elsevier, Pennsylvania, pp. 411–440.

CHAPTER 29

PRESSURE ULCERS

Jessica S. Suber, Rajiv P. Parikh and Deniz Dayicioglu

Illustrative Case

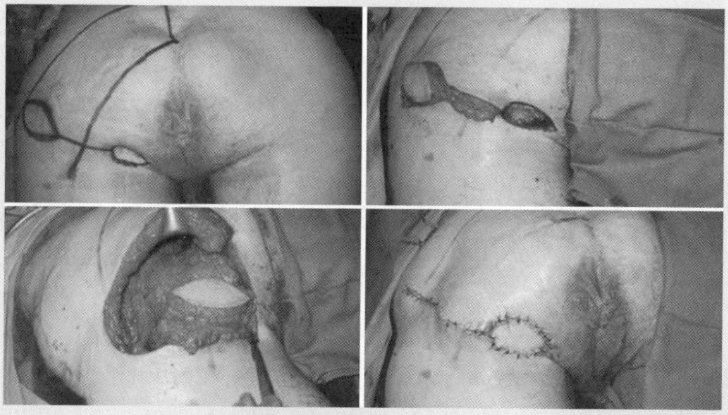

Fig. 1. Gluteal island perforator flap utilizing only musculocutaneous perforators from the inferior gluteal vessels (Design; Incision; Elevation; Inset/Closure).

A 49 year old man is referred to the plastic surgery service with a left ischial wound. He was recently involved in an automobile accident that resulted in a spinal cord injury, transient paraplegia and a pelvic fracture, for which he was confined to strict bed rest. He now uses a wheelchair and has limited mobility with frequent muscle spasms secondary to the sustained injuries; however, he is in rehabilitation with full recovery expected. He has no other medical comorbidities, but does report active, 1 pack/day, tobacco use. He has been treating the wound with moist dressings and notes some purulent wound drainage. A comprehensive evaluation is performed, including an assessment of nutritional status and the presence of wound infection. His serum albumin is 2.5 g/dL and leukocyte count is 13.4/mm^3. Physical examination reveals a 4 × 2 cm, partially necrotic, wound that does not extend to the ischial bone. Following classification of the wound as a stage 3 ischial pressure ulcer (Table 1), it is operatively excised and debrided for removal of devitalized tissue and wound bed preparation. Culture results are quantitatively $<10^5$ organisms/gram of tissue and negative for *Beta Hemolytic Streptococcus*. A multidisciplinary team approach is taken to optimize the patient's medical status, with an emphasis on nutritional supplementation, smoking cessation, relief of ongoing sources of pressure, and control of spasticity. After successful medical intervention, it is determined that the patient is an appropriate candidate for surgical closure.

Given the patient's future expected ambulatory status and low risk of ulcer recurrence, a gluteal island fasciocutaneous perforator flap is chosen for closure (for details, see: Operative Techniques → Ischial ulcers → Gluteal flap). This approach offers several advantages for the patient, including an augmented vascular supply to withstand potential ischemia from wheelchair induced pressure and minimal donor site morbidity which will benefit future ambulation. Figure 1 illustrates the operative procedure. A Doppler probe is used to mark the dominant musculocutaneous perforator arising from the inferior gluteal artery and an elliptical skin island is marked. The flap is elevated subfascially to include the underlying deep fascia, until encountering a large perforator of the inferior gluteal vessels. The perforator is dissected to the pivot point, taking care to maintain a distance of 1–2 cm from the perforator to retain soft tissue around the pedicle. The flap is islanded and the incision is deepened with precision to avoid violating other perforators. Further flap elevation is performed to improve mobilization and provide tension-free flap transposition. Primary tension-free closure of the skin is performed after insetting the flap in the recipient deficit. The patient is followed post-operatively by a multidisciplinary team, including specialists from physical therapy, physical medicine and rehabilitation, nutrition, wound care and plastic surgery. He is educated on his condition and followed as an outpatient. His post-operative course is without complication.

Introduction

Pressure ulcers result from prolonged ischemia and subsequent tissue injury incited by unrelieved pressure occurring over bony prominences. A pressure ulcer is often referred to as a "decubitus ulcer," terminology derived from the latin word *decumbere*, meaning "to lie down." However, in addition to lying down, pressure ulcers can occur in several other positions, including sitting. Thus, pressure ulcer is a more appropriate term than decubitus ulcer.

Epidemiology[1]

- 1.3 to 3 million people are affected annually in the United States
- Overall prevalence estimated at 15%

Incidence[2–8]

- Acute care setting: 1–8%
- Nursing home setting: 3–26%
- Paraplegic patients: 16–37%
- ICU setting: 14–41%
- Elderly patients with Hip Fractures: 66%

Prevalence[2–8]

- Acute care/hospital setting: 3–14%
- Nursing home setting: 1.2–28%

> Patients with highest incidences: quadriplegics, elderly orthopedic patients, acutely ill and young patients with SCI or neurological impairment

Costs[1,2]

- Cost to heal 1 full thickness ulcer as high as $70,000 (Avg = $30,000)
- Estimated annual cost for management: 5.0 to 8.5 billion dollars

- Surgical closure[9]
  - $17,000 more expensive than conservative therapy
  - Probability of living at least 1 year is 0.64 compared with 0.26 for conservative therapy

Locations[10,11]

- 70% on the buttock region (*Ischial > Trochanter > Sacrum*)
- 30% on the lower extremities (heel, malleolus, patella, pretibial) or other areas that sustain ongoing pressure such as occiput, nose, elbows, chin, forehead, chest or back

Pathophysiology[12]

Sir James Paget described the pathophysiology behind pressure ulcers in 1873. He reported when external pressure exceeds capillary pressure, ischemia occurs and subsequently causes necrosis and ulceration. An inverse relationship exists between pressure and time to ulceration.[13] This external pressure results from surface contact and positioning. When that contact occurs between an external surface and human soft tissue overlying bony prominences, it has the potential to incite pressure ulcer formation. When an applied load is evenly distributed, human tissue can withstand a high degree of pressure with normal capillary pressure being between 12–32 mmHg. However, that is not typically the case in positions such as supine and prone:

- Supine position: points of highest pressure are sacrum, buttocks, heel and occiput, ranging from 40–60 mmHg
- Prone: pressures at knees and chest can be 40–50 mmHg
- Sitting: pressures up to 100 mmHg applied to ischial tuberosities (kenkel)

"Tip of the Iceberg" Phenomenon

- Muscle initially affected because of the larger need for oxygen and higher metabolic requirements
- Muscle and surrounding tissue suffers irreversible changes after 2 hours of uninterrupted pressure
- The skin, however, can withstand direct pressure for up to 12 hours

- Ulceration evident at the skin level is usually indicative of significant damage to the underlying tissue and muscle, occurring in the shape of an inverted cone[14]

Etiology

Extrinsic factors include: pressure, shear, friction, and moisture. Intrinsic factors include: sensory loss, diminished muscle strength or mobility, incontinence, infection, anemia, protein malnutrition, and advancing age.

Extrinsic/Environmental[11,15]

- Pressure: perpendicular load that causes tissue deformation, mechanical damage and blockage of blood vessels
- Shear: mechanical stress parallel to the plane that causes injury by stretching and compressing the muscle-perforating vessels to skin leading to ischemia
- Friction: resistance of two surfaces moving across one another. This resistance can act directly on the epidermis by rubbing off the outermost layer, increasing transepidermal water loss which then allows moisture to accumulate on the surface of the body. This type of trauma is often related to patient transfers[8]
- Moisture: exacerbates detrimental effects of both friction and shear. Primary causes of moisture include sweating and incontinence. Primary effect is skin maceration

Intrinsic/Systemic[2,4,15]

All factors that result in prolonged periods of pressure-induced tissue ischemia or reduce the capacity for tissue repair, including:

- Infection: causes skin and soft tissue breakdown and delays wound healing
- Ischemia: decreases tissue perfusion or subcutaneous tissue oxygen tension, increases necrosis and delays wound healing
- Diminished sensory perception: prolongs soft tissue to external surface contact time
- Spasticity: prolongs immobility and delays surgical intervention

- Malnutrition: nutrient, mineral and vitamin deficiencies: delays wound healing
- Increased age: delays wound healing
- Low BMI: delays wound healing
- Anemia: delays wound healing and prolongs immobilization
- Metabolic disturbances: delays wound healing
- Prolonged immobility: prolongs soft tissue to surface contact and leads to ongoing pressure

Any medical comorbidity that results in one of the above factors significantly increases a patient's risk for pressure ulcers. Comorbidities that impair wound healing: diabetes, smoking, peripheral vascular disease and cardiovascular. Most common comorbidities associated with pressure ulcers: stroke, SCI, paralysis, hip fracture or dementia

Risk factor assessment scales (Norton, Waterlow, and Braden scales) have not gained wide acceptance due to concerns over sensitivity, specificity, reliability, and validity (Source: Kuzin 2011)

Classification[16]

Table 1. Classification System.

Stage	Lesion Description
Deep Tissue Injury	Purple or maroon localized area of discolored intact skin or blood-filled blister due to damage of underlying soft tissue from pressure and/or shear
I	Skin intact but reddened for >1 hour after pressure relief. The erythema indicates reactive hyperemia. This can present with warmth and induration
II	Blister or partial thickness loss of skin involving the epidermis and dermis
III	Full thickness loss of skin with extension into the subcutaneous tissue
IV	Full thickness loss of skin with extension into muscle, bone, tendon or joint capsule. Sinus tracts are common
Unstageable	Full-thickness tissue loss in which the base of the ulcer is covered by slough or eschar. Depth cannot be appreciated until debrided

Patient Evaluation and Medical Management[1,12]

Infection control

- Treat all infections including UTI, cardiac valves, sinus cavities
- Debride wound and eliminate all devitalized tissue
- Quantitative cultures must reveal $<1 \times 10^5$ CFU/gram of bacteria with no *Beta Hemolytic Streptococcus*
- If osteomyelitis is suspected, perform bone biopsy. If positive, wound must be debrided, covered with fascia or muscle flap with antibiotic treatment for 3 weeks

> For diagnosing OM, clinical exam, CT and plain films are only 33%, 50% and 88% sensitive, respectively.[17] Bone biopsy is the definitive diagnostic method.

Nutrition

- Protein 1.25–1.50 g/kg/day
- Non-protein 30–35 cal/kg/day
- Calorie counts
- Supplementation with Vitamin A, C, Ca, Fe, Copper (only for patients with vitamin deficiencies)
- Albumin levels <3.5 g/dL have been associated with poor wound healing and higher recurrence rates

Pressure relief

- Relief for 5 minutes every 2 hours allows adequate perfusion and prevents breakdown
- Turn Q2 hours in bed or lift up for 10 seconds Q10 minutes if seated
- Proper mattress
    - Low air loss
    - Air fluidized

Muscle spasms[18]

- Valium, baclofen or dantrolene
- Invasive methods: nerve blocks, epidural stimulators or rhizotomy

Wound care and dressings[11,19]

There are two main categories of dressings: passive and active dressings. Passive dressings are synthetic polymers that customize in absorbency, physical form and gas permeability. Their main action is control of moisture levels. Active dressings are targeted for wounds with higher bacterial counts to decrease the bacterial load and control moisture levels.

- *Passive dressings*
    - Hydrocolloid: an occlusive barrier that covers the ulcer while maintaining a moist wound environment and preventing bacterial contamination. Gel forms when wound exudate comes in contact. Ideal for light to moderate exudate in shallow full-thickness defects
    - Alginate: a fibrous product derived from brown seaweed and forms a gel on contact with wound drainage. Ideal for moderate to heavy exudate. Should not be applied to dry or minimally draining wounds, because it may lead to dehydration
    - Hydrogels: glycerin or water based cross-linked polymer gels or sheets used for minimal to moderate exudate and superficial to deep wounds for re-hydration
    - Foams: air bubbles in a matrix of polyurethane or silicone capable of holding or releasing fluid for moderate to heavy exudate
    - Transparent film: a thin sheet of polyurethane film for dry wounds to maintain moisture
- *Active dressings*
    - Antimicrobial dressings
        - Chlorhexidine
        - Povidone-iodine
        - Cadexomer iodine
        - Alcohol

  - Acetate
  - Hydrogen peroxide
  - Silver Sulfadiazine
  - Silver nitrate
  - Dakin's solution (Sodium hypochlorite (0.45–0.5%) and boric acid (4%).

> Topical antimicrobial use can be limited by patient sensitization, allergic reactions and systemic toxicity. A special awareness is necessary when treating large wounds that require frequent applications. Dakin's solution is locally toxic and should not be used for an extended period of time (> 2–3 days)

  - Collagenase: goal is enzymatic debridement. Collagen dressings are 55% bovine collagen and 45% oxidized regenerated cellulose that provide a scaffold for growth of tissue; they are hydrophilic in nature, chemotactic to fibroblasts, granulocytes and macrophages for moderate to heavy exudate, infected wounds, skin grafts or donor sites
  - Wound VAC: stimulates wound contracture while removing exudate and edema

> Hyperbaric oxygen therapy has not been shown to have a statistically significant effect on pressure ulcer healing

Operative Techniques[20–24]

General principles

- Excise entire ulcer, surrounding scar, underlying bursa and soft-tissue calcification. Paint the wound with methylene blue to help identify all of the tissue that needs to be excised
- Explore and unroof all sinus cavities
- Remove all prominent, soft, necrotic or heterotopic bone
- Smooth all bony edges with rasp or file

- Resurface with a regional, axial, pedicled flap, which provides vascularized tissue, fills anatomical dead space, and pads bony stumps to offload pressure
- Establish hemostasis and place drains, if necessary
- Tension-free closure
- Graft donor site if applicable
- Primary closure and skin grafting not generally recommended due to the high recurrence rates and insignificant bulk/padding provided

> Patient's ambulatory status, comorbid medical conditions and risk of recurrence must be taken into consideration when planning flap reconstruction. If patient is at high risk for recurrence, care must be taken to choose reusable flaps and to not violate or destroy anatomic territory that may become necessary in the future[6]

Reconstruction by Wound Location

Ischial pressure ulcers[11,20–23]

- Total ischectomy: minimizes ipsilateral ischial recurrence but secondary problems are frequent
- Unilateral ischiectomy: transfers weight to the opposite ischium in the sitting position which leads to an increased risk of a contralateral ischial ulcer
- Bilateral ischiectomies: transfers weight to the pubic rami and perineum which leads to increased risk of perineal ulcers and urethrocutaneous fistula: Avoid this approach

> After any type of ischiectomy or bone resection: patient must undergo seat mapping to observe changes in pressure dynamics so appropriate adjustments can be made to seat cushions or wheelchairs

***Flap options*:** fasciocutaneous or musculocutaneous

- Lateral thigh[22]
- Size 7 × 20 cm

- Fasciocutaneous
- Sensory: lateral cutaneous nerve of thigh (L2–3)
- Dominant pedicles: First, second and third perforating branches of profunda fermoris artery and venae comitantes
- Prep: draw line from greater trochanter to lateral condyle of femur to outline lateral intermuscular septum. The skin island is designed along the line from the trochanter to the knee with 2/3 of flap width anterior to this line. Pedicle enters flap just below insertion of gluteus maximus through the lateral intermuscular septum
- Technique: initial incision is located at the anterior flap border to level of fascia lata, but the fascia lata is not included with the flap. Flap is elevated from anterior to posterior. Continue dissection to intermuscular septum until pedicle is observed. Elevate the remaining portion of the skin island with the flap isolated on the vascular pedicle. Dissect in the plane superficial to the fascia lata. You can rotate the flap 90 degrees for trochanteric and/or ischial pressure ulcer defects
- Gluteus maximus[22,25,26]

    - Size 24 × 24cm
    - Type III
    - Motor: inferior gluteal nerve (L5–S1–2)
    - Sensory: branches of posterior division of S1–3 medially and the posterior division of the L1–3 laterally. Posterior cutaneous nerve (S1–2) supplies skin of inferior buttocks and posterior thigh
    - Vascular supply

        - Dominant pedicle: superior gluteal artery and inferior gluteal artery and venae comitantes
        - Minor pedicle: first perforator of profunda femoris artery and two to three intermuscular branches of lateral circumflex femoral artery and venae comitantes

    - Technique # 1

        - The gluteal flap can be raised with superior half, inferior half or complete muscle for use as a turnover flap.

    - In general, a linear incision is made of the cutaneous territory of the gluteus maximus muscle needed parallel to its muscle fibers
    - The insertion is identified and fibers of insertion are divided
    - The deep surface is dissected away from piriformis and care is taken to avoid the pedicle, which enters the deep surface

  - Technique # 2 (26): Perforator sparing technique with a Gluteal Rotation Flap (can be used for sacral and trochanteric as well):

    - The perforator incorporated into the rotation flap can be from the superior or inferior gluteal vessels
    - Undermining from cranially to raise an inferiorly based flap (for sacral or trochanteric ulcers), the superior gluteal perforators would be encountered and incorporated into the rotation flap. Elevating the flap from caudally to raise a superiorly based flap (for ischial sores), the inferior gluteal perforators would be encountered and then preserved
    - A subfascial dissection is performed and musculocutaneous perforators are located, with dissection of the dominant perforator through the gluteus maximus muscle to its origin at the superior or inferior gluteal arteries
    - These arteries are in turn further mobilized to the emergent point above and below the piriformis muscle, respectively
    - A part of the gluteus muscle can be transposed or advanced to fill deadspace in the wound
    - Finally, the flap is rotated into the defect carrying the perforator and closed in a tension-free manner. Drains are placed and the wound is closed

- V-Y with posterior hamstring muscle[18,22]

  - 3 muscles occupy posterior thigh: biceps femoris, semimembranosus and semitendinosus
  - Size 15 × 45 cm
  - Type II

- Nerve: branches of sciatic for motor, postcutaneous nerve of thigh (S1–3) for sensory
- Vascular supply
    - Dominant pedicle of long head of biceps femoris: first perforating branch of profunda femoris artery and venae comitantes
    - Minor pedicles of long head: second perforating branch of profunda femoris artery and venae comitantes and branch of inferior gluteal artery and venae comitantes
    - Dominant pedicle of short head: second or third perforating branch of profunda femoris artery and venae comitantes
    - Minor pedicle of short head: superior lateral genicular artery and venae comitantes
    - Dominant pedicle of semimembranosus: first perforating branch of profunda femoris artery and venae comitantes
    - Minor pedicles of semimembranosus: second or third perforating branch of profunda fermoris artery, branch of inferior gluteal artery and branch of superficial femoral artery with venae comitantes
    - Dominant pedicle of semitendinosus: first perforating branch of profunda femoris artery and venae comitantes
    - Minor pedicles of semitendinosus: muscular branch of inferior gluteal, descending branch of medial circumflex femoral artery, and inferior medial genicular artery with venae comitantes
- The posterior thigh skin is elevated to expose the muscles
- Muscles are divided at musculotendinous junction and are mobilized from below upward toward their origin
- Distal pedicles are ligated and muscles can be turned over on proximal pedicle
- For V-Y advancement, the biceps can be divided at the junction of the muscle with its tendon while the semimembranosus and semitendinosus are divided medially which allows excellent advancement
- Muscle layer is sutured to gluteus maximus and skin island is sutured to overlying skin

- Tensor fascia lata[22]
    - Size 12 × 20 cm
    - Fasciocutaneous Type B and C circulation
    - Nerve: lateral femoral cutaneous (L2–3)
    - Vascular supply
        - Dominant pedicle: Septocutaneous branches of descending branch of lateral circumflex femoral artery and venae comitantes
        - Minor pedicle: Musculocutaneous branches of descending branch of lateral circumflex femoral artery as well as branches of transverse branch of lateral circumflex femoral artery and venae comitantes
    - Incise the medial vertical border of the flap through deep fascia
    - The deep and overlying skin are elevated laterally until lateral edge of rectus femoris muscles are identified
    - Dissect fascia septum between rectus femoris and vastus lateralis at midpoint of thigh to locate vascular pedicle
    - After identification of suitable septocutaneous or musculocutaneous perforator branch, inferior and lateral borders of the flap are outlined centered on the faciocutaneous pedicle
    - Incise flap edges through subcutaneous tissue and deep fascia
    - Elevate flap from lateral border toward medial border with subfascial dissection
    - Transpose flap to defect and close

Sacral pressure ulcers[2,4,6,10]

- May treat ambulatory patients who have superficial wound with split thickness skin graft; however, flap reconstruction strongly preferred for any Stage III or Stage IV defect

Flap options

- Gluteus maximus: can be rotational, advancement or turn-over flap, based superiorly or inferiorly with use of partial or all of the muscle. Recent techniques have focused on island-type perforator flaps or perforator-preserving rotational flaps[22–26]
    - See Ischial Ulcer → Flap Options → Gluteus Maximus

- Transverse lumbosacral flap: significantly less bulky so only for superficial wounds[22]
    - Size 20 × 7 cm
    - Fasciocutaneous
    - Sensory: T12–L1
    - Vascular supply:
        - Segmental pedicle: branches of lumbar artery passing through lateral edge of quadratus lumborum to erector spinae (sacrospinalis) and 2–4 branches of posterior intercostal arteries
    - Flap dissection begins at posterior axillary line and includes deep fascia overlying the inferior latissimus dorsi muscle and superior aspect of the gluteus maximus muscle
    - Lumbosacral fascia is encountered at this point but is not routinely included with the flap
    - The segmental perforating vessels are divided as they penetrate the midpoint of the ipsilateral paraspinous muscle entering the flap
    - As the flap is raised, care is taken to avoid division of the perforating vessels through the paraspinous fascia on the contralateral side
    - Flap elevation is completed 2 cm across the posterior midline or at the level where the segmental pedicle is visualized
    - Flap is rotated 90 degrees directly into sacral or posterior midline trunk defect

Trochanteric pressure ulcers[11,20–23,27]

Pressure ulcers in this region are closely associated with prolonged Lateral decubitus positioning and wheelchair use

Flap options

- Tensor fasciae latae: sensation from the nerve roots of L1, L2 and L3 by the lateral femoral cutaneous nerve makes this a potentially sensate flap in patients with spinal cord injury below L3
    - See: Ischial Pressure Ulcers → Flap Options → TFL

- Vastus lateralis is often used to fill dead space after Girdlestone procedure (resection of femoral head)
  - Size 10 × 26 cm
  - Muscle and musculocutaneous Type I
  - Motor: muscular branch of femoral nerve
  - Sensory: lateral femoral cutaneous nerve (L2–3)
  - Vascular supply
    - Dominant pedicle: descending branch of lateral circumflex femoral artery and venae comitantes
    - Minor pedicle: transverse branch of lateral circumflex femoral artery, posterior branches from profunda femoris artery, Superficial branch of lateral superior genicular artery and venae comitantes
  - Expose the muscle through a lateral thigh incision from a point 10 cm below the anterior superior iliac spine at the level of the greater trochanter to the lateral condyle of the femur
  - Extend through the deep fascia at the medial edge of the tensor fascia lata muscle in the proximal one fourth of the leg and the iliotibial tract distally
  - Retract rectus femoris medially to expose adjacent vastus lateralis.
  - Divide the muscle at origin and elevate proximally for inset

Post-Operative Care[1,11,15]

- Pressure relief / proper mattress
- Bed rest 2–3 weeks minimal
- Culture-directed antibiotics
- Bowel regimen / ostomy care
- Aggressive nutritional repletion
- Active or passive ROM of uninvolved extremity
- Sitting protocol
  - Wound/flap with complete re-epithelialization with dry surface and no open area for minimum of 96 hours
  - Change from Clinitron to Low Air Loss mattress

- Sit for 30 minutes in bed
- Once tolerating 30 minutes BID in bed may move to wheelchair
- Increase by 15 minutes every 2 days
- After each sitting session check skin for erythema and/or drainage from site of flap/wound. If skin doesn't tolerate progression, as evidenced by erythema fading which takes longer than 20 minutes, time of sitting should be reduced

Post-Operative Complications[18,24,28]

- Hematoma: 7%
- Seroma: 2.3 to 12.5%
- Infection (sepsis): 6.6 to 11%
- Wound dehiscence: 4.2 to 51%
- Partial flap loss: 2.7 to 22.9%
- Flap necrosis: 4.3 to 6.3%
- ***Recurrence***[15]
  - 15–43% with fasiocutaneous flaps
  - 13–42% with musculocutaneous flaps
  - Overall: 19–69%, depending on length of F/U
  - Young posttraumatic paraplegics: 79% at 11 months
  - Cerebrally compromised elderly: 69% at 8 months
  - Paraplegics: 82% recurrence at same location at mean 18.2 months and 64% "recurrence" or new occurrence at a different site

> All rates are dependent on length of follow-up, reconstructive technique and postoperative care. It is important to simply note that recurrence rates, for certain patient populations, are very high and care must be taken to choose the appropriate reconstructive option

Summary

- Comprehensive evaluation is critical
- Multidisciplinary team approach essential for management

- Emphasis should be placed on prevention for patients with the following high risk factors: spinal cord injury, older age, prolonged immobility, chronic illness and multiple comorbidities
- Management goals: prevention of ulcer progression, prevention of additional ulcers, prevention of complications and wound closure in appropriately selected patients utilizing surgical principles for flap selection to minimize risk of recurrence
- Flap selection should incorporate patient dependent factors
- Adhere to surgical principles when selecting flaps. Given overall high recurrence rates, favor rotation or advancement flaps that can be re-rotated or re-advanced
- Post-operatively: emphasis should be placed on rehabilitation, minimizing risk factors for recurrence and patient education

References

1. Whitney J, Phillips L, Aslam R, Barbul A, Gottrup F, Gould L, Robson MC, Rodeheaver G, Thomas D, Stotts N. (2006) Guidelines for the treatment of pressure ulcers. *Wound Repair Regen* **14**: 663–679.
2. National Pressure Ulcer Advisory Panel. (1999) Pressure ulcers prevalence, cost and risk adjustment: consensus development conference statement. *Decubitus* **2**: 24–28.
3. Bergstrom N, Braden B, Kemp M, Champagne M, Ruby E. (1996) Multi-site study of incidence of pressure ulcers and the relationship between risk level, demographic characteristics, diagnoses, and prescription of preventive interventions. *J Am Geriatr Soc* **44**: 22–30.
4. Allman RM. (1997) Pressure ulcer prevalence, incidence, risk factors, and impact. *Clin Geriatr Med* **13**: 421–436.
5. Brandeis GH, Morris JN, Nash DJ, Lipsitz LA. (1990) The epidemiology and natural history of pressure ulcers in elderly nursing home residents. *JAMA* **264**: 2905–2909.
6. Gusenoff JA, Redett RJ, Nahabedian MY. (2002) Outcomes for surgical coverage of pressure sores in nonambulatory, nonparaplegic, elderly patients. *Ann Plast Surg* **48**: 633–640.
7. Keller BP, Wille J, van Ramshorst B, van der Werken C. (2002) Pressure ulcers in intensive care patients: a review of risks and prevention. *J Intensive Care Med* **28**: 1379–1388.

8. Vangilder C, Macfarlane GD, Meyer. (2008) Results of nine international pressure ulcer prevalence surverys: 1989 to 2005. *Ostomy Wound Manage* **54**: 40–54.
9. Siegler EL, Lavizzo–Mourey R. (1991) Management of stage III ulcers in moderately demented nursing home residents. *J Gen Intern Med* **6**: 507–513.
10. Dansereau JG, Conway H. (1964) Closure of decubiti in paraplegics. Report on 2000 cases. *Plast Reconstr Surg* **33**: 474–480.
11. Kenkel JM. (1998) Pressure sores. *Sel Read Plast Surg* **8**(39): 1–29.
12. Bauer J, Phillips L. (2008) MOC-PS CME article: pressure sores. *Plast Reconstr Surg* **121**: 1–10.
13. Dinsdale SM. (1974) Decubitus ulcers: role of pressure and friction in causation. *Arch Phys Med Rehabil* **55**: 147–152.
14. Daniel RK, Priest DL, Wheatley DC. (1981) Etiologic factors in pressure sores: an experimental model. *Arch Phys Med Rehabil* **62**: 492–498.
15. Janis J. (2007) Pressure sores. In: Janis J (ed.), *Essentials of Plastic Surgery*. Quality Medical Publishing, St. Louis, pp. 449–457.
16. National Pressure Sore Advisory Panel. Consensus Development Conference Staging System. (2007) Available at: http://www.npuap.org/pr2.htm. Accessed April 24, 2011.
17. Larson DL, Gilstrap J, Simonelic K, Carrera GF. (2011) Is there a simple, definitive, and cost-effective way to diagnose osteomyelitis in the pressure ulcer patient? *Plast Reconstr Surg* **127**(2): 670–676.
18. Yildirim S, Taylan G, Akoz T. (2007) Freestyle perforator-based V-Y advancement flap for reconstruction of soft tissue defects at various anatomic regions. *Ann Plast Surg* **58**: 501–506.
19. Fan K, Tang J, Escandon J, Kirsner RS. (2011) State of the art in topical wound-healing products. *Plast Reconstr Surg* **127:** 44S–55S.
20. Thorne C, Beasley R, Aston S, Bartlett SP, Gurtner GC, Spear SL. (2006) *Grabb and Smith's Plastic Surgery*. Lippincott Williams & Wilkins, New York.
21. Ahluwalia R, Martin D, Mahoney J. (2010) The operative treatment of pressure wounds; a 10 year experience in flap selection. *Int Wound J* **7**: 103–106.
22. Mathes S, Nahai F. (1997) *Reconstructive Surgery Principles, Anatomy and Technique*. Quality Medical Publishing, St. Louis.
23. Schryvers OI, Stranc MF, Nance PW. (2000) Surgical treatment of pressure ulcers: 20-year experience. *Arch Phys Med Rehabil* **81**: 1556–1562.
24. Tchanque-Fossuo CN, Kuzon WM Jr. (2011) An evidence-based approach to pressure sores. *Plast Reconstr Surg* **127**(2): 932–939.

25. Kim JT, Kim YH, Naidu S. (2010) Gluteus maximus perforator-based island flap for coverage of buttock defects. *Plast Reconstr Surg* **125**(6): 1744–1751.
26. Wong CH, Tan BK, Song C. (2007) The perforator-sparing buttock rotation flap for coverage of pressure sores. *Plast Reconstr Surg* **119**(4): 1259–1266.
27. Evans G, Lewis V, Manson P, Loomis M, Vander Kolk CA. (1993) Hip joint communication with pressure sore: the refractory wound and the role of girdlestone arthroplasty. *Plast Reconst Surg* **91**: 288–294.
28. Goodman CM, Cohen V, Armenta A, Thornby J, Netscher DT. (1999) Evaluation of results and treatment variables for pressure ulcers in 48 veteran spinal cord-injured patients. *Ann Plast Surg* **42**: 665–672.

CHAPTER 30

VASCULAR ANOMALIES

Harvey Chim and Arun K. Gosain

Illustrative Case

- A 10 year old boy presents with a persistently enlarging mass of the right lower lip. What is the next step in management?
- This is an arteriovenous malformation involving the right lower lip.
- The patient was treated with superselective arterial embolization followed by surgical resection.

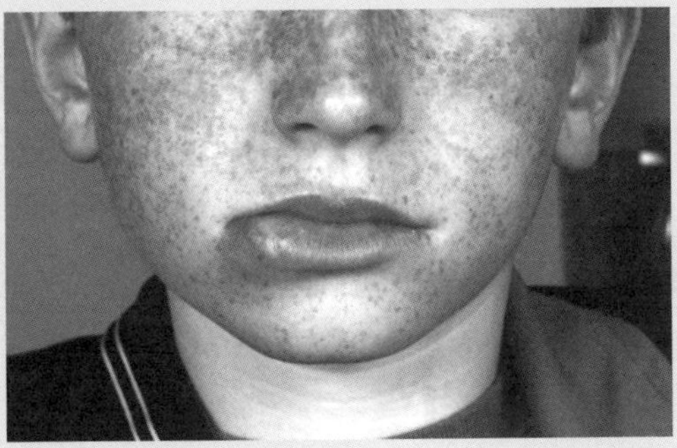

Classification

- ISSVA classification divides vascular anomalies into vascular tumors and vascular malformations.
- Vascular tumors include hemangiomas[1] and other proliferative lesions.

- Vascular malformations include capillary (CM), venous (VM), lymphatic (LM) and arterial (AM) malformations.
- Vascular malformations can also be combined, e.g. AVM, CLVM, LVM or arteriovenous fistula (AVF).

Vascular Tumors

Characteristics, Preoperative Tests, Management

- Varies by type of vascular anomaly.
- ***Hemangioma:*** Management is observation for majority of lesions.[2–4]
- Three phases: proliferative, involutional, involuted.
- Majority of proliferative growth occurs during rapid growth phase in first 5 months of age with growth ceasing by 1 year of age.
- Involution continues for 2 to 10 years.
- Indications for intervention prior to involution include high risk areas with tendency for complications (eyelids, ear, airway) or local wound complications, e.g. ulceration, bleeding.
- Medical management options include steroids, interferon alfa-2, propranolol.
- Lasers used include pulsed dye, Nd:YAG and KTP.
- Surgery is reserved for failure of medical management or risk of life-threatening or functional complications, e.g. eyelid hemangioma at risk of amblyopia.
- MRI can be used to better define lesion if uncertain of depth or extent.
- Surgery is also indicated for residual scarring or fibrofatty tissue, mostly in school age children.

Vascular Malformations

Characteristics, Preoperative Tests, Management

- Multidisciplinary management key to successful management.[5]
- Imaging helps to evaluate and better define lesion.
- First line imaging modality is plain radiographs, which show skeletal growth disturbances and phleboliths in vascular malformations.
- Color Doppler ultrasound useful for assessment of superficial lesions and blood flow velocity to define type of malformation.

- CT not so useful for characterization of soft tissue.
- MRI is better for characterizing vascular malformations. MRA and MRV can differentiate between slow-flow and fast-flow malformations.
- MRI is often used as initial diagnostic test for workup of vascular malformations.
- ***Capillary Malformations:*** Treatment of choice is the 585 nm flash-lamp-pulsed pulsed dye laser (PDL).
- PDL selectively targets oxyhemoglobin and results in intravascular thrombosis.
- Other treatment options include alexandrite laser (755 nm), Nd:YAG (1064 nm) or intense pulsed light (IPL).
- Multiple treatment sessions are often required.
- ***Venous Malformations:*** First line treatment is percutaneous sclerotherapy.
- VMs are slow-flow lesions.
- VMs most common in the head and neck.
- MRV most useful investigation to confirm the diagnosis and define extent of involvement.
- Coagulation profile to exclude underlying coagulopathy.
- Surgery may be used for lesions in head and neck where cosmesis is of concern.
- Surgery also indicated for lesions complicated by bleeding and pain.
- ***Arteriovenous Malformations:*** Treatment consists of primary arterial embolization, resection or superselective arterial embolization followed by resection 24 to 48 hours after embolization.
- AVMs are high-flow lesions with direct connections between artery and vein.
- Schobinger staging system describes 4 stages.
    - Stage I (quiescent phase): Asymptomatic, typically from birth till adolescence
    - Stage II (progressive phase): Enlarged, palpable thrill or pulse, murmur on auscultation; typically at adolescence
    - Stage III: Destructive lesions with pain, bleeding, ulceration or bony erosion; typically after many years
    - Stage IV: Cardiac decompensation with high-output cardiac failure

- MRA is useful to confirm diagnosis of fast-flow malformation.
- Ligation or embolization of feeding vessels to an AVM should be avoided, as this causes recruitment of collateral vessels from adjacent arteries, and limits access to the nidus for superselective arterial embolization.
- ***Lymphatic Malformations:*** Treatment consists of sclerotherapy for macrocystic lesions, while microcystic lesions often require surgical excision.
- Lymphatic malformations most often occur in the cervical region, followed by the axilla, trunk and extremities.
- Cervicofacial malformations can have skeletal distortion and overgrowth leading to malocclusion; as well as macroglossia and macrochilia.
- Extremity malformations can result in gigantism from bone and soft tissue overgrowth.
- Magnetic resonance lymphangiography can detail anatomy of diseased lymphatics.
- Sclerosing agents used include hypertonic saline, sodium tetradecyl sulfate, absolute ethanol, bleomycin and OK-432.
- Indications for surgery include symptomatic lesions, functional limitations and for cosmesis.

Operative Techniques

- Surgery is effective for symptomatic hemangiomas, arteriovenous malformations and microcystic lymphatic malformations.
- Large arteriovenous malformations are best managed by superselective arterial embolization for temporary occlusion of the nidus, followed by surgical resection 24 to 48 hours after embolization.
- Lesions should be excised and closed primarily where possible.
- Other reconstructive options include skin grafts, local or regional flaps and free tissue transfer.
- Staged surgical excision may be used for very large lesions.
- Tissue expansion provides a useful reconstructive modality.
- Combined medical and surgical management may be the best option for extensive lesions.

Postoperative Care

- Lymphatic malformations often require prolonged suction drainage and prophylactic antibiotics, to prevent seroma formation and infection.
- Elastic compression garments are useful adjuncts to surgical excision of extremity lesions.
- Orthodontic treatment of orthognathic surgery may be used to correct malocclusion or skeletal changes resulting from skeletal lesion.
- Lymphatic malformations have a high rate of recurrence (40% with incomplete excision and 17% with macroscopically complete excision). Post-surgical follow-up is essential.

References

1. Drolet BA, Esterly NB, Frieden IJ. (1999) Hemangiomas in children. *N Engl J Med* **341**: 173–181.
2. Jacobs AH, Walton RG. (1976) The incidence of birthmarks in the neonate. *Pediatrics* **58**: 218–222.
3. Holmdahl K. (1995) Cutaneous hemangiomas in premature and mature infants. *Acta Paediatr* **44**: 370–379.
4. Chiller KG, Passaro D, Frieden IJ. (2002) Hemangiomas of infancy: clinical characteristics, morphologic subtypes, and their relationship to race, ethnicity, and sex. *Arch Dermatol* **138**: 1567–1576.
5. Jackson IT, Carreno R, Potparic Z, *et al.* (1993) Hemangiomas, vascular malformations, and lymphovenous malformations: classification and methods of treatment. *Plast Reconstr Surg* **91**: 1216–1230.

INDEX